Toxicology and Immunology

Toxicology and Immunology

Edited by Jim Wang

hayle medical
New York

Hayle Medical,
750 Third Avenue, 9th Floor,
New York, NY 10017, USA

Visit us on the World Wide Web at:
www.haylemedical.com

ISBN: 978-1-63241-447-2

The publisher's policy is to use permanent paper from mills that operate a sustainable forestry policy. Furthermore, the publisher ensures that the text paper and cover boards used have met acceptable environmental accreditation standards.

Printed in the United States of America.

Cataloging-in-Publication Data

Toxicology and immunology / edited by Jim Wang.
p. cm.
Includes bibliographical references and index.
ISBN 978-1-63241-447-2
1. Toxicology. 2. Immunology. 3. Toxicity testing. I. Wang, Jim.
RA1216 .T69 2017
615.9--dc23

Table of Contents

Preface

Toxicology is the study of substances that can cause physical damage to living organisms. This book on toxicology and immunology discusses the principles of toxicology spread and immune response and therapy. Toxicology diagnosis seeks to determine the level of toxicology acuteness and exposure to lethal substances. Topics included in this text will contribute to the advancement of these fields. The extensive content of this book provides the readers with a thorough understanding of the subject. It brings forth some of the most innovative concepts and elucidates the unexpected aspects of this field. This book is a vital tool for all researching or studying toxicology and immunology as it gives incredible insights into emerging trends and concepts.

The information shared in this book is based on empirical researches made by veterans in this field of study. The elaborative information provided in this book will help the readers further their scope of knowledge leading to advancements in this field.

Finally, I would like to thank my fellow researchers who gave constructive feedback and my family members who supported me at every step of my research.

Editor

Preface

Editor

1

[6]-Gingerol Induces Caspase-Dependent Apoptosis and Prevents PMA-Induced Proliferation in Colon Cancer Cells by Inhibiting MAPK/AP-1 Signaling

EK Radhakrishnan[1☯], Smitha V. Bava[2☯], Sai Shyam Narayanan[2¶], Lekshmi R. Nath[2¶], Arun Kumar T. Thulasidasan[2], Eppurathu Vasudevan Soniya[1*], Ruby John Anto[2*]

1 Division of Plant Molecular Biology, Rajiv Gandhi Centre for Biotechnology, Thiruvananthapuram, Kerala, India, **2** Division of Cancer Research, Rajiv Gandhi Centre for Biotechnology, Thiruvananthapuram, Kerala, India

Abstract

We report mechanism-based evidence for the anticancer and chemopreventive efficacy of [6]-gingerol, the major active principle of the medicinal plant, Ginger (*Zingiber officinale*), in colon cancer cells. The compound was evaluated in two human colon cancer cell lines for its cytotoxic effect and the most sensitive cell line, SW-480, was selected for the mechanistic evaluation of its anticancer and chemopreventive efficacy. The non-toxic nature of [6]-gingerol was confirmed by viability assays on rapidly dividing normal mouse colon cells. [6]-gingerol inhibited cell proliferation and induced apoptosis as evidenced by externalization of phosphatidyl serine in SW-480, while the normal colon cells were unaffected. Sensitivity to [6]-gingerol in SW-480 cells was associated with activation of caspases 8, 9, 3 &7 and cleavage of PARP, which attests induction of apoptotic cell death. Mechanistically, [6]-gingerol down-regulated Phorbol Myristate Acetate (PMA) induced phosphorylation of ERK1/2 and JNK MAP kinases and activation of AP-1 transcription factor, but had only little effects on phosphorylation of p38 MAP kinase and activation of NF-kappa B. Additionally, it complemented the inhibitors of either ERK1/2 or JNK MAP kinase in bringing down the PMA-induced cell proliferation in SW-480 cells. We report the inhibition of ERK1/2/JNK/AP-1 pathway as a possible mechanism behind the anticancer as well as chemopreventive efficacy of [6]-gingerol against colon cancer.

Editor: Rana Pratap Singh, Jawaharlal Nehru University, India

Funding: The authors have no support or funding to report.

* Email: evsoniya@rgcb.res.in (EVS); rjanto@rgcb.res.in (RJA)

☯ These authors contributed equally to this work.

¶ These authors also contributed equally to this work.

Introduction

Colon cancer is the third most diagnosed type of cancer and the third leading cause of cancer-related mortality in United States. Globally, it is the fourth most common cause of mortality due to cancer. The variations in dietary pattern and increased consumptions of red and processed meat contribute to this increase in incidence of colon cancer [1,2].Surgical procedures and chemotherapy constitutes the major therapeutic regimens for colon cancer [3]. The increase in drug resistance impedes the treatment of colon cancer and the problems associated with metastasis increases its severity. Search is on for novel therapeutic agents that targets molecular signaling pathways in colon cancer in order to arrest its growth and metastasis.

Ginger (*Zingiber officinale*) has long been used in traditional medicine and is called as "*Maha-aushadhi*" in Ayurveda, meaning "*the great medicine*" [4]. The rhizome from ginger contains many pungent phenolic compounds like [6]-gingerol, [6]-shagol, [6]-paradol and zingerone [5].These compounds have been studied for their anti-bacterial, anti-oxidant, anti-inflammatory and anti-tumor properties [6,7]. Many studies have proved the anti-cancer properties of these phenolics against cancers of various origins. The rhizome of ginger is an ingredient of daily diets in many countries and is an active ingredient in many traditional systems of herbal medicines, like Oriental medicine and Ayurveda, for managing many ailments including indigestion and other gastro-intestinal disorders. This traditional knowledge triggers a particular interest in characterizing the chemo-preventive and anti-cancerous nature of these phenolics against gastric cancers like colorectal cancer or pancreatic cancers.

Among these phenolic compounds, [6]-gingerol (1-[4′-hydroxy-3′-methoxyphenyl]-5-hydroxy-3-decanone) has been studied for its cytotoxic effects in various cancer cell lines, including colorectal cancer. [6]-gingerol was shown to induce cell death in cervical cancer cell line, HeLa, by caspase-3 dependent apoptosis and autophagy [8]. It could inhibit the metastasis of MDA-MB-231 breast cancer cells and induce apoptosis in LNCaP prostate cancer cells [9,10]. Administration of [6]-gingerol inhibited the growth of several types of murine tumors such as melanomas, renal cell carcinomas and colon carcinomas by enhancing the infiltrations of tumor-infiltrating lymphocytes CD4 and CD8 T-cells and $B220^+$ B-cells [11]. [6]-gingerol was also shown to inhibit the progression of phorbol ester-induced skin tumor in ICR mice [12]. Only limited numbers of studies have been published on the anti-cancer properties of [6]-gingerol and its mechanism of action against colon cancer [13,14,15].

In this study the cytotoxic effects of [6]-gingerol on SW-480 colon cancer cells were compared with its effects on rapidly dividing normal intestinal epithelial cells from mouse. The study also performed an *in vitro* mechanistic evaluation on the inhibitory effects of [6]-gingerol on phorbol 12-myristate 13-acetate (PMA) induced anti-apoptotic signals in SW-480 cells.

Materials and Methods

2.1. Materials

Dulbecco's modified Eagle's medium (DMEM) was obtained from Life Technologies (Grand Island, NY, USA); Fetal bovine serum (FBS) from PAN Biotech (GmbH, Aidenbach, Germany); Hank's Balanced Salt Solution (HBSS), Epidermal Growth Factor (EGF) and Insulin, Transferrin, Selenium, Sodium Pyruvate solution (ITS-A) from Invitrogen; Antibodies against phospho-p38, phospho-ERK1/2, phospho-JNK, beta-actin and caspases were purchased from Cell Signaling (Beverly, MA, USA) and antibodies against poly ADP ribose polymerase (PARP) was from Santa Cruz Biotechnology (Santa Cruz, CA). [6]-gingerol was purchased from Biomol (Hamburg, Germany). The MAP kinase inhibitors U0126, SP600125, SB203580 and NF-kappaB inhibitor SN50 were procured from Calbiochem (San Diego, CA). All other chemicals, including Phorbol 12-myristate 13-acetate (PMA) were purchased from Sigma Chemicals (St. Louis, MO, USA).

2.2. Cell culture

Human colon cancer cell lines, SW-480 and HCT116 were obtained from National Centre for Cell Sciences (NCCS), Pune, India. Cells were cultured in Dulbecco's Modified Eagle's Medium (DMEM) supplemented with 10% Fetal Bovine Serum (FBS) along with 100 U/ml penicillin, 50 microgram/ml streptomycin and 1 microgram/ml of amphotericin B. The cell lines were maintained at 37°C in a humidified atmosphere of 5% CO2 and were sub-cultured twice weekly.

Normal intestinal epithelial cells (IECs) were isolated from mouse colon as per established protocol [16,17], with appropriate modifications, as approved by the Institutional Animal Ethical Committee, Rajiv Gandhi Centre for Biotechnology as per rules of the *Committee for the Purpose of Control and Supervision of Experiments on Animals*, Ministry of Environment and Forest, Government of India (Sanction No: IAEC/151/RUBY/2012). Briefly, mouse (*Swiss albino*, 7 weeks old, IAEC sanction No: IAEC/151/RUBY/2012) colon was dissected out and cleaned aseptically with 1× Hank's Balanced Salt Solution (HBSS) to remove fecal matter. The intestine was longitudinally opened and cut into 1 cm pieces and were incubated in presence of type 1 collagenase (200 U/ml) for 30 min with vigorous shaking. The dislodged epithelial cells were isolated by centrifuging the supernatant. These cells were cultured in high glucose DMEM with 10% FBS and 2× antibiotics, containing 10 ng/ml epidermal growth factor (EGF) and 5 µg/ml Insulin-Transferrin-Selenium-Sodium Pyruvate (ITS-A) (Invitrogen, USA). This cell line was maintained at 37°C in a humidified atmosphere of 5% CO_2 and was sub-cultured once in a month.

2.3. Drug treatment

[6]-gingerol stock (20 mg/ml) was prepared in ethanol and the working concentrations were prepared by diluting this stock in dimethyl sufoxide (DMSO). For MTT assay, 5×10^3 cells/well of human colon cancer cells and 10^4 cells/well of mouse IECs were seeded in 96-well plates. Cells were treated with [6]-gingerol for 48 h,72 h or 96 h before performing MTT assay and for 16 h before Annexin-V staining. PMA (5 mg/ml) was prepared in DMSO and stored at −20°C. In all combination treatments [6]-gingerol was added 2 h before treating with PMA. In cell viability assay/Western blot for combination treatments with MAP kinase inhibitors (2.5 micromolar U0126, 5 micromolar SP600125, 1′micromolar SB203580) or NF-kappaB inhibitor (18 micromolar SN50), cells were first treated with the inhibitor for 1 h and subsequently pre-treated with [6]-gingerol for 2 h, followed by exposure to PMA for 48 h before performing MTT assay. For Electrophoretic Mobility Shift Assay (EMSA), 10^6 cells of SW-480 were seeded in 60 mm plates and cells were pretreated with [6]-gingerol for 2 h and then with PMA for 30 min.

2.4. Cell viability assay

Cytotoxic effects of [6]-gingerol was determined by MTT assay as described earlier [18] and the relative cell viability percentage is expressed as [A_{570} of treated wells/A_{570} of untreated wells ×100].

2.5. Annexin V-Propidium Iodine staining

The membrane flip-flop induced by 16 h treatment with [6]-gingerol was analyzed by staining the cells with fluorescein isothiocyanate-conjugated Annexin V/PI (Santa Cruz Biotechnology) according to the manufacturer's instructions and the apoptotic cells were photographed under fluorescent microscope [19]. The total number of cells in the microscopic field was counted under a phase contrast microscope and the number of fluorescent cells in the same field was counted under a fluorescent microscope. The fraction of fluorescent cells to total number of cells is represented as percentage of apoptotic cells. This was repeated in several fields of the same well and the average was taken for plotting.

2.6. Immunoblotting

The total protein isolated from cells following treatments, with or without PMA/[6]-gingerol, were subjected to Western blotting as described previously [20]. In short, 60 microgram of whole cell lysate was separated on a 10–15% polyacrylamide gel, blotted on to a PVDF membrane, probed with corresponding antibody and detected using ECL (Millipore, Billerica, MA, USA).

2.7. Electrophoretic Mobility Shift Assay (EMSA)

EMSA was performed to evaluate DNA-binding activity of NF-kappa B or AP-1 transcription factors in cells treated with PMA and/or [6]-gingerol, as described earlier [21]. In brief, 10 microgram of nuclear proteins, isolated from cells following drug treatments, were incubated for 30 min with ^{32}P-end-labeled double-stranded 45-mer oligonucleotide for NF kappaB (5′TTGTTACAAGGGACTT-TCCGCTGGGGACTTTCCAGGGAGGCGTGG-3′; at 37°C) or 21-mer oligonucleotide for AP-1 (5′-CGCTTGATGACT-CAGCCGGAA-3′;at 30°C) and the DNA protein complex was resolved on 6.6% non-denaturing polyacrylamide gel, which was dried and visualized on Phosphor Imager (Personal Molecular Imager FX; Bio-Rad Laboratories, Hercules, CA, USA).

2.8. Statistical Analysis

All the experiments were performed at least in triplicates (n = 3). The error bars represent ± standard deviation (S.D) of the experiments. The statistical analysis was carried out using Student's t-test and the symbols *, ** and *** represents P-values, $p \leq 0.05$, $p \leq 0.005$, and $p \leq 0.001$ respectively.

Results

3.1. [6]-gingerol induces dose dependent cytotoxicity in colon cancer cells while normal intestinal epithelial cells are unaffected

[6]-gingerol was screened for its cytotoxic effects on SW-480 and HCT116 cells at various concentrations ranging from 5 micromolar to 300 micromolar, for 72 h, using MTT assay. Dose-dependent changes in cellular morphology were clearly evident under phase contrast microscope (Fig. 1A). The results shows [6]-gingerol to be cytotoxic towards both SW-480 and HCT116 cells in a dose-dependent manner, with prominent cytotoxicity at higher concentrations producing an IC_{50} value of 205±5 micromolar and 283±7 micromolar, respectively (Fig. 1B and Fig. 1C).The effect was more prominent in case of SW-480 than HCT116 and thus the former was used in all further studies. On the contrary, the results from MTT assay with mouse normal IECs revealed only 10–15% cytotoxicity even at twice the IC_{50} concentration of [6]-gingerol against SW-480.The cellular morphology and cell number was seen largely unaffected even at 500 micromolar of [6]-gingerol (Fig. 2A). Studying the time-dependent effect of [6]-gingerol at the effective concentrations revealed an increase in cytotoxicity of SW-480 cells over time from 48 h to 96 h, although the cell viability of mouse normal IECs remained unchanged (Fig. 2B).These results suggest the specificity of [6]-gingerol in inducing cytotoxicity in cancerous cells without being toxic to normal cells even at higher concentrations.

3.2. [6]-gingerol induces apoptosis in colon cancer cells, but not in normal intestinal epithelial cells

In order to assess whether the induction of cytotoxicity by [6]-gingerol is mediated by apoptosis, the membrane flip-flop and externalization of phosphotedylserine were monitored in [6]-gingerol treated SW-480 cells by performing Annexin-V/PI staining. The results from Annexin-V/PI staining confirmed the early events of apoptotis in [6]-gingerol treated SW-480 cells, as evident from the dose-dependent increase in the fluorescent cells (Fig. 3A).The results from similar study performed on mouse IECs showed only negligible number of fluorescent cells, even at 500 micromolar of [6]-gingerol treatment.100 micromolar 5-Fluro Uracil (5-FU) served as positive control for Annexin V staining on normal IECs (Fig. 3B).

We also analyzed the cell extracts from SW-480 cells treated with [6]-gingerol for the activation of caspases-8, 9, 3, 7 and cleavage of PARP using immunoblotting experiments. Caspases are a family of cysteine proteases which are activated during the apoptotic program. We observed a significant cleavage of pro-caspase 8 to its active fragments (p43/41) and procaspase-9 to its active fragments (p35/37) (Fig. 4A and 4B). The activation of the effector caspases 3 and 7 were also induced by [6]-gingerol in a dose-dependent manner, cleaving procaspase-3 to its active fragments (p17/19) and enhancing the cleavage of procaspase-7 to its active fragment (p20) (Fig. 4C and 4D). Finally, we examined cleavage of the DNA repairing protein, PARP, which is a substrate of caspase-3.Upon treating the cells with 200 and 300 micromolar of [6]-gingerol, the 116-kDa form of PARP was cleaved to the 89 kDa fragment (Fig. 4E), confirming a caspase mediated apoptosis. Since 200 micromolar of [6]-gingerol was efficiently activating caspases leading to PARP cleavage and apoptosis, this concentration was used in further signaling studies.

3.3. [6]-gingerol inhibits PMA-induced activation of the MAP kinases in SW-480 cells

PMA is a well- known tumor promoter that activates almost all protein kinase C (PKC) isozymes, which are prominent upstream regulators of mitogen-activated protein (MAP) kinase pathway [22,23].The kinetics of phosphorylation of Ras/Raf/extracellular signal-regulated kinase (ERK1/2), c-jun NH 2 -terminal kinase (JNK) and p38 MAP kinase in SW-480 cells in response to treatment with 50 ng/ml (80 nM) PMA for different time intervals were studied. Western blot analysis revealed a time dependant phosphorylation of ERK1/2, JNK and p38.In all three cases, phosphorylation was evident at 5 min from PMA treatment and it peaked at 30 min and then receded by 120 min (Fig. 5A). The effect of [6]-gingerol on the PMA-induced transient phosphorylation of MAP kinases was studied on 30 min PMA-treated SW-480 cells, pretreated with 200 micromolar [6]-gingerol for 2 h. Interestingly, [6] - gingerol pretreatment abolished the PMA-induced transient phosphorylation of ERK1/2 and JNK almost completely, but only partially abolished the phosphorylation of p38 MAP kinase in SW-480 cells (Fig. 5B).

3.4. [6]-gingerol inhibits the transcriptional binding activity of PMA-induced AP-1, but not NF-kappaB, in SW-480

PMA is a well known activator of the transcription factors AP-1 and NF-kappaB in different cancer cells [24,25,26,27]. To determine the transcriptional binding activity of AP-1 in SW-480, induced in response to PMA, nuclear extract from the cells treated with 50 ng/microlitre PMA for 1 h was used for EMSA. A clear dose dependent activation of AP-1 was observed in SW-480 cells upon PMA treatment (Fig. 5C; Lane 5).A dose-dependent down-regulation of this PMA-induced AP-1 binding was observed upon 2 h pre-treatment with [6]-gingerol (Fig. 5C; Lane 6–8). [6]-gingerol pretreatment did not show a drastic effect on the transcriptional binding property of NF-kappaB, even though there was a significant inhibition of its DNA binding at 300 micromolar [6]-gingerol (Fig. 5D; Lane 6–8).

3.5. [6]-gingerol inhibits the PMA-induced cell proliferation in SW-480 through inhibition of ERK1/2 and JNK MAP kinase pathways

In order to further understand the mechanistic details behind the inhibitory effects of [6]-gingerol on PMA-activated signal pathways in SW-480, the viability and proliferation of SW-480 cells were monitored by MTT assay after treating them with various combinations of PMA, [6]-gingerol and inhibitors of MAP kinases or NF-kappaB. Primarily, PMA treatment enhanced the proliferation of SW-480 cells significantly. But, [6]-gingerol pre-treatment of the cells brought down the PMA-induce proliferation drastically. However, viability of SW-480 cells after [6]-gingerol treatment were comparatively higher in presence of PMA (Fig. 6A).

Next, we performed the same experiments on SW-480 cells pre-treated with inhibitors of members of MAP kinase family and NF-kappaB. U0126 was used as a specific inhibitor of ERK1/2 pathway, SP600125 as an inhibitor of JNK activation and SB203580 as the inhibitor of p38 MAP kinase pathway.SN50 was used as an inhibitor of NF-kappaB transcription factor. None

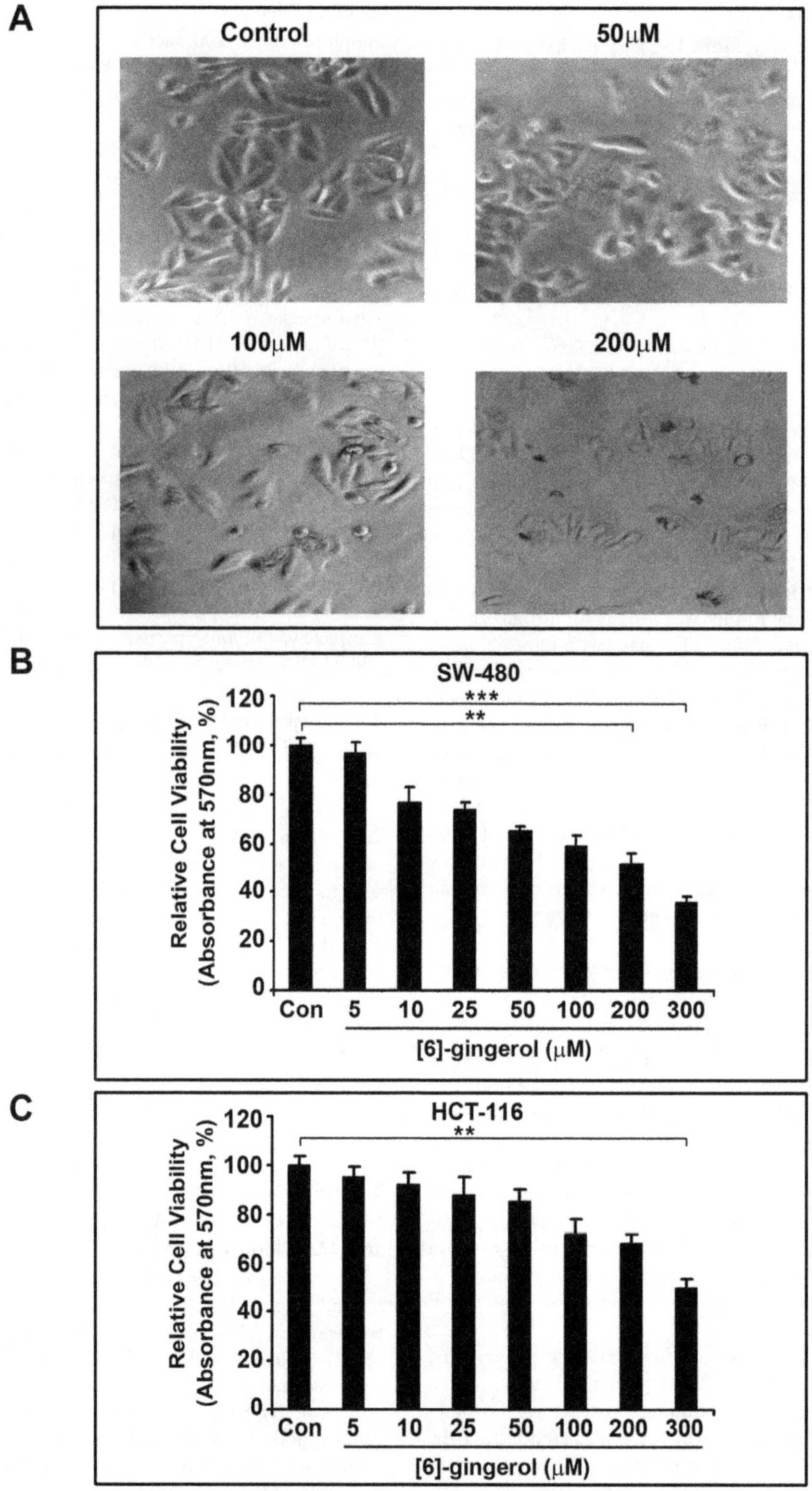

Figure 1. Cytotoxic effects of [6]-gingerol on SW-480 colon cancer cells. (A) Phase contrast microscopy images of morphological changes in SW-480 cells when treated with indicated concentrations of [6]-gingerol for 72 h. (B) Relative cell viability of SW-480 cells after [6]-gingerol treatment, determined by MTT assay and expressed as percentage of the untreated control. 5000 cells/well of SW-480 cells were treated with the indicated concentration of [6]-gingerol for 72 h prior to MTT assay.(C) Relative cell viability of HCT-116 cells after [6]-gingerol treatment. The results are represented as mean of triplicate experiments ± standard deviation (SD).

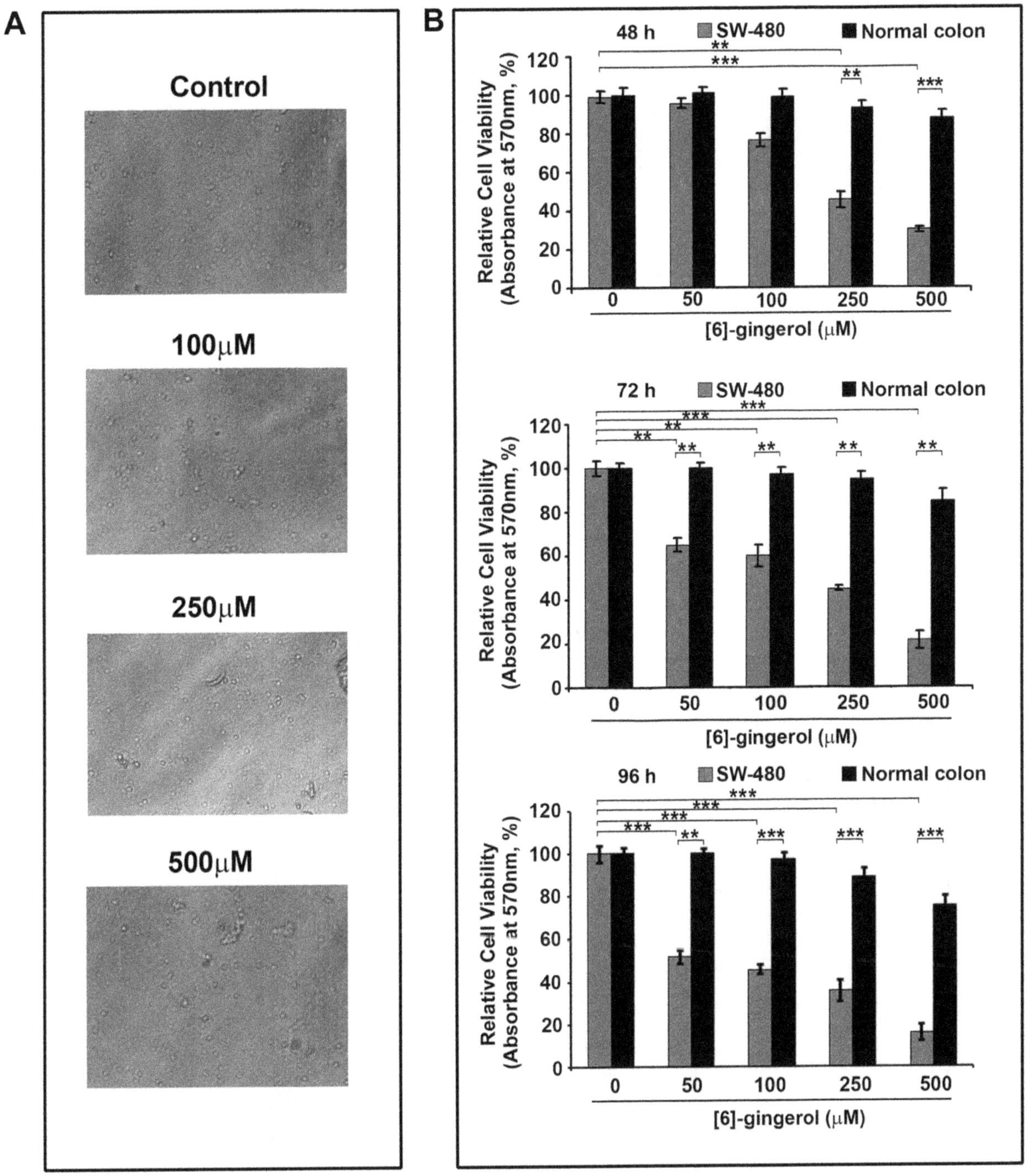

Figure 2. Comparison of cytotoxic effects of [6]-gingerol on SW-480 colon cancer cells with mouse normal intestinal epithelial cells (IECs). (A) Phase contrast microscopy images of IECs treated with indicated concentrations of [6]-gingerol for 72 h. (B) Time dependent cytotoxic effects of [6]-gingerol on SW-480 and IECs at 48, 72 and 96 h. 5000 cells/well of SW-480 and 10,000 cells/well of IECs were treated for 48 to 96 h with indicated doses of [6]-gingerol prior to MTT assay. The results are represented as mean ± SD from triplicate experiments.

of the above inhibitors had any cytotoxic effect on SW-480 cells at the tested concentration (Fig. 6A). But, pre-treatment with U0126 and SP600125 significantly reduced the PMA-induced proliferation of SW-480 cells to the same extend, even though to a lesser extend compared to [6]-gingerol pre-treatment (Fig. 6A). These results prove the essential role of ERK1/2 and JNK MAP kinases pathways in inducing proliferation of SW-480 cells in presence of PMA. Pre-treatment with SB203580 and SN50 had little effect on PMA-induced proliferation of SW-480 cells (Fig. 6A), proving the lack of involvement of p38 MAP kinase pathway and NF-kappaB transcription factor in this process.

Finally, [6]-gingerol treatment was performed on SW-480 cells pre-treated with each of the above inhibitors prior to induction with PMA. Surprisingly, in each case the cell viability was reduced to a level similar to that of pre-treatment with only [6]-gingerol prior to PMA treatment. This result suggests that, in presence of

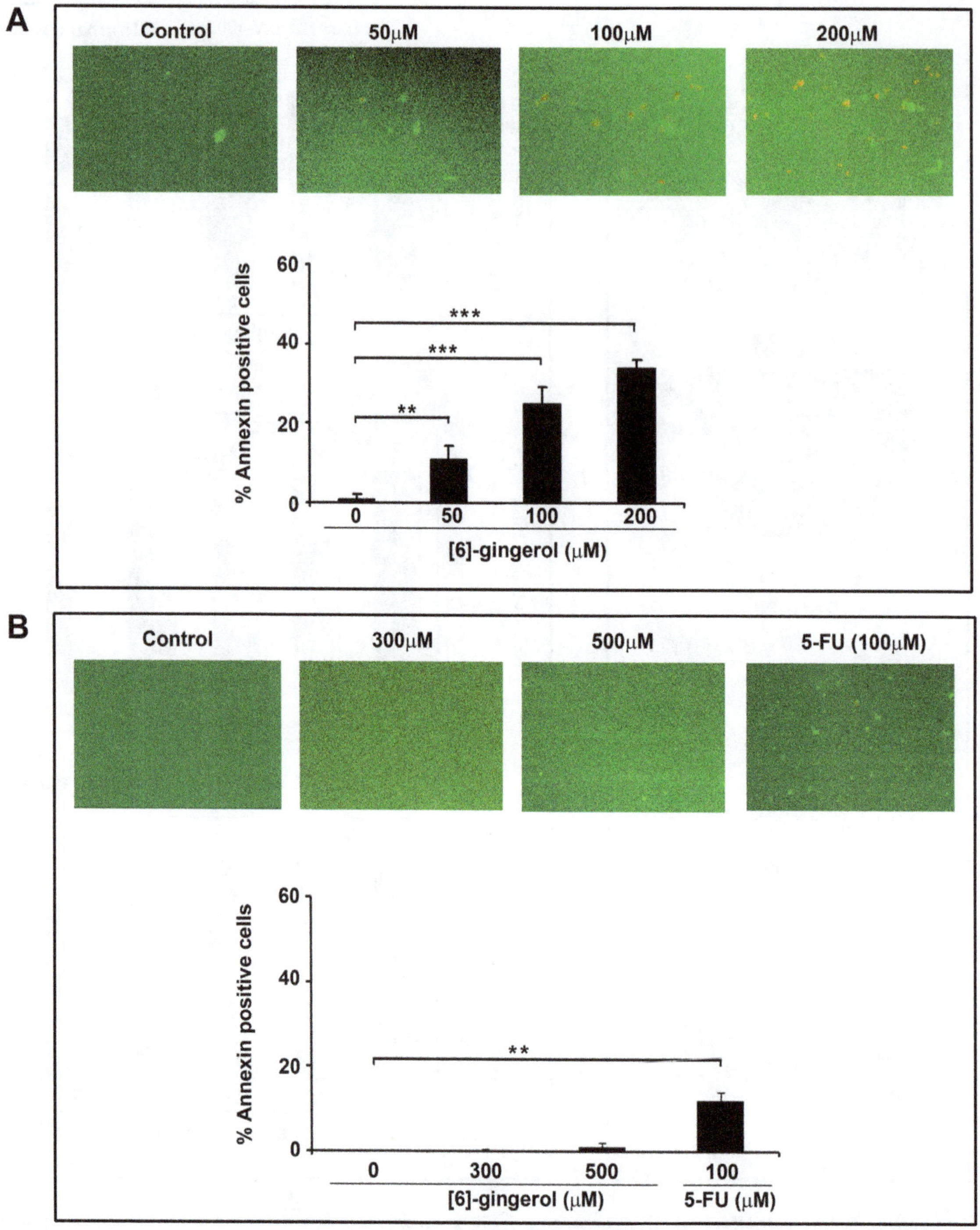

Figure 3. Effects of [6]-gingerol on induction of apoptosis in SW-480 cells and IECs. (A, upper panel) SW-480 cells were treated with indicated concentrations of [6]-gingerol for 16 h and stained for Annexin V/propidium iodide (PI) positivity. Green-fluorescence indicates Annexin V binding to the damaged cell membrane during early apoptosis and the red fluorescence indicates PI binding to the exposed DNA during late apoptosis. (A, lower panel) Graphical representation of the percentage of Annexin V/PI positive SW-480 cells in relation to [6]-gingerol concentration. (B, upper panel) IECs were treated with up to 500 μM of [6]-gingerol for 16 h before performing Annexin V-PI staining. Treatment with 100 μM 5-FU was used as positive control for apoptosis induction. (B, lower panel) Representative histogram of the percentage of Annexin/PI positive IECs following [6]-gingerol/5-FU treatment. The results are represented as mean from triplicate experiments ± SD.

U0126, [6]-gingerol complements this ERK1/2 inhibitor by abrogating the activation of JNK MAP kinase and, in presence of SP600125 it inhibits the ERK1/2 activation, thus reducing cell viability to the same level in both these cases. In presence of SB203580 and SN50 inhibitors [6]-gingerol exerts its inhibitory effects on both ERK1/2 and JNK MAP kinase pathways, thus brings down the cell viability to the same level as above. These results attest the equal contribution of both ERK1/2 and JNK

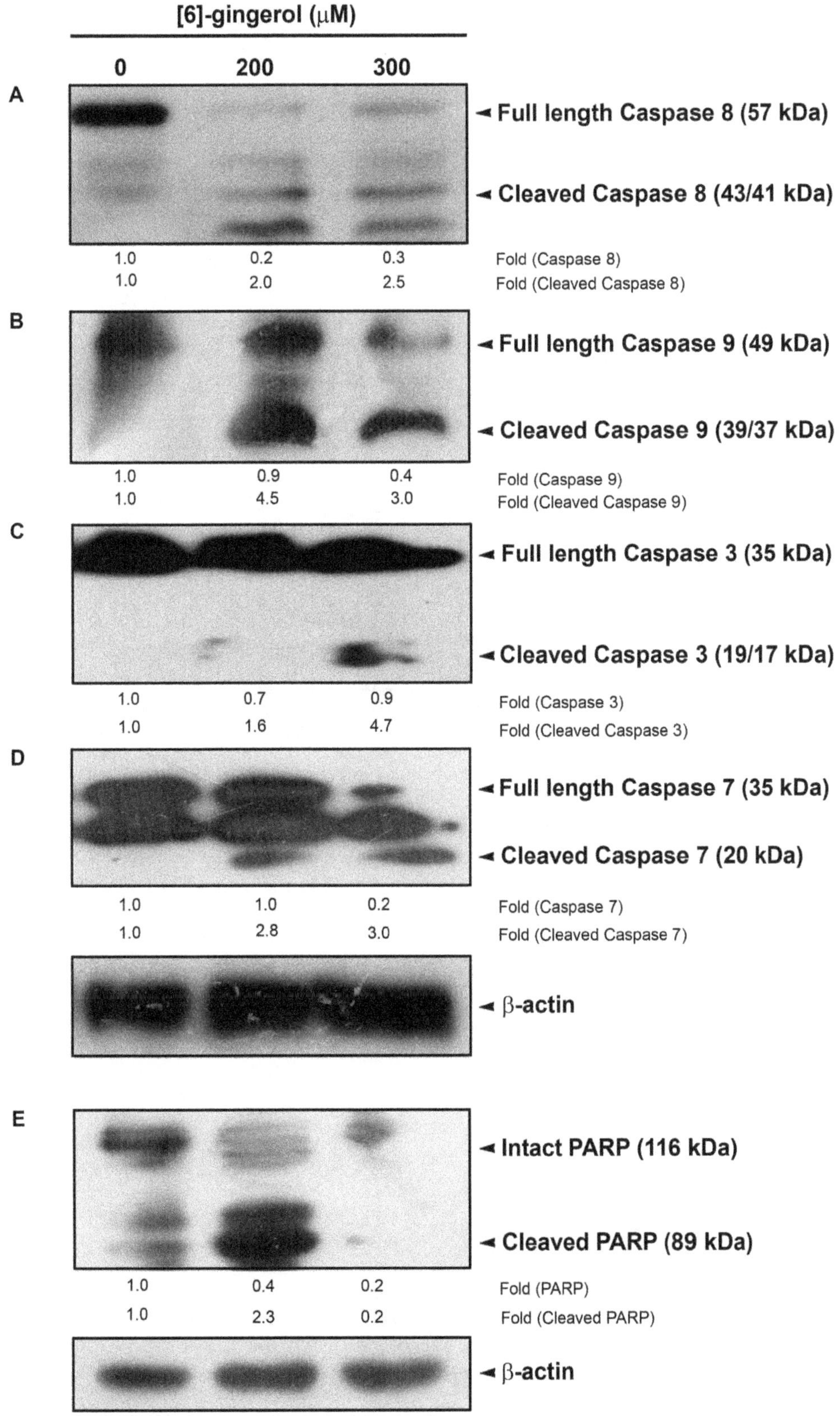

Figure 4. Effects of [6]-gingerol on activation of caspases and PARP cleavage in SW-480 cells. SW-480 cells (10^6 cells/well) were treated with the indicated concentrations of [6]-gingerol for 48 h and the whole cell extracts were Western blotted on to PVDF membrane. The activation of caspases and PARP cleavage were detected by probing the blotted membrane with antibodies against Caspase-3, 7, 8, 9 and against PARP. The blots were developed using Enhanced Chemiluminescence (ECL). The relative fold differences of bands with control treatments were quantified from volume analysis of the bands using Biorad- Quantity One software. β-actin served as the loading control in each case.

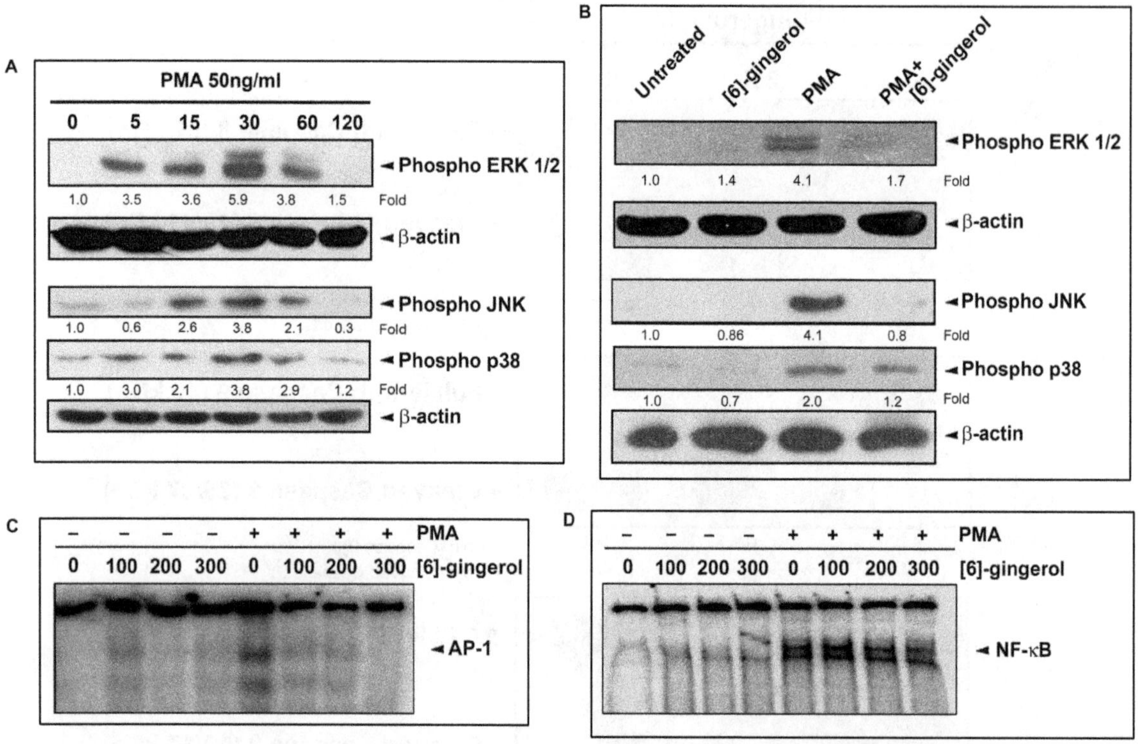

Figure 5. Effect of [6]-gingerol on PMA-induced phosphorylation of MAP kinases and activation of AP-1 and NF-kappaB in SW-480 cells. (A) Overnight grown SW-480 cells were treated with 50 ng/ml of PMA for different time intervals (0–120 min) and the whole cell lysate was immunoblotted onto PVDF membrane, probed using antibodies against phospho-ERK1/2, phospho-JNK and phospho-p38, developed by ECL. The kinetics of PMA-induced phosphorylation of these MAP kinases were followed from this blot (B) SW-480 cells were pre-treated with 200 μM [6]-gingerol before treating with 50 ng/ml of PMA for 30 min and the whole cell lysates were immunoblotted, probed and detected as above. The relative fold difference of bands with control treatments are indicated below each lane. β-actin served as the loading control in each case. (C) SW-480 cells, pre-treated with indicated concentrations of [6]-gingerol for 2 h, were treated with PMA (50 ng/ml) for 30 min. The nuclear extracts from each treatment were analysed for the activation of AP-1 or (D) NF-kappaB, by performing the transcriptional binding assay on isotope labelled AP-1/NF-kappaB specific DNA binding probe and analysing it on electrophoretic mobility shift assay (EMSA). The arrowhead in each case indicates complexes between AP-1/NF-kappaB and DNA probe.

MAP kinase pathways in [6]-gingerol mediated inhibition of PMA-induced cell proliferation of SW-480. Since there is no additive or synergistic inhibitory effects on proliferation of PMA-treated SW-480 cells resulting from pre-treatment with the combination of [6]-gingerol with U0126 or SP600125, compared to pre-treatment with [6]-gingerol alone, ERK1/2 and JNK MAP kinase pathway seems to be the key signaling pathways affected by [6]-gingerol during inhibition of PMA-induced cell proliferation in SW-480.

In order to test whether the inhibitory effects on the PMA-induced cell proliferation of SW-480 cells by [6]-gingerol and U0126 or SP600125 were apoptosis mediated, we monitored the activation of caspase 3 from each of these treatments by Western blotting. We observed cleavage of procaspase 3 in all the treatments involving [6]-gingerol, U0126 or SP600125 and in combination of [6]-gingerol and these inhibitors (Fig. 6B and 6C). It was also interesting to note that no additional degradation of the caspase 3 mother band was produced when the inhibitors and the gingerol were used together. This attests that down-regulation of ERK1/2/JNK/AP-1 pathway induced by PMA, is responsible for the inhibitory effects of [6]-gingerol on PMA-induced cell proliferation in SW-480.

Discussion

Anti-cancer and anti-inflammatory properties of [6]-gingerol has been recognized since long and many studies have reported different molecular mechanisms behind these properties. The inhibitory effects of [6]-gingerol against cancers of various origins were reported previously. [6]-gingerol has been shown to be particularly effective against skin carcinoma and in inhibiting of angiogenesis in endothelial cells [28,29]. Ginger being a dietary supplement and a major ingredient in many traditional medicines, it is logical to study the effects of [6]-gingerol on cancer of gastro-intestinal tract such as colon cancer. Moreover, the pharmacokinetic studies on the active components of ginger from orally administered ginger extracts in human beings detected a significant levels of [6]-gingerol, either in free or conjugated form, in plasma and colon tissues [30,31]. Another study on bioavailability of [6]-gingerol in rats suggested that when orally administered it is detected at concentrations of 4.3 μg/ml in plasma at ten minutes post-administration. The same study also determined its high distribution in tissues with highest concentration in tissues of gastrointestinal tract. The tissue to plasma ratio of [6]-gingerol was reported to be >1 and was attributed to its lipophilicity [32]. All these facts support a study on anti-cancer effects of [6]-gingerol on colon cancer.

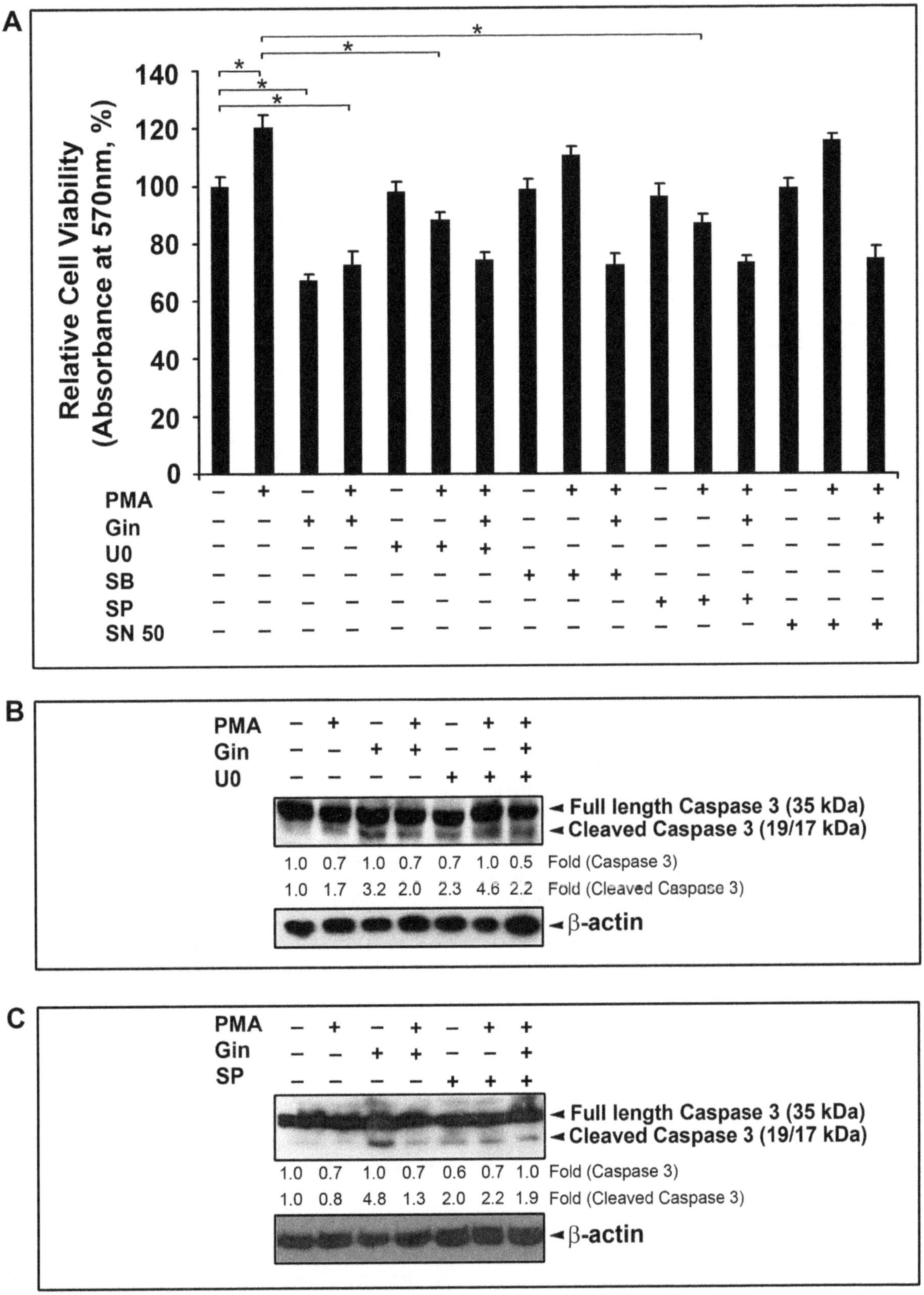

Figure 6. Effects of [6]-gingerol on PMA-induced cell proliferation in SW-480 in presence of inhibitors of MAP kinases and NF-kappaB. (A) Overnight grown SW-480 cells were pre-treated with inhibitors (U0126, SP600125, SB203580 for ERK1/2, JNK and p38 MAP kinases, respectively or SN50 for NF-kappaB) for 1 h and then treated with [6]-gingerol for 2 h, followed by exposure to PMA for 48 h, before performing cell viability assay using MTT. The relative viability of SW-480 cells in each treatment represented as percentage of untreated control. The values presented are mean of triplicate experiments ± SD. Total lysates from cells treated with combination of [6]-gingerol with (B) U0126 and (C) SP600125

inhibitors and from appropriate control treatments were Western blotted and probed with anti-caspase-3 antibody and the blots were developed using ECL. Beta-actin served as the loading control.

The first decade of 21st century had an increased number of studies on characterizing the mechanisms behind the anti-cancer effects of phytochemicals. Studies on the mechanistic evaluation of anti-cancer properties of [6]-gingerol against different kinds of cancers provided valuable insights into its multiple mechanisms of action in bringing about cytotoxic or pro-apoptotic effects in cancer cells. Some recent reports on the anti-cancer activities of [6]-gingerol against colon cancer presented different mechanisms for its action on different colon cancer cell lines [13,14,15,33]. The present study on SW-480 cell line demonstrates the *in vitro* cytotoxicity of [6]-gingerol with an IC_{50} value of 205 micromolar. The previous study on *in vitro* cytotoxic effects of [6]-gingerol on SW-480 cell line reported only 17% cell death at this concentration [13].These differences in the magnitude of effects might be due to the variations in the method used in studying cytotoxicity. It is also noteworthy that the same study reported only 13% cytotoxicity in LoVo cells when treated with 200 micromolar of [6]-gingerol for 72 h, which was later reported in a different study as 75% at 50 micromolar in the same cell line after 48 h treatment [15]. The dose-dependent increase in apoptotic cells (Annexin-V/PI positive cells) in SW-480 cells upon treatment with [6]-gingerol, upto 25-folds at 300 μM concentration, proved that the cytotoxicity was induced mainly by apoptosis. Previous studies reported both cell cycle arrest and apoptosis as the mechanism of action of [6]-gingerol [13,34]. Two-fold increase in apoptosis was reported at similar conditions in SW-480 by [13], but they also demonstrated significant G2/M arrest in cell cycle in response to [6]-gingerol treatment. Many previous reports suggested that [6]-gingerol induces apoptosis only at or near 300 micromolar in cancer cells [13,34,35,36] and below this concentration it induces cytotoxicity mainly by other mechanisms. However, we observed fluorescent cells in SW-480 treated with even 100 micromolar [6]-gingerol, clearly suggesting early apoptosis events even at lower concentrations. Furthermore, the dose-dependent activation of caspases-8,9, 3 and 7 in our study further confirmed apoptosis as the major mechanism of cell death in SW-480 cells treated with [6]-gingerol. Activation of caspase-9 by [6]-gingerol confirms the involvement of mitochondrial pathway in [6]-gingerol-mediated apoptotis. However, the cleavage of caspase-8 induced by [6]-gingerol may not essentially suggest the involvement of receptor-mediated pathway, as mitochondrial pathway could also lead to cleavage of caspase-8 through cleavage of BH3 interacting-domain death agonist (BID) [37]. Induction of apoptosis in SW-480, a p53-mutant colon cancer cell line, by [6]-gingerol is particularly interesting as p53-mutant cells are considered to be more resistant to standard chemotherapeutics and radiation [13,36]. p53-independent induction of apoptosis by [6]-gingerol was reported previously in pancreatic cancer cell lines, where the expression of Cyclin-dependent kinase inhibitor, p21^{cip1}, was increased independent of p53 expression leading to decrease in Cyclin A and Cyclin-dependent kinase expression and cell cycle arrest [36].

Even though [6]-gingerol is generally considered as non-toxic to normal cells, some of the recent studies reported otherwise. Genotoxic effects of [6]-gingerol at higher doses was demonstrated in human hepatoma G2 cells [38]. Another recent study reported that [6]-gingerol treatment leads to a significant dose-dependent inhibition of proliferation of the dermal papilla cells of human hair follicles and elongation of hair shaft [39].They were successful in demonstrating apoptosis in dermal papilla cells at less than 50 micromolar [6]-gingerol. In light of these studies we studied the cytotoxic effects of [6]-gingerol on cultured mouse intestinal epithelial cells. As seen from our results, [6]-gingerol did not induce any significant cytotoxicity even at 500 micromolar. Lack of induction of apoptosis at these concentrations proved [6]-gingerol to be non-toxic to the normal cells of gastro-intestinal tract. Our results go in hand with a previous report where 900 micromolar [6]-gingerol produced only 50% growth inhibition in rat intestinal epithelial cells [36].Thus [6]-gingerol might be showing differential effects on proliferation of normal cells from different origins, but certainly seems to be safe for use in treating gastro-intestinal disorders.

Protein kinase C (PKC) are group of kinases known to regulate cell growth, differentiation and apoptosis mainly through their ability to phosphorylate and activate their substrates, including the members of MAP kinase family [40,41]. Phorbol esters such as phorbol-12-myristate-13-acetate (PMA) are known tumor promoters by virtue of their role in activating PKC as substitutes to their physiological activators like diacylglycerol and phosphatidylserine [22,42]. MAP kinase pathways are involved in regulating proliferation, invasion and metastasis in colon cancer cells [43,44]. As presented in the results, PMA treatment in SW-480 cells activated the members of MAP kinase family, like ERK1/2, JNK and p38 MAPK, as evident from the transient increase in their phosphorylated forms in Western blotting. Remarkable suppression of this activation upon pre-treatment with [6]-gingerol was very evident in case of ERK1/2 and JNK MAP kinases, but less in the case of p38 MAPK. The results from Western blotting were further confirmed from the cell proliferation assay in presence of the inhibitors of MAP kinases. Reversal of PMA-induced proliferation of SW-480 cells in presence of U0126 and SP600125 provides evidence for the role of ERK1/2 and JNK in the cell proliferation. Also the lack of effect of p38 MAP kinase inhibitor, SB203580, rules out the role of p38 MAP kinase in the process. The combination treatment with [6]-gingerol and inhibitors of ERK1/2 or JNK shows that PMA-induced activation of each of these MAP kinase pathways are down-regulated independent to each other by [6]-gingerol and the additive effects of their down-regulation results in the inhibitory effects seen with [6]- gingerol. Although we have not performed the inhibition of both ERK1/2 and JNK pathways together in SW-480 cells, we speculate that a double-inhibition would result in inhibition of PMA-induce cell proliferation typically like that with [6]-gingerol alone. Since no additional inhibitory effects of [6]-gingerol were seen in combination with the inhibitors of ERK1/2 or JNK, we believe that no other additional factors up-regulated by PMA in SW-480 cells are affected by [6]-gingerol. Stimulation of MEK-ERK1/2 pathway by growth factors and induction of both ERK1/2 and JNK pathways by oncogenic proteins like Src and Ras, leading to the activation of their downstream targets, like AP-1, have been found crucial in the development of colon cancer [45,46]. Inhibition of the constituents of MAP kinase pathway has long been recognized as ideal approach to arrest the progression of colon cancer [46].There are reports on other natural compounds like epicatechin gallate, curcumin, silibinin and red ginseng of inducing apoptosis in colon cancer cells via inhibition of MAP kinases [15,47,48,49]. [6]-gingerol was previously shown to inhibit the phosphorylation of ERK1/2, JNK and p38 MAP kinases in mouse skin cancer cell lines, hepatocarcinoma cells and pancreatic cancer cells [28,34,36,50]. But, to the best of our knowledge present study reports for the first time the inhibition of ERK1/2 and JNK MAP kinases as the mechanism of action of [6]-gingerol in reversing the PMA induced proliferation in colon cancer cells.

There are increasing evidence which establish the role of transcription factors like NF-kappB and AP-1 in tumourigenesis, progression, invasion and metastasis of cancer of colon epithelium [46]. In colon cancer, NF-kappaB plays an anti-apoptosis role by many means like, by inhibiting the ROS pathways, by inhibiting JNK cascade and by inducing the expression of anti-apoptotic genes Bcl-2, Bcl-x and cIAPs [51,52]. NF-kappaB is also known to facilitate angiogenesis, invasion and metastasis in colon cancer tumor cells by up-regulating vascular endothelial growth factor (VEGF), cyclooxygenase 2 (COX-2), interleukine (IL)-6 and matrix metalloproteinases (MMPs) [52,53]. AP-1 group of transcription factors have a more direct role in tumorogensis of colon cancer. Enhanced activity of AP-1 has been demonstrated in human colon adenocarcinoma and the immune-histochemical analysis of majority of colon adenocarcinoma has revealed high-level expression of AP-1 correlating with the high expression of its downstream targets like EGFR and COX-2 [46]. AP-1 also mediates the anti-apoptotic response to the hypoxic conditions encountered in the solid tumors which contributed to their resistance to chemotherapy and radiotherapy [54]. AP-1 is under the direct regulatory control of MAP kinases, which phosphorylate the Jun and Fos components of AP-1 protein and facilitate their target binding [46,54].The presence of high concentrations of bile acids also induces the AP-1 expression in colon cells via PKC and ERK1/2 signaling, resulting in tumor promotion [55].Treatment with PMA activates both NF-kappaB and AP-1 transcription factors through Ras/Raf/ERK1/2, JNK and phosphoinositise-3-kinase/Akt signaling pathways [56,57]. In our study too PMA treatment up-regulated both NF-kappaB and AP-1 in SW-480 cells, as evident from the increase in their transcriptional binding. Pre-treatment with [6]-gingerol drastically reduced the up-regulated AP-1, almost completely abolishing their transcriptional binding at 300 μM concentration. On the contrary [6]-gingerol had only a little effect on the transcriptional binding of NF-kappaB. Inhibition of NF-kappa B with SN50 did not have any significant effects on the PMA-induced cell proliferation of SW-480, suggesting no direct role of the PMA-induced NF-kappaB in enhancing proliferation of SW-480 cells. This goes together with the fact that [6]- ginerol had little effect on PMA-induced NF-kappaB while bringing about cytotoxicity in SW-480 cells. Similar effects were reported previously for inhibitory properties of caffeic acid 3, 4-dihydroxy-phenethyl ester (CADPE) on PMA-stimulated gastric carcinoma cells [57]. CADPE was reported to inhibit the phosphorylation of ERK1/2, with little effects on JNK and p38 MAP kinases, inhibiting the transcriptional binding of AP-1, but with no effect on DNA binding of NF-kappaB. Even though we did not include any inhibitors of AP-1 in studying the inhibition of PMA-induced cell proliferation of SW-480, taken together, our results suggests that AP-1 is down-regulated by [6]-gingerol via the inhibition of phosphorylation of ERK1/2 and JNK MAP kinase in SW80 cells. It is well known that ERK1/2 pathway is involved in activation of the c-Fos component and JNK pathway is involved in activation of both c-Jun and c-Fos components of AP-1 [54]. Also we have seen activation of caspase-3 with inhibition of ERK1/2, JNK MAP kinase and with [6]-gingerol while bringing about inhibition of PMA-induced proliferation of SW-480 cells. Thus, [6]-gingerol must be exerting its effect inhibiting the activation of Ras/Raf/ERK1/2/JNK/AP-1 pathway activated by PMA in SW-480 cells. Compounds and small molecules inhibiting the MAP kinases, AP-1 dimerization or AP-1 transcriptional binding are considered ideal candidates for treatment of colon cancer [46]. Thus [6]-gingerol could be an ideal candidate to be developed as an anti-cancer agent against colon cancer.

Previous works on effect of [6]-gingerol on colon cancer cells describe molecular mechanisms different from the present study. Lee et al., 2008 [13] revealed the inhibition of Cyclin D1 and the activation of NAG-1 as mechanism behind cell cycle arrest and pro- apoptotic effect of [6]-gingerol. Another interesting study from Jeong et al, 2009 [14], demonstrated the inhibition of Leukotriene A4 hydrolase, the terminal enzyme in the Leukoteriene B4 synthesis, as the site of action of [6]-gingerol in inhibiting the anchorage dependent growth of HCT116 colon cancer cells in culture and in xenograft model. Another recent study on inhibitory effect on [6]-gingerol on LoVo cells describes down-regulation of cell cycle regulators Cyclin A, B1 and CDK1 along with the increase in the generation of intracellular reactive oxygen species (ROS) as the mechanism of action [15].The present study identifies a totally different mechanism of action for [6]-gingerol in colon cancer cells.

Down-regulation of AP-1 transcriptional binding by [6]-gingerol directly implies to its therapeutic potential against colon cancer, as AP-1 is known to be the transcription factor responsible for transcription of effectors like COX-2, MMPs and VEGF, which are responsible for invasiveness, metastasis and angiogenesis in colon cancer tumors [46,54]. [6]-gingerol was previously shown to inhibit COX-2 expression in skin cancer model [28,29], but till date their effects on COX-2 in colon cancer has not been studied. In the present study, SW-480 being a COX-2 negative cell line [58] might have other down-stream effectors of AP-1, like MMP-9 or VEGF, affected by [6]-gingerol. Down-regulation of MMP-9 and MMP-2 by [6]-gingerol has been reported previously in hepatic cancer and breast cancer cell lines respectively [9,50].Components of ginger were also shown to inhibit angiogenesis by inhibiting VEGF in ovarian cancer cells [29,59].Even though the present study has not explored the effect of [6]-gingerol on down-stream targets of AP-1, it calls for attention in exploring its effects on these effectors molecules in colon cancer cells. Extending the results from present study into an *in vivo* study would further provide valuable insights on the bioavailability of [6]-gingerol and its mechanistic role in prevention of colon tumorogenesis.

Acknowledgments

We thank Dr. K. B. Harikumar for his valuable guidance in the isolation of normal mouse colon cells and Dr. Vinod V, Dr. Vineshkumar TP and Dr. Vinod Balachandran for technical help.

Author Contributions

Conceived and designed the experiments: EVS RJA. Performed the experiments: REK SVB SSN LRN AKTT. Analyzed the data: EVS RJA. Contributed reagents/materials/analysis tools: EVS RJA. Contributed to the writing of the manuscript: SSN RJA.

References

1. Chan DS, Lau R, Aune D, Vieira R, Greenwood DC, et al. (2011) Red and processed meat and colorectal cancer incidence: meta-analysis of prospective studies. PLoS One 6: e20456.
2. Magalhaes B, Peleteiro B, Lunet N (2012) Dietary patterns and colorectal cancer: systematic review and meta-analysis. Eur J Cancer Prev 21: 15–23.
3. Mayer RJ (2009) Targeted therapy for advanced colorectal cancer–more is not always better. N Engl J Med 360: 623–625.
4. Krell J, Stebbing J (2012) Ginger: the root of cancer therapy? Lancet Oncol 13: 235–236.
5. Surh YJ, Lee E, Lee JM (1998) Chemoprotective properties of some pungent ingredients present in red pepper and ginger. Mutat Res 402: 259–267.
6. Baliga MS, Haniadka R, Pereira MM, D'Souza JJ, Pallaty PL, et al. (2011) Update on the chemopreventive effects of ginger and its phytochemicals. Crit Rev Food Sci Nutr 51: 499–523.
7. Shukla Y, Singh M (2007) Cancer preventive properties of ginger: a brief review. Food Chem Toxicol 45: 683–690.
8. Chakraborty D, Bishayee K, Ghosh S, Biswas R, Mandal SK, et al. (2012) [6]-Gingerol induces caspase 3 dependent apoptosis and autophagy in cancer cells: drug-DNA interaction and expression of certain signal genes in HeLa cells. Eur J Pharmacol 694: 20–29.
9. Lee HS, Seo EY, Kang NE, Kim WK (2008) [6]-Gingerol inhibits metastasis of MDA-MB-231 human breast cancer cells. J Nutr Biochem 19: 313–319.
10. Shukla Y, Prasad S, Tripathi C, Singh M, George J, et al. (2007) In vitro and in vivo modulation of testosterone mediated alterations in apoptosis related proteins by [6]-gingerol. Mol Nutr Food Res 51: 1492–1502.
11. Ju SA, Park SM, Lee YS, Bae JH, Yu R, et al. (2012) Administration of 6-gingerol greatly enhances the number of tumor-infiltrating lymphocytes in murine tumors. Int J Cancer 130: 2618–2628.
12. Park KK, Chun KS, Lee JM, Lee SS, Surh YJ (1998) Inhibitory effects of [6]-gingerol, a major pungent principle of ginger, on phorbol ester-induced inflammation, epidermal ornithine decarboxylase activity and skin tumor promotion in ICR mice. Cancer Lett 129: 139–144.
13. Lee SH, Cekanova M, Baek SJ (2008) Multiple mechanisms are involved in 6-gingerol-induced cell growth arrest and apoptosis in human colorectal cancer cells. Mol Carcinog 47: 197–208.
14. Jeong CH, Bode AM, Pugliese A, Cho YY, Kim HG, et al. (2009) [6]-Gingerol suppresses colon cancer growth by targeting leukotriene A4 hydrolase. Cancer Res 69: 5584–5591.
15. Lin CB, Lin CC, Tsay GJ (2012) 6-Gingerol Inhibits Growth of Colon Cancer Cell LoVo via Induction of G2/M Arrest. Evid Based Complement Alternat Med 2012: 326096.
16. Whitehead RH, Demmler K, Rockman SP, Watson NK (1999) Clonogenic growth of epithelial cells from normal colonic mucosa from both mice and humans. Gastroenterology 117: 858–865.
17. Weigmann B, Tubbe I, Seidel D, Nicolaev A, Becker C, et al. (2007) Isolation and subsequent analysis of murine lamina propria mononuclear cells from colonic tissue. Nat Protoc 2: 2307–2311.
18. Anto RJ, Mukhopadhyay A, Shishodia S, Gairola CG, Aggarwal BB (2002) Cigarette smoke condensate activates nuclear transcription factor-kappaB through phosphorylation and degradation of IkappaB(alpha): correlation with induction of cyclooxygenase-2. Carcinogenesis 23: 1511–1518.
19. Bava SV, Sreekanth CN, Thulasidasan AK, Anto NP, Cheriyan VT, et al. (2011) Akt is upstream and MAPKs are downstream of NF-kappaB in paclitaxel-induced survival signaling events, which are down-regulated by curcumin contributing to their synergism. Int J Biochem Cell Biol 43: 331–341.
20. Bava SV, Puliappadamba VT, Deepti A, Nair A, Karunagaran D, et al. (2005) Sensitization of taxol-induced apoptosis by curcumin involves down-regulation of nuclear factor-kappaB and the serine/threonine kinase Akt and is independent of tubulin polymerization. J Biol Chem 280: 6301–6308.
21. Puliyappadamba VT, Cheriyan VT, Thulasidasan AK, Bava SV, Vinod BS, et al. (2010) Nicotine-induced survival signaling in lung cancer cells is dependent on their p53 status while its down-regulation by curcumin is independent. Mol Cancer 9: 220.
22. Rickard KL, Gibson PR, Young GP, Phillips WA (1999) Activation of protein kinase C augments butyrate-induced differentiation and turnover in human colonic epithelial cells in vitro. Carcinogenesis 20: 977–984.
23. Kudınov Y, Wiseman CL, Kharazi AI (2003) Phorbol myristate acetate and Bryostatin 1 rescue IFN-gamma inducibility of MHC class II molecules in LS1034 colorectal carcinoma cell line. Cancer Cell Int 3: 4.
24. Yu R, Hebbar V, Kim DW, Mandlekar S, Pezzuto JM, et al. (2001) Resveratrol inhibits phorbol ester and UV-induced activator protein 1 activation by interfering with mitogen-activated protein kinase pathways. Mol Pharmacol 60: 217–224.
25. Mowla S, Pinnock R, Leaner VD, Goding CR, Prince S (2011) PMA-induced up-regulation of TBX3 is mediated by AP-1 and contributes to breast cancer cell migration. Biochem J 433: 145–153.
26. Lallena MJ, Diaz-Meco MT, Bren G, Paya CV, Moscat J (1999) Activation of IkappaB kinase beta by protein kinase C isoforms. Mol Cell Biol 19: 2180–2188.
27. Park KA, Byun HS, Won M, Yang KJ, Shin S, et al. (2007) Sustained activation of protein kinase C downregulates nuclear factor-kappaB signaling by dissociation of IKK-gamma and Hsp90 complex in human colonic epithelial cells. Carcinogenesis 28: 71–80.
28. Kim SO, Kundu JK, Shin YK, Park JH, Cho MH, et al. (2005) [6]-Gingerol inhibits COX-2 expression by blocking the activation of p38 MAP kinase and NF-kappaB in phorbol ester-stimulated mouse skin. Oncogene 24: 2558–2567.
29. Kim EC, Min JK, Kim TY, Lee SJ, Yang HO, et al. (2005) [6]-Gingerol, a pungent ingredient of ginger, inhibits angiogenesis in vitro and in vivo. Biochem Biophys Res Commun 335: 300–308.
30. Yu Y, Zick S, Li X, Zou P, Wright B, et al. (2011) Examination of the pharmacokinetics of active ingredients of ginger in humans. AAPS J 13: 417–426.
31. Zick SM, Djuric Z, Ruffin MT, Litzinger AJ, Normolle DP, et al. (2008) Pharmacokinetics of 6-gingerol, 8-gingerol, 10-gingerol, and 6-shogaol and conjugate metabolites in healthy human subjects. Cancer Epidemiol Biomarkers Prev 17: 1930–1936.
32. Jiang SZ, Wang NS, Mi SQ (2008) Plasma pharmacokinetics and tissue distribution of [6]-gingerol in rats. Biopharm Drug Dispos 29: 529–537.
33. Brown AC, Shah C, Liu J, Pham JT, Zhang JG, et al. (2009) Ginger's (Zingiber officinale Roscoe) inhibition of rat colonic adenocarcinoma cells proliferation and angiogenesis in vitro. Phytother Res 23: 640–645.
34. Bode AM, Ma WY, Surh YJ, Dong Z (2001) Inhibition of epidermal growth factor-induced cell transformation and activator protein 1 activation by [6]-gingerol. Cancer Res 61: 850–853.
35. Lee E, Surh YJ (1998) Induction of apoptosis in HL-60 cells by pungent vanilloids, [6]-gingerol and [6]-paradol. Cancer Lett 134: 163–168.
36. Park YJ, Wen J, Bang S, Park SW, Song SY (2006) [6]-Gingerol induces cell cycle arrest and cell death of mutant p53-expressing pancreatic cancer cells. Yonsei Med J 47: 688–697.
37. Anto RJ, Mukhopadhyay A, Denning K, Aggarwal BB (2002) Curcumin (diferuloylmethane) induces apoptosis through activation of caspase-8, BID cleavage and cytochrome c release: its suppression by ectopic expression of Bcl-2 and Bcl-xl. Carcinogenesis 23: 143–150.
38. Yang G, Zhong L, Jiang L, Geng C, Cao J, et al. (2010) Genotoxic effect of 6-gingerol on human hepatoma G2 cells. Chem Biol Interact 185: 12–17.
39. Miao Y, Sun Y, Wang W, Du B, Xiao SE, et al. (2013) 6-Gingerol inhibits hair shaft growth in cultured human hair follicles and modulates hair growth in mice. PLoS One 8: e57226.
40. Azzi A, Boscoboinik D, Hensey C (1992) The protein kinase C family. Eur J Biochem 208: 547–557.
41. Nishizuka Y (1992) Intracellular signaling by hydrolysis of phospholipids and activation of protein kinase C. Science 258: 607–614.
42. Meyer E, Vollmer JY, Bovey R, Stamenkovic I (2005) Matrix metalloproteinases 9 and 10 inhibit protein kinase C-potentiated, p53-mediated apoptosis. Cancer Res 65: 4261–4272.
43. Masur K, Lang K, Niggemann B, Zanker KS, Entschladen F (2001) High PKC alpha and low E-cadherin expression contribute to high migratory activity of colon carcinoma cells. Mol Biol Cell 12: 1973–1982.
44. Heider I, Schulze B, Oswald E, Henklein P, Scheele J, et al. (2004) PAR1-type thrombin receptor stimulates migration and matrix adhesion of human colon carcinoma cells by a PKCepsilon-dependent mechanism. Oncol Res 14: 475–482.
45. Ashida R, Tominaga K, Sasaki E, Watanabe T, Fujiwara Y, et al. (2005) AP-1 and colorectal cancer. Inflammopharmacology 13: 113–125.
46. Vaiopoulos AG, Papachroni KK, Papavassiliou AG (2010) Colon carcinogenesis: Learning from NF-kappaB and AP-1. Int J Biochem Cell Biol 42: 1061–1065.
47. Cordero-Herrera I, Martin MA, Bravo L, Goya L, Ramos S (2013) Epicatechin gallate induces cell death via p53 activation and stimulation of p38 and JNK in human colon cancer SW480 cells. Nutr Cancer 65: 718–728.
48. Collett GP, Campbell FC (2004) Curcumin induces c-jun N-terminal kinase-dependent apoptosis in HCT116 human colon cancer cells. Carcinogenesis 25: 2183–2189.
49. Seo EY, Kim WK (2011) Red ginseng extract reduced metastasis of colon cancer cells in vitro and in vivo. J Ginseng Res 35: 315–324.
50. Weng CJ, Chou CP, Ho CT, Yen GC (2012) Molecular mechanism inhibiting human hepatocarcinoma cell invasion by 6-shogaol and 6-gingerol. Mol Nutr Food Res 56: 1304–1314.
51. Bubici C, Papa S, Pham CG, Zazzeroni F, Franzoso G (2006) The NF-kappaB-mediated control of ROS and JNK signaling. Histol Histopathol 21: 69–80.
52. Chen F, Castranova V (2007) Nuclear factor-kappaB, an unappreciated tumor suppressor. Cancer Res 67: 11093–11098.
53. Basseres DS, Baldwin AS (2006) Nuclear factor-kappaB and inhibitor of kappaB kinase pathways in oncogenic initiation and progression. Oncogene 25: 6817–6830.
54. Shaulian E, Karin M (2002) AP-1 as a regulator of cell life and death. Nat Cell Biol 4: E131–136.
55. Debruyne PR, Bruyneel EA, Li X, Zimber A, Gespach C, et al. (2001) The role of bile acids in carcinogenesis. Mutat Res 480–481: 359–369.
56. Cho HJ, Kang JH, Kwak JY, Lee TS, Lee IS, et al. (2007) Ascofuranone suppresses PMA-mediated matrix metalloproteinase-9 gene activation through

the Ras/Raf/MEK/ERK- and Ap1-dependent mechanisms. Carcinogenesis 28: 1104–1110.
57. Han H, Du B, Pan X, Liu J, Zhao Q, et al. (2010) CADPE inhibits PMA-stimulated gastric carcinoma cell invasion and matrix metalloproteinase-9 expression by FAK/MEK/ERK-mediated AP-1 activation. Mol Cancer Res 8: 1477–1488.
58. Shao J, Sheng H, Inoue H, Morrow JD, DuBois RN (2000) Regulation of constitutive cyclooxygenase-2 expression in colon carcinoma cells. J Biol Chem 275: 33951–33956.
59. Rhode J, Fogoros S, Zick S, Wahl H, Griffith KA, et al. (2007) Ginger inhibits cell growth and modulates angiogenic factors in ovarian cancer cells. BMC Complement Altern Med 7: 44.

2

Heat-Stable Molecule Derived from *Streptococcus cristatus* Induces APOBEC3 Expression and Inhibits HIV-1 Replication

Ziqing Wang[1,¶,¤a], Yi Luo[1,¶], Qiujia Shao[1], Ballington L. Kinlock[1], Chenliang Wang[1,3], James E. K. Hildreth[1,¤b], Hua Xie[2]*, Bindong Liu[1]*

1 Center for AIDS Health Disparities Research, School of Medicine, Meharry Medical College, Nashville, Tennessee, United States of America, **2** Department of Oral Biology and Research, School of Dentistry, Meharry Medical College, Nashville, Tennessee, United States of America, **3** Institute of Gastroenterology and Institute of Human Virology, Sun Yat-sen University, Guangzhou, Guangdong, Peoples of Republic of China

Abstract

Although most human immunodeficiency virus type 1 (HIV-1) cases worldwide are transmitted through mucosal surfaces, transmission through the oral mucosal surface is a rare event. More than 700 bacterial species have been detected in the oral cavity. Despite great efforts to discover oral inhibitors of HIV, little information is available concerning the anti-HIV activity of oral bacterial components. Here we show that a molecule from an oral commensal bacterium, *Streptococcus cristatus* CC5A can induce expression of APOBEC3G (A3G) and APOBEC3F (A3F) and inhibit HIV-1 replication in THP-1 cells. We show by qRT-PCR that expression levels of A3G and A3F increase in a dose-dependent manner in the presence of a CC5A extract, as does A3G protein levels by Western blot assay. In addition, when the human monocytic cell line THP-1 was treated with CC5A extract, the replication of HIV-1 IIIB was significantly suppressed compared with IIIB replication in untreated THP-1 cells. Knock down of A3G expression in THP-1 cells compromised the ability of CC5A to inhibit HIV-1 IIIB infectivity. Furthermore, SupT1 cells infected with virus produced from CC5A extract-treated THP-1 cells replicated virus with a higher G to A hypermutation rate (a known consequence of A3G activity) than virus used from untreated THP-1 cells. This suggests that *S. cristatus* CC5A contains a molecule that induces A3G/F expression and thereby inhibits HIV replication. These findings might lead to the discovery of a novel anti-HIV/AIDS therapeutic.

Editor: Roberto F. Speck, University Hospital Zurich, Switzerland

Funding: This work was supported by NIH grants SC1GM089269, U54RR019192, G12MD007586, P30AI054999 and UL1TR000445 to BL and NIH grant U54RR019192 to HX. BLK is supported by NIH training grant T32HL007737. NIH website is www.nih.gov. The funders had no role in study design, data collection and analysis, decision to publish, or preparation of the manuscript.

Competing Interests: The authors have declared that no competing interests exist.

* Email: bliu@mmc.edu (BL); hxie@mmc.edu (HX)

¶ These authors contributed equally to this work.

¤a Current address: Department of Integrative Biology and Pharmacology, University of Texas Health Science Center at Houston, Houston, Texas United States of America
¤b Current address: College of Biological Sciences, University of California Davis, Davis, California, United States of America

Introduction

HIV-1 can be transmitted through intravenous contact with contaminated blood products, from infected mothers to offspring *in utero* or through lactation after birth. However, the predominant mode of HIV transmission is by sexual contact through broken mucosal or epidermal epithelia. In contrast, oral transmission of HIV is an extremely rare event [1–3]. This is true despite the fact that a recent study reported that cell-associated proviral HIV-1 DNA was detected in gingival crevicular fluid of 49% of HIV-1 infected patients [4]. Moreover, hyper-excretion of HIV-1 RNA in saliva has been reported [5]. Normally HIV-1 infected patients have plasma titers exceeding those found in saliva, but in one study, 7% of 67 tested individuals had a four-fold or higher viral load in saliva compared to plasma [5]. Therefore, it has been suggested that certain oral components are capable of inactivating HIV-1. Several endogenous components have been proposed as contributors to HIV inactivation, either when found alone or in combination [6]. Among them, secretory leucocyte protease inhibitor (SLPI) has been extensively studied [7]. Another known class of proteins with innate immunity capacity in the oral cavity is the β-defensins, which are secreted by epithelial cells [8].

More than 700 bacterial species have been detected in the oral cavity [9]. Despite great effort to uncover oral inhibitors of HIV, little information is available on the anti-HIV activity of oral bacterial components. Our previous work revealed that the binding domains (HGP17 and 44) of *Porphyromonas gingivalis'* gingipains can block HIV infection by interacting with the viral glycoprotein, gp120 [10]. One mechanism by which products from oral bacteria could block HIV infection that has not been considered is their role in the production of host cell restriction factors. One such factor is APOBEC3. Here we report that *S. cristatus* expresses a small molecular weight heat-stable molecule with apparent anti-HIV activity via its ability to induce expression of the human HIV-restriction factor APOBEC. This ability is previously unreported in bacteria.

S. cristatus is a member of the mitis group of streptococci and has been detected on the surfaces of the buccal epithelium and the teeth of healthy individuals [9]. It has not been associated with oral infectious diseases, although it has been documented that noninvasive *S. cristatus* can be transferred into human epithelial cells by *F. nucleatum* [11]. Interestingly, a small study of 14 HIV-1 positive patients by the Forsyth Institute examined the presence/absence of 109 oral bacterial species. The patients suffered from gingivitis, periodontitus or linear gingival erythema. The authors found detectable levels of *S. cristatus* in 2 of 9 HIV-positive patients who had a low viral load and high CD4 counts, while *S. cristatus* was undetectable in all of the 5 patients with high viral load and low CD4 counts [12]. However at this time it is premature to make any conclusions about the correlation between specific bacterial species and the different immune states of HIV-positive patients.

Members of the APOBEC3 family of proteins that mediate cytidine deaminase activity, serve as potent restriction factors to HIV-1 infection [13–15]. Among them, APOBEC3G (A3G) and ABOPEC3F (A3F) show potent anti-HIV-1 activity [15–20]. HIV-1 Vif is a 23 kD small regulatory protein which is essential for HIV-1 replication [21,22]. HIV-1 Vif hijacks human ubiquitin E3 ligase Cullin 5 [23] to promote the proteosome mediated degradation of A3G [23–28]. Degradation of A3G depletes A3G from the cytoplasm of virus-producing cells thereby preventing A3G from being incorporated into virions to perform its antiviral function. In the absence of Vif, A3G is packaged into the HIV-1 virion [23,25–29]. Upon infecting the target cells, A3G drastically restricts HIV-1 replication by causing G to A hypermutations in the newly synthesized cDNA. Recent reports show that A3G also inhibits the production of HIV-1 reverse transcription products [30–33] and viral DNA integration [32] and that antiviral activity found in A3G could also be independent of its deaminase activity [33,34]. In addition to inhibition of HIV-1, A3G restricts replication of other retroviruses including simian immunodeficiency virus, equine infectious anemia virus and murine leukemia virus. Similar in activity to A3G, [17,19,20,35] A3F is also packaged into HIV-1ΔVif virions and induces G to A hypermutations, although it differs with respect to the target sequence motif [19].

A3G gene expression is upregulated in response to multiple regulatory factors. Treatment of H9 T cell lines with phorbol myristate acetate (PMA) increases expression of A3G. This increased expression of A3G is mediated by the protein kinase C/mitogen-activated protein/ERK signaling cascade [36]. Similarly, treatment of resting peripheral blood lymphocytes (PBLs) with phytohemagglutinin (PHA) plus IL-2 or particular cytokines when each are added alone (IL-2, IL-7 and IL-15) increases expression of A3G through the JAK/MAPK signaling pathway [24,37]. Interferon also plays a role in upregulating A3G in primary macrophages, CD4 T cells and primary hepatocytes or in laboratory-adapted hepatocellular carcinoma cell lines such as Hep3B, HepG2 and Huh 7 [38–40]. Here we will show evidence that a molecule associated with *S. cristatus* can induce expression of A3G and A3F and inhibit HIV-1 replication.

Materials and Methods

Cell culture and reagents

The cell lines THP-1, SupT1, TZM-bl and H9/HTLV- IIIB along with anti-human APOBEC3G and anti-human APOBEC3F antibody were obtained from the NIH AIDS Research and Reference Reagent Program. THP-1 and Sup T1 were cultured in regular RPMI medium with 10% fetal calf serum (FBS). TZM-bl was grown in DMEM supplemented with 10% fetal calf serum. Immortalized human keratinocytes OKF6/TERT-2, provided by Dr. James G. Rheinwald (Harvard Medical School, MA) [41], were cultured in Keratinocyte-SFM (Invitrogen) supplemented with 0.2 ng/ml recombinant epidermal growth factor (rEGF; Invitrogen), 25 μg/ml bovine pituitary extract (BPE) and 0.4 mM CaCl2 (final). Immortalized human vaginal epithelial cells VK2/E6E7, purchased from ATCC and cultured as described [42]. Lipopolysaccharide (LPS-EK Ultrapure) and lipoteichoic acid (LTA-SA) were purchased from Invivogen. MEK inhibitor U0126 was purchased from Calbiochem. Anti p-ERK (E-4) (sc-7383) and anti-ERK2 (D-2) (sc-1647) were purchased from Santa Cruz, USA.

Preparation of sonicated bacterial cell extracts

Oral bacteria, including *Actinomyces naeslundii* NC-3, *Streptococcus gordonii* DL1, *S. cristatus* CC5A, *S. mutans* KPSK2, *Actinomyces viscosus* EG4, and *Porphyromonas gingivalis* 33277, which were from our laboratory collection at Meharry Medical College School of Dentistry, were grown in appropriate media aerobically or anaerobically at 37°C for 16 h. Bacterial cells were harvested by centrifugation at 6,000×*g* for 10 min at 4°C. Bacterial cells were washed twice with cold PBS. The cell extracts were then prepared by sonication at Power 15 (10×30 sec) using a Misonix XL-2000. The supernatants were collected and filtered through a 0.22 μm PVDF filter (Millipore). The bacterial extracts were stored in −20°C freezers if long term storage were needed.

Preparation of the *S. cristatus* PBS solution

S. cristatus CC5A cells were incubated in PBS at 37°C for 4 h without sonication, and the supernatant of the cell mixture (hereafter termed CC5A/PBS) was collected following centrifugation at 6,000*g*, 4°C, for 15 min and filtration through a 0.22 μm PVDF filter (Millipore). For separate experiments, some *S. cristatus* CC5A cells were also boiled in 2% SDS for 1 h. After washing them six times with PBS, the cells were either incubated in PBS at 37°C for 4 h for preparation of a CC5A/PBS solution or they were sonicated as described to prepare a sonicated bacterial cell extracts.

To treat THP-1 cells, 25 μg (or as indicated) equivalent protein content measured by BCA assay (Pierce) of bacterial extracts was added to 5×10^5 cells in 12-well-plates (Celltreat Scientific Products) containing 1 ml of complete medium and incubated at 37°C, 5% CO_2 for 16 h. After treatment, THP-1 cells were subjected to total RNA isolation as indicated in the qRT-PCR procedure. For the MEK inhibitor treatment, 5×10^5 THP-1 cells were treated with 20 μM U0126 for 1 h prior to CC5A/PBS treatment. After U0126 treatment, THP-1 cells were washed twice with PBS and subjected to CC5A/PBS treatment.

To treat OKF6 or VK2 cells, 100% confluent cells in a 12-well-plate (around 5×10^5 cells per well) were treated with the indicated amount of CC5A/PBS for the indicated times. After treatment, cells were analyzed by either qRT-PCR or Western-blot as described previously [43].

qRT-PCR

Real-time quantitative reverse transcription PCR (qRT-PCR) was performed with a Bio-Rad MyiQ Single-Color Real-Time PCR Detection System using Bio-Rad iQ SYBR Green Supermix reagent. Total RNA was extracted using a TRizol plus PureLink Micro-to-Midi Total RNA Purification System (Invitrogen) following the manufacturer's protocol. DNA was further removed by on-column digestion using RQI RNase free DNase (Promega). An equal amount of RNA was reverse transcribed using random hexamer primers and M-MLV RT reverse transcriptase (Promega). Expression of A3F, A3G and GAPDH were analyzed by qRT-PCR using the following primers A3G: 5′-TCAGAGGACGGCATGAGACTTA-3′, 5′-AGCAGGACCCAGGTGTCATT-3′; A3F: 5′-CCTACGCAAAGCCTATGGTCGG-3′, 5′-CCAGGAGACAGGTGAGTGGTGC-3′; GAPDH: 5′-GAAGGTGAAGGTCGGAGT-3′, 5′-GAAGATGGTGATGGGATTTC-3′ as described previously [44]. qRT-PCR result was normalized using GAPDH amplification levels and calculated by $2^{-\Delta\Delta CT}$ comparative method. All experiments were independently repeated at least three times. The variation was expressed by calculating the standard deviation (SD) from the three independent experiments and presented as the mean values ± SD.

Gel filtration chromatography

D-Salt Polyacrylamide Desalting Columns (6KMWCO, Pierce) were used to estimate the molecular weight of the active molecule of *S. cristatus*. The column was mounted on a LKB FPLC system. The column was calibrated by a gel-filtration standard (Bio-rad Cat #151-1901); 100 μg CC5A/PBS was loaded onto the column. The chromatography was performed under the following conditions: elution buffer: PBS; flow rate: 1 ml/min; and UV monitoring: 220 nm. Fractions (1.5 ml) were collected and the induction effect of these fractions on A3G mRNA was measured by qRT-PCR.

Viral infectivity assay

HIV-1 IIIB virus was obtained from the cell cultural supernatant of H9/HTLV-IIIB cell line. THP-1 cells were infected by HIV-1 IIIB virus and cultured for two weeks to generate a chronically infected THP-1 cell line (THP-1/IIIB). Equal numbers of these cells were treated with PBS or 40 μg CC5A/PBS overnight. After washing cells twice with PBS, cells were cultured in complete medium at 37°C, 5% CO_2 for 24 h. After 24 h of culture, the cells were washed twice again with PBS, then cultured in the fresh complete medium for another 24 h. The culture supernatants were harvested. The released virus was measured by standard p24 ELISA assay. The viral infectivity of released virus was measured by a MAGI assay using TZM-bl cells as described [45]. Briefly, TZM-bl cells were infected with serial dilutions of released virus in complete medium with 20 μg/ml of DEAE-Dextran in a 37°C, 5% CO_2 incubator. After 3 h incubation, the culture volume was increased 1 fold by complete medium. After 48 h incubation, viral infectivity was measured by a Promega Luciferase Kit. The luciferase result was normalized to the p24 input for each sample.

Viral replication assay

THP-1 cells (5×10^5) were treated with only PBS or 40 μg CC5A/PBS overnight. After washing twice with PBS, the treated cells were infected with equal amounts of HIV-1 IIIB (containing 100 ng p24 protein content) for 3 h. The cells were washed twice with PBS and cultured in complete medium for 8 days at 37°C, 5% CO_2. Every other day, a 50 μl sample of supernatant was collected and p24 content determined using a standard p24 ELISA assay. A viral replication curve was generated by plotting p24 concentration against replication days.

Establishment of A3G knockdown THP-1 cells using CRISPR/Case9 system

Oligos: CACCGCGAAGCGCCTCCTGGTAATC and AAACGATTACCAGGAGGCGCTTCGC were annealed together to form short dsDNA 1; oligos: CACCGTAACCTTCGGGTCCTCGGCC and AAACGGCCGAGGACCCGAAGGTTAC were annealed together to form short dsDNA 2. dsDNA 1 and dsDNA 2 were designed to target A3G genome exon 3. pX330 (Addgene 42230) was digested by BssI. dsDNA1 and dsDNA2 were cloned into pX330 respectively to form pX330-A3G1 and pX330-A3G2. pX330-A3G1 and pX330-A3G2 (3 μg each) were transfected into 1×10^6 THP-1 cells using Neon Transfection System (Invitrogen). The transfection condition is voltage: 1300 V; width: 30 ms; pulse: 1 pulse. Three days post transfection, the transfected THP-1 cells were cloned by limited dilution method. Single clones were screen by Western-blot and qRT-PCR for A3G expression analysis.

DNA hypermutation assay

Equal numbers of THP-1/IIIB cells were treated with PBS or 40 μg CC5A/PBS overnight. After washing with PBS twice, the cells were cultured in complete medium at 37°C, 5% CO_2 for two days. Culture supernatants containing released virus (containing 100 ng p24 protein content) were used to infect 1×10^6 Sup T1 cells for 4 h. The infected SupT1 cells were washed twice with PBS then incubated at 37°C, 5% CO_2 for 16 h. DNA was isolated using DNeasy DNA isolation kit (Qiagen). A 650 bp DNA fragment covering a portion of nef, U3 and R of HIV-1 was amplified with platinum Taq DNA polymerase (Invitrogen) using the primers HIV-1-F, 5′-AGGCAGCTGTAGATATTAGCCAC, and HIV-1-R, 5′-GTATGAGGGATCTCTAGCTACCA. The PCR products were cloned into the TOPO TA-cloning vector (Invitrogen). The nucleotide sequences of individual clones from each infected culture sample were determined [46]. Statistical significance was determined by Mann Whitney U test using GraphPad Prism software.

Cytotoxicity assay

The cytotoxicity of CC5A/PBS and Sonicated CC5A treatment was measured by a Live/Dead Cell Vitality Assay Kit (Invitrogen). The kit provides a two-color fluorescence assay that distinguishes metabolically active cells from injured cells and dead cells. THP-1 cells were treated with the indicated dose of protein from sonicated CC5A or unsonicated CC5A/PBS respectively. PBS treated THP-1 was used as untreated control. Sixteen h post treatment, the samples were subjected to Live/Dead Cell Vitality Assay Kit following the product manual. The samples were analyzed by BD FACSCalibur.

Results

Bacterial extract from *S. cristatus* CC5A induces A3F and A3G expression

To determine the role of oral bacteria on the expression of innate intracellular immune factors A3G and A3F, we utilized a group of oral bacteria, including *A. naeslundii* NC-3, *S. gordonii* DL1, *S. cristatus* CC5A, *S. mutans* KPSK2, *A. viscosus,* and *P. gingivalis* 33277. The sonicated bacterial extracts (25 μg equivalent protein content) were added to THP-1 growth medium. PBS treated cells were used as controls and GAPDH was used as a normalization control. Expression of A3F and A3G was measured using qRT-PCR. As shown in Fig. 1A, the expression of A3F and A3G mRNA was enhanced in the presence of the *S. cristatus*

CC5A sonicated cell extract. Expression of A3F was increased as high as around 8 fold above baseline (set = 1), and expression of A3G was increased around 6 fold. In contrast, the extracts from the other oral bacteria tested and *E coli* DH5α (DH5A) had little or no effect on the expression of A3F and A3G. This experiment and all other experiments throughout this study were independently repeated at least three times. The variation was expressed by calculating the standard deviation (SD) from the three independent experiments and presented as the mean values ± SD. For the results of Western-blot analysis, one image representing the consent of the data will be shown.

We also tested several other oral *S. cristatus* strains such as CR311, CR3, CH34110 and pSH11a and pSH11b. CR3, CR311 and CH34110, which are closely related to CC5A, were as efficient as CC5A at inducing A3F and A3G expression, whereas pSH11b and pSH11a had almost no effect on APOBEC induction (Fig. 1B). Thus CC5A is not the only *S. cristatus* strain that is active, in terms of containing a molecule that induces APOBEC expression. We also treated THP-1 cells with different doses of CC5A in order to identify whether the induction of mRNA and protein expression levels was dose dependent. After a 16 h treatment, total RNA was isolated and induction of A3G and A3F measured by qRT-PCR. The induction of A3F and A3G mRNA gradually increased in response to the increasing amount of CC5A/PBS (Fig. 1C). By Western blot analysis, we also showed that A3G and A3F protein levels increased when THP-1 cells were treated with increasing amounts of CC5A/PBS (Fig. 1D). The dose response of APOBEC mRNA and protein further confirmed the effect of CC5A on A3F and A3G induction.

CC5A/PBS contains a small active molecule, which covalently conjugates to the cell wall

Interestingly, we found that the active molecule appeared to be released from S. cristatus CC5A when the bacterial cells were simply incubated in PBS for 4 h at 37°C without sonication (Fig. 2A). When the process of 4 h incubation in PBS was done at 4°C (Fig. 2A) or after CC5A cells were boiled in 2% SDS for 1 h (Fig. 2B), the activity of inducing A3G expression was dramatically compromised. However, if sonication was used to treat the SDS treated CC5A cells, the active molecule was released into the

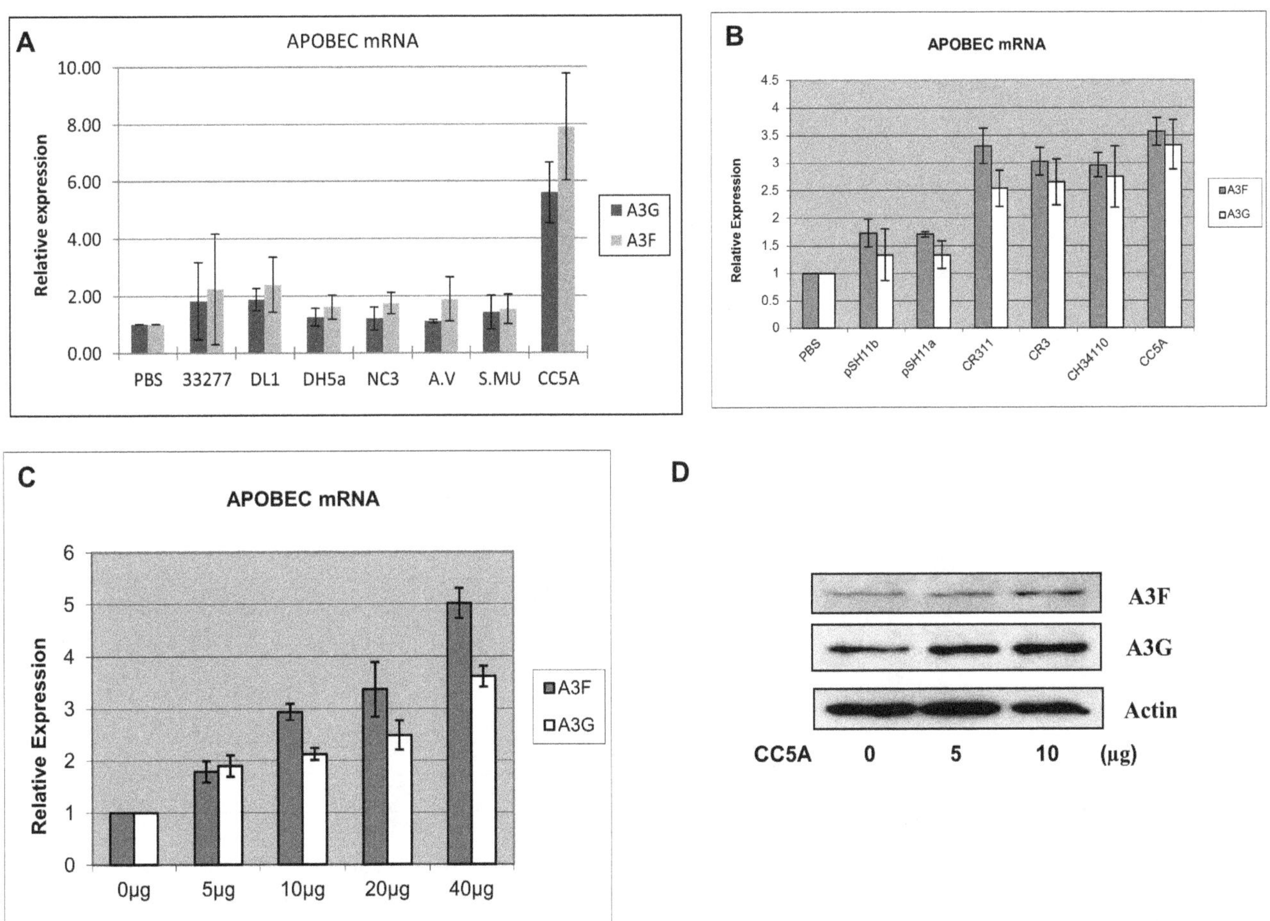

Figure 1. A molecule derived from oral *Streptococcus cristatus* induces APOBEC3F/G expression. (A) Cell extracts from NC3 (*Actinomyces naeslundii* NC-3), DL1 (*Streptococcus gordonii* DL1) and DH5a, CC5A (*S. cristatus* CC5A), A.V (*Actinomyces viscosus*), 33277 (*Porphyromonas gingivalis* 33277) and S.MU (*S. mutans* KPSK2) were used to treat THP-1 cells. THP-1 cells treated by PBS were used as a control. After 16 h of exposure, total RNA was isolated and the expression of A3G and A3F quantified by qRT-PCR. (B) CC5A and different strains of *S. cristatus* (pSH11b, pSH11a, CR311, CR3, and CH34110) were used to treat THP-1. The induction of A3G and A3F was measured by qRT-PCR. (C) Different doses (0–40 μg) of CC5A/PBS were used to treat THP-1 cells for 16 h. A3G and A3F expression was measured by qRT-PCR. (D) A3G and A3F expression following a 48 h exposure to 0–10 μg CC5A was tested by Western blot assay. Values shown in (A), (B) and (C) are given as means ± SD of three independent experiments compared to normalized to 1.0 for controls. The Western-blot data is representative of three independent experiments.

supernatant (Fig. 2C). This indicates that the active molecule could not be removed from the cell (or destroyed) by boiling in 2% SDS, yet sonicating these cells released the active molecule into the PBS. This data implies that the active molecule may be covalently conjugated to the cell wall and an enzymatic reaction is necessary to release the active molecule from the CC5A cells when CC5A cells are simply incubated, for example, in PBS at 37°C for 4 h. These findings also show that the active molecule is very heat-stable.

To help identify the molecular weight of the active molecule, we used D-Salt Polyacrylamide Desalting Columns from Pierce with molecular weight cut-off of 6 kD. We first calibrated the column using Bio-Rad gel filtration standards, which contain equine myoglobin (17 kD) and vitamin B12 (1.3 kD). Equine myoglobin appears yellow and vitamin B12 appears pink in eluates. These two molecules eluted in fractions 3 and 5, respectively (Fig. 2D, indicated by arrows). When 100 μg CC5A/PBS was analyzed using this column, the peak A3G induction activity appeared in fractions 3 (17 kD) and 8 (Fig. 2D). A similar result was also observed for A3F induction (data not shown). Despite the fact that the molecular weight of fraction 8 must be <1.3 kD, this fraction is capable of inducing A3G mRNA. As the molecular weight cut-off of this column is 6 kD, the active molecule in fraction 3 is bigger than 6 kD and most likely represents the partially enzymatically digested cell wall component which is covalently conjugated to the small molecule found in fractions 8 and 9. This suggestion will be further addressed during our process of identifying this molecule. Nonetheless, the data shows that a small, heat stable molecule from CC5A is able to induce A3F and A3G expression.

CC5A/PBS induces APOBEC through an MEK1/2 pathway

It has been reported that A3G is regulated through PKC and the JAK/MAPK signaling pathways in response to stimulation by PMA and cytokines [36,37]. Stimulation of cell surface CCR5 and CD40 molecules by their ligands or by HSP70 up-regulates APOBEC3G expression in $CD4^+$ T cells and dendritic cells through the p38 and ERK dependent signaling pathway [47]. A3G is also regulated through a STAT1-independent pathway when liver cells are treated with IFNα [39]. To test the signaling events involved in CC5A/PBS regulation of APOBEC expression, THP-1 cells were pretreated with the MEK inhibitor U0126. U0126 strongly inhibited CC5A/PBS mediated up-regulation of A3F and A3G mRNA (Fig. 3A). To confirm that CC5A/PBS

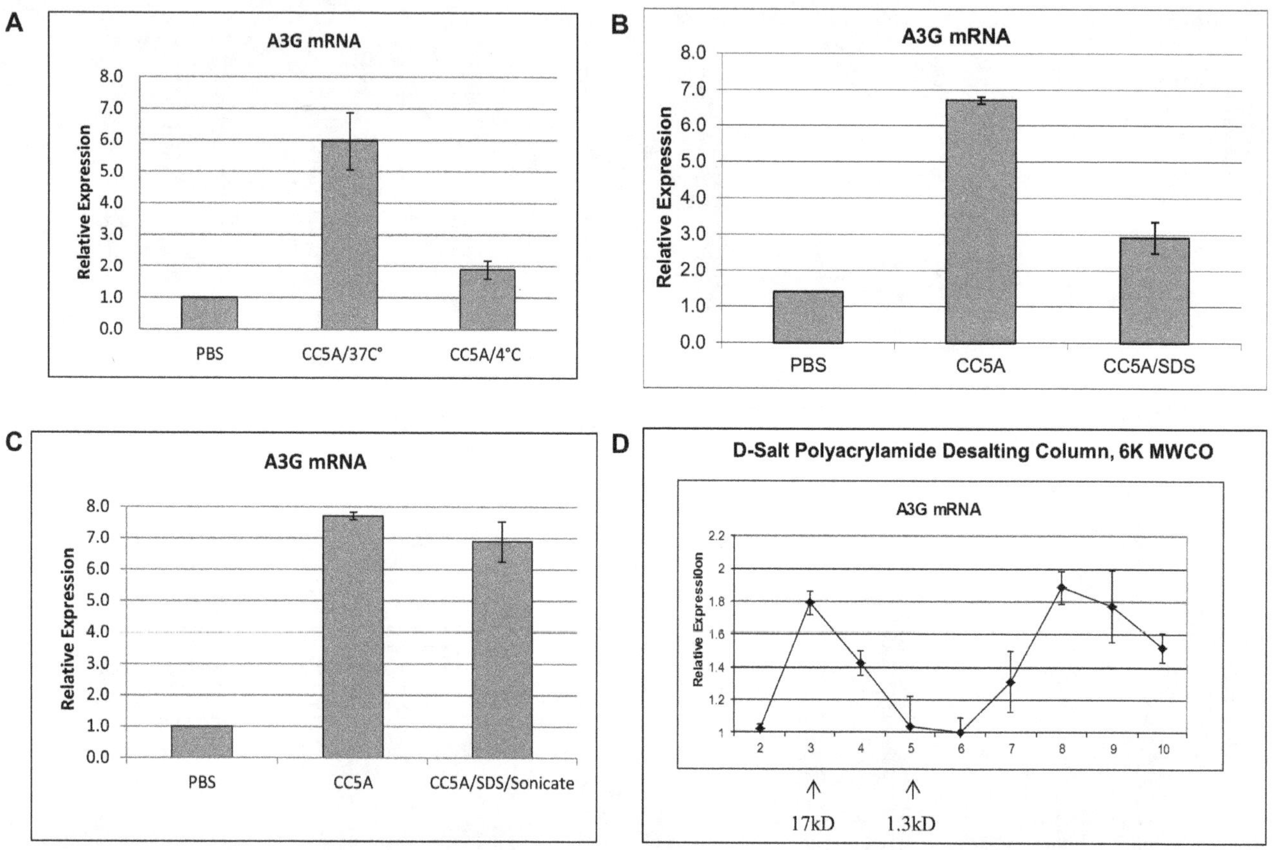

Figure 2. CC5A/PBS contains a small active heat-stable molecule, which may be covalently conjugated to the cell wall. (A) CC5A cells were incubated in PBS at 37°C or 4°C respectively. After 4 h of incubation, CC5A/PBS was prepared as described in Material and Methods. The CC5A/37°C and CC5A/4°C were used to treat THP-1 and the relative expression of A3G mRNA was measured by qRT-PCR. (B) CC5A cells were boiled in 2% SDS for 1 h. After being extensively washed with PBS, the SDS-treated CC5A cells were incubated in PBS at 37°C for 4 h for the preparation of CC5A/SDS. CC5A/SDS was used to treat THP-1 cells. The relative expression of A3G mRNA was measured by qRT-PCR. (C) After CC5A cells were treated with 2% SDS, the cells were sonicated to collect the CC5A extract as described in Material and Methods. The sonicated CC5A molecules were used to treat THP-1 cells. The relative expression of A3G mRNA was measured by qRT-PCR. (D) CC5A/PBS (100 μg) was subjected to a D-Salt Polyacrylamide Desalting Column (with a molecular weight cut-off of 6 kD). Two standards are shown by arrows: myoglobin (17 kD) and vitamin b12 (1.3 kD); 1.5 ml fractions were collected. The A3G induction response to eluate samples was measured by qRT-PCR. In all the qRT-PCR assays, the expression of A3G mRNA from untreated THP-1 cells was set as one.

activates the MAPK pathway, we analyzed the expression of phospho-ERK1/2 by using Western blot analysis. After THP-1 cells were treated with CC5A/PBS, phospho-ERK1/2 (Fig. 3B lane 3) was significantly increased compared with PBS treated THP-1 cells (lane 1). When U0126 was used to pretreat THP-1 cells, phospho-ERK1/2 was undetectable (lane 2) even with CC5A/PBS treatment. We noticed that the phosphorylation of ERK1/2 in lane 2 was even lower than that in lane 1 in Fig. 3B, indicating that U0126 not only inhibited the phosphorylation of ERK1/2 induced by CC5A, but also the phosphorylation caused by the endogenous mechanisms. Taken together, these results indicate that CC5A/PBS regulates A3G and A3F through a MEK1/2 dependent pathway.

CC5A/PBS reduces HIV-1 infectivity and inhibits HIV-1 replication

A3G is a potent host restriction factor of HIV-1 replication. It reduces HIV-1 infectivity once it is packaged into HIV-1 particles [15]. Since CC5A/PBS induces A3G expression, we next asked whether CC5A/PBS can reduce HIV infectivity in the THP-1 cell system. THP-1/IIIB cells, chronically infected by HIV-1 IIIB, were treated with PBS or CC5A/PBS (40 μg) for 16 h. Post-treatment, THP-1 cells were washed twice by PBS and cultured for 24 h. After 24 h, the cells were washed with PBS again and cultured for another 24 h. The culture supernatant was collected for a MAGI infectivity assay as describe previously [48]. The amount of virus for the infectivity assay was normalized by p24 ELISA [48]. After CC5A/PBS treatment, HIV infectivity was reduced approximately 70% compare to untreated cells (Fig. 4A). To determine if CC5A/PBS was capable of inhibiting HIV-1 replication throughout multiple rounds of infection, THP-1 cells were pretreated overnight with CC5A/PBS (40 μg) or PBS before infection with HIV-1 IIIB. After 3 h of infection, the cells were washed twice with PBS and put back into culture for eight days. Viral-containing supernatants were collected every two days and viral replication was monitored by p24 ELISA. Viral replication in CC5A/PBS-treated THP-1 cells was significantly inhibited (Fig. 4B). This data suggests that CC5A/PBS is able to inhibit HIV-1 replication.

A3G knockdown compromised the effect of CC5A in reducing HIV infectivity

CC5A induced A3G expression (Fig. 1) and inhibits HIV infectivity (Fig. 4). This suggests that A3G may play a role in mediating the effect of CC5A in inhibiting HIV infectivity. To prove this, we established an A3G knockdown cell line using CRISP/Case 9 system. CRISPR stands for Clustered Regularly Interspaced Short Palindromic Repeats. The CRISPR/Case system is currently the most commonly used RNA-Guided Endonuclease technology for genome engineering [49,50]. We constructed plasmids pX300-A3G1 and pX300-A3G2, which targeted A3G genome exon 3. We established A3G knockdown cell line after one round screening as described in the material and methods section. As shown in Fig. 5A and 5B, the expression level of A3G mRNA and protein levels decreased more than 50% in THP-1 A3GKD cell line compared with wild-type THP-1. Both THP-1 and THP-1 A3GKD cell lines were infected with HIV-1 IIIB to generate chronically infected cell lines. The effects of CC5A on reducing HIV infectivity were measured in both cell lines as described earlier for Fig. 4A. As shown in Fig. 5C, the viral infectivity of PBS treated THP-1/A3GKD/PBS is about two fold higher than the infectivity of PBS treated wild-type THP-1. This data is consistent with the function of A3G in which lower expression of A3G will render higher viral infectivity. When the infectivity of CC5A treated THP-1 A3GKD was compared with wild-type THP-1, we demonstrate that the infectivity of THP-1 A3GKD was about two fold higher than the infectivity of CC5A treated wild-type THP-1. The data showed that A3G knockdown reduced CC5A's effects in reducing HIV infectivity, suggesting that A3G played a role in mediating the effects of CC5A in inhibiting HIV infectivity.

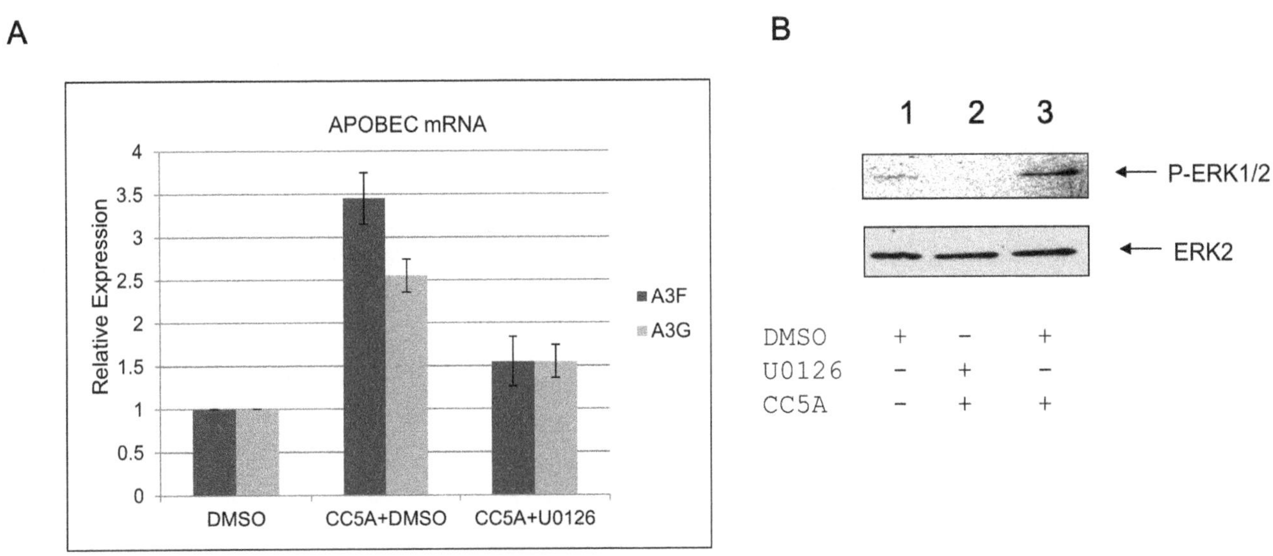

Figure 3. A3F and A3G are regulated through the MEK1/2 dependent pathway. (**A**) Prior to treatment with CC5A/PBS for 16 h, THP-1 cells were pre-treated by DMSO alone or the ERK1/2 inhibitor U0126 in DMSO for 1 h. The induction of A3G and A3F was measured by qRT-PCR. (B) Lysates from THP-1 cells pre-treated DMSO or U0126 in DMSO, following by CC5A/PBS (40 μg) are subjected to Western blot analysis. Phosphorylated ERK1/2 and ERK1/2 were probed by anti-p-ERK1/2 and anti-ERK2, respectively.

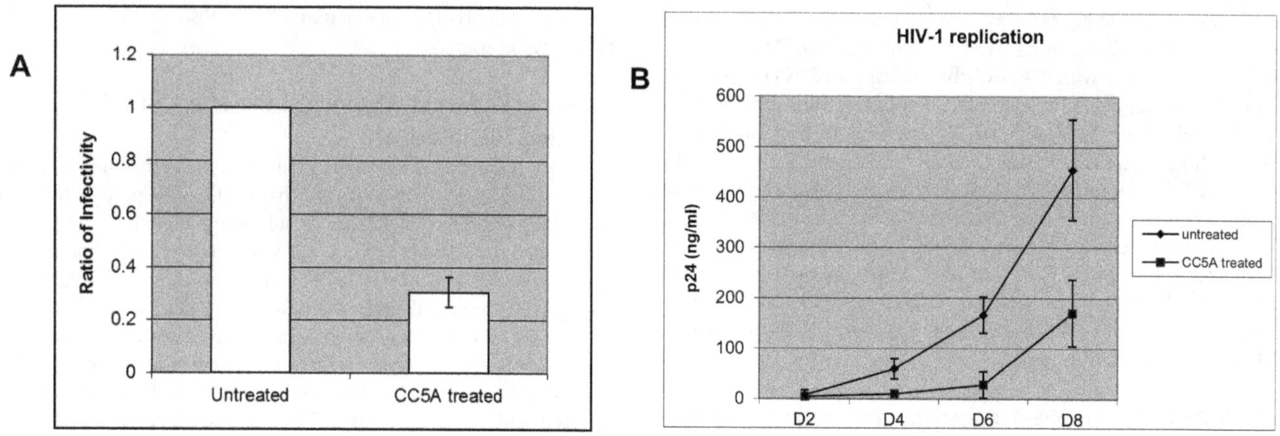

Figure 4. The active CC5A molecule inhibits HIV-1 replication. (A) THP-1/IIIB cells were treated with PBS or CC5A/PBS for 16 h. Post-treatment, THP-1 cells were washed twice by PBS and cultured for 24 h. The cells were then washed with PBS and cultured for another 24 h. The culture supernatants were collected for infectivity assays. The amount of input virus for the infectivity assay was normalized by p24 ELISA. (B) THP-1 cells were pre-treated overnight with CC5A/PBS or PBS before IIIB infection. After 3 h of infection, the cells were washed twice with PBS and put back into culture for eight days. Viral samples were collected every other day and viral replication was monitored by p24 assay.

CC5A enhances HIV G to A hypermutation rate

A G to A hypermutation is a hallmark of APOBEC antiviral activity. We therefore performed a G to A hypermutation analysis to determine if this function of APOBEC contributes to CC5A mediated inhibition of HIV replication. As mentioned in the material and methods, culture supernatants were used to infect SupT1 cells for a DNA hypermutation assay. Only 2 G to A hypermutation was detected in 24 clones from SupT1 cells infected with virus taken from the untreated THP-1/IIIB cell line. Infection of the SupT1 cells with virus obtained from the CC5A/PBS-treated THP-1/IIIB cell line resulted in 9 hypermutations in 13 clones upon examination of viral DNA (Fig. 6). Mann Whitney U test calculated a p-value of 0.023. Thus CC5A/PBS significantly increased G to A hypermutations in HIV-1 IIIB viral DNA. The data suggest that APOBEC plays a role in CC5A/PBS mediated-inhibition of HIV-1 replication.

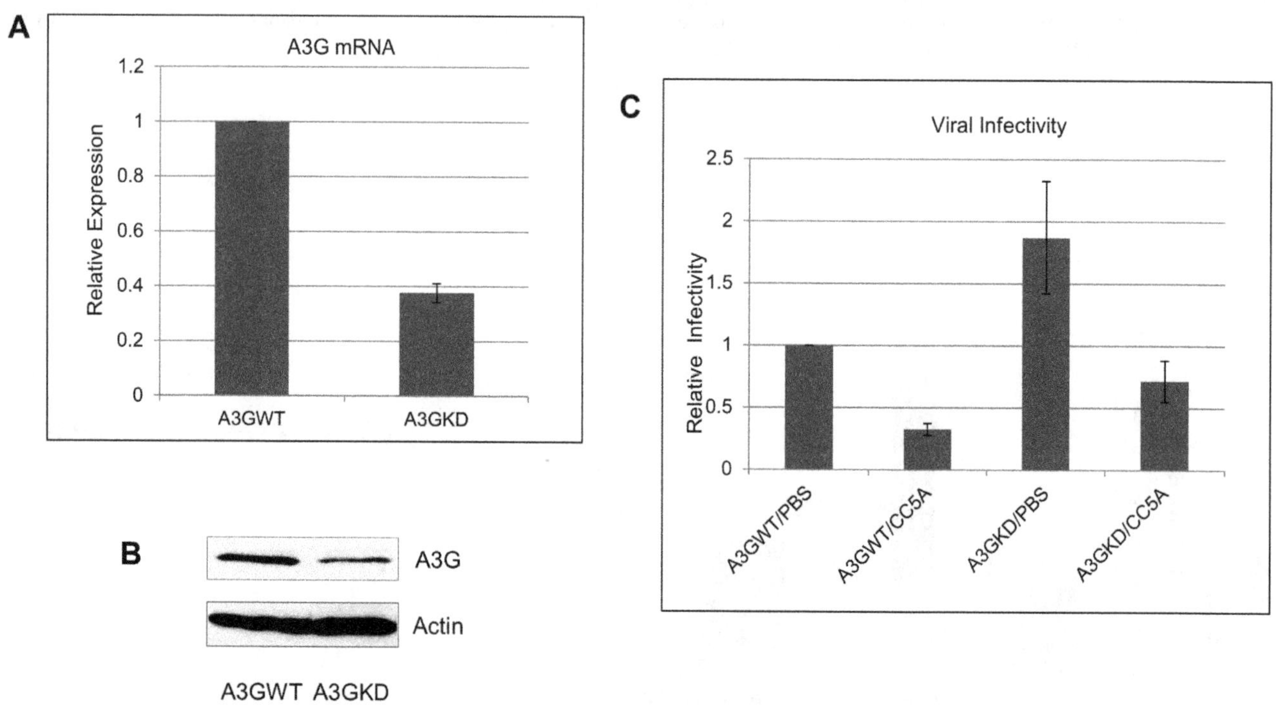

Figure 5. A3G knockdown compromised the effect of CC5A in reducing HIV infectivity. pX330-A3G1 and pX330-A3G2 (3 μg each) were transfected into 1×10^6 THP-1 cells using Neon Transfection System (Invitrogen). Three days post transfection, the transfected THP-1 cells were cloned by limited dilution method. Single clones were screen by Western-blot and qRT-PCR for A3G expression analysis. A3GKD was selected as A3G knockdown cell line for further experiment. A3G expression was tested by Western-blot (A) and qRT-PCR (B) analysis. THP-1/IIIB and THP-1 A3GKD/IIIB were treated with CC5A or PBS to measure the effects of CC5A on reducing HIV infectivity in THP-1 and THP-1 A3GKD cell line (B).

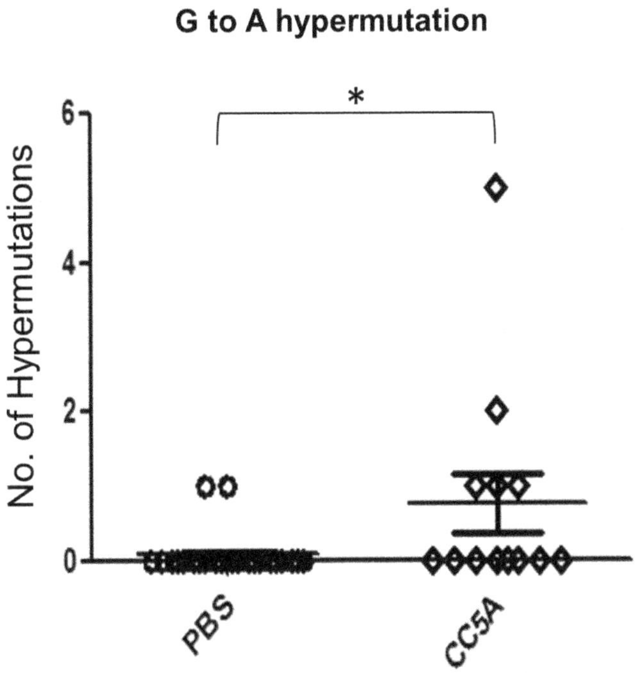

Figure 6. CC5A enhances HIV G to A hypermutation rate. HIV from CC5A or PBS treated THP-1 culture supernatants were used to infect SupT1 cells. The infected SupT1 cells were washed twice with PBS then incubated at 37°C, 5% CO2 for 16 h. HIV cDNA was isolated using DNeasy DNA isolation kit (Qiagen). A 650 bp DNA fragment covering a portion of nef, U3 and R of HIV-1 was amplified by PCR. The PCR products were cloned into the TOPO TA-cloning vector. The nucleotide sequences of individual clones from each infected culture sample were determined. Statistical significance was determined by Mann Whitney U test using GraphPad Prism software. Mann Whitney U test was used to calculate p-value.

CC5A/PBS induces A3G and A3F expression in human oral OKF6 keratinocytes and human vaginal VK2 epithelial cells

Vaginal epithelial cells and oral keratinocytes are the first line of defense after vaginal or oral exposure of HIV-1 to females. It has been shown that mouse APOBEC3 plays a role in blocking the transmission of mouse mammary tumor virus [51] and murine acquired immunodeficiency virus [52]. Therefore, we determined if CC5A/PBS also induced A3G and A3F expression in VK2 and OKF6 cells. In a pilot study, we found OKF6 cells were very sensitive to CC5A treatment. We therefore used a low dose of CC5A/PBS (5 μg) to treat OKF6 cells. Cells were harvested at the indicated time points (Fig. 7A) and the relative APOBEC mRNA levels measured by qRT-PCR. CC5A/PBS increased the APOBEC A3F and A3G mRNA levels up to 2.5 fold at 48 h post treatment compare to untreated cells. The values at 72 h were similar to those at 48 h. Untreated samples in Fig. 6A were normalized to 1.0. The effect of 2.5 and 5 μg of CC5A/PBS on A3G protein levels at 72 h is shown in Fig. 7B. Therefore as little as 2.5 μg was as effective as 5 μg in these cells. Similarly, CC5A/PBS (40 μg) also increased A3F and A3G mRNA (Fig. 7C) in VK2 cells compared to controls (set at a comparative value of 1.0). The effect of CC5A appears to some degree, cell specific, as the sensitivity to CC5A/PBS with respect to induction of A3G protein levels was greatest in THP-1>VK2>OKF6 cells (Fig. 7). In addition, 40 μg CC5A incubated for 16 h with THP-1 cells produced an 8 fold increase in A3G mRNA, the same dose of CC5A produced a<2.5 fold difference at 16 h in VK2 cells.

CC5A/PBS and Sonicated CC5A do not cause cytotoxicity in THP-1 cells

The cytotoxicity of CC5A/PBS and Sonicated CC5A treatment was measured by a Live/Dead Cell Vitality Assay Kit (Invitrogen). The kit provides a two-color fluorescence assay that distinguishes metabolically active cells from injured cells and dead cells. THP-1 cells were treated with PBS (untreated control), 25 μg sonicated CC5A or 40 μg CC5A/PBS respectively (Fig. 8). Cells were harvested 16 h post-treatment. The cytotoxicity effect of CC5A treatment was measured by a Live/Dead Cell Vitality Assay kit following the manufacturer's directions. While untreated controls indicated the presence of around 85% live cells, when treated with sonicated CC5A or CC5A/PBS, the percent of live THP-1 cells was still 85% (Fig. 8). In addition, percentage of the injured and dead cells are all similar among the three samples (Fig. 8). In summary, the treatment of sonicated CC5A or CC5A/PBS does not cause appreciably cytotoxicity to THP-1 cells.

Discussion

Although most HIV-1 is transmitted through mucosal surfaces, the transmission through the oral mucosa is uncommon. Further HIV from the saliva of an HIV-seropositive individual is less infectious than that from plasma or vaginal fluid. The recovery rate of infectious HIV from saliva is low (1–2%) in HIV-seropositive individuals, although the DNA and RNA detection frequency of HIV by PCR is higher (20–50%) [53], suggesting there are innate inhibitory factors in saliva and/or in the oral epithelium that function to reduce HIV infectivity. Numerous studies have shown that oral transmission is not an independent risk factor for an HIV-seronegative individual (see review in [54]). In the oral cavity, HIV host restriction factors, such as secretory

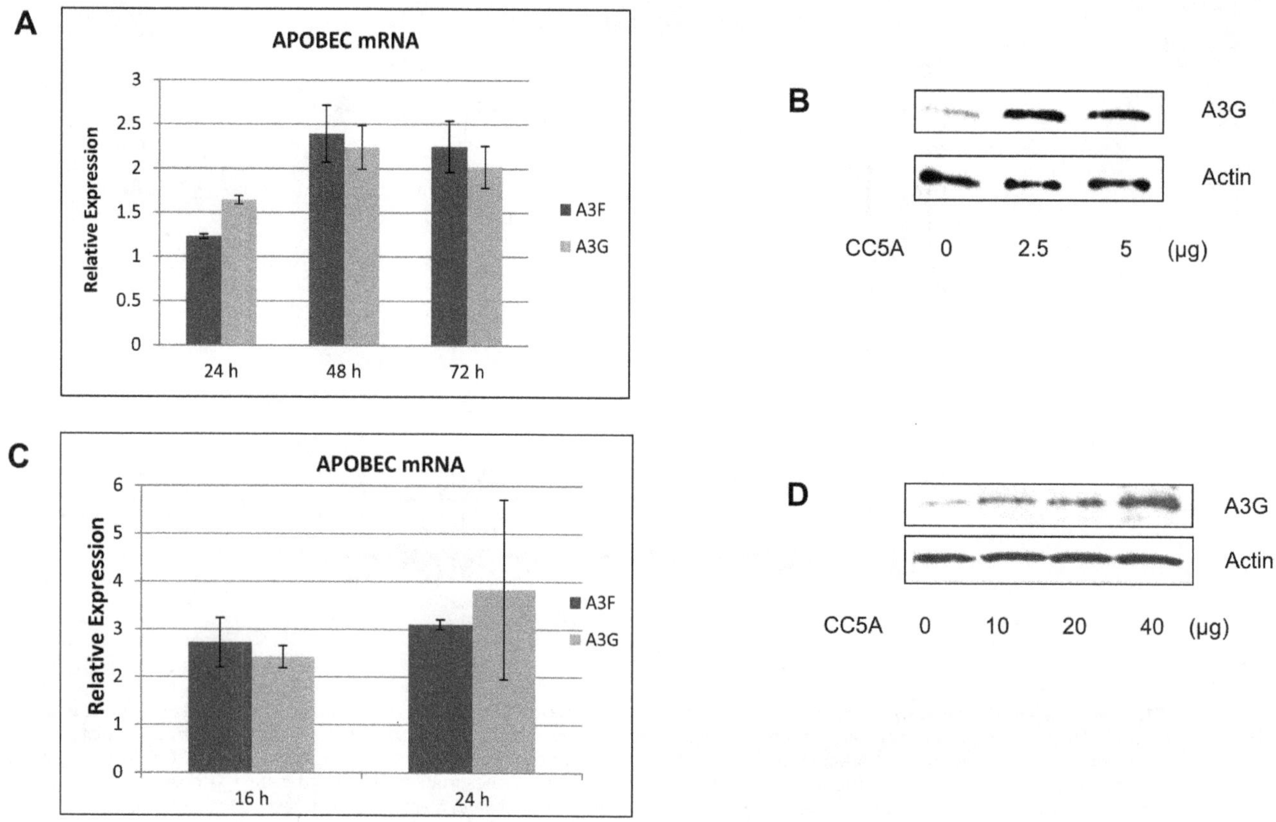

Figure 7. CC5A/PBS induces A3G and A3F expression in human oral keratinocyte (OKF6) and human vaginal VK2 epithelial cells. (A) CC5A/PBS (5 µg) was used to treat OKF6 cells. The cells were harvested at the indicated time points, and qRT-PCR was used to measure the relative expression of A3F and A3G mRNA. The expression levels shown represent the ratio of CC5A/PBS treated cells compared to the untreated cells at each given time point. **(B)** Different doses (0–5 µg) of CC5A/PBS were used to treat OKF6 cells for 72 h, and A3G expression was measured by Western-blot analysis. **(C)** VK2 cells were treated with 40 µg CC5A/PBS or vehicle for the time periods shown. qRT-PCR was used to measure the relative expression of A3F and A3G mRNA in these cells. The expression levels shown represent the ratio of the levels found in CC5A/PBS treated cells compared to untreated cells at each time point. **(D)** Different doses (0–40 µg) of CC5A/PBS were used to treat VK2 cells for 48 h. A3G protein expression was measured by Western-blot analysis.

leukocyte protease inhibitor (SLPI), lysozyme, defensins, ribonuclease and thrombospondin-1, may be contributors to the extremely low risk of oral transmission of the virus [54]. In this study, we show that a molecule from *S. cristatus* up-regulates expression levels of A3G and A3F. This molecule also inhibits HIV-1 replication in an APOBEC-related manner (Figs. 4, 5, 6). Indeed, the fold-reduction of HIV infectivity in CC5A -treated A3GKD cells relative to PBS-treated A3GKD cells is approximately the same as that in CC5A-treated A3GWT cells relative to PBS-treated A3GWT cells (Fig. 5C). However, considering the fact that the infectivity of CC5A treated THP-1 A3GKD was about two fold higher than the infectivity of CC5A treated wild-type THP-1, we think the A3G knockdown data demonstrated that A3G played a role in mediating the effects of CC5A in inhibiting HIV infectivity. Similar data was obtained when Peng et al. tried to prove that A3G played a role in IFN induced ant-HIV-1 activity [55]. These findings support the idea that APOBEC3 proteins may represent an additional set of host restriction factors that work to block the oral transmission of HIV. Indeed, it has been shown that mouse APOBEC3 plays a role in blocking the transmission of mouse mammary tumor virus (46) and murine acquired immunodeficiency virus (47). In addition, our data demonstrate that the CC5A-derived molecule is able to induce A3G and A3F expression in oral keratinocytes (OKF6) and vaginal epithelial cells (VK2). Studies in relevant primary cells and using an HIV-1 transmission assay will bolster the clinical relevance of our results to date.

Previous reports show that A3G expression is regulated by PMA, PHA and certain cytokines through the PKC/JAK/ERK/MAPK signaling pathway [24,36,37]. Stimulation of cell surface CCR5 and CD40 molecules by their ligands or by HSP70 up-regulates APOBEC3G expression in $CD4^+$ T cells and dendritic cells through the p38 and ERK dependent signaling pathway [47]. In our study, we show that a molecule from *S. cristatus* up-regulates A3G and A3F through the same pathway. To our knowledge, this is the first report showing that A3G and A3F expression may be regulated by an oral bacterial component. In response to bacterial exposure, host immune systems rapidly induce the expression of a variety of genes involved in producing interferons and proinflammatory cytokines to generate protection against bacterial invasion. The reason why A3G and A3F are also up-regulated and whether they play a role in the protection against bacterial invasion are still open questions.

This active molecule could be a potential candidate for developing novel anti-HIV drugs to prevent or treat HIV infection. *S. cristatus* CC5A is a gram positive bacterium. It exists in normal, healthy oral cavities. It has not been associated with any oral infectious disease. Therefore, it is highly possible that this

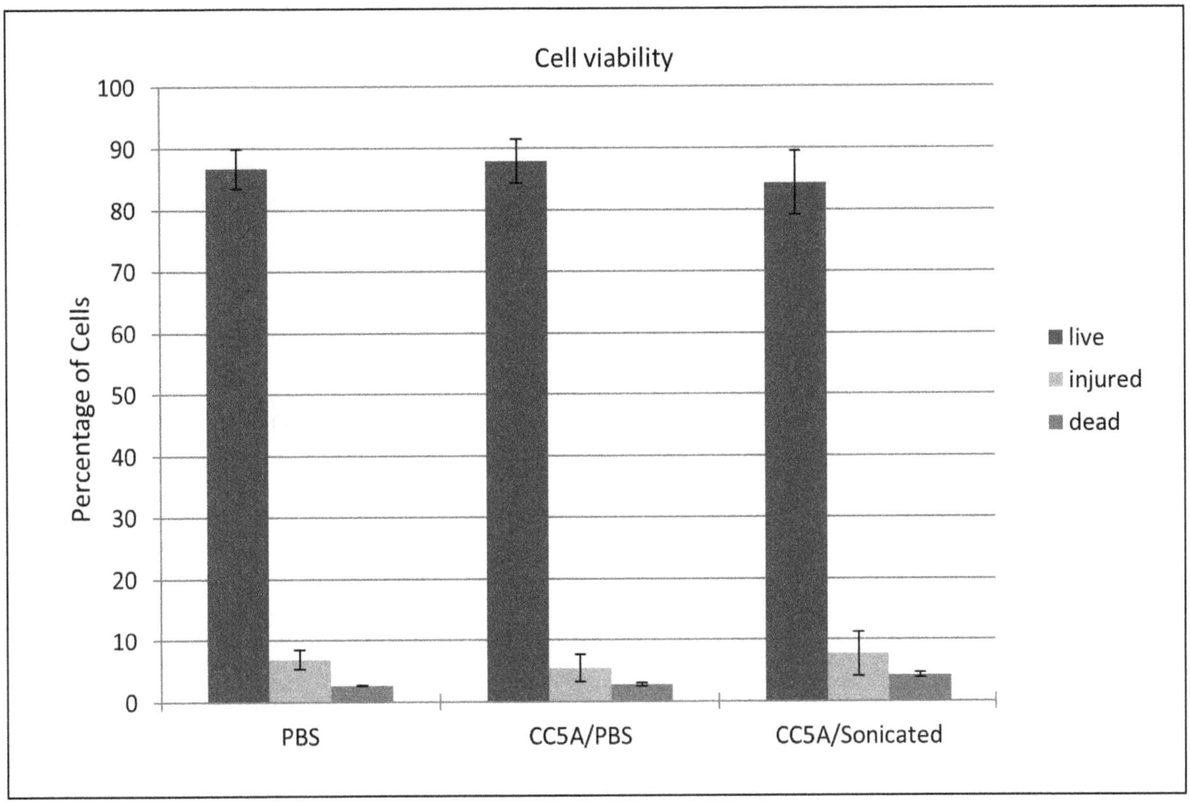

Figure 8. CC5A/PBS and sonicated CC5A do not cause cytotoxicity in THP-1 cells. The cytotoxicity of CC5A/PBS and sonicated CC5A treatment was measured by a Live/Dead Cell Vitality Assay Kit (Invitrogen). THP-1 cells were treated with PBS, 40 µg CC5A/PBS and 25 µg sonicated CC5A for 16 h then subjected to the Live/Dead Cell Vitality Assay Kit analysis.

active molecule could be useful because of its low toxicity. In fact, our cytotoxicity data showed there was no obvious cytotoxicity after THP-1 cells were treated for 16 h with preparations containing the *S. cristatus* CC5A active molecule. Boiling in 2% SDS was not able to inactive the molecule suggests that the active molecule is heat-stable. In addition given the fact that the active molecule is smaller than 1.3 kD, we argue that *S. cristatus* CC5A contains a small, heat-stable molecule, which has the effect to enhance innate immunity and inhibit HIV-1 replication. The idea of promoting A3G and A3F as anti-HIV/AIDS agents is distinct from conventional anti-HIV drugs, such as reverse transcriptase and protease inhibitors, wherein HIV is prone to generating drug-resistant mutations. A3G interacts with the HIV nucleocapsid and is incorporated into the virion [56–63]. The domain on nucleocapsid with which A3G interacts is critical for HIV assembly, implying the impossibility of HIV to exclude A3G by mutation. On the other hand, it has been suggested that HIV actively recruits a small amount of A3G to promote its diversification, escape immune pressure and generate drug resistance [64–66]. This HIV reliance on low-levels of APOBEC can be exploited by designing an anti-HIV/AIDS drug based on this CC5A extract that amplifies A3G and A3F expression beyond what the virus can sustain. Continuation of these studies may result in an entirely new class of antiretroviral drugs.

Acknowledgments

The following reagents were obtained through the NIH AIDS Research and Reference Reagent Program, Division of AIDS, NIAID, NIH: THP-1 from Drs. Li Wu and Vineet N. KewalRamani; SupT1 from Dr. James Hoxie; TZM-bl from Dr. John C. Kappes; anti-human APOBEC3G antibody Cat #10201 from Dr. Jaisri Lingappa and Cat #9968 from Dr. Warner C. Greene; Rabbit Anti-Human APOBEC3F (C-18) from Dr. Michael Malim; H9/HTLV-IIIB from Dr. Robert Gallo.

We thank Dr. Diana Marver for a critical reading of the manuscript and Jared Elzey and Robin Broughton for editorial assistance.

Author Contributions

Conceived and designed the experiments: HX BL. Performed the experiments: ZW YL QS BLK. Analyzed the data: CW HX BL. Contributed reagents/materials/analysis tools: JEKH. Wrote the paper: ZW YL QS BLK CW JEKH HX BL.

References

1. Yassi A, McGill M (1991) Determinants of blood and body fluid exposure in a large teaching hospital: hazards of the intermittent intravenous procedure. Am J Infect Control 19: 129–135.
2. Figueiredo JF, Borges AS, Martinez R, Martinelli Ade L, Villanova MG, et al. (1994) Transmission of hepatitis C virus but not human immunodeficiency virus type 1 by a human bite. Clin Infect Dis 19: 546–547.
3. Baron S (2001) Oral transmission of HIV, a rarity: emerging hypotheses. J Dent Res 80: 1602–1604.
4. Maticic M, Poljak M, Kramar B, Tomazic J, Vidmar L, et al. (2000) Proviral HIV-1 DNA in gingival crevicular fluid of HIV-1-infected patients in various stages of HIV disease. J Dent Res 79: 1496–1501.
5. Shugars DC, Patton LL, Freel SA, Gray LR, Vollmer RT, et al. (2001) Hyper-excretion of human immunodeficiency virus type 1 RNA in saliva. J Dent Res 80: 414–420.
6. Shugars DC, Alexander AL, Fu K, Freel SA (1999) Endogenous salivary inhibitors of human immunodeficiency virus. Arch Oral Biol 44: 445–453.

7. Wahl SM, McNeely TB, Janoff EN, Shugars D, Worley P, et al. (1997) Secretory leukocyte protease inhibitor (SLPI) in mucosal fluids inhibits HIV-I. Oral Dis 3 Suppl 1: S64–69.
8. Sun L, Finnegan CM, Kish-Catalone T, Blumenthal R, Garzino-Demo P, et al. (2005) Human beta-defensins suppress human immunodeficiency virus infection: potential role in mucosal protection. J Virol 79: 14318–14329.
9. Aas JA, Paster BJ, Stokes LN, Olsen I, Dewhirst FE (2005) Defining the normal bacterial flora of the oral cavity. J Clin Microbiol 43: 5721–5732.
10. Xie H, Belogortseva NI, Wu J, Lai WH, Chen CH (2006) Inhibition of Human Immunodeficiency Virus Type 1 Entry by a Binding Domain of Porphyromonas gingivalis Gingipain. Antimicrob Agents Chemother 50: 3070–3074.
11. Edwards AM, Grossman TJ, Rudney JD (2006) Fusobacterium nucleatum transports noninvasive Streptococcus cristatus into human epithelial cells. Infect Immun 74: 654–662.
12. Aas JA, Barbuto SM, Alpagot T, Olsen I, Dewhirst FE, et al. (2007) Subgingival plaque microbiota in HIV positive patients. J Clin Periodontol 34: 189–195.
13. Wedekind JE, Dance GS, Sowden MP, Smith HC (2003) Messenger RNA editing in mammals: new members of the APOBEC family seeking roles in the family business. Trends Genet 19: 207–216.
14. Jarmuz A, Chester A, Bayliss J, Gisbourne J, Dunham I, et al. (2002) An anthropoid-specific locus of orphan C to U RNA-editing enzymes on chromosome 22. Genomics 79: 285–296.
15. Sheehy AM, Gaddis NC, Choi JD, Malim MH (2002) Isolation of a human gene that inhibits HIV-1 infection and is suppressed by the viral Vif protein. Nature 418: 646–650.
16. Dang Y, Wang X, Esselman WJ, Zheng YH (2006) Identification of APOBEC3DE as another antiretroviral factor from the human APOBEC family. J Virol 80: 10522–10533.
17. Zheng YH, Irwin D, Kurosu T, Tokunaga K, Sata T, et al. (2004) Human APOBEC3F is another host factor that blocks human immunodeficiency virus type 1 replication. J Virol 78: 6073–6076.
18. Wiegand HL, Doehle BP, Bogerd HP, Cullen BR (2004) A second human antiretroviral factor, APOBEC3F, is suppressed by the HIV-1 and HIV-2 Vif proteins. Embo J 23: 2451–2458.
19. Liddament MT, Brown WL, Schumacher AJ, Harris RS (2004) APOBEC3F properties and hypermutation preferences indicate activity against HIV-1 in vivo. Curr Biol 14: 1385–1391.
20. Bishop KN, Holmes RK, Sheehy AM, Davidson NO, Cho SJ, et al. (2004) Cytidine deamination of retroviral DNA by diverse APOBEC proteins. Curr Biol 14: 1392–1396.
21. Fisher AG, Ensoli B, Ivanoff L, Chamberlain M, Petteway S, et al. (1987) The sor gene of HIV-1 is required for efficient virus transmission in vitro. Science 237: 888–893.
22. Strebel K, Daugherty D, Clouse K, Cohen D, Folks T, et al. (1987) The HIV 'A' (sor) gene product is essential for virus infectivity. Nature 328: 728–730.
23. Yu X, Yu Y, Liu B, Luo K, Kong W, et al. (2003) Induction of APOBEC3G ubiquitination and degradation by an HIV-1 Vif-Cul5-SCF complex. Science 302: 1056–1060.
24. Stopak K, de Noronha C, Yonemoto W, Greene WC (2003) HIV-1 Vif blocks the antiviral activity of APOBEC3G by impairing both its translation and intracellular stability. Mol Cell 12: 591–601.
25. Sheehy AM, Gaddis NC, Malim MH (2003) The antiretroviral enzyme APOBEC3G is degraded by the proteasome in response to HIV-1 Vif. Nat Med 9: 1404–1407.
26. Mehle A, Strack B, Ancuta P, Zhang C, McPike M, et al. (2003) Vif overcomes the innate antiviral activity of APOBEC3G by promoting its degradation in the ubiquitin-proteasome pathway. J Biol Chem 279: 7792–7798.
27. Marin M, Rose KM, Kozak SL, Kabat D (2003) HIV-1 Vif protein binds the editing enzyme APOBEC3G and induces its degradation. Nat Med 9: 1398–1403.
28. Conticello SG, Harris RS, Neuberger MS (2003) The Vif protein of HIV triggers degradation of the human antiretroviral DNA deaminase APOBEC3G. Curr Biol 13: 2009–2013.
29. Liu B, Yu X, Luo K, Yu Y, Yu XF (2004) Influence of primate lentiviral Vif and proteasome inhibitors on human immunodeficiency virus type 1 virion packaging of APOBEC3G. J Virol 78: 2072–2081.
30. Mariani R, Chen D, Schrofelbauer B, Navarro F, Konig R, et al. (2003) Species-Specific Exclusion of APOBEC3G from HIV-1 Virions by Vif. Cell 114: 21–31.
31. Yang Y, Guo F, Cen S, Kleiman L (2007) Inhibition of initiation of reverse transcription in HIV-1 by human APOBEC3F. Virology.
32. Mbisa JL, Barr R, Thomas JA, Vandegraaff N, Dorweiler IJ, et al. (2007) HIV-1 cDNAs Produced in the Presence of APOBEC3G Exhibit Defects in Plus-Strand DNA Transfer and Integration. J Virol.
33. Holmes RK, Koning FA, Bishop KN, Malim MH (2007) APOBEC3F can inhibit the accumulation of HIV-1 reverse transcription products in the absence of hypermutation. Comparisons with APOBEC3G. J Biol Chem 282: 2587–2595.
34. Newman EN, Holmes RK, Craig HM, Klein KC, Lingappa JR, et al. (2005) Antiviral function of APOBEC3G can be dissociated from cytidine deaminase activity. Curr Biol 15: 166–170.
35. Pintard L, Willems A, Peter M (2004) Cullin-based ubiquitin ligases: Cul3-BTB complexes join the family. Embo J 23: 1681–1687.
36. Rose KM, Marin M, Kozak SL, Kabat D (2004) Transcriptional regulation of APOBEC3G, a cytidine deaminase that hypermutates human immunodeficiency virus. J Biol Chem 279: 41744–41749.
37. Stopak KS, Chiu YL, Kropp J, Grant RM, Greene WC (2007) Distinct patterns of cytokine regulation of APOBEC3G expression and activity in primary lymphocytes, macrophages, and dendritic cells. J Biol Chem 282: 3539–3546.
38. Chen K, Huang J, Zhang C, Huang S, Nunnari G, et al. (2006) Alpha interferon potently enhances the anti-human immunodeficiency virus type 1 activity of APOBEC3G in resting primary CD4 T cells. J Virol 80: 7645–7657.
39. Sarkis PT, Ying S, Xu R, Yu XF (2006) STAT1-independent cell type-specific regulation of antiviral APOBEC3G by IFN-alpha. J Immunol 177: 4530–4540.
40. Tanaka Y, Marusawa H, Seno H, Matsumoto Y, Ueda Y, et al. (2006) Anti-viral protein APOBEC3G is induced by interferon-alpha stimulation in human hepatocytes. Biochem Biophys Res Commun 341: 314–319.
41. Dickson MA, Hahn WC, Ino Y, Ronfard V, Wu JY, et al. (2000) Human keratinocytes that express hTERT and also bypass a p16(INK4a)-enforced mechanism that limits life span become immortal yet retain normal growth and differentiation characteristics. Mol Cell Biol 20: 1436–1447.
42. Kinlock BL, Wang Y, Turner TM, Wang C, Liu B (2014) Transcytosis of HIV-1 through Vaginal Epithelial Cells Is Dependent on Trafficking to the Endocytic Recycling Pathway. PLoS One 9: e96760.
43. Timmons CL, Shao Q, Wang C, Liu L, Liu H, et al. (2013) GB virus type C E2 protein inhibits human immunodeficiency virus type 1 assembly through interference with HIV-1 gag plasma membrane targeting. J Infect Dis 207: 1171–1180.
44. Rose KM, Marin M, Kozak SL, Kabat D (2005) Regulated production and anti-HIV type 1 activities of cytidine deaminases APOBEC3B, 3F, and 3G. AIDS Res Hum Retroviruses 21: 611–619.
45. Wei X, Decker JM, Liu H, Zhang Z, Arani RB, et al. (2002) Emergence of resistant human immunodeficiency virus type 1 in patients receiving fusion inhibitor (T-20) monotherapy. Antimicrob Agents Chemother 46: 1896–1905.
46. Luo K, Wang T, Liu B, Tian C, Xiao Z, et al. (2007) Cytidine deaminases APOBEC3G and APOBEC3F interact with human immunodeficiency virus type 1 integrase and inhibit proviral DNA formation. J Virol 81: 7238–7248.
47. Pido-Lopez J, Whittall T, Wang Y, Bergmeier LA, Babaahmady K, et al. (2007) Stimulation of cell surface CCR5 and CD40 molecules by their ligands or by HSP70 up-regulates APOBEC3G expression in CD4(+) T cells and dendritic cells. J Immunol 178: 1671–1679.
48. Wang Y, Shao Q, Yu X, Kong W, Hildreth JE, et al. (2011) N-terminal hemagglutinin tag renders lysine-deficient APOBEC3G resistant to HIV-1 Vif-induced degradation by reduced polyubiquitination. J Virol 85: 4510–4519.
49. Mali P, Yang L, Esvelt KM, Aach J, Guell M, et al. (2013) RNA-guided human genome engineering via Cas9. Science 339: 823–826.
50. Cong L, Ran FA, Cox D, Lin S, Barretto R, et al. (2013) Multiplex genome engineering using CRISPR/Cas systems. Science 339: 819–823.
51. Okeoma CM, Huegel AL, Lingappa J, Feldman MD, Ross SR (2010) APOBEC3 proteins expressed in mammary epithelial cells are packaged into retroviruses and can restrict transmission of milk-borne virions. Cell Host Microbe 8: 534–543.
52. Jones PH, Mehta HV, Okeoma CM (2012) A novel role for APOBEC3: susceptibility to sexual transmission of murine acquired immunodeficiency virus (mAIDS) is aggravated in APOBEC3 deficient mice. Retrovirology 9: 50.
53. Liuzzi G, Chirianni A, Clementi M, Bagnarelli P, Valenza A, et al. (1996) Analysis of HIV-1 load in blood, semen and saliva: evidence for different viral compartments in a cross-sectional and longitudinal study. Aids 10: F51–56.
54. Campo J, Perea MA, del Romero J, Cano J, Hernando V, et al. (2006) Oral transmission of HIV, reality or fiction? An update. Oral Dis 12: 219–228.
55. Peng G, Lei KJ, Jin W, Greenwell-Wild T, Wahl SM (2006) Induction of APOBEC3 family proteins, a defensive maneuver underlying interferon-induced anti-HIV-1 activity. J Exp Med 203: 41–46.
56. Burnett A, Spearman P (2007) APOBEC3G multimers are recruited to the plasma membrane for packaging into human immunodeficiency virus type 1 virus-like particles in an RNA-dependent process requiring the NC basic linker. J Virol 81: 5000–5013.
57. Zennou V, Perez-Caballero D, Gottlinger H, Bieniasz PD (2004) APOBEC3G incorporation into human immunodeficiency virus type 1 particles. J Virol 78: 12058–12061.
58. Svarovskaia ES, Xu H, Mbisa JL, Barr R, Gorelick RJ, et al. (2004) Human apolipoprotein B mRNA-editing enzyme-catalytic polypeptide-like 3G (APOBEC3G) is incorporated into HIV-1 virions through interactions with viral and nonviral RNAs. J Biol Chem 279: 35822–35828.
59. Schafer A, Bogerd HP, Cullen BR (2004) Specific packaging of APOBEC3G into HIV-1 virions is mediated by the nucleocapsid domain of the gag polyprotein precursor. Virology 328: 163–168.
60. Luo K, Liu B, Xiao Z, Yu Y, Yu X, et al. (2004) Amino-terminal region of the human immunodeficiency virus type 1 nucleocapsid is required for human APOBEC3G packaging. J Virol 78: 11841–11852.
61. Douaisi M, Dussart S, Courcoul M, Bessou G, Vigne R, et al. (2004) HIV-1 and MLV Gag proteins are sufficient to recruit APOBEC3G into virus-like particles. Biochem Biophys Res Commun 321: 566–573.
62. Cen S, Guo F, Niu M, Saadatmand J, Deflassieux J, et al. (2004) The interaction between HIV-1 Gag and APOBEC3G. J Biol Chem 279: 33177–33184.

63. Alce TM, Popik W (2004) APOBEC3G is incorporated into virus-like particles by a direct interaction with HIV-1 Gag nucleocapsid protein. J Biol Chem 279: 34083–34086.
64. Jern P, Russell RA, Pathak VK, Coffin JM (2009) Likely role of APOBEC3G-mediated G-to-A mutations in HIV-1 evolution and drug resistance. PLoS Pathog 5: e1000367.
65. Kim EY, Bhattacharya T, Kunstman K, Swantek P, Koning FA, et al. (2010) Human APOBEC3G-mediated editing can promote HIV-1 sequence diversification and accelerate adaptation to selective pressure. J Virol 84: 10402–10405.
66. Mulder LC, Harari A, Simon V (2008) Cytidine deamination induced HIV-1 drug resistance. Proc Natl Acad Sci USA 105: 5501–5506.

3

Brain-Targeted Delivery of Trans-Activating Transcriptor-Conjugated Magnetic PLGA/Lipid Nanoparticles

Xiangru Wen[1,5]⁹, Kai Wang[2]⁹, Ziming Zhao[3]⁹, Yifang Zhang[2], Tingting Sun[2], Fang Zhang[4], Jian Wu[4], Yanyan Fu[4], Yang Du[4], Lei Zhang[6], Ying Sun[6], YongHai Liu[6], Kai Ma[5,7], Hongzhi Liu[4]*, Yuanjian Song[1,4]*

1 Jiangsu Key Laboratory of Brain Disease Bioinformation, Xuzhou Medical College, Xuzhou, Jiangsu Province, China, **2** College of Animal Science and Technology, Yunnan Agricultural University, Yunnan, Kunming Province, China, **3** School of Pharmacy, Xuzhou Medical College, Xuzhou, Jiangsu Province, China, **4** Research Center for Neurobiology and Department of Neurobiology, Xuzhou Medical College, Xuzhou, Jiangsu Province, China, **5** School of Basic Education Sciences, Xuzhou Medical College, Xuzhou, Jiangsu Province, China, **6** Department of Neurology, Affiliated Hospital of Xuzhou Medical College, Xuzhou, Jiangsu Province, China, **7** Department of Medical Information, Xuzhou Medical College, Xuzhou, Jiangsu Province, China

Abstract

Magnetic poly (D,L-lactide-co-glycolide) (PLGA)/lipid nanoparticles (MPLs) were fabricated from PLGA, L-α-phosphatidylethanolamine (DOPE), 1,2-distearoyl-sn-glycero-3-phosphoethanolamine-N-amino (polyethylene glycol) (DSPE-PEG-NH_2), and magnetic nanoparticles (NPs), and then conjugated to trans-activating transcriptor (TAT) peptide. The TAT-MPLs were designed to target the brain by magnetic guidance and TAT conjugation. The drugs hesperidin (HES), naringin (NAR), and glutathione (GSH) were encapsulated in MPLs with drug loading capacity (>10%) and drug encapsulation efficiency (>90%). The therapeutic efficacy of the drug-loaded TAT-MPLs in bEnd.3 cells was compared with that of drug-loaded MPLs. The cells accumulated higher levels of TAT-MPLs than MPLs. In addition, the accumulation of QD-loaded fluorescein isothiocyanate (FITC)-labeled TAT-MPLs in bEnd.3 cells was dose and time dependent. Our results show that TAT-conjugated MPLs may function as an effective drug delivery system that crosses the blood brain barrier to the brain.

Editor: Bing Xu, Brandeis University, United States of America

Funding: This work was supported by Jiangsu Key Laboratory of Brain Disease Bioinformation (Jsbl1102), the Priority Academic Program Development of Jiangsu Higher Education Institutions, the Education Departmental Natural Science Research Funds of Jiangsu Provincial Higher School of China (13KJB310021), the National Natural Science Foundation of China (31100762, 81371300), the Foundation of President of Xuzhou Medical College (2012KJZ06), and the Qing Lan Project of Jiangsu Province. The funders had no role in study design, data collection and analysis, decision to publish, or preparation of the manuscript.

Competing Interests: The authors have declared that no competing interests exist.

* Email: xzmclhz@126.com (HL); biosongyuanjian@126.com (YJS)

⁹ These authors contributed equally to this work.

Introduction

Developing an effective drug delivery system with the ability of crossing the blood brain barrier (BBB) is the crucial point in treating diseases of the human central nervous system (CNS) effectively. Many potential drugs have been abandoned during their development for their poor ability to cross the BBB in sufficient quantities to produce a therapeutic effect [1]. The BBB is not only an anatomical barrier to the free movement of solutes between the blood and brain, but also a transport and metabolic barrier [2]. Consequently, developing tools and methods that allow the therapeutic agents to delivery to the brain safely and effectively *in vivo* is important.

Nanocarrier systems, such as micelles, liposomes [3,4], and polymeric nanoparticles [5,6], have been investigated for delivering therapeutic agents to the brain [7]. Magnetically driven Nanocarrier drug delivery systems are powerful tools for delivering drugs, genes and cells to a target organ, and may be suitable for delivering drugs to the brain. These systems have many unique characteristics, including the delivery of a range of biomolecules *in vivo*, such as DNA and siRNA [8]; non-invasive magnetic targeting with therapeutic biomolecules by using external magnetic fields over the target organ or injury site, and trackability *in vivo* with various imaging systems [9–11]. Furthermore, carrying capacity could be improved by magnetic guidance to target the drug to the brain parenchyma. In order to increase the uptake efficiency, magnetic nanoparticles can be modified with specific ligands such as cationic albumin [12], thiamine [13], or transferrin [14], surfactant coatings [15], proteins and peptides [16–18]. The HIV-1 trans-activating transcriptor (TAT) peptide [19], which is a cell penetrating peptide, has been widely used to increase the transport efficiency of drug-loaded NPs across the BBB to the CNS [20]. TAT has been used to form the Chitosan-PEG-TAT nanoparticles for complexing siRNA to be delivered in neuronal cells [21]. TAT-GS nanoparticle-mediated calcitonin gene-related peptide (CGRP) gene delivery has been proposed to be an innovative strategy for cerebral vasospasm [22]. Therefore, normal brain drugs combining with peptides, nanotechnology and magnetic targeting may greatly improve the treatment of brain disorders [23].

Magnetic poly (D,L-lactide-co-glycolide) (PLGA)/lipid NPs (MPLs) combine the advantages of PLGA and magnetic liposomes, such as a well-defined biocompatible coating and

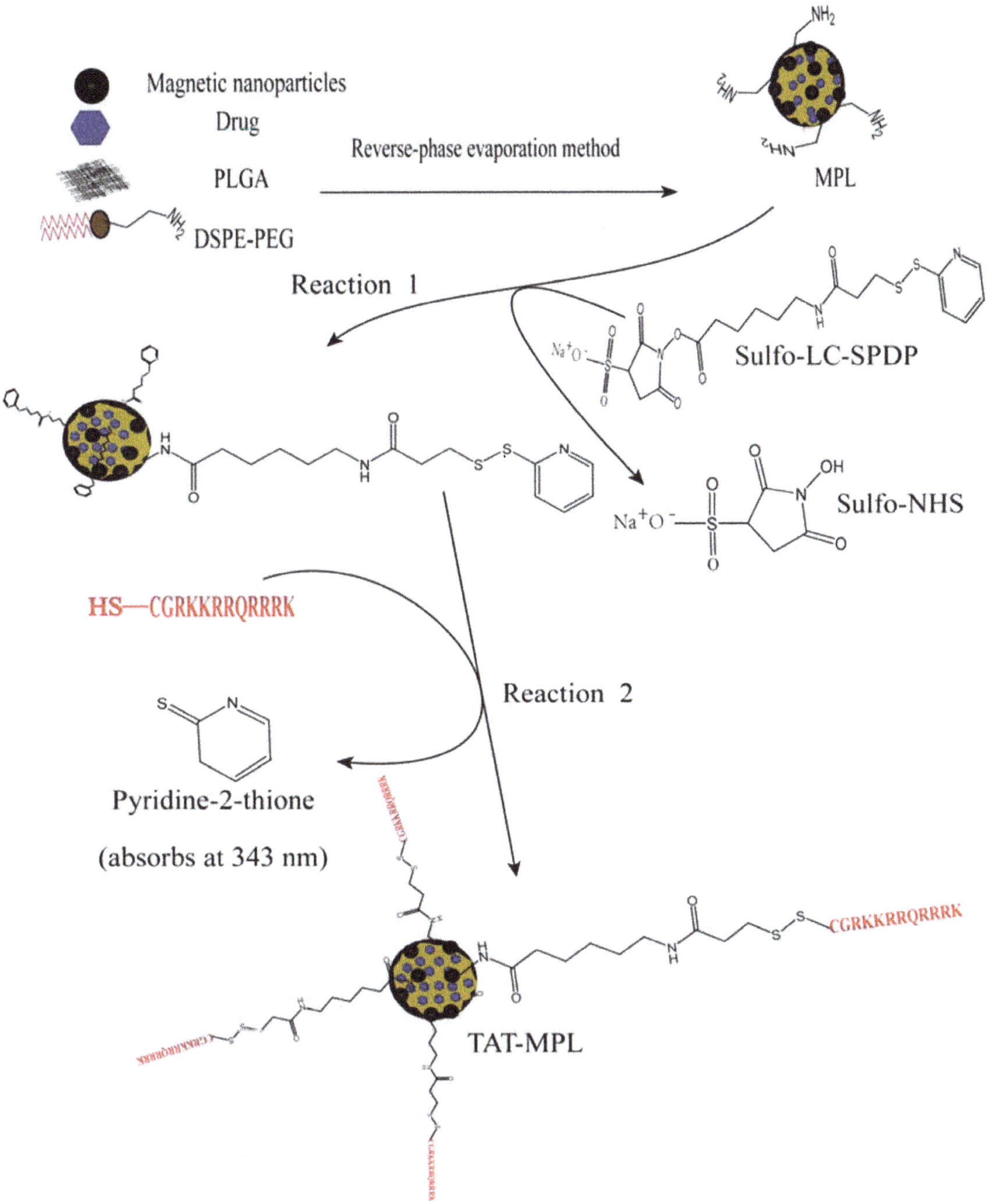

Figure 1. Schematic of the preparation of stealth MPLs and the conjugation of TAT peptide to MPLs.

simple fabrication [24], and have broad applications, including drug delivery and biodetection [25–27]. Monodispersed superparamagnetic magnetite/lipid nanospheres have been studied extensively [28–30]. Compared with conventional stealth liposomes [31,32], the surface of MPLs can be easily modified by groups, including functional amino (-NH_2) headgroups. In this work, we combine magnetic guidance and cell penetrating peptides to improve the delivery of drugs by TAT-conjugated MPLs.

Materials and Methods

Materials

Cholesterol and 1,2-distearoyl-sn-glycero-3-phosphoethanolamine-N-[amino (polyethylene glycol)-2000] (DSPE-PEG2000-NH_2) were purchased from Avanti Polar Lipids (USA). Quantum Dot (QD) were purchased from Wuhan Jiayuan Quantum Dots Co., Ltd (China). TAT-peptide with the sequence CGRKKRRQRRRK was purchased from ShineGene (China). Chitosan (deacetylation >90%, $M_w = 50{,}000$) was supplied by Yuhuan Aoxing (China). Octadecyl quaternized carboxymethyl

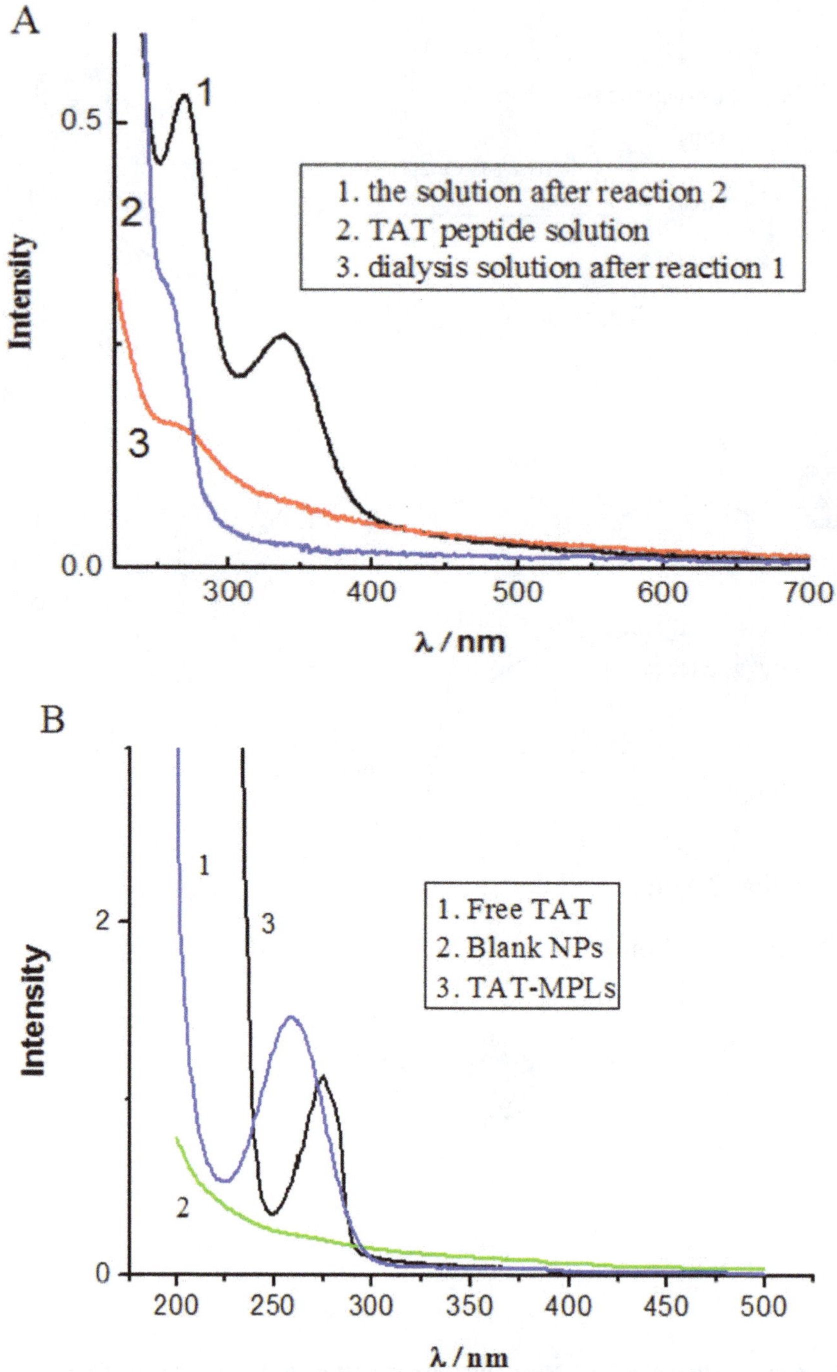

Figure 2. UV/Vis spectra. (A) UV/Vis spectra of the reaction solutions (conjugation of TAT to MPLs). (B) UV/Vis spectra of blank NPs and TAT-MPLs.

chitosan (OQCMC) and hydrophobic magnetic nanoparticles (HMNs) were prepared according to a previously published method [26], [28]. Poly (D,L-lactic-co-glycolic acid) (M_w = 10,000, lactic/glycolic acid ratio = 50/50) was purchased from Shandong Key Laboratory of Medical Polymer Material (China). L-α-Phosphatidylethanolamine (DOPE), N-succinimidyl 3-(2-pyridyldithio) propionate (SPDP), 2-iminothiolane, disuccinimidyl suberate (DSS), PD-10 columns were purchased from Sigma-Aldrich (USA). All other chemicals were of reagent grade and were used as received.

Preparation of MPLs

The MPLs were prepared by the reverse-phase evaporation (REV) method. For blank MPLs, PLGA, OQCMC, HMNs, DOPE, and DSPE-PEG-NH_2 (weight ratio = 1:0.2:0.3:0.2:0.2, total weight 30 mg) were dissolved in chloroform (4.0 mL) at room temperature to obtain the organic phase. The aqueous deionized water phase (6.0 mL) was mixed with the organic phase under sonication for 120 s at an output of 100 W. The organic solvents were evaporated on a rotary evaporator to form a gel-like MPL suspension. The MPLs were then separated by using a magnet and

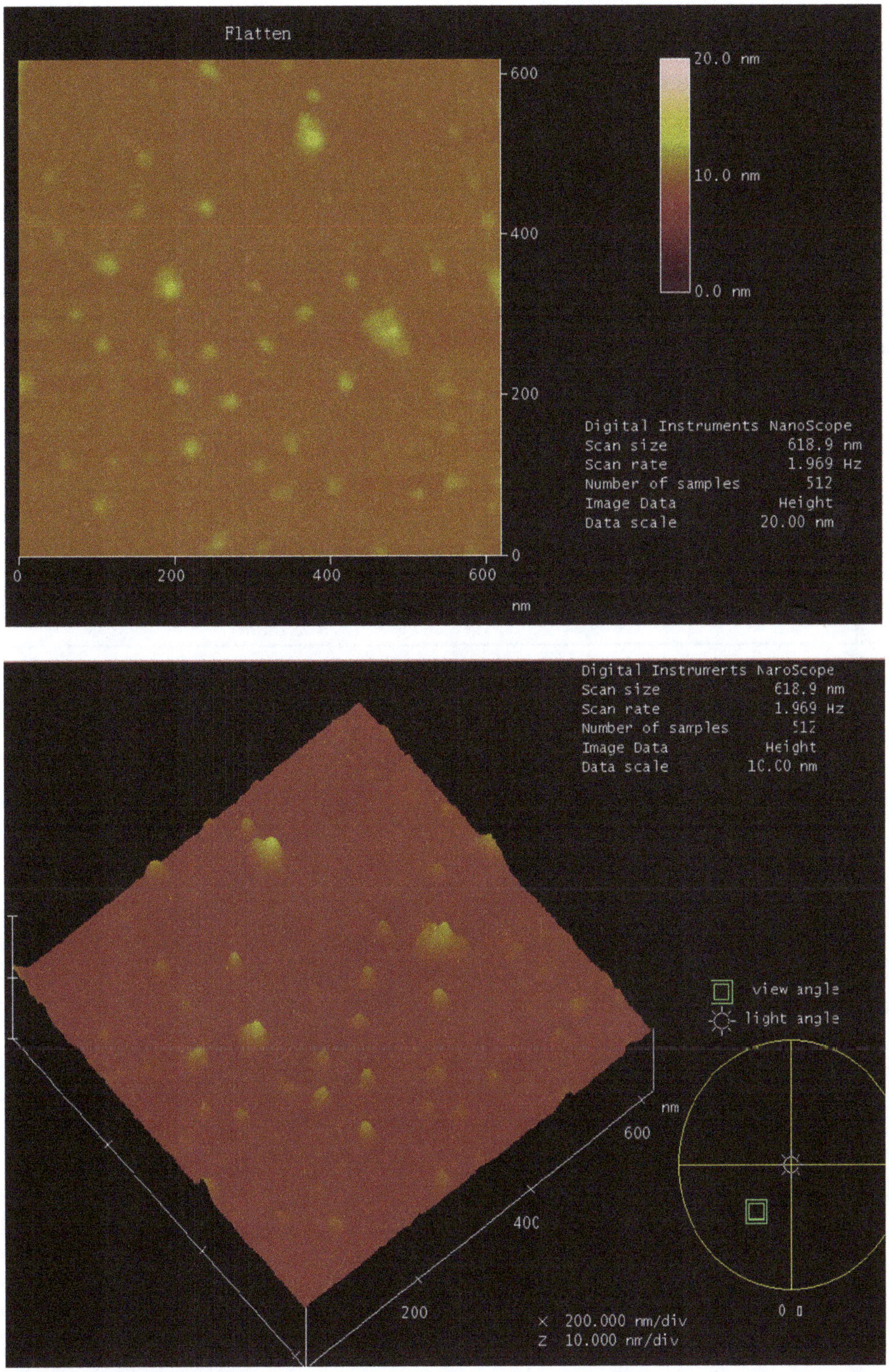

Figure 3. AFM micrographs of TAT-MPLs.

were washed with deionized water for three times. The collected product was freeze-dried and stored at 4°C.

For drug-loaded MPLs, the appropriate drug PLGA, OQCMC, HMNs and DSPE-PEG-NH_2 were dissolved in chloroform. Hesperidin (HES) and naringin (NAR) were soluble in the organic phase whereas glutathione (GSH) was dissolved in aqueous solution. The weight ratio of the drug to PLGA was adjusted according to experimental requirements.

TAT conjugation via a disulfide linkage

The MPLs were reacted with SPDP to install a 2-pyridyldithiol-end group on the surface of the NPs. A 0.1 M phosphate-buffered

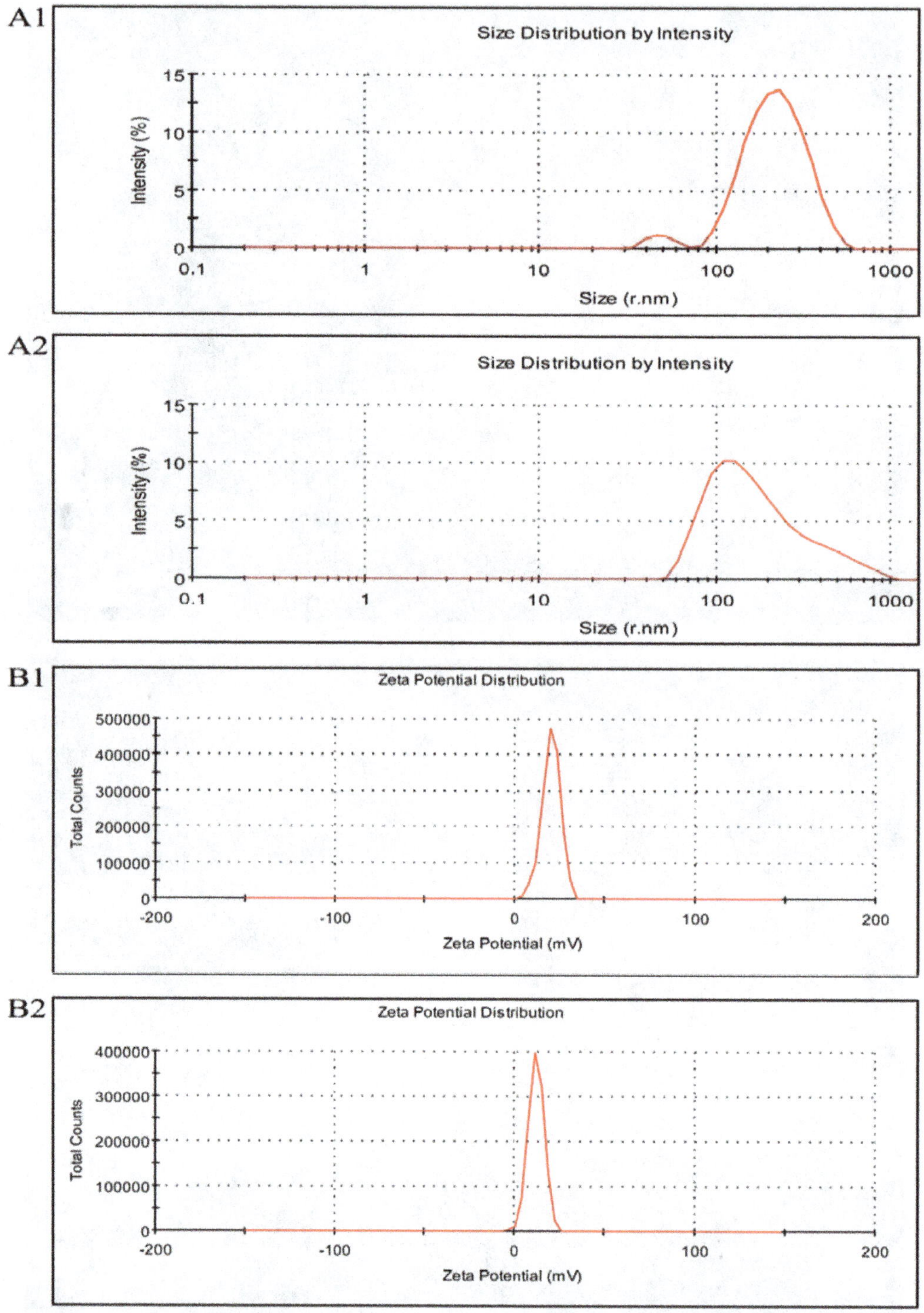

Figure 4. XRD spectrum and Magnetization curve. (A) XRD spectrum of TAT-MPLs. (B) Magnetization curve of Fe_3O_4 ferrofluid (1) and TAT-MPLs (2).

saline (PBS; pH 7.4) solution of MPL (5 mg/mL, 2.0 mL) was added to SPDP (2.0 mg) in DMSO (0.32 mL). The mixture was incubated at room temperature for 60 min. Low molecular weight impurities were dialyzed against 0.1 M PBS for 5 h with a dialysis bag (M_w = 12,000–14,000).

The 2-pyridyl disulfide-conjugated MPL solution was added to a 0.1 M PBS solution of TAT (5 mg/mL, 1.0 mL). The mixture was incubated overnight at 4°C to form a disulfide linkage between the surface of the MPLs and the TAT peptide. The excess TAT peptide was not removed and the TAT-conjugated MPL solution was stored at 4°C. The P2T method was used to verify the conjugation of the 2-pyridyl disulfide groups to the MPLs. The TAT-conjugated MPL solution was separated with a magnet and the supernatant solution was collected. The supernatant (300 μL) was diluted to 3 mL with PBS. UV-Visible Spectrophotometer

Table 1. Physical characterization of TAT-conjugated MPLs.

Formulation	Mean diameter (nm)	Polydispersity (μ/Γ^2)	Zeta potential (mV)
MPLs	102.6±1.3	0.202	20.7±3.62
TAT-MPLs	102.0±0.7	0.304	12.7±1.82
GSH-loaded TAT-MPLs	131.8±11.2	0.556	31.7±4.53
HES-loaded TAT-MPLs	112.9±1.1	0.220	5.39±0.42
NAR-loaded TAT-MPLs	93.1±1.6	0.237	32.8±2.43

was used to measure the absorbance of the MPL samples at 343 nm.

Characterization of MPLs

The particle size of the MPLs in solution was measured by quasielastic laser light scattering with a zeta potential analyzer. The MPL concentration in PBS was 0.3 mg/mL. Each measurement was repeated three times, and an average value was used. The size measurements were performed by multimodal analysis.

The morphologies of MPLs were observed by atomic force microscopy. For the AFM observations, droplets of the samples (approximately 30 μL) were deposited onto freshly cleaved mica and left for 10 min. Images were captured with scan rates between 0.5 and 1 Hz. The magnetic properties of magnetic TAT-MPLs were determined with a vibrating sample magnetometer.

Drug loading efficiency and release *in vitro*

The concentration of the three drugs was determined by UV/Vis spectroscopy at a fixed wavelength. The calibration curve was obtained in the concentration range of 0.5–50 μg/mL and the detection limit was 0.05 μg/mL.

After preparing the drug-loaded MPLs, the solution was centrifuged to remove any unencapsulated drug (4,000 rpm for 10 min). Drug content was determined by calculating the weight of the drug encapsulated in the MPLs.

The drug encapsulation efficiency (EE) and drug loading efficiency (LE) of the process were calculated using the following equation:

$$EE(\%) = \frac{A-B}{A} \times 100,\ LE(\%) = \frac{C}{D} \times 100,$$

where A is the total amount of drug; B is the amount of unencapsulated drug; C is the weight of drug in vesicle; D is the weight of vesicle.

In vitro drug release experiments of drug-loaded MPLs were carried out under shaking at 100 rpm and 37±0.5°C. The drug-loaded samples were enclosed in a dialysis membrane and then incubated in Phosphate buffer saline (10 mL, pH = 7.4). The buffer solution was exchanged completely at regular time points. The amount of drug release was determined by UV-Visible Spectrophotometer at set times, with PBS as a reference.

Cell culture and cytotoxicity studies

Bend.3 cells were grown in Dulbecco Modified Eagle Medium supplemented with 10% (v/v) fetal bovine serum and 1% (v/v) penicillin/streptomycin. The cytotoxicity was evaluated by MTT assays. bEnd.3 cells were seeded at a density of 1×10^4 cells/well in 96-well flat-bottomed microassay plates and incubated for 24 h at 37°C, in a fully humidified atmosphere of 5% CO_2. An increasing amount of drug-loaded MPLs and TAT-MPLs (1–100 μg/mL) were added and incubated for 12 h, 24 h and 48 h at 37°C. MTT saline solution (5 mg/mL, 100 μL/well) was added to the cells and formazan crystals were allowed to form over 3 h, then the crystals were dissolved with DMSO. The absorbance was measured at 490 nm with a Multi-Mode Microplate Reader.

Uptake studies

The uptake and intracellular distribution of QD-loaded fluorescein isothiocyanate (FITC)-TAT-MPLs in bEnd.3 cells were determined qualitatively using confocal fluorescence microscopy (Leica TCS SP8 MP, Leica Micosystems, Germany). bEnd.3 cells were seeded at a density of 8×10^4 cells/well in a 24-well plate with a pre-sterilized cover glass at the bottom and the cells were allowed to attach overnight. The following day, the cells were treated with QD-loaded FITC-MPLs and QD-loaded FITC-TAT-MPLs in the medium at a concentration of 20 μg/mL. At 0.5, 3, and 12 h after treatment, the cells were washed three times with PBS and fixed with 4% (w/w) paraformaldehyde in PBS for 15 min. The cells were counterstained with 4′,6-diamidino-2-phenylindole (DAPI) and rinsed three times. The images were captured with a confocal laser scanning microscope with appropriate filters for the red QD fluorescence (excitation at 560–575 nm and emission at 605 nm), green FITC fluorescence (excitation at 480–495 nm and emission at 525 nm) and blue DAPI fluorescence (excitation at 358 nm and emission at 461 nm). Finally, images captured using red and blue filters were overlain to determine the localization and association of red QD fluorescence in the cytoplast or nucleus, respectively.

Qualitative images and quantification of drug-loaded MPLs internalization

To measure the internalization of QD-loaded TAT-MPLs quantitatively, bEnd.3 cells were cultured on 24-well plates for 24 h to achieve approximately 80% confluence. Free FITC, free QDs, QD-loaded FITC-MPLs, or QD-loaded FITC-TAT-MPLs were then added to the wells. After incubation for 0.5, 3, or 12 h the cells were collected for fluorescence measurements (FITC and QDs). The fluorescence from individual cells was detected with a flow cytometer (FACS Calibur, BD Biosciences, USA). To detect the green FITC fluorescence, excitation was with the 488 nm line of an argon laser, and the emission fluorescence was measured at 525 nm. To detect red QD fluorescence, excitation was with the 570 nm line of an argon laser, and the emission fluorescence was measured at 605 nm.

For quantitative analysis, the uptake of FITC and QDs in bEnd.3 cells was determined by using fluorescence and the bicinchoninic (BCA) method. At the end of the treatment period,

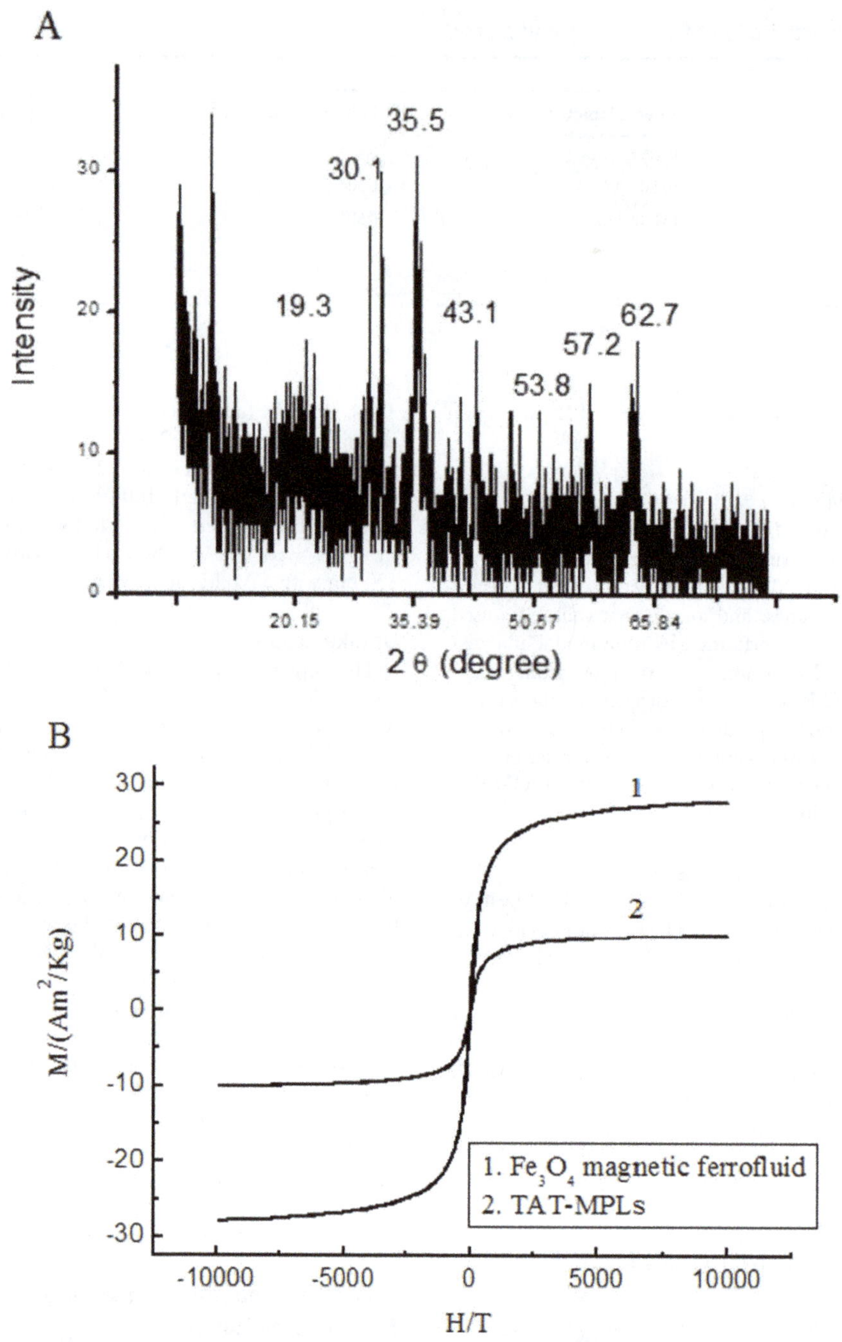

Figure 5. Particle-size-distribution and Zeta potential. (A) Particle-size-distribution based intensity of MPLs (1) and TAT-conjugated MPLs (2) in PBS. (B) Zeta potential of MPLs (1) and TAT-conjugated MPLs (2) in PBS.

the cells were washed three times with PBS (pH 7.4) and then incubated with cell culture lysis reagent (50 μL) for 10 min at 37°C. The protein content of the cell lysate was determined using the Pierce BCA protein assay. Cell lysates were harvested by adding PBS (50 μL, pH 7.4) and shaking at 37°C for 2 h. Samples were centrifuged at 10,000 rpm for 10 min at 4°C. The concentrations of the fluorescent materials (FITC and QDs) in the PBS extract were determined by a microplate spectrophotometer. Data are expressed as the amount of fluorescence material normalized to the total cell protein.

Statistical analysis

All data are expressed as mean±standard error of means. Statistical analyses were performed using Student's T-test. The differences were considered significant for p values<0.05.

Results and Discussion

Formulation of magnetic PLGA/lipids NPs

PLGA/lipid complexes have many advantages as delivery vehicles. They combine the properties of liposomes and PLGA and can be modified with molecular targeting factors. Multifunc-

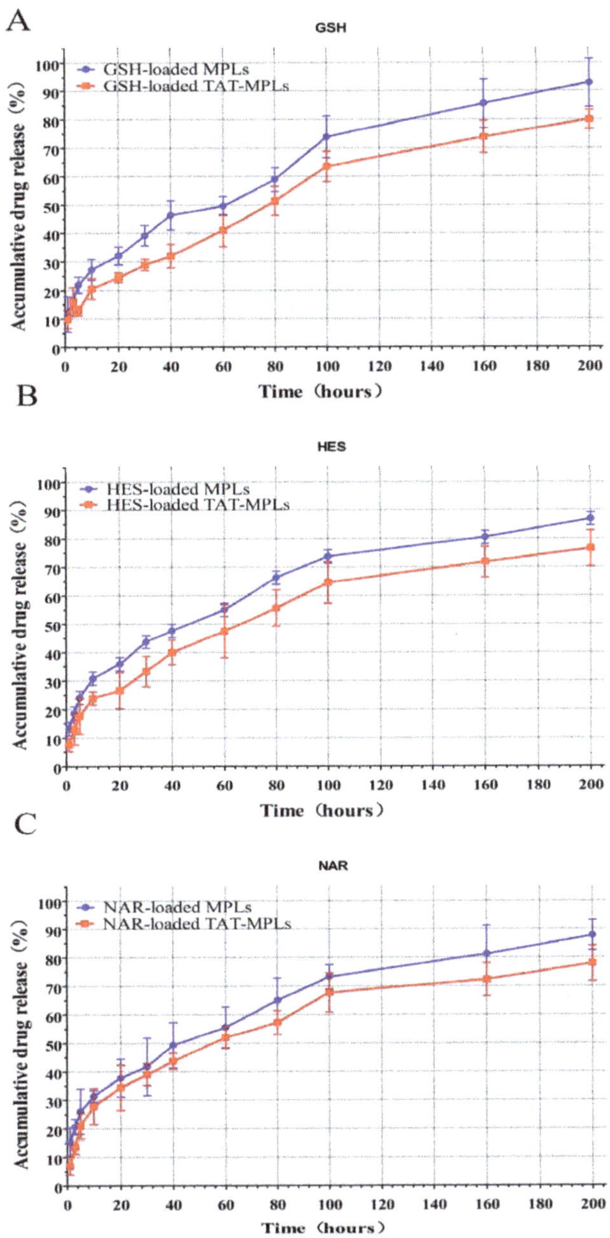

Figure 6. Drug release profiles of the TAT-conjugated MPLs in PBS (pH 7.4) at 37±0.5°C *in vitro.*

tional targeted drug delivery systems, such as magnetic cationic liposomes [30] and PEG- and TAT-conjugated MPLs, can be fabricated from DSPE-PEG or DOPE. Attaching flexible PEG polymers to the liposome surface increases the blood circulation time significantly. These PEG-coated liposomes are referred to as stealth liposomes [31,32]. A schematic illustration of the preparation of stealth TAT-conjugated MPLs is presented in Figure 1. PEGylated MPLs can be assembled by the REV method from DSPE-PEG-NH_2, OQCMC, and DOPE. The DSPE-PEG-NH_2 and OQCMC components of MPLs mean that amine groups are present on the surface of stealth MPLs [33–35]. In this study, SPDP reagents, which are a unique group of amine- and sulfhydryl-reactive heterobifunctional cross-linkers, were used to form amine-to-sulfhydryl cross-links between molecules. Because TAT peptide contains sulfhydryl groups (-SH), the MPLs are modified by the SPDP reagent in reaction 1. Reaction 2 results in the displacement of a pyridine-2-thione group, the concentration of which may be determined by measuring the absorbance at 343 nm.

UV/Vis spectra of the reaction solutions are shown in Figure 2A. An absorbance peak at 343 nm was clearly visible after reaction 2, which confirmed the presence of pyridine-2-thione. In addition, the peak at 343 nm was not observed for the dialyzed solution after reaction 1 and the TAT peptide solution, indicating that pyridine-2-thione must be the product of reaction 2. The results also suggest that amine groups were present on the surface of MPLs. UV/Vis spectroscopy was also used to determine the content of TAT peptide on the MPLs (Figure 2B). Differences were observed in the UV absorption of MPLs and TAT-MPLs. TAT had an absorption peak at 275 nm. The UV spectrum of the TAT-MPLs was similar to that of TAT, although it also contained a bathochromic shift at 277.5 nm, which was attributed to the addition of TAT to the MPLs. These results indicate that the modification of the TAT unit was responsible for the differences between the UV spectra of MPLs and TAT-MPLs.

Characterization of MPLs

The TAT-MPLs generally had irregular spherical shapes (Figure 3) and were about 80 nm in size. The hydrodynamic diameter of TAT-conjugated MPLs was 102.0±0.7 nm, with a corresponding polydispersity index (PDI) of 0.304, which was greater than the AFM diameter because of the hydration of MPLs in aqueous solution. The TAT conjugation decreased the zeta potential of NPs (Figure 4 and Table 1). HES were encapsulated effectively in the TAT-conjugated MPLs, and the drug encapsulation efficiency and loading capacity were above 90% and 10%, respectively. The size of the HES-loaded TAT-conjugated MPLs in PBS solution was 112.9±1.1 nm with a narrow size distribution and a polydispersity index of 0.220 (Table 1). The AFM images also show the spherical shape and homogeneous size distribution of the magnetic NPs.

X-ray powder diffraction analysis (XRD) is a kind of useful method to demonstrate the structure of magnetic nanoparticles. The XRD pattern of TAT-MPLs was detected as illustrated in Figure 5a. The characteristic peaks of Fe_3O_4 ferrofluid are at $2\theta = 30.1°$, 35.5°, 43.1°, 53.7° and 62.7°, which corresponding to crystal face of (220), (311), (400), (422), (511) and (440). The results indicated that TAT-MPLs has the same crystalline structure with Fe_3O_4 ferrofluid. The broad peak in the $2\theta = 15°–25°$ region approve the existence of PLGA polymer. Figure 5b shows the room-temperature magnetization curves of Fe_3O_4 ferrofluid (1) and TAT-MPLs. As shown in the figure, both the samples show a typical superparamagnetic behavior at room temperature without any hysteresis loop. The saturation magnetization value of TAT-MPLs is 10.1 emu/g at 300 K, which is about 36.2% of the magnetization of Fe_3O_4 ferrofluid.

The drug release profiles of TAT-conjugated MPLs showed a high burst release during the first 24 h followed by slower release (Figure 6). During the initial burst release, 20%–40% of the encapsulated drug was released from the TAT-conjugated MPLs. After 8 days, 70%–90% of the total drug was released. The surface conjugation of the TAT-MPLs meant that they had a slower drug release than the MPLs.

Cytotoxicity and growth inhibition of bEnd.3 cells *in vitro*

The cytotoxicity of MPLs and TAT-MPLs in bEnd.3 cells was examined with an MTT assay. Figure 7 shows the cytotoxicity of MPLs and TAT-MPLs at concentrations of less than 100 μg/mL.

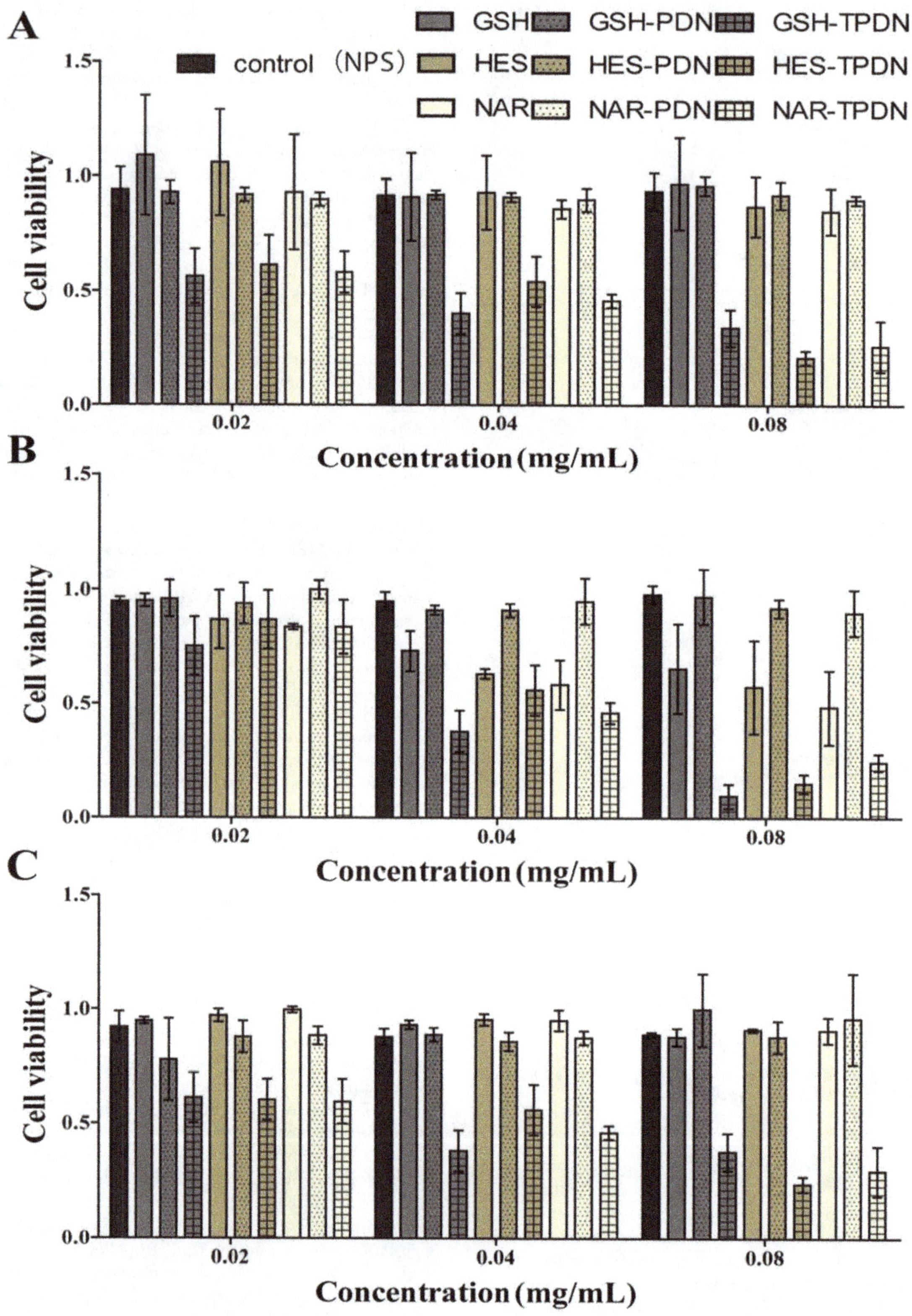

Figure 7. Cytotoxicity of MPLs and drug-loaded TAT-MPLs measured using MTT assays after. (A) 12, (B) 24, and (C) 48 h incubation with bEnd.3 cells. (GSH: glutathione, HES: hesperidin, NAR: naringin).

The bEnd.3 cells treated with MPLs at concentrations of 20.0, 40.0, and 80.0 μg/mL showed good viability (>85%), whereas the cells treated with TAT-MPLs showed poor viability (<75%) after incubation for 12, 24, and 48 h. As the concentration of NPs increased, the drug-loaded TAT-MPLs were more cytoxic than the MPLs. This was because the TAT conjugation delivered a

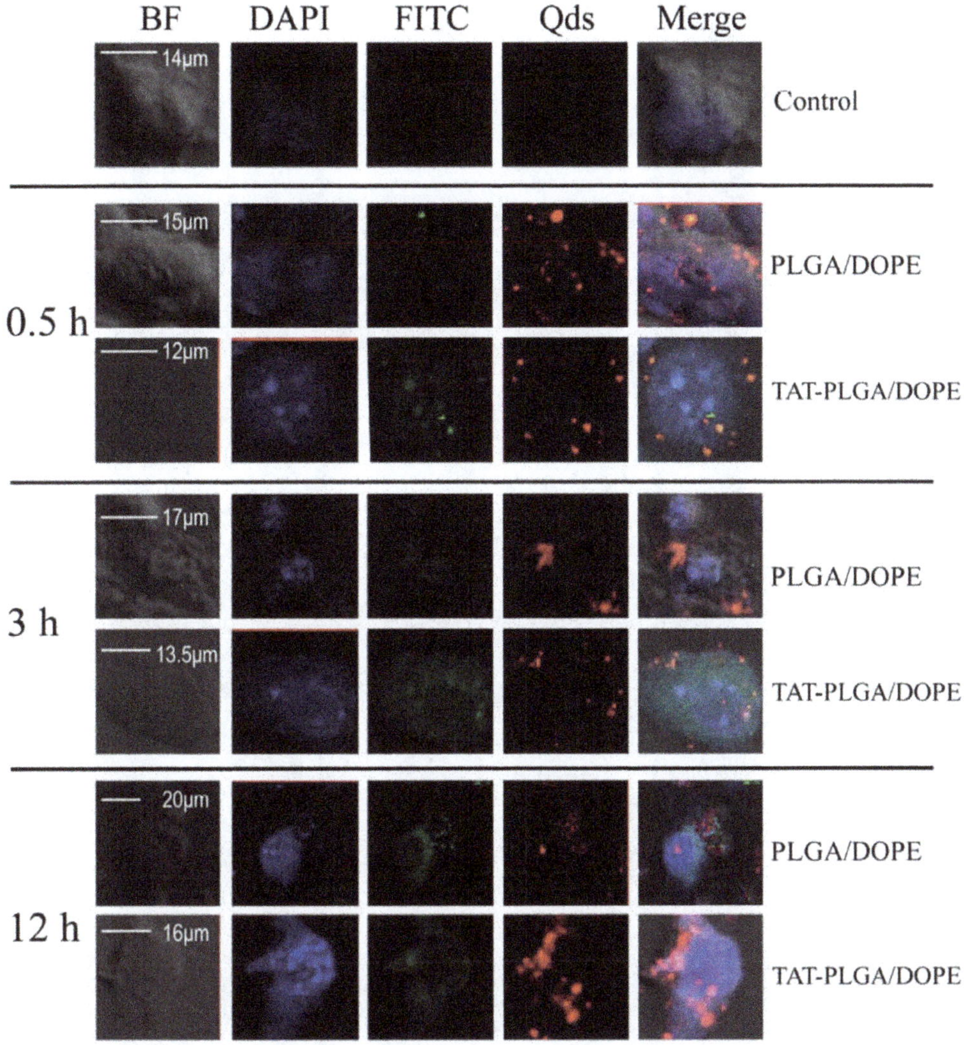

Figure 8. Localization and distribution of QDs encapsulated in TAT-MPLs in bEnd.3 cells. Cells were cultured in FITC-labeled NP-containing medium (1 μM QDs) on a glass-bottomed culture plate for 0.5, 3, and 12 h, treated with DAPI for 5–10 min, and then examined by confocal microscopy.

greater amount of the drugs into cells. Furthermore, the cytotoxicity of the blank TAT-MPLs was low and this was confirmed by observing morphological changes in the cells by microscopy. These results demonstrate that TAT-MPLs has low cellular toxicity and were suitable for use in experimental concentrations.

Figure 7 also shows the growth inhibition of bEnd.3 cells by GSH, HES, and NAR in MPLs, TAT-MPLs, and in solution after 48 h at concentrations of GSH, HES, and NAR from 20 to 80 μg/mL. The cell growth inhibition rate was dose-dependent in all the experiments. At GSH, HES, and NAR concentrations of 20 μg/mL, there was no difference in the growth inhibition of bEnd.3 cells treated with the drug solutions and drug-loaded NPs. As the concentration of the drugs increased, the cytotoxicity of the TAT-MPLs was significantly higher ($P<0.05$ for NPs concentrations of 40 and 80 μg/mL). The cell growth inhibition rate of the TAT-MPLs was also greater than that of the MPLs without TAT, indicating that a greater number of drug-loaded TAT-MPLs entered the cells because TAT increased the cell membrane penetration.

Intracellular distribution of QD-loaded NPs

To verify whether encapsulating different drugs in the NPs affected their trafficking in tumor cells, we evaluated the intracellular distribution of free FITC/QDs, QD-loaded FITC-MPLs, and QD-loaded FITC-TAT-MPLs in bEnd.3 cells with a nuclear stain. The intracellular trafficking of FITC and QDs was studied by laser confocal microscopy to clarify the mechanism of efficacy of drug-loaded NPs. The QD-loaded FITC-NPs showed a diffuse distribution within the cells, with a significant fraction appearing in the cytoplasm near the cell nucleus at 0.5 h. A significant proportion of QD-loaded FITC-NPs also appeared in the cytoplasm. Therefore, the strong fluorescence of TAT-MPLs in the cytoplasm and cell nucleus demonstrates that they can deliver QDs efficiently to bEnd.3 cells. In addition, the FITC-TAT-MPLs were concentrated in the perinuclear region rather than at the cell periphery at 12 h. QDs were also present in the nuclei of cells treated with FITC-TAT-MPLs at 12 h. (Figure 8).

Interestingly, the cells treated with FITC-TAT-MPLs accumulated QDs in the nucleus, whereas cells treated with FITC-MPLs did not. The nuclear delivery of QDs by TAT-MPLs was greater

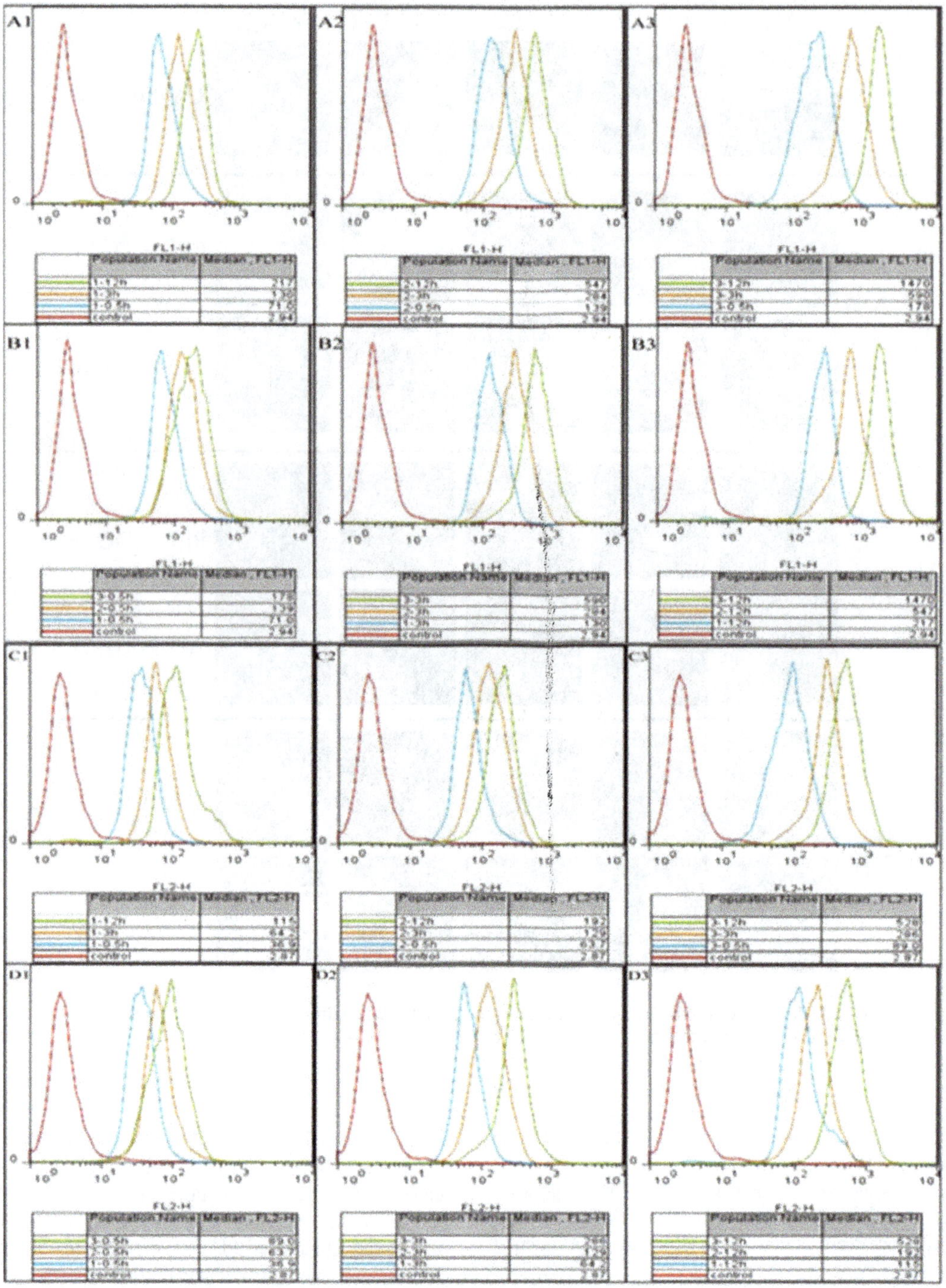

Figure 9. Flow cytometry analysis of bEnd.3 cells. Cells incubated with free FITC and QDs (1), MPLs (2), and TAT-MPLs (3) for 0.5 h, 3 h and 12 h at a NP concentration of 20 μg/mL. The NPs were labeled with FITC. The FITC (A and B) and QD fluorescence intensity (C and D) are shown.

than that by MPLs, which is also consistent with the greater cytotoxicity observed in the MTT assay. These results were further verified by quantitative analysis of accumulation of FITC and QDs.

Quantitative analysis of accumulation in bEnd.3 cells

To determine the efficacy of cellular drug delivery by TAT-MPLs, the cellular accumulation of equivalent doses of FITC and QDs was quantitatively analyzed in bEnd.3 cells. Figure 9 and Figure 10 show that cells treated with QD-loaded TAT-MPLs accumulated higher levels of QDs than those treated with QD-loaded MPLs. Furthermore, bEnd.3 cells treated with TAT-MPLs accumulated a significantly higher level of QDs and FITC than those treated with QDs and FITC in MPLs and in solution ($P < 0.05$) at 3 h and 12 h. Thus, the accumulation of QDs and FITC in bEnd.3 cells is enhanced by TAT conjugation.

Our results show that NPs enhance QDs accumulation considerably in bEnd.3 cells compared with free QDs, and that

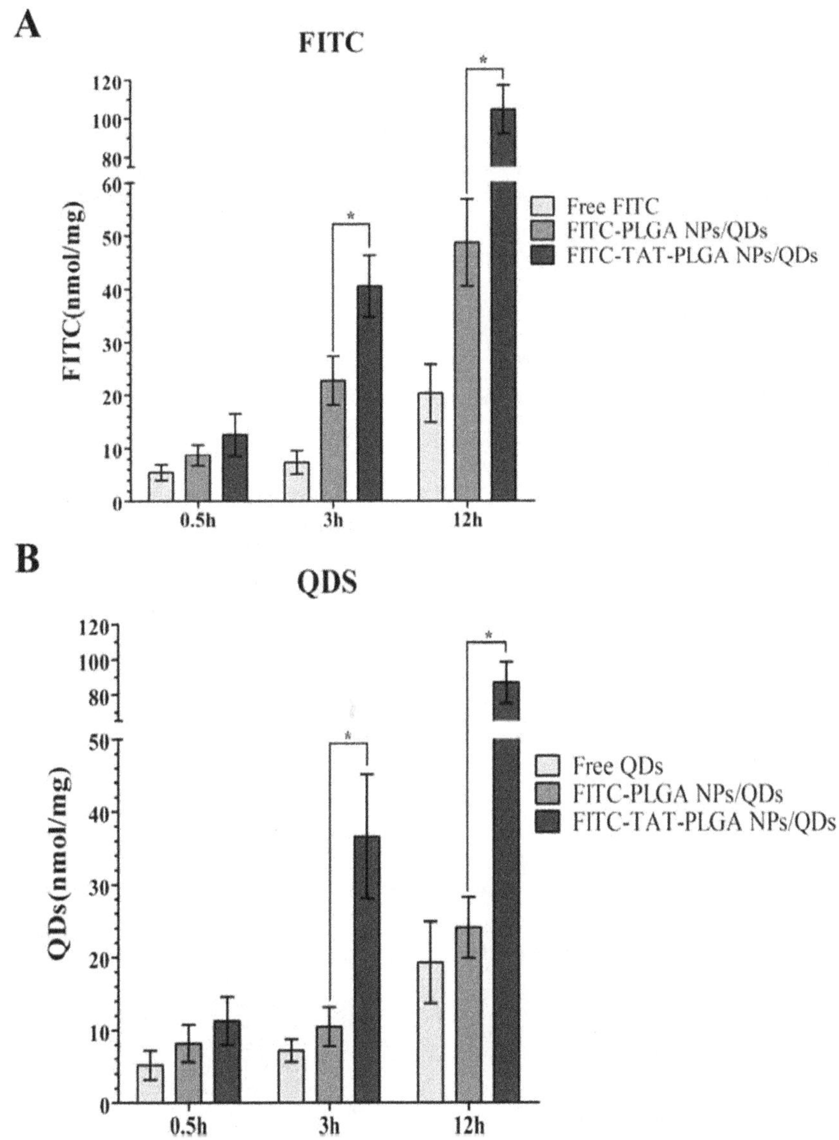

Figure 10. Quantitative analysis of QD-loaded FITC-MPLs and FITC-TAT-MPLs in bEnd.3 cells. Cells were cultured in a 24-well plate for 0.5 h, 3 h and 12 h, lysed, and the FITC and QDs fluorescence were measured by a microplate spectrophotometer to determine FITC (A) and QDs (B) contents in the cells.

TAT-MPLs increase QDs accumulation more efficiently than MPLs. These results were confirmed by laser confocal microscopy. Many studies have shown that the increased level of drug accumulation in cells treated with MPLs contributes to the enhanced therapeutic efficacy of drug-loaded NPs [15]. Thus, our method of fabricating TAT-conjugated magnetic NPs successfully produced TAT-MPLs that may be effective for delivering drugs across the BBB.

Conclusion

Previous studies indicate that there are many applications of magnetic nanoparticles for cells and bacteria [36–38]. In this study, we fabricated TAT-conjugated MPLs from OQCMC, DOPE, and magnetic NPs. The size of the HES-loaded TAT-MPLs in aqueous solution was close to 112.9±1.1 nm with a narrow size distribution with a polydispersity index of 0.220. AFM images showed the TAT-MPLs were spherical and had a homogeneous size distribution. The TAT-MPLs showed very strong fluorescence in the cytoplasm and cell nucleus, and delivered QDs to bEnd.3 cells efficiently. The levels of QDs and FITC that accumulated in bEnd.3 cells were dose- and time-dependent for MPLs and TAT-MPLs. The TAT conjugation of MPLs could significantly enhance the cellular delivery and the therapeutic efficacy of drugs in bEnd.3 cells by penetrating the cell membrane. This may be useful in designing drug-loaded NPs for crossing the BBB and delivering drugs to the brain.

Author Contributions

Conceived and designed the experiments: HZL YJS XRW YFZ. Performed the experiments: KW ZMZ YFZ. Analyzed the data: FZ JW YYF YD LZ KM. Contributed reagents/materials/analysis tools: TTS YS YHL. Wrote the paper: KW.

References

1. Liu L, Guo K, Lu J, Venkatraman SS, Luo D, et al. (2008) Biologically active core/shell nanoparticles self-assembled from cholesterol-terminated PEG-TAT for drug delivery across the blood-brain barrier. Biomaterials 29: 1509–1517.
2. Abbott NJ, Patabendige AA, Dolman DE, Yusof SR, Begley DJ (2010) Structure and function of the blood-brain barrier. Neurobiol Dis 37: 13–25.
3. Andreu A, Fairweather N, Miller AD (2008) Clostridium neurotoxin fragments as potential targeting moieties for liposomal gene delivery to the CNS. Chembiochem 9: 219–231.
4. Aichberger KJ, Herndlhofer S (2007) Liposomal cytarabine for treatment of myeloid central nervous system relapse in chronic myeloid leukaemia occurring during imatinib therapy. Eur J Clin Invest 37: 808–813.
5. Rao KS, Reddy MK, Horning JL, Labhasetwar V (2008) TAT-conjugated nanoparticles for the CNS delivery of anti-HIV drugs. Biomaterials 29: 4429–4438.
6. Mika P, Jere P, Thomas W, Tommy T (2008) Three-step tumor targeting of paclitaxel using biotinylated PLA-PEG nanoparticles and avidin-biotin technology: Formulation development and in vitro anticancer activity. Eur J Pharm Biopharm 70: 66–74.
7. Tiwari SB, Amiji MM (2006) A review of nanocarrier-based CNS delivery systems. Curr Drug Deliv 3: 219–232.
8. Pan BF, Cui DX, Sheng Y (2007) Dendrimer-modified magnetic nanoparticles enhance efficiency of gene delivery system. Cancer Res 67: 8156–8163.
9. Choi KM, Choi SH, Jeon H (2011) Chimeric capsid protein as a nanocarrier for siRNA delivery: stability and cellular uptake of encapsulated siRNA. ACS Nano 5: 8690–8699.
10. Dobson J (2006) Gene therapy progress and prospects: magnetic nanoparticle-based gene delivery. Gene Ther 13: 283–287.
11. Akhtari M, Bragin A, Cohen M (2008) Functionalized magnetonanoparticles for MRI diagnosis and localization in epilepsy. Epilepsia 49: 1419–1430.
12. Lu W, Tan YZ, Hu KL, Jiang XG (2005) Cationic albumin conjugated pegylated nanoparticle with its transcytosis ability and little toxicity against blood-brain barrier. Int J Pharm 295: 247–260.
13. Salman HH, Gamazo C, Agüeros M, Irache JM (2007) Bioadhesive capacity and immunoadjuvant properties of thiamine-coated nanoparticles. Vaccine 25: 8123–8132.
14. Kievit FM, Zhang M (2011) Cancer Nanotheranostics: Improving Imaging and Therapy by Targeted Delivery Across Biological Barriers. Adv Mater 23: H217–247.
15. Chavanpatil MD, Khdair A, Gerard B, Bachmeier C, Miller DW, et al. (2007) Surfactant-polymer nanoparticles overcome P-glycoprotein-mediated drug efflux. Mol Pharm 4: 730–738.
16. Torchilin VP (2008) Cell penetrating peptide-modified pharmaceutical nanocarriers for intracellular drug and gene delivery. Biopolymers 90: 604–610.
17. Lazar AN, Mourtas S, Youssef I, Parizot C, Dauphin A, et al. (2013) Curcumin-conjugated nanoliposomes with high affinity for Aβ deposits: possible applications to Alzheimer disease. Nanomedicine 9: 712–721.
18. Costantino L, Gandolfi F, Tosi G, Rivasi F, Vandelli MA, et al. (2005) Peptide-derivatized biodegradable nanoparticles able to cross the blood-brain barrier. J Control Release 108: 84–96.
19. Schwarze SR, Ho A, Vocero-Akbani A, Dowdy SF (1999) In vivo protein transduction: delivery of a biologically active protein into the mouse. Science 285: 1569–1582.
20. Santra S, Yang H, Stanley JT, Holloway PH, Moudgil BM, et al. (2005) Rapid and effective labeling of brain tissue using TAT-conjugated CdS: Mn/ZnS quantum dots. Chem Commun 25: 3144–3156.
21. Malhotra M, Tomaro-Duchesneau C, Prakash S (2013) Synthesis of TAT peptide-tagged PEGylated chitosan nanoparticles for siRNA delivery targeting neurodegenerative diseases. Biomaterials 34: 1270–1280.
22. Tian XH, Wang ZG, Meng H, Wang YH, Feng W, et al. (2013) Tat peptide-decorated gelatin-siloxane nanoparticles for delivery of CGRP transgene in treatment of cerebral vasospasm. Int J Nanomedicine 8: 865–876.
23. Teixidó M, Giralt E (2008) The role of peptides in blood-brain barrier nanotechnology. J Pept Sci 14: 163–173.
24. Sophie L, Delphine F, Marc P (2008) Magnetic Iron Oxide Nanoparticles: Synthesis, Stabilization, Vectorization, Physicochemical Characterizations, and Biological Applications. Chem Rev 108: 2064–2110.
25. Cui Y, Xu Q, Chow PK, Wang D, Wang CH (2013) Transferrin-conjugated magnetic silica PLGA nanoparticles loaded with doxorubicin and paclitaxel for brain glioma treatment. Biomaterials 34: 8511–8520.
26. Krack M, Hohenberg H, Kornowski A, Lindner P, Weller H, et al. (2008) Nanoparticle-loaded magnetophoretic vesicles. J Am Chem Soc 130: 7315–7320.
27. Liang XF, Wang HJ, Luo H, Tian H, Zhang BB, et al. (2008) Characterization of novel multifunctional cationic polymeric liposomes formed from octadecyl quaternized carboxymethyl chitosan/cholesterol and drug encapsulation. Langmuir 24: 7147–7153.
28. Liang X, Li X, Chang J, Duan Y, Li Z (2013) Properties and Evaluation of Quaternized Chitosan/lipid Cation Polymeric Liposomes for Cancer Targeted Gene Delivery. Langmuir 29: 8683–8693.
29. Zhao AJ, Yao P, Kang CS (2005) Synthesis and characterization of tat-mediated O-CMC magnetic nanoparticles having anticancer function. J Magn Magn Mater 295: 37–43.
30. Liang XF, Wang HJ (2010) Development of monodispersed and functional magnetic nanospheres via simple liposome method. J Nanopart Res 12: 1723–1732.
31. Gabizon AA (2001) Stealth Liposomes and Tumor Targeting: One Step Further in the Quest for the Magic Bullet. Clin Cancer Res 7: 223–225.
32. Garbuzenko O, Barenholz Y, Priev A (2005) Effect of grafted PEG on liposome size and on compressibility and packing of lipid bilayer. Chem Ph Lipids 135: 117–129.
33. Liang X, Tian H, Luo H, Wang H, Chang J (2009) Novel quaternized chitosan and polymeric micelles with cross-linked ionic cores for prolonged release of minocycline. J Biomater Sci Polym Ed 20: 115–131.
34. Yu Z, Schmaltz RM, Bozeman TC, Paul R, Rishel MJ, et al. (2013) Selective tumor cell targeting by the disaccharide moiety of bleomycin. J Am Chem Soc 135: 2883–2886.
35. Yamanouchi D, Wu J, Lazar AN, Kent KC, Chu CC, et al. (2008) Biodegradable arginine-based poly(ester-amide)s as non-viral gene delivery reagents. Biomaterials 29: 3269–3277.
36. Pan Y, Du X, Zhao F, Xu B (2012) Magnetic nanoparticles for the manipulation of proteins and cells. Chem Soc Rev 41: 2912–2942.
37. Shin J, Lee KM, Lee JH, Lee J, Cha M (2014) Magnetic manipulation of bacterial magnetic nanoparticle-loaded neurospheres. Integr Biol (Camb) 6: 532–539.
38. Liu F, Mu J, Wu X, Bhattacharjya S, Yeow EK, et al. (2014) Peptide-perylene diimide functionalized magnetic nano-platforms for fluorescence turn-on detection and clearance of bacterial lipopolysaccharides. Chem Commun (Camb) 50: 6200–6203.

4

Inhibition of c-Abl Kinase Activity Renders Cancer Cells Highly Sensitive to Mitoxantrone

Kemal Alpay[1], **Mehdi Farshchian[2]**, **Johanna Tuomela[3]**, **Jouko Sandholm[4]**, **Kaappo Aittokallio[1]**, **Elina Siljamäki[2]**, **Marko Kallio[5]**, **Veli-Matti Kähäri[2]**, **Sakari Hietanen[1]***

1 Department of Obstetrics and Gynecology and Joint Clinical Biochemistry Laboratory of Turku University Hospital, Medicity Research Laboratory, University of Turku, Turku, Finland, **2** Department of Dermatology and MediCity Research Laboratory, University of Turku and Turku University Hospital, Turku, Finland, **3** Department of Cell Biology and Anatomy, University of Turku, Turku, Finland, **4** Cell Imaging Core, Turku Centre for Biotechnology, University of Turku and Åbo Akademi University, Turku, Finland, **5** VTT Health, VTT Technical Research Centre of Finland, Turku, Finland

Abstract

Although c-Abl has increasingly emerged as a key player in the DNA damage response, its role in this context is far from clear. We studied the effect of inhibition of c-Abl kinase activity by imatinib with chemotherapy drugs and found a striking difference in cell survival after combined mitoxantrone (MX) and imatinib treatment compared to a panel of other chemotherapy drugs. The combinatory treatment induced apoptosis in HeLa cells and other cancer cell lines but not in primary fibroblasts. The difference in MX and doxorubicin was related to significant augmentation of DNA damage. Transcriptionally active p53 accumulated in cells in which human papillomavirus E6 normally degrades p53. The combination treatment resulted in caspase activation and apoptosis, but this effect did not depend on either p53 or p73 activity. Despite increased p53 activity, the cells arrested in G2 phase became defective in this checkpoint, allowing cell cycle progression. The effect after MX treatment depended partially on c-Abl: Short interfering RNA knockdown of c-Abl rendered HeLa cells less sensitive to MX. The effect of imatinib was decreased by c-Abl siRNA suggesting a role for catalytically inactive c-Abl in the death cascade. These findings indicate that MX has a unique cytotoxic effect when the kinase activity of c-Abl is inhibited. The treatment results in increased DNA damage and c-Abl–dependent apoptosis, which may offer new possibilities for potentiation of cancer chemotherapy.

Editor: Stephan Neil Witt, Louisiana State University Health Sciences Center, United States of America

Funding: This study was financially supported by grants from Finnish Medical Society, Turku University Foundation and Cancer Society of South-Western Finland, the Academy of Finland (projects 137687 and 268360), the Finnish Cancer Research Foundation, Sigrid Juselius Foundation, Turku University Hospital EVO grant (project 13336). The funders had no role in study design, data collection and analysis, decision to publish, or preparation of the manuscript.

Competing Interests: The authors have declared that no competing interests exist.

* Email: sakari.hietanen@utu.fi

These authors contributed equally to this work.

Introduction

Chemotherapy in tumor treatment works mainly through causing DNA damage that induces a complex network of cellular responses ultimately leading to cancer cell death. At the core of the response are pathways that recognize the damage, halt the cell cycle, and enact the death cascade. In cancer therapy, radiotherapy and most chemotherapy agents function by directly damaging DNA or interfering with DNA replication. The DNA damage response of malignant and normal cells determines the efficacy and side effects of the treatment. The fate of the cell lies in the complex DNA repair pathways evoked by numerous types of DNA damage that can arise after genotoxic treatment [1]. Successful repair is critical for normal tissue to overcome the side effects of the therapy but in the tumor can result in treatment resistance. Cancer cells usually have accumulated mutations in genes involved in DNA repair, offering a variety of therapeutic opportunities for agents that modulate the remaining functional repair pathways. After DNA damaging treatment, damaged bases, mismatches, or DNA adducts are usually tolerated up to a certain quantitative threshold but can give rise to mutations if they remain unrepaired [2].

c-Abl inhibition has been recently proposed to lead to an altered DNA damage response [3]. c-Abl is a non–receptor tyrosine kinase that plays a role in differentiation, adhesion, cell division, death, and stress responses and binds to several proteins involved in apoptosis pathways [4]. The changes in c-Abl protein conformation vary, and the binding partners consequently differ [4–6]. Several proteins such as ATM, DNA-PK, BRCA1, and the transcription factors p73 and RFX1 interact with c-Abl [5]. Most notably, c-Abl has been reported to interact with the homologous recombination-repair protein Rad51, elevate [7] its expression at the gene level, and activate it by phosphorylation. Active c-Abl can be inhibited by the small molecule drug imatinib (Gleevec; STI-571), which was developed against the aberrant BCR/Abl fusion protein found in chronic myeloid leukemia (CML) [8]. In CML cells, the first exon of c-Abl is replaced by the BCR gene sequence, resulting in constitutively active c-Abl expression. This aberrant kinase activity results in enhanced proliferation, which can be inhibited with imatinib. Imatinib is an ATP-competitive inhibitor stabilizing inactive c-Abl conformation [8]. The kinase activity of c-Abl is increased after DNA damage and then increases the activity of Atm and Atr [9]. Treatment with imatinib decreases the level of elevated RAD51 involved in double-strand break (DSB) repair and sensitizes several cell types to chemotherapy [10–13]. Direct interaction has also been demonstrated between c-Abl and DNA-PK, which regulates non-homologous end joining [14].

The development of uterine cervical cancer is a multistep process that involves cervical mucosal cell transformation by oncogenic human papillomavirus (HPV) E6 and E7 proteins. E7 inactivates the cell cycle regulator pRb, inhibiting cell cycle arrest, while E6 inactivates the tumor suppressor protein p53, the key regulator of apoptosis and genotoxic stress response [15]. Because cervical cancer cells almost always carry wild-type p53, which is degraded by high-risk HPV, p53 was formerly regarded as completely non-functional in cervical cancer cells. However, the work of several groups has recently made evident that p53 inactivation may be reverted in HPV E6–carrying cells and that p53 status in cervical cancer cells is not equal to that of cancer cells with a mutated p53 gene [16]. We previously observed that chemoradiation reactivates p53 in cervical cancer cells and promotes cell death synergistically. However, when analyzed in detail, the p53 protein may either enhance or inhibit the cytotoxicity of the chemotherapy drug [17,18]. Mouse embryonic fibroblasts null for c-Abl are defective in p53 phosphorylation and resistant to death after genotoxic damage. Inhibition of c-Abl by imatinib diminishes hydroxyurea-induced p53 phosphorylation [9]. We hypothesized that the active p53 may enhance DNA repair and thus wanted to study the effect on cell death of repair modulation. c-Abl is generally believed to relay pro-apoptotic signaling from Atm and Atr to p53 and p73, among other targets [3]. We studied here the effect of c-Abl inhibition on p53 activity in HPV-positive cells and how it relates to the damage and death responses.

A comprehensive panel of drugs representing alkylating agents, platinum drugs, and topoisomerase I and II inhibitors was studied together with imatinib in cervical cancer cells carrying HPV and in HPV-negative cell lines. We report here that c-Abl inhibition by imatinib in combination with MX genotoxic treatment results in impaired DNA repair, abrogation of the G2 phase checkpoint, and massive apoptosis.

Materials and Methods

Cell lines and cytotoxicity assays

The human cervical cancer cell lines SiHa (HPV 16+), CaSki (HPV16+), and HeLa (HPV 18+), breast cancer cell line MCF7, and vulvar cancer cell line A431 were obtained from the American Type Culture Collection (Manassas, VA, USA). The primary human fibroblasts have been described before [19]. The cells were grown as monolayers in DMEM supplemented with 10% fetal bovine serum, 2 mM L-glutamine, non-essential amino acids (Euroclone, Wetherby, UK), and 50 μg/ml gentamycin (Calbiochem, San Diego, CA, USA). The HeLa p53 reporter cell line, carrying the p53 reporter plasmid ptkGC3p53-luc, has been described previously [18]. Despite the presence of HPV E6, even the HPV-positive cell lines show some p53 activity after genotoxic stress, but the activity can be degraded by dominant-negative p53 (DDp53) or ectopic E6 driven by a strong promoter. The SiHa DDp53, SiHa CMV, HeLa DDp53, HeLa CMV (empty vector), and SiHa E6 cell lines have also been described previously [18].

The dominant-negative p53–expressing HeLa cell line (HeLa DD) was derived by transfecting the parental cell line with a plasmid that expresses a truncated mouse p53 containing amino acid residues 1–14 and 302–390 under the control of the CMV promoter. Stable transfectants were selected with 0.8 mg/ml G418.

In short-term cell viability assays, $1–2\times10^4$ cells per well (depending on cell line) were seeded into 96-well plates, and the medium was replaced with drugs diluted with medium. The cell viability was measured by WST-1 agent (Roche, Mannheim, Germany) or MTT agent (Sigma-Aldrich Inc., St. Louis, MO, USA), and absorbance was measured at 450 nm (Multiskan plate microreader; Labsystems, Finland) or at 570 nm (Tecan multiplate reader; Tecan, Switzerland), respectively.

For clonogenic growth assays, SiHa and HeLa cells were seeded into 6-well plates 48 hours before treatment. The cells were exposed to treatment for 6 hours and then trypsinized and suspended in fresh medium and seeded into 6-well plates with 3 μM imatinib. SiHa cells were incubated for 14 days and HeLa cells for 7 days. Following incubation, cells were fixed with 1:1 acetone–methanol and stained with Giemsa (Merck, Whitehouse Station, NJ, USA). Then clones were either counted manually or analyzed as described previously [20]. Caspase 3/7 activity of cells undergoing apoptosis was determined using the Apo-ONE Caspase-3/7 homogenous caspase assay (Promega).

Reagents, drugs, and antibodies

The chemotherapy compounds mitoxantrone (MX) (Wyeth-Lederle, Finland), doxorubicin (DXR) (Nycomed, Roskilde, Denmark), cyclophosphamide (Orion Pharma, Espoo, Finland), topotecan (GlaxoSmithKline, Uxbridge, Middlesex, UK), etoposide (Pfizer), cisplatin (Bristol-Myers Squibb, Princeton, NJ, USA), docetaxel (Aventis), and carboplatin (Bristol-Myers Squibb, Princeton, NJ, USA) were stored and prepared as described [17]. Imatinib was a gift from Novartis Pharmaceuticals (Basel, Switzerland). The stock solution of imatinib at 200 mM was prepared by dissolving the compound in DMSO. The c-kit and PDGF-α and β receptor blocker AG1296 was purchased from Calbiochem (cat. no. 658551). PDGF-BB was purchased from Sigma-Aldrich. The following antibodies were used for Western blotting: mouse monoclonal DO-1 for p53 (Santa Cruz Biotechnology, Santa Cruz, CA, USA), rabbit polyclonal anti-GADD45α (Cell Signaling, cat. no. 3518), rabbit polyclonal anti-phospho-PDGF β receptor (Cell Signaling, cat. no. 3161), monoclonal mouse anti-RAD51 (Invitrogen, Carlsbad, CA, USA; cat. No. 35-6500), monoclonal mouse anti-cyclin B1 (BD Biosciences, cat. no. 554178) and monoclonal anti-p73 (Santa Cruz Biotechnology, Santa Cruz, CA, USA). The RNA was isolated using the RNeasy kit (Qiagen, Hilden, Germany).

Short interfering RNAs and transfections

The c-Abl short interfering RNAs (siRNAs) were obtained from Invitrogen (Stealth, Carlsbad, CA, USA; cat. no. 1299003), and non-targeting siRNA (Qiagen, cat. no. 1027281) was used as control. Transfection of the cells was performed with 75 nM of three individual siRNAs targeting c-Abl and control siRNA using the siLentFect Lipid Reagent (Bio-Rad).

p53 reporter assay

Stable ptkGC3p53luc-bsd SiHa, CaSki, and HeLa cell lines as well as the composition of the p53 reporter plasmid ptkGC3p53-luc have been described earlier [17]. The cells were seeded into 96-well plates (10^4 cells/well). After allowing for cell attachment for 24 hours, the treatments were begun for the indicated durations. The living cells in each well were determined colorimetrically with the WST-1 assay. Thereafter, the cells were rinsed with PBS and overlaid with 100 μl of a mixture containing 50% PBS and 50% Bright-Glo luciferase assay reagent (Promega, Madison, WI, USA). The luciferase activity was quantified with the aid of a hybrid capture luminometer (Digene, Gaithersburg,

MD, USA). Luciferase readings were divided by WST-1 value to obtain normalized reporter activity.

Western blotting

The cells were harvested using 200 µl of standard 1×SDS sample buffer. The resulting whole cell extracts were boiled and then separated by 10% SDS-PAGE and transferred to Immobilon-P polyvinylidene fluoride membranes (Millipore, Billerica, MA, USA). The membranes were probed with the indicated primary antibodies, and secondary detection was done with anti-mouse horseradish peroxidase (HRP) (GE Healthcare, NJ, USA), anti-rabbit HRP (DAKO, Glostrup, DK), and ECL (GE healthcare, NJ, USA). Beta-actin was used as a loading control. The Western blot films were digitized with a ChemiDoc MP gel analysis platform (Bio-Rad, Hercules, CA, USA). and analyzed with Fiji (ImageJ) ver 1.47q (Wayne Rasband, NIH, USA) using the Gels option.

Flow cytometry

Cell cycle analysis was performed by flow cytometry. Cells were harvested with trypsinization together with floating non-viable cells. The cells were washed once with PBS and suspended in sodium citrate buffer (40 mM Na-Citrate, 0.3% Triton X-100, 0.05 mg/ml propidium iodide, PBS) 20 minutes prior to analysis. Cell cycle analysis was performed using FACSCalibur (Becton Dickinson, CA, USA) and CellQuest Pro software (Becton Dickinson). Cell cycle and apoptosis analyses were performed with ModFit LT (Verity Software House, Inc., Topsham, ME, USA) and Flowing Software ver. 2.5 (Mr. Perttu Terho, Turku Centre for Biotechnology, Finland, www.flowingsoftware.com), respectively. To further analyze the apoptosis induction after MX and MX + imatinib treatment HeLa cells were grown on 6-well plates and treated with indicated drugs for 24 and 48 hours. Medium and cells were collected and the samples were stained with Annexin-V-FITC kit (ab14085; Abcam, Cambridge, UK) according to manufacturer's instructions. Data were acquired with a FACSCalibur flow cytometer, and analyzed with Flowing Software.

Real-time quantitative reverse transcription PCR

The RT-PCR method has been described before [18]. The primers were HPV 18 E6, forward, 5′-TGGCGCGCTTTGAGGA-3′, and reverse, 5′-TGTTCAGTTCCGTGCACAGATC-3′; and EF1α, forward, 5′-CTGAACCATCCAGGCCAAAT-3′, and reverse, 5′-GCCGTGTGGCAATCCAAT-3′. The amounts of HPV 18 E6 transcripts were normalized against the readings for EF1α.

Comet assay

DNA damage was studied with a single cell gel electrophoresis kit (Trivigen, Gaithersburg, MD, USA). The assay was performed in alkaline conditions to detect both single- and double-stranded DNA damage. The single-cell gel electrophoresis of DNA was performed as described by the manufacturer. Images were captured using an Olympus BX60 fluorescence microscope (Zeiss AxioVert 200 M) at ×20 magnification.

Time-lapse microscopy

Images were captured in one hour interval for 72 hours with IncuCyte ZOOM kinetic imaging system (Essen Bioscience, Michigan, USA). Representative wells were selected and movies were constructed with ImageJ ver 1.47d (Wayne Rasband, NIH, USA). Bar represents 200 µm.

Statistics

To evaluate differences between groups, we used Student's t-tests. A p value below 0.05 was considered to indicate statistical significance.

Results

Inhibition of c-Abl by imatinib potentiates the cytotoxic effect of mitoxantrone in cancer cells but not in primary fibroblasts

The potency of imatinib in enhancing cytotoxicity was screened in a large panel of chemotherapy drugs. In the short-term cytotoxicity assays, imatinib alone was not cytotoxic to any of the cell lines at 3 µM to 10 µM. When HeLa, CaSki, and SiHa cells were treated with the topoisomerase I inhibitors (topotecan and etoposide), nucleoside analogues (gemcitabine, fluorouracil, and cytarabine), alkylating agents (cyclophosphamide and dacarbazine), or cisplatin, imatinib did not enhance cytotoxicity (data not shown). Neither did it affect anthracycline-(doxorubicin,DXR) treated cells (Figure 1A). The effect of carboplatin was enhanced two fold by addition of imatinib for 48 hours (data not shown). In contrast to all the other chemotherapy drugs tested, imatinib showed a dramatic effect together with mitoxantrone (MX), a topoisomerase II inhibitor (Figure 1A). The effect of imatinib was equal between 3 µM and 10 µM indicating that the kinase activity is blocked in the studied cell lines even at 3 µM.

The enhanced effect was also seen in CaSki and SiHa cells although to a lesser extent (Figure S1). The cell lines that we primarily wanted to test were derived from HPV-positive cervical cancer. However, the effect appears to not have been restricted to these cells. The drugs were tested with two cancer cell lines of different origin: The vulvar carcinoma cell line A431 has a missense mutation in the p53 gene, and the MCF7 breast cancer cell line has a wild-type p53. The survival was strikingly similar to the HPV-positive cell lines (Figure 1B). In contrast, primary non-transformed fibroblasts were not more sensitive when imatinib was added to MX treatment (Figure 1B). This result indicates that the observed effect is not restricted to HPV-positive cancer cells but can occur more broadly regardless of p53 status. However, non-transformed cells may exhibit resistance to this treatment.

The enhanced effect of imatinib was also seen in native and differently modified HeLa and SiHa cells in a manner independent of either p53 or E6 (Figure S2). MX was further studied in clonogenic growth assays to monitor the long-term recovery capacity of the cells. MX concentrations as low as 1 nM together with 3 µM imatinib inhibited HeLa cell clonal growth completely, both p53-null and empty vector–carrying cells (Figure 1C). In SiHa cell lines, 3 µM imatinib alone did not affect clonal growth. The sensitivity of CaSki cells for imatinib addition was between that of SiHa and HeLa cells (Figure S3).

Mitoxantrone induces caspase 3/7, which is enhanced by blocking c-Abl with imatinib

The treatment with MX increases the release of caspase 3 and 7 from the mitochondria indicative of apoptosis. Imatinib alone is not able to alter these levels (Figure 2). Cells treated with 0.6 µM MX and 0.8 µM DXR increased the caspase activity 2.5 fold, whereas the MX + imatinib combination treatment increased the activity 4 fold. Imatinib did not increase the activity induced by DXR alone.

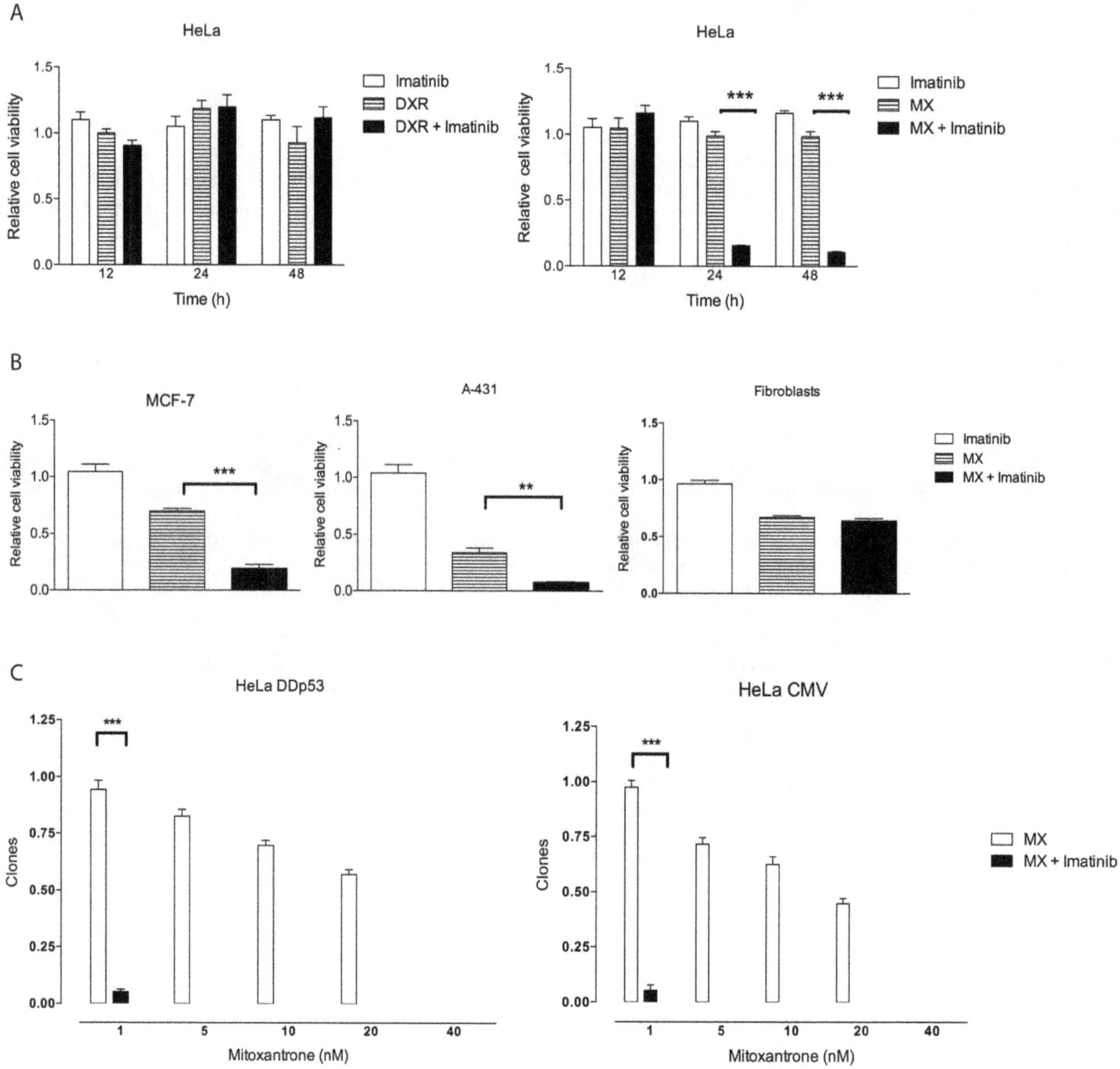

Figure 1. Imatinib increases cytotoxicity of mitoxantrone (MX) but not doxorubicin (DXR) in HeLa cells and this effect is not specific for cervical cancer cell lines or dependent on p53 status. (A) Human cervical cancer (HeLa) cells were treated with MX (0.6 μM), DXR (0.8 μM), imatinib (10 μM) or their combinations. WST cell viability assay was performed at 12 h, 24 h and 48 h. The results were normalized with cell number in medium only containing wells. *** $p<0.001$ independent samples T-test. (B) Both A-431 vulvar carcinoma cell line which has a missense mutation in the p53 gene and MCF-7 breast cancer cell line which has a wild type p53 gene show an enhanced effect when MX and imatinib are combined. Imatinib does not increase the cytotoxicity of MX in primary fibroblasts. Measurements were performed at 48 h using WST cell viability assay. ** $p<0.01$, *** $p<0.001$ independent samples T-test. (C) Clonogenic assay. Imatinib enhances MX cytotoxicity both in in HeLa CMV cell line with wild-type p53 and empty vector and HeLa DDp53 cell line carrying a dominant negative p53. Cells were treated with each drug for 12 h. Then, medium was replaced with fresh medium without drugs. The concentration of imatinib was 3 μM whereas MX was used in different concentrations ranging from 1 nM to 40 nM. Clones were counted under microscope. Experiment was done in triplicate, mean ± SD. *** $p<0.001$.

Inhibition of c-Abl kinase activity increases DNA damage in MX-treated cells

Adding imatinib to MX increased comet tailing in HeLa cells whereas imatinib alone did not have any effect (Figure 3A). Imatinib did not induce tailing in DXR-treated cells. The amount of GADD45α protein increased slightly even in the whole cell lysates with MX + imatinib (5 fold, Figure 3B). This increase seems to be regulated at the transcriptional level because we also have observed a marked increase in GADD45α transcript levels after the combination therapy in microarray RNA analyses (unpublished data). Like p53 protein accumulation in cell stress, GADD45α transcription increases under stress, including with DNA damage. Both DXR and MX increased RAD51 levels (10 fold), and imatinib pretreatment inhibited the increase equally (20%) but enhanced the accumulation of p53 when added to MX (13 fold, Figure 4).

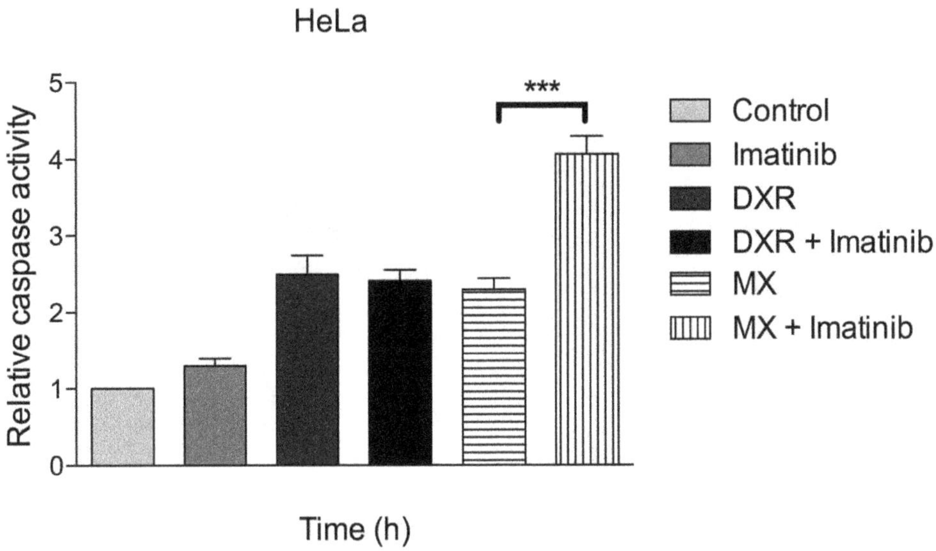

Figure 2. Combination of MX and imatinib activates caspase cascades. HeLa cells were treated with indicated drugs for 48 h. Then, fresh medium was replaced and caspase 3/7 activity was measured using ELISA assay. Experiment was done in triplicate, mean ± SD. *** $p<0.001$ T-test.

Mitoxantrone-induced p53 activation is enhanced by inhibiting c-Abl kinase activity

The chemotherapy drugs used in this study induce various forms of DNA damage, which p53 in the target cells senses. p53 is activated in cervical cells despite the degradation activity of E6 [16,19]. We measured p53 reporter activity in HeLa, CaSki, and SiHa cell lines with DXR, MX, and cisplatin. When the drugs were compared, cisplatin induced the reporter more than MX in HeLa and CaSki cells but similarly in SiHa cells, and 0.6 μM MX alone did not activate the reporter at all in HeLa cells at 48 hours. DXR induced the reporter more than cisplatin and MX in all cell lines (Table 1). Imatinib alone did not significantly alter the activity in any of the cell lines. Adding imatinib to cisplatin slightly reduced the activity, but there was no effect for DXR. In contrast, adding imatinib to 0.6 μM MX increased the activity in all cell lines, by 50% in SiHa cells but four fold in HeLa cells and eight fold in CaSki cells. The limitation of this approach is that a direct comparison between cell lines cannot be made because of different amounts of integrated reporter plasmid. Consistent with the reporter assays, p53 protein level was also significantly increased in Western blot analyses (Figure 4). We saw no decrease in p53 level with imatinib alone, results that were in accordance with the reporter analysis outcomes.

p73 is a member of the p53 protein family and interacts with c-Abl directly and can also induce apoptosis. The p73 protein levels did not change after the treatments (Figure S4).

Imatinib does not alter HPV E6 levels

Most of the chemotherapy drugs reduce the amount of E6 mRNA [17]. We wanted to know whether imatinib causes reduction in E6 expression in HeLa cells either alone or combined with MX. We found that 1 μM MX decreases E6 mRNA levels in HeLa cells by approximately 50% and that 5 μM imatinib alone does not reduce the level of E6 mRNA in these cells. A combination of 5 μM imatinib and 1 μM MX did not reduce the level of E6 mRNA in HeLa cells more than 1 μM MX alone.

Imatinib abrogates S-phase arrest caused by MX and increases apoptosis

In HeLa cells treated with imatinib alone, at 24 hours, cell cycle distribution was the same as in cells with medium alone, but there were slightly more cells in S phase after 48 hours (Figure 5A). At 24 hours and especially 48 hours, DXR accumulated the cells at G2 phase. Adding imatinib induced S phase arrest in the software analysis; however, at 48 hours with DXR + imatinib, there appeared to be a small G2 population that the analysis software failed to detect. MX-treated cells progressed at 24 hours to S and G2, but the extended incubation after 48 hours showed a clear G2 arrest. Adding imatinib to MX showed at 24 hours a population progressing to G1, indicating abrogation of the arrest. At 48 hours, there were no cells beyond S phase but still also a clear G1 population. This finding suggests that the cells had prematurely entered directly from S phase to mitosis and that the imatinib drove this effect. Alternatively, MX + imatinib may induce a delay from G1/S to G2. However, several unsuccessful mitoses were detected in the time-lapse video of MX+imatinib-treated cells favoring the interpretation that the cell cycle arrest was abrogated (Video S1). We also determined the cyclin B1 levels, a well-acknowledged mitotic marker, in the drug treated cell populations to collect further evidence for the notion that the MX+imatinib co-treated cells are capable of proceeding in cell cycle and entering M-phase. We found that treatment of HeLa cells with DXR, DXR+imatinib, MX and MX+imatinib leads to accumulation of cyclin B1. The protein level of imatinib treated cells was under level of detection similarly to the non-treated controls exhibiting basal level cyclin B1 expression (Figure S5).

Imatinib increased the sub G1 events in MX-treated HeLa cells, partly indicative of apoptosis. The sub G1 population was the largest (38.6%) in the MX + imatinib group at 48 hours. Imatinib also increased DXR-induced sub G1 but to a lesser extent (17.8%) at 48 hours (Table S1). To further analyze the possible apoptosis we stained the cells with annexin V which is a marker of early apoptosis. We found that imatinib significantly increases the proportion of apoptotic cells in MX-treated cells, but failed to detect any increase when imatinib was added to DXR (Figure 5B)

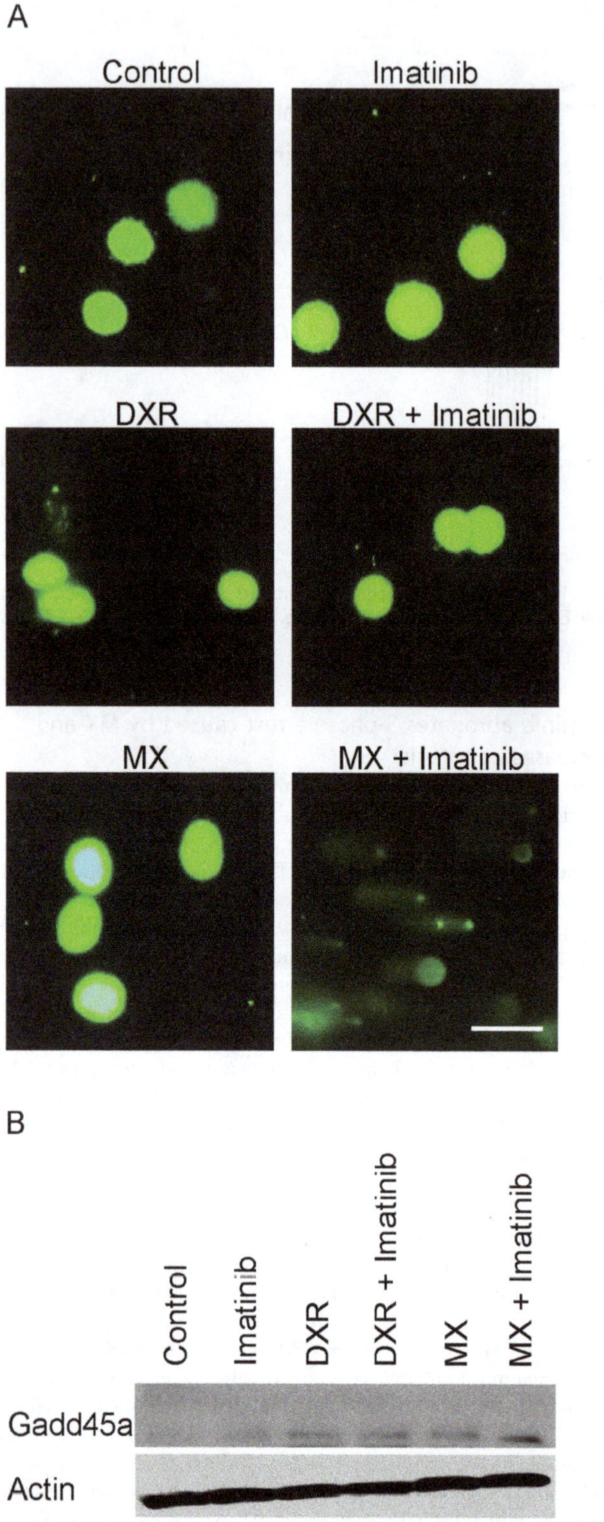

Figure 3. Imatinib increases DNA-damage induced by MX but not by DXR. (A) DNA damage in the HeLa cells was studied using Comet assay after treatment with MX (0.6 μM), DXR (0.8 μM) and imatinib (5 μM), or their combinations. Cometting (tailing) indicates DNA damage. (B) Imatinib combined with MX increases the level of GADD45α. Western blot of GADD45α protein levels from whole cell lysates. HeLa cells were treated with MX (0.6 μM), DXR (0.8 μM), imatinib (5 μM), or their combinations for 30 h.

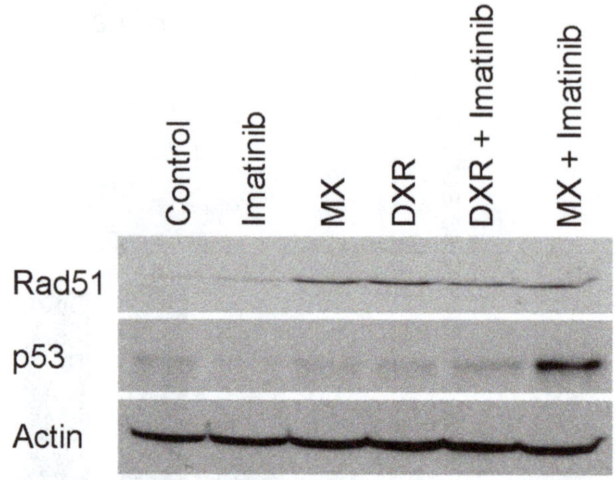

Figure 4. Imatinib increases p53 levels when combined with MX, but not with DXR. Western blot of p53 and RAD 51 in HeLa cells. Imatinib combined with MX increases p53 protein levels in HeLa cells. RAD51 level was slightly reduced in cells treated with imatinib and MX. Cells were treated with MX (0.6 μM), DXR (0.8 μM), imatinib (5 μM) or their combinations for 30 hours.

Flow cytometry results are in line with the caspase experiment supporting the notion that imatinib with MX is more potent inducer of cell death than with DXR. Imatinib has been previously reported to cause G1 arrest in head and neck cancer cell lines [21] whereas MX and DXR cause G2 arrest [22]. We saw no G1 arrest with imatinib alone.

Downregulation of c-Abl with siRNA impedes the cytotoxicity of MX + imatinib

Imatinib and MX showed an additive effect in reducing the number of control siRNA HeLa cells. When c-Abl was knocked down with siRNA, we found that the proliferation of untreated cells was reduced by 30–50% in repeated experiments (Figure 6, Video S2). Both the growth curves and time-lapse microscopy data show a slight growth inhibition in c-Abl siRNA HeLa cells. However, neither control siRNA nor c-Abl siRNA alone induced cell death. This result suggests that c-Abl is required for the normal proliferation of these cells. Targeting of c-Abl in HeLa cells by siRNA rendered the cells less sensitive to MX. CaSki cells were also less sensitive to MX when c-Abl was downregulated with siRNA, but no inhibition of proliferation was observed. These cells were harder to transfect with siRNA and only 40% efficacy was achieved. This may also explain why the proliferation was not inhibited in these cells. Moreover, the combinatory effect of imatinib was significantly reduced, implicating c-Abl as the pivotal target of imatinib in this outcome. The latter finding is also in line with experiments with other targets of imatinib, PDGF and c-Kit. AG1296 is known to potently inhibit signaling of human PDGF α- and β-receptors as well as of the related stem cell factor receptor c-Kit, at 1 μM and 5 μM concentrations, respectively. AG1296 could not mimic the action of imatinib with MX (Figure 7A). Moreover MX does not have any effect on phosphorylation of PDGF receptor (Figure 7B). Furthermore, the siRNA experiment implied that the kinase-active c-Abl is responsible for cell survival after MX damage. Of importance, this experiment points to different roles for kinase-active and kinase-inactive c-Abl. Kinase-inactive c-Abl appears to be required for apoptosis with MX, but kinase-active c-Abl is a key player for DNA damage repair after MX in HeLa cells.

Table 1. p53 reporter activity changes in HeLa, SiHa and CaSki cells.

	Hela	SiHa	CaSki
Cisplatin	2.7±0.2	3.6±0.3	14.7±0.6
Cisplatin + Imatinib	1.9±0.1	2.6±0.1	10.3±0.0
Doxorubicin	4.3±0.2	9.5±0.3	32.6±0.6
Doxorubicin + Imatinib	4.2±0.23	8.6±0.35	31.1±0.4
Mitoxantrone	0.9±0.1	3.8±0.1	3.0±0.2
Mitoxantrone + Imatinib	4.1±0.0	4.7±0.2	24.0±0.2
Imatinib	1.0±0.0	1.2±0.1	1.2±0.1

The results are given in fold-change. The concentrations used were MX 0.6 μM, 1 μM and 1 μM in HeLa, SiHa and CaSKi cell lines, respectively; DXR 0.8 μM, 1.4 μM and 1 μM in HeLa, SiHa and CaSKi cell lines, respectively; Cisplatin 40 μM, 70 μM and 40 μM in HeLa, SiHa and CaSKi cell lines respectively. Imatinib 10 μM in each cell line.

Discussion

One of the major findings in this study is that the synergizing effect of imatinib was specifically seen with MX. Previous studies have shown that imatinib may enhance the cytotoxicity of a wide range of chemotherapy drugs in solid tumor–derived cells [13,23]. Nevertheless, one group found that colon cancer cells become less sensitive to TRAIL-induced apoptosis after imatinib [24]. These reports did not involve testing the possible sensitivity differences between chemotherapeutics in this context. Interestingly, Pinto et al. very recently found in a comparable screening setting that imatinib and MX additively inhibit the proliferation of PC-3 prostate cancer cells [25,26].

MX is an anthracenedione that targets topoisomerase II. It can also induce DNA intercalation and free radical generation [27]. The effect of imatinib with MX observed in the present study cannot merely be explained by topoisomerase II inhibition because DXR (also a topoisomerase II inhibitor) did not have similar activity with imatinib. The effect of imatinib is linked to its ability to increase DNA damage in target cells, but it did not notably increase the DNA damage induced by DXR in HeLa cells. The difference in these closely related compounds is not entirely clear, but there are some reported differences in these drugs that may be related to the multi-drug resistance (MDR) clearance of the drug.

Several tyrosine kinase inhibitors can selectively modulate MDR-dependent drug efflux [28]. Imatinib has been reported to reverse the resistance to topotecan and SN-38, an active metabolite of irinotecan, and this activity has been attributed to inhibition of the ABCG2 transporter [29]. MX resistance is additionally mediated by transport proteins MRP-1 and ABCB1 [30]. Nilotinib, an imatinib derivative, inhibits the activity of both ABCG2 and ABCB1, leading to enhanced DXR accumulation. Different cells may behave in opposite ways because imatinib has been reported to increase DXR concentration and synergize cytotoxicity in breast cancer cells [31] but not in sarcoma cells [28,32]. The concentration of the drug in the cell is not likely solely to explain the outcome, because, for example, raising the concentration of the drug does not lead to such a profound p53 accumulation and activity as seen with the MX + imatinib combination (data not shown). Moreover, the cells can be rescued by knocking down c-Abl. Therefore, without c-Abl commitment, the effect is profoundly hampered.

c-Abl knockdown by siRNA rendered HeLa cells resistant to MX. Taken together with the fact that kinase-inactive c-Abl sensitized the cells to MX, this finding indicates that maximal MX cytotoxicity depends on kinase-inactive c-Abl. The results suggest that either 1) kinase-active c-Abl is a direct inhibitor of apoptosis in these cells or 2) kinase-inactive c-Abl is pro-apoptotic in stress conditions. Of relevance, kinase-inactive c-Abl has an important function that is not present in knocked-down cells. It has been shown that in addition to BCR/Abl cell lines, even in solid tumor–derived cells that have increased c-Abl activity, imatinib may inhibit aberrant growth. Moreover, c-Abl activation may either enhance or decrease cell cycle progression in a cell type–specific way or inhibit apoptosis and induce cell death [23,33]. We saw no difference in cell proliferation or clonogenic growth after imatinib treatment, but c-Abl knockdown diminished proliferation of HeLa cells. This finding suggests that kinase-inactive c-Abl supports cell cycle progression in these cells in unstressed conditions. In fact, a positive mitogenic role for c-Abl has been shown in studies exploiting *abl*-deficient cells [34,35]. When DNA is damaged, c-Abl is activated, and the cell cycle is stalled. If the catalytic activity is inhibited, the lack of c-Abl enhances cell cycle progression, allowing no time for repair, highlighting the key role of c-Abl in cell cycle control in these cells. These results suggest that kinase activity of c-Abl may either enhance or inhibit proliferation depending on either cell type–specific differences or protein conformation properties and is not simply a binary choice.

c-Abl facilitates a repair checkpoint following moderate DNA damage but promotes death after severe damage. This checkpoint depends on the catalytic activity of c-Abl and is ruptured by imatinib [3]. Checkpoint activation and mitosis block occur especially in cells that have defective replication. Cells lacking the S phase checkpoint with disordered replication eventually die [36]. HeLa cells were arrested in G2 phase after 48 hours of exposure to MX and DXR. Of importance, we found that inhibition of c-Abl kinase activity repressed the G2 phase arrest induced by MX, but not that induced by DXR G1 and the number of annexin positive cells also increased significantly, indicating defective replication that was followed by apoptosis with enhanced caspase 3/7 activation. This finding, together with the comet assay results, suggests a different form of DNA damage recognition that depends on active c-Abl function in the case of MX damage. Consistently, microarray analyses exploring the different outcomes of MX and DXR reveal that there are differences in MX and DXR damage responses (unpublished data). The cell cycle analyses hint at an important connection between c-Abl and cell cycle control for certain chemotherapy drugs. This possibility is in line with c-Abl being a binding partner to a number of substrates linked to cell cycle checkpoint control [4].

After DNA damage, RAD51 is centrally involved in homologous recombination repair and mediates the DNA strand-pairing step. Russell et al. have previously shown that imatinib reduces

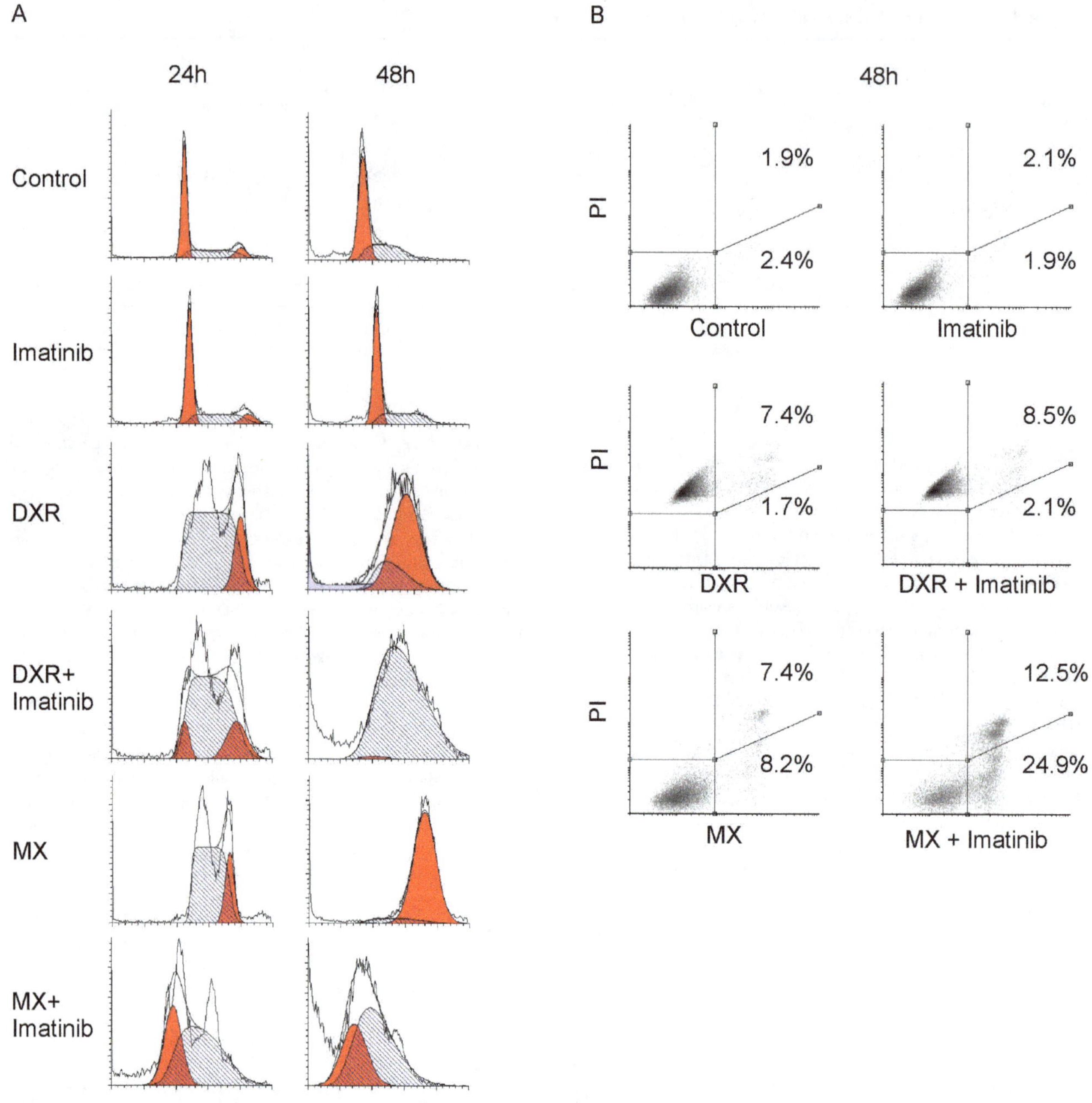

Figure 5. Adding imatinib to MX results in abrogation of G2 phase arrest in HeLa cells and significant increase in apoptosis induction. (A) Cells were treated with MX (0.6 μM), DXR (0.8 μM), imatinib (5 μM) or their combinations for 24 and 48 hours. After treatment, cells were harvested and stained with propidium iodide to quantify DNA content using flow cytometry. Histograms show cell cycle distributions.(B) Annexin-V (X-axis) vs. PI (Y-axis) staining of HeLa cells treated with indicated drugs for 48 h. Percentages indicate the early (lower right quadrant) and late (upper right quadrant) apoptotic fraction. MX and imatinib show a clear synergistic effect in apoptosis induction. The emission spectra of PI and DXR coincide at the FL2 channel, making it impossible to distinguish the early apoptotic population from the late apoptotic population in DXR-treated cells. However, when the right quadrants were added together, there was no difference between DXR and DXR + imatinib populations.

RAD51 levels in glioma cells, but not in fibroblast cells exposed to X-rays [12]. In the present study, both DXR and MX increased RAD51 levels, and imatinib pretreatment inhibited the increase equally. A similar effect on RAD51 levels suggest that other targets are responsible for the observed c-Abl effect on MX-induced lesions.

p53 is a core node in DNA damage signaling. In HPV-positive cells, its function is knocked down by HPV E6-induced degradation, but it can still be activated after genotoxic insult and play a role in DNA repair and apoptosis [16,20,37]. Imatinib alone did not affect p53 reporter activity or alter the protein levels. Imatinib activity also did not increase with cisplatin or DXR. Recently, Chan et al. reported that active c-Abl protects p53 from E6AP-mediated degradation and that imatinib reduces p53 levels [38]. In the present study, we saw no p53 reduction in unstressed conditions, which was supported by the unchanged reporter

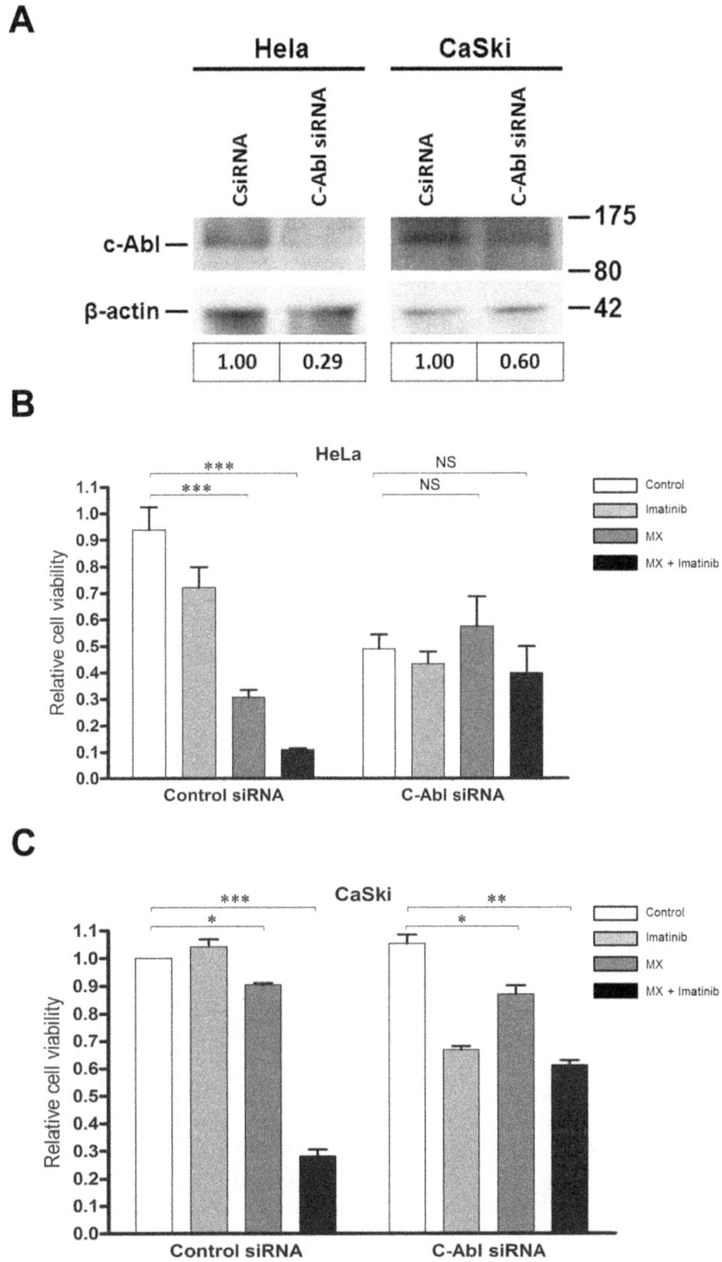

Figure 6. Down-regulation of c-Abl by siRNA counteracts MX induced apoptosis in HeLa and CaSki cells. (A) HeLa and CaSki Cells were transfected with non-targeting or c-Abl siRNA (75 nM). Western blot analysis was performed to examine the effect of siRNA. Level of c-Abl was quantitated and corrected for β-actin level. Values are proportioned to levels of control siRNA for each cell line. (B) HeLa, and (C) CasKi cells were transfected with control or c-Abl siRNA. After treansfection cells were treated with MX (0.6 μM), imatinib (5 μM) and their combination for 48 h. Relative amount of surviving cells was determined by WST-1 assay. Results are from two independent experiments in triplicates. Data are shown as mean ± SD. * $p<0.05$, ** $p<0.01$, *** $p<0.001$. NS, not significant.

activity. In contrast, the potentiating effect of imatinib for p53 was profound after MX treatment. These findings indicate a difference between cell lines treated with different chemotherapy drugs in respect to p53 activity after c-Abl kinase inhibition. Second, p53 activation is in line with the observation in comet assays that c-Abl inhibition by imatinib added DNA tailing after MX but not after DXR. Despite the accumulation of transcriptionally active p53, cell survival and clonogenic growth did not alter when p53 was inactivated by overexpression of dominant-negative p53. p73 is a direct substrate of c-Abl and is phosphorylated upon DNA damage [1,39]. We found no evidence that p73 was responsible for the combined effect in HeLa cells in Western analyses. Upon DNA damage, p73 accumulates in an active c-Abl-dependent manner [40]. We blocked the c-Abl kinase activity by imatinib; therefore, it is not surprising that we saw no p73 dependence for the MX + imatinib effect. Taken together, these results implicate pathways other than p53 or p73 as being involved here in the kinase-inactive c-Abl–mediated apoptosis. The more detailed gene level determi-

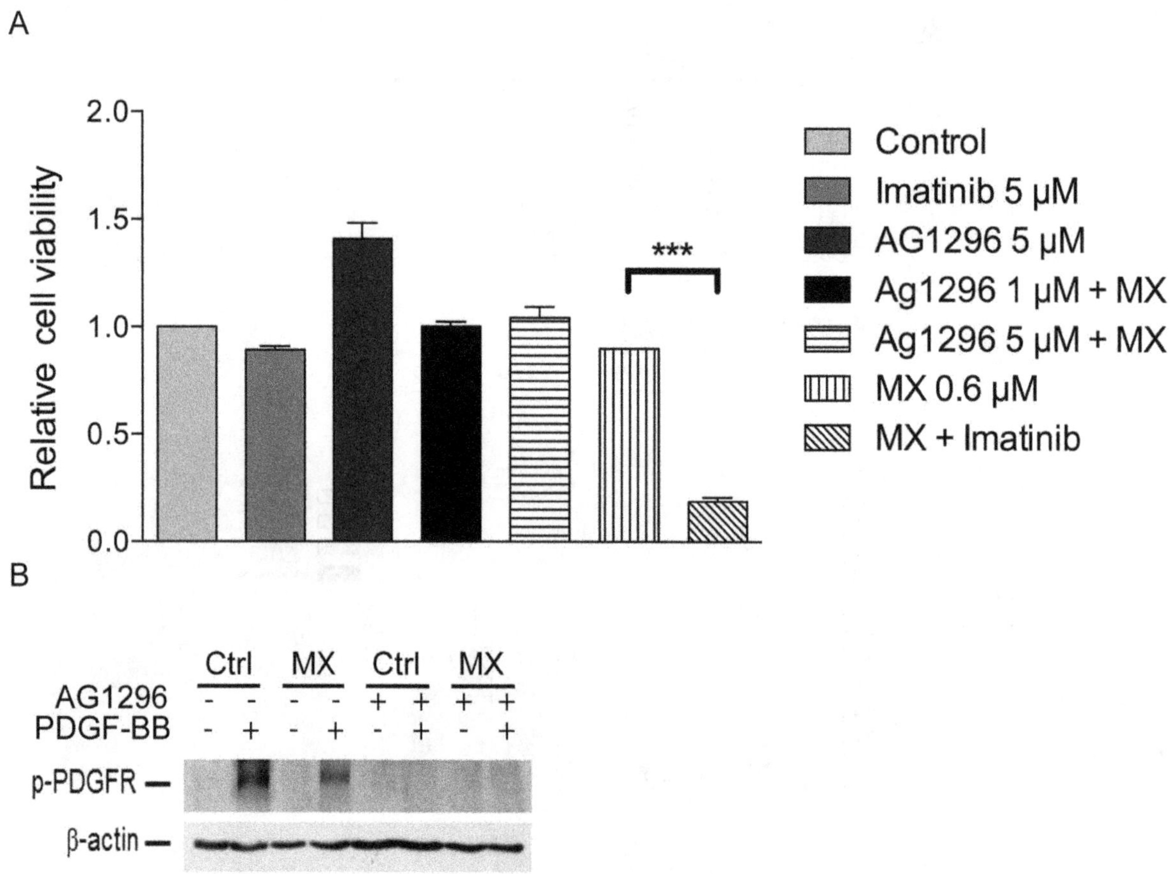

Figure 7. C-kit and PDGF receptor kinase inhibitor AG1296 does not modify the effect of MX. (A) Cells were treated with MX and AG1296 or their combinations for 48 hours and measured with WST-1 assay. Results are from three independent experiments, mean ± SD. *** $p<0.001$. (B) The effect of AG1296 on PDGFR phosphorylation. HeLa cells were first treated with either medium alone (Ctrl) or 0.6 µM MX for 48 h. Cells were then treated with 5 µM AG1296 for 15 min. Phosphorylation of PGDF receptor was induced by 0.1 µM of PDGF-BB for 10 min.

nants for the observed cell cycle effects and DNA damage potentiation are of key importance and the work is currently underway.

The role of c-Abl after genotoxic treatment has been very inconsistent. The initial report on mouse embryonic oocytes after cisplatin treatment showed that inhibition of c-Abl activity results in survival [41], although contradicting results have been presented [42]. Wang et al. [9] have reported that Atm-mediated c-Abl activation in response to DSBs further activates both Atm and Atr and their downstream effects, enhancing DNA repair. In contrast, Meltser et al. have reported that inhibition of c-Abl kinase activation after irradiation of mouse embryonic fibroblasts results in higher DSB rejoining and higher survival [43]. It may seem that the form of genotoxic treatment - i.e., chemotherapy or irradiation - may explain the difference in outcomes. However, Fanta et al. have previously shown that inhibition of c-Abl results in genetic instability as a consequence of diminished DNA repair [44]. Our results clearly favor the role of c-Abl as a critical factor in DNA repair and survival in MX-induced damage. Chen et al. have found that ultraviolet irradiation that does not lead to c-Abl activation induces a CUL-4A-dependent ubiquitination and degradation of the DNA-binding proteins DDB1 and DDB2. This process is c-Abl-independent [45]. They then showed that kinase-inactive c-Abl may negatively regulate nucleotide excision repair. This activity would explain the dual role of c-Abl in MX-treated cells, an intriguing possibility that needs validation in subsequent experiments. It is also important to note that the cellular background has a profound influence in this context; therefore, it is relevant that we did not see the effect in primary fibroblasts. c-Abl has a plethora of binding partners and sits at the crossroads of several crucial cellular pathways. Alterations in these genes may have a pivotal impact on c-Abl catalytic activity modulation. The difference in primary cells vs. cancer cells in this respect may also offer unique therapeutic opportunities.

Conclusion

In this study, we show that c-Abl has a dual role in the damage response after chemotherapy exposure depending on its kinase activity. Furthermore, c-Abl may be a key player in MX-induced genotoxic stress but might be dispensable after several other drug treatments. The kinase-active c-Abl facilitates the repair of the damaged DNA whereas the catalytically inactive c-Abl triggers apoptosis in the afflicted cells. This finding has not been reported before in cells treated with c-Abl-activating damage including chemotherapy or ionizing radiation. The obscure role of c-Abl in BCR/Abl-negative cells has hampered the use of antagonists in solid tumor treatment. It remains to be seen whether different tumor subsets with specific molecular signatures respond to the combined treatment with specific chemotherapy drugs together with c-Abl inhibition.

Supporting Information

Figure S1 Imatinib enhances MX induced cytotoxicity also in CaSKi and SiHa cell lines. Short-term cytotoxicity assay. Results were from three independent experiments, mean ± SD. *** $p<0.001$.

Figure S2 Enhancement of MX induced cytotoxicity by imatinib is not p53 dependent. p53 activity was abolished with either dominant negative p53 (DDp53) or ectopic HPVE6. CMV depicts the empty vector. Treatment duration 48 h. A. Stably transfected HeLa cells B. Stably transfected SiHa cells.

Figure S3 Imatinib enhances MX induced cytotoxicity in CaSKi and SiHa cell lines with growing in clonal densities. Targeting of residual p53 activity with ectopic E6 does not rescue SiHa cells from the imatinib enhanced cytotoxicity. Cells were treated in the clonogenic assay with each drug for 12 h. Then, fresh medium was replaced. The concentration of imatinib was 3 µM whereas MX was used in concentrations from 1 nM to 32 nM in experiments done with CaSKi cell line and from 1 nM to 15 nM with SiHa CMV cell line. Results were from three independent experiments, mean ± SD. *** $p<0.001$.

Figure S4 p73 protein levels after indicated treatments. Western blot image from whole cell lysates at 48 h after treatment.

Figure S5 Cyclin B1 accumulation in HeLa cells treated with imatinib, DXR, DXR+imatinib, MX, and MX+imatinib. Cyclin B1 protein level was examined with Western blot analysis 48 h after the treatment.

Table S1 Cell cycle distributions of HeLa cells. Cell cycle distribution percentages from experiment shown in Fig. 5. Cells were treated with indicated drugs for 24 and 48 h. Cell cycle phase percentages were calculated using ModFit LT cell cycle modelling software. Results are shown as percentages of G1, S and G2/M populations.

Video S1 Combination of MX (0.6 µM) and imatinib (5 µM) induces more abnormal mitoses than MX alone in HeLa cells. Cells were seeded on 96-well plates and images were acquired at 1 hour interval. Bar represents 200 µm.

Video S2 c-Abl siRNA induces mild growth inhibition but not cell death in HeLa cells. Cells were seeded on 96-well plates and images were acquired at 1 hour interval. Bar represents 200 µm.

Acknowledgments

We thank Mr. Jaakko Lehtimäki, Ms. Johanna Markola-Wärn, and Ms. Sari Pitkänen for skillfull technical assistance.

Author Contributions

Conceived and designed the experiments: SH MF K. Alpay JS JT. Performed the experiments: K. Alpay MF JT JS K. Aittokallio ES. Analyzed the data: SH JS JT MF MK K. Alpay VMK. Contributed reagents/materials/analysis tools: SH VMK MK. Wrote the paper: SH MF JT JS VMK K. Alpay. Conceived and supervised the study: SH.

References

1. Agami R, Blandino G, Oren M, Shaul Y (1999) Interaction of c-Abl and p73alpha and their collaboration to induce apoptosis. Nature 399: 809–813.
2. Hoeijmakers JH (2007) Genome maintenance mechanisms are critical for preventing cancer as well as other aging-associated diseases. Mech Ageing Dev 128: 460–462.
3. Maiani E, Diederich M, Gonfloni S (2011) DNA damage response: the emerging role of c-Abl as a regulatory switch? Biochem Pharmacol 82: 1269–1276.
4. Colicelli J (2010) ABL tyrosine kinases: evolution of function, regulation, and specificity. SciSignal 139. re6. doi: 10.1126/scisignal.3139re6
5. Wang JY (2004) Controlling Abl: auto-inhibition and co-inhibition? Nat Cell Biol 6: 3–7.
6. Nagar B (2007) c-Abl tyrosine kinase and inhibition by the cancer drug imatinib (Gleevec/STI-571). J Nutr 137: 1518S–1523S.
7. Slupianek A, Schmutte C, Tombline G, Nieborowska-Skorska M, Hoser G, et al. (2001) BCR/ABL regulates mammalian RecA homologs, resulting in drug resistance. Mol Cell 8: 795–806.
8. Buchdunger E, O'Reilly T, Wood J (2002) Pharmacology of imatinib (STI571). Eur J Cancer 38 Suppl 5: S28–S36.
9. Wang X, Zeng L, Wang J, Chau JF, Lai KP, et al. (2011) A positive role for c-Abl in Atm and Atr activation in DNA damage response. Cell Death Differ 18: 5–15.
10. Chen G, Yuan SS, Liu W, Xu Y, Trujillo K, et al. (1999) Radiation-induced assembly of Rad51 and Rad52 recombination complex requires ATM and c-Abl. J Biol Chem 274: 12748–12752.
11. Kubler HR, van Randenborgh H, Treiber U, Wutzler S, Battistel C, et al. (2005) In vitro cytotoxic effects of imatinib in combination with anticancer drugs in human prostate cancer cell lines. Prostate 63: 385–394.
12. Russell JS, Brady K, Burgan WE, Cerra MA, Oswald KA, et al. (2003) Gleevec-mediated inhibition of Rad51 expression and enhancement of tumor cell radiosensitivity. Cancer Res 63: 7377–7383.
13. Choudhury A, Zhao H, Jalali F, Al Rashid S, Ran J, et al. (2009) Targeting homologous recombination using imatinib results in enhanced tumor cell chemosensitivity and radiosensitivity. Mol Cancer Ther 8: 203–213.
14. Kharbanda S, Yuan ZM, Weichselbaum R, Kufe D (1997) Functional role for the c-Abl protein tyrosine kinase in the cellular response to genotoxic stress. Biochim Biophys Acta 1333: O1–O7.
15. zur Hausen H (2002) Papillomaviruses and cancer: from basic studies to clinical application. Nat Rev Cancer 2: 342–350.
16. Hietanen S (2009) Apoptosis in Carcinogenesis and Chemoherapy of the Uterine Cervix. In: Chen GG, Lai PBS, editors. Apoptosis in Carcinogenesis and Chemotherapy: Springer Netherlands. pp.51–73.
17. Koivusalo R, Hietanen S (2004) The cytotoxicity of chemotherapy drugs varies in cervical cancer cells depending on the p53 status. Cancer Biol Ther 3: 1177–1183.
18. Koivusalo R, Krausz E, Ruotsalainen P, Helenius H, Hietanen S (2002) Chemoradiation of cervical cancer cells: targeting human papillomavirus E6 and p53 leads to either augmented or attenuated apoptosis depending on the platinum carrier ligand. Cancer Res 62: 7364–7371.
19. Hietanen S, Auvinen E, Syrjanen K, Syrjanen S (1998) Anti-proliferative effect of retinoids and interferon-alpha-2a on vaginal cell lines derived from squamous intra-epithelial lesions. Int J Cancer 78: 338–345.
20. Koivusalo R, Krausz E, Helenius H, Hietanen S (2005) Chemotherapy compounds in cervical cancer cells primed by reconstitution of p53 function after short interfering RNA-mediated degradation of human papillomavirus 18 E6 mRNA: opposite effect of siRNA in combination with different drugs. Mol Pharmacol 68: 372–382.
21. Wang-Rodriguez J, Lopez JP, Altuna X, Chu TS, Weisman RA, et al. (2006) STI-571 (Gleevec) potentiates the effect of cisplatin in inhibiting the proliferation of head and neck squamous cell carcinoma in vitro. Laryngoscope 116: 1409–1416.
22. Potter AJ, Rabinovitch PS (2005) The cell cycle phases of DNA damage and repair initiated by topoisomerase II-targeting chemotherapeutic drugs. Mutat Res 572: 27–44.
23. Lin J, Arlinghaus R (2008) Activated c-Abl tyrosine kinase in malignant solid tumors. Oncogene 27: 4385–4391.
24. Huang DY, Chao Y, Tai MH, Yu YH, Lin WW (2012) STI571 reduces TRAIL-induced apoptosis in colon cancer cells: c-Abl activation by the death receptor leads to stress kinase-dependent cell death. J Biomed Sci 19: 35.
25. Pinto AC, Angelo S, Moreira JN, Simoes S (2011) Schedule treatment design and quantitative in vitro evaluation of chemotherapeutic combinations for metastatic prostate cancer therapy. Cancer Chemother Pharmacol 67: 275–284.

26. Pinto AC, Moreira JN, Simoes S (2011) Liposomal imatinib-mitoxantrone combination: formulation development and therapeutic evaluation in an animal model of prostate cancer. Prostate 71: 81–90.
27. Hande KR (2008) Topoisomerase II inhibitors. Update Cancer Ther 3: 13–26.
28. Tiwari AK, Sodani K, Wang SR, Kuang YH, Ashby CR Jr, et al. (2009) Nilotinib (AMN107, Tasigna) reverses multidrug resistance by inhibiting the activity of the ABCB1/Pgp and ABCG2/BCRP/MXR transporters. Biochem Pharmacol 78: 153–161.
29. Houghton PJ, Germain GS, Harwood FC, Schuetz JD, Stewart CF, et al. (2004) Imatinib mesylate is a potent inhibitor of the ABCG2 (BCRP) transporter and reverses resistance to topotecan and SN-38 in vitro. Cancer Res 64: 2333–2337.
30. Morrow CS, Peklak-Scott C, Bishwokarma B, Kute TE, Smitherman PK, et al. (2006) Multidrug resistance protein 1 (MRP1, ABCC1) mediates resistance to mitoxantrone via glutathione-dependent drug efflux. Mol Pharmacol 69: 1499–1505.
31. Sims JT, Ganguly SS, Bennett H, Friend JW, Tepe J, et al. (2013) Imatinib reverses doxorubicin resistance by affecting activation of STAT3-dependent NF-kappaB and HSP27/p38/AKT pathways and by inhibiting ABCB1. PLoS One 8: e55509.
32. Villar VH, Vogler O, Martinez-Serra J, Ramos R, Calabuig-Farinas S, et al. (2012) Nilotinib counteracts P-glycoprotein-mediated multidrug resistance and synergizes the antitumoral effect of doxorubicin in soft tissue sarcomas. PLoS One 7: e37735.
33. Srinivasan D, Sims JT, Plattner R (2008) Aggressive breast cancer cells are dependent on activated Abl kinases for proliferation, anchorage-independent growth and survival. Oncogene 27: 1095–1105.
34. Plattner R, Kadlec L, DeMali KA, Kazlauskas A, Pendergast AM (1999) c-Abl is activated by growth factors and Src family kinases and has a role in the cellular response to PDGF. Genes Dev 13: 2400–2411.
35. Furstoss O, Dorey K, Simon V, Barila D, Superti-Furga G, et al. (2002) c-Abl is an effector of Src for growth factor-induced c-myc expression and DNA synthesis. EMBO J 21: 514–524.
36. Labib K, De Piccoli G (2011) Surviving chromosome replication: the many roles of the S-phase checkpoint pathway. PhilosTrans R Soc Lond B Biol Sci 366: 3554–3561.
37. Hietanen S, Lain S, Krausz E, Blattner C, Lane DP (2000) Activation of p53 in cervical carcinoma cells by small molecules. Proc Natl Acad Sci USA 97: 8501–8506.
38. Chan AL, Grossman T, Zuckerman V, Campigli DG, Moshel O, et al. (2013) c-Abl phosphorylates E6AP and regulates its E3 ubiquitin ligase activity. Biochemistry 52: 3119–3129.
39. White E, Prives C (1999) DNA damage enables p73. Nature 399: 734–735, 737.
40. Yuan ZM, Shioya H, Ishiko T, Sun X, Gu J, et al. (1999) p73 is regulated by tyrosine kinase c-Abl in the apoptotic response to DNA damage. Nature 399: 814–817.
41. Gonfloni S, Di Tella L, Caldarola S, Cannata SM, Klinger FG, et al. (2009) Inhibition of the c-Abl-TAp63 pathway protects mouse oocytes from chemotherapy-induced death. Nat Med 15: 1179–1185.
42. Kerr JB, Hutt KJ, Cook M, Speed TP, Strasser A, et al. (2012) Cisplatin-induced primordial follicle oocyte killing and loss of fertility are not prevented by imatinib. Nat Med 18: 1170–1172.
43. Meltser V, Ben Yehoyada M, Reuven N, Shaul Y (2010) c-Abl downregulates the slow phase of double-strand break repair. Cell Death Dis 1: e20.
44. Fanta S, Sonnenberg M, Skorta I, Duyster J, Miething C, et al. (2008) Pharmacological inhibition of c-Abl compromises genetic stability and DNA repair in Bcr-Abl-negative cells. Oncogene 27: 4380–4384.
45. Chen X, Zhang J, Lee J, Lin PS, Ford JM, et al. (2006) A kinase-independent function of c-Abl in promoting proteolytic destruction of damaged DNA binding proteins. Mol Cell 22: 489–499.

5

Gold(I)-Triphenylphosphine Complexes with Hypoxanthine-Derived Ligands: *In Vitro* Evaluations of Anticancer and Anti-Inflammatory Activities

Radka Křikavová[1], Jan Hošek[1], Ján Vančo[1], Jakub Hutyra[1], Zdeněk Dvořák[2], Zdeněk Trávníček[1]*

1 Regional Centre of Advanced Technologies and Materials & Department of Inorganic Chemistry, Faculty of Science, Palacký University, Olomouc, Czech Republic,
2 Regional Centre of Advanced Technologies and Materials & Department of Cell Biology and Genetics, Faculty of Science, Palacký University, Olomouc, Czech Republic

Abstract

A series of gold(I) complexes involving triphenylphosphine (PPh_3) and one *N*-donor ligand derived from deprotonated mono- or disubstituted hypoxanthine (HL_n) of the general composition $[Au(L_n)(PPh_3)]$ (**1–9**) is reported. The complexes were thoroughly characterized, including multinuclear high resolution NMR spectroscopy as well as single crystal X-ray analysis (for complexes **1** and **3**). The complexes were screened for their *in vitro* cytotoxicity against human cancer cell lines MCF7 (breast carcinoma), HOS (osteosarcoma) and THP-1 (monocytic leukaemia), which identified the complexes **4–6** as the most promising representatives, who antiproliferative activity was further tested against A549 (lung adenocarcinoma), G-361 (melanoma), HeLa (cervical cancer), A2780 (ovarian carcinoma), A2780R (ovarian carcinoma resistant to *cisplatin*), 22Rv1 (prostate cancer) cell lines. Complexes **4–6** showed a significantly higher *in vitro* anticancer effect against the employed cancer cells, except for G-361, as compared with the commercially used anticancer drug *cisplatin*, with $IC_{50} \approx 1–30$ μM. Anti-inflammatory activity was evaluated *in vitro* by the assessment of the ability of the complexes to modulate secretion of the pro-inflammatory cytokines, i.e. tumour necrosis factor-α (TNF-α) and interleukin-1β (IL-1β), in the lipopolysaccharide-activated macrophage-like THP-1 cell model. The results of this study identified the complexes as auspicious anti-inflammatory agents with similar or better activity as compared with the clinically applied gold-based antiarthritic drug Auranofin. In an effort to explore the possible mechanisms responsible for the biological effect, the products of interactions of selected complexes with sulfur-containing biomolecules (L-cysteine and reduced glutathione) were studied by means of the mass-spectrometry study.

Editor: Swati Palit Deb, Virginia Commonwealth University, United States of America

Funding: The authors gratefully thank the Operational Program Research and Development for Innovations - European Regional Development Fund (CZ.1.05/2.1.00/03.0058), the National Program of Sustainability I (LO1305) of the Ministry of Education, Youth and Sports of the Czech Republic and Palacký University in Olomouc (IGA_PrF_2014009). The funders had no role in study design, data collection and analysis, decision to publish, or preparation of the manuscript.

Competing Interests: The authors have declared that no competing interests exist.

* Email: zdenek.travnicek@upol.cz

Introduction

Gold-based medication was used for a wide range of ailments already in the distant history of ancient China 2500 BC [1,2]. Thus, it is quite extraordinary that even current clinical practice still recognizes chrysotherapy (*chrysos*, gold in Greek), i.e. the treatment of diseases by the administration of gold-based therapeutic agents, as an integral part of modern medicine [3,4]. During the last eighty years of clinical use of gold-based metallotherapeutics, two major groups of complexes have been introduced. The first one is represented by the parenteral preparations, containing relatively simple gold(I)-complexes, such as sodium aurothiomalate (Myochrysin, sodium ((2-carboxy-1-carboxylatoethyl)thiolato)gold(I)) and aurothioglucose (Solganol, {(2 *S*,3*R*,4 *S*,5 *S*,6*R*)-3,4,5-trihydroxy-6-(hydroxymethyl)-oxane-2-thiolato}gold(I)) [5], and the second one comprises the orally administered drug Auranofin (Ridaura) [6–8] (triethylphosphine-(2,3,4,6-tetra-*O*-acetyl-1-D-thiopyranosato-*S*)gold(I)) (See Figure 1). Nowadays, the gold-based metallotherapeutics do not represent antiarthritic agents of the first choice, since new highly potent and more specific anti-rheumatic compounds have been developed (i.e. biopharmaceuticals, novel non-steroidal anti-inflammatory drugs, NSAIDs, or corticosteroids), however, they are still indicated in specific conditions, including moderately to severely active rheumatoid arthritis [8,9]. Although the clinical application of Auranofin has declined in recent years, there are several attempts for repurposing it in other significant indications, such as cytoprotective agents and in the treatment of HIV, severe microbial infections and cancer [1,2,4,8,10].

Several Auranofin inspired gold(I)-complexes have been studied for significant anti-inflammatory, and/or antitumor activities. Among linear gold(I) phosphine complexes, those involving ligands as e.g. dithiocarbamates [1], sulfanylpropenoates [11], naphthalimide derivatives [12], imidazole, pyrazole [13,14] as well as purine derivatives [15,16] have been investigated. It has been

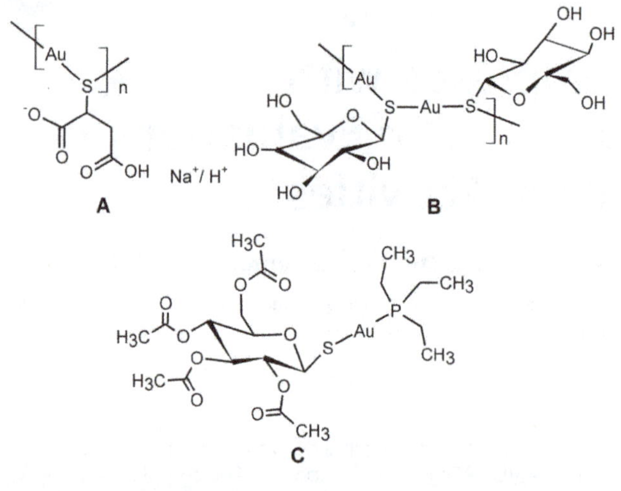

Figure 1. Schematic representations of gold(I) complexes used as anti-inflammatory drugs. A: Sodium aurothiomalate (Myochrysin, sodium {(2-carboxy-1-carboxylatoethyl)thiolato}gold(I)); **B:** Aurothioglucose (Solganol, {(2 *S*,3*R*,4 *S*,5 *S*,6*R*)-3,4,5-trihydroxy-6-(hydroxymethyl)-oxane-2-thiolato}gold(I)); **C:** Auranofin (Ridaura, triethylphosphine-(2,3,4,6-tetra-*O*-acetyl-1-D-thiopyranosato-*S*)gold(I)).

established that the gold(I)-phosphine moiety is responsible for the actual interactions [3,17] with the target sites of the biological molecules, i.e. mostly the selanyl-groups of enzymes [1,18], while the other, weaker bonded ligand influences the kinetic profile of the compounds. This principle has been employed by our group in several recently published works, describing highly antitumor active as well as anti-inflammatory potent gold(I) complexes of the type $[Au(L)(PPh_3)]$ involving various *N*6-benzyladenine derivatives (L) [15,16].

In this work, we report a series of gold(I) complexes of the general formula $[Au(L_n)(PPh_3)]$, where HL_n represents variously mono- and disubstituted derivatives of hypoxanthine (See Figure 2). The rationale for the selection of these *N*-donor ligands is based on the fact that variously substituted derivatives of hypoxanthine have been identified as promising inhibitors of diverse essential enzymes, as cyclin-dependent kinases [19,20] and *O*6-alkylguanine-DNA-alkyltransferase [21,22], and therefore in combination with the $\{Au\text{-}PPh_3\}$ moiety could bring additional means of influencing the cellular metabolism both on the level of cell division, and modulation of cellular responses to the inflammatory stimuli.

The complexes were fully characterized, including high resolution NMR spectroscopy and single crystal X-ray analysis (for complexes **1** and **3**), and were evaluated for their cytotoxicity against a panel of nine human cancer cell lines (MCF7, HOS, THP-1, A549, G361, HeLa, A2780, A2780R (*cisplatin* resistant), and 22Rv1, and also for their *in vitro* anti-inflammatory effect on the model of LPS-stimulated human monocytic leukaemia (THP-1) macrophage-like cell line and the mechanisms of interaction of the complexes with sulfur-containing biomolecules (i.e. L-cysteine and reduced glutathione) were studied by means of mass spectrometry. Moreover, this work fits within the focus of our long term study dedicated to research and development of new transition metal complexes showing various types of biological effects, represented dominantly by the anticancer {Pt(II) [23], Pd(II) [24], Cu(II) [25,26] or Ru(III) [27]}, anti-inflammatory {Au(I/III)} [15,16,28], antidiabetic and cytoprotective {Cu(II) [29]} activities.

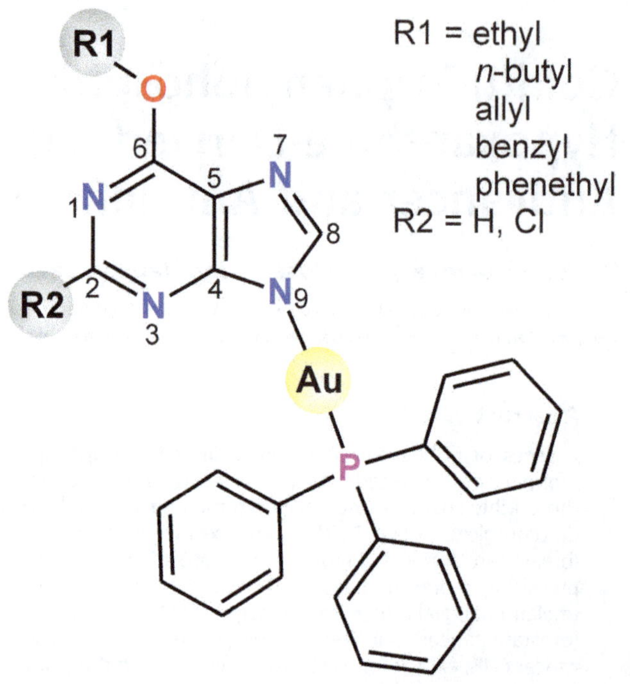

Figure 2. Schematic representation of the prepared gold(I) complexes 1–9.

Materials and Methods

Chemicals and Biochemicals

All the chemicals, involving $H[AuCl_4]\cdot 3H_2O$ (Acros Organics, Pardubice, Czech Republic), triphenylphosphine (PPh_3; Sigma-Aldrich Co., Prague, Czech Republic), NaOH (Sigma-Aldrich Co., Prague, Czech Republic) and used solvents (acetone, diethyl ether, dimethyl sulfoxide (DMSO), toluene, *n*-hexane and *N, N'*-dimethylformamide (DMF); Fisher-Scientific, Pardubice, Czech Republic) were obtained from the commercial sources and were used without any further purification. The *N*-donor ligands derived from hypoxanthine, HL_{1-9} (HL_1 = 6-ethoxy-9*H*-purine; HL_2 = 6-butyloxy-9*H*-purine; HL_3 = 6-allyloxy-9*H*-purine; HL_4 = 6-benzyloxy-9*H*-purine; HL_5 = 6-phenetyloxy-9*H*-purine; HL_6 = 2-chloro-6-ethoxy-9*H*-purine; HL_7 = 2-chloro-6-butyloxy-9*H*-purine, HL_8 = 2-chloro-6-allyloxy-9*H*-purine, HL_8 = 2-chloro-6-benzyloxy-9*H*-purine) were prepared according to the previously published procedure [19] and characterized by elemental analysis, FT-IR and ^1H and ^{13}C NMR spectroscopy, which gave evidence about their composition and purity. The starting $[AuCl(PPh_3)]$ complex was synthesized as described previously [30,31].

The RPMI 1640 medium and penicillin-streptomycin mixture (Lonza, Verviers, Belgium), phosphate-buffered saline (PBS), foetal bovine serum (FBS), phorbol myristate acetate (PMA), prednisone (≥98%), Auranofin (≥98%), erythrosin B, and *Escherichia coli* 0111:B4 lipopolysaccharide (LPS) (Sigma-Aldrich, Steinheim, Germany), as well as a Cell Proliferation Reagent WST-1, and cOmplete Proteinase Inhibitor Cocktail (Roche, Mannheim, Germany) were obtained from commercial sources.

A RealTime Ready Cell Lysis Kit (Roche, Mannheim, Germany) served for isolation of RNA from cells and Transcriptor Universal cDNA Master (Roche, Mannheim, Germany) was used for reverse transcription of RNA to cDNA. Specific primers and probes (Gene Expression assays) for polymerase chain reaction

Table 1. ^{1}H and ^{13}C NMR coordination shifts ($\Delta\delta = \delta_{complex} - \delta_{ligand}$; ppm) of calculated for **1–9**.

	^{1}H NMR		^{13}C NMR				
	C2 H	**C8 H**	**C2**	**C4**	**C5**	**C6**	**C8**
1	-0.05	-0.08	-0.90	4.80	-1.14	-1.04	4.40
2	-0.05	-0.10	-0.60	4.82	-0.59	-0.21	3.57
3	-0.11	-0.23	0.98	2.20	-0.56	-0.24	5.11
4	-0.13	-0.23	0.86	3.00	-0.81	0.50	5.03
5	-0.12	-0.25	-0.01	2.16	-1.29	-0.32	5.85
6	n.a.	-0.27	-0.16	2.02	-1.17	0.05	6.02
7	n.a.	-0.10	-0.04	4.01	-0.54	-0.73	6.89
8	n.a.	-0.12	-0.49	2.38	-0.74	-0.35	4.89
9	n.a.	-0.24	-0.53	3.22	-1.01	-0.18	5.70

n.a. - not available.

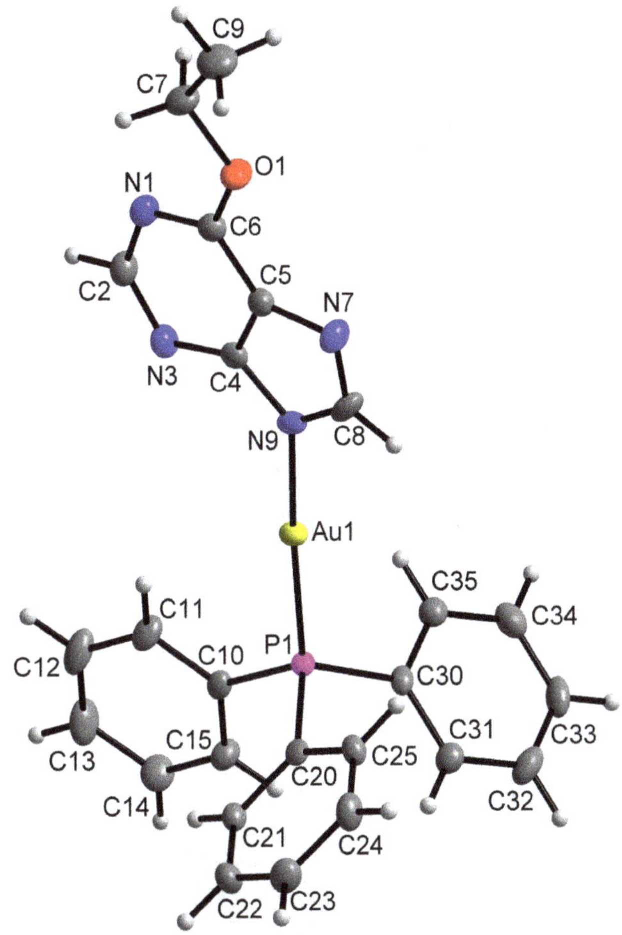

Figure 3. Molecular structure of [Au(L$_1$)(PPh$_3$)] (1). The molecular structure of **1** showing the atom numbering scheme. Non-hydrogen atoms are displayed as ellipsoids at the 50% probability level.

(PCR) were obtained from Applied Biosystems (Foster City, CA, USA). The following assays were chosen for the quantification of gene expression: Hs00174128_ml for tumour necrosis factor-α (TNF-α), Hs01555410_ml for interleukin-1β (IL-1β), and 4326315E for β-actin, which served as an internal control of gene expression. Quantitative PCR (qPCR) was performed with Fast Start Universal Probe Master (Roche, Mannheim, Germany). Instant ELISA Kits (eBioscience, Vienna, Austria) were used to evaluate the production of TNF-α and IL-1β by the enzyme linked immunosorbent assay (ELISA). The Immun-Blot PVDF (polyvinylidene fluoride) membrane 0.2 μm (Bio-Rad, Hercules, CA, USA) and albumin bovine fraction V (BSA) (Serva, Heidelberg, Germany) were used for Westernblot. Murine monoclonal anti-IκB-α (Cell Signaling, Danvers, MA, USA), murine monoclonal anti-β-actin (Abcam, Cambridge, UK) and goat polyclonal anti-mouse IgG (with the conjugated peroxidase) antibodies (Sigma-Aldrich, Saint Louis, MO, USA) were applied for immunodetection. The activity of the conjugated peroxidase was detected by an Opti-4CN Substrate Kit (Bio-Rad, Hercules, CA, USA).

Chemistry

Gold(I) complexes of the general formula [Au(L$_n$)(PPh$_3$)] (**1**–**9**), where L$_n$ stands for a deprotonated form of a hypoxanthine-derived compound, were prepared by a slight modification of the previously reported procedure for the synthesis of similar

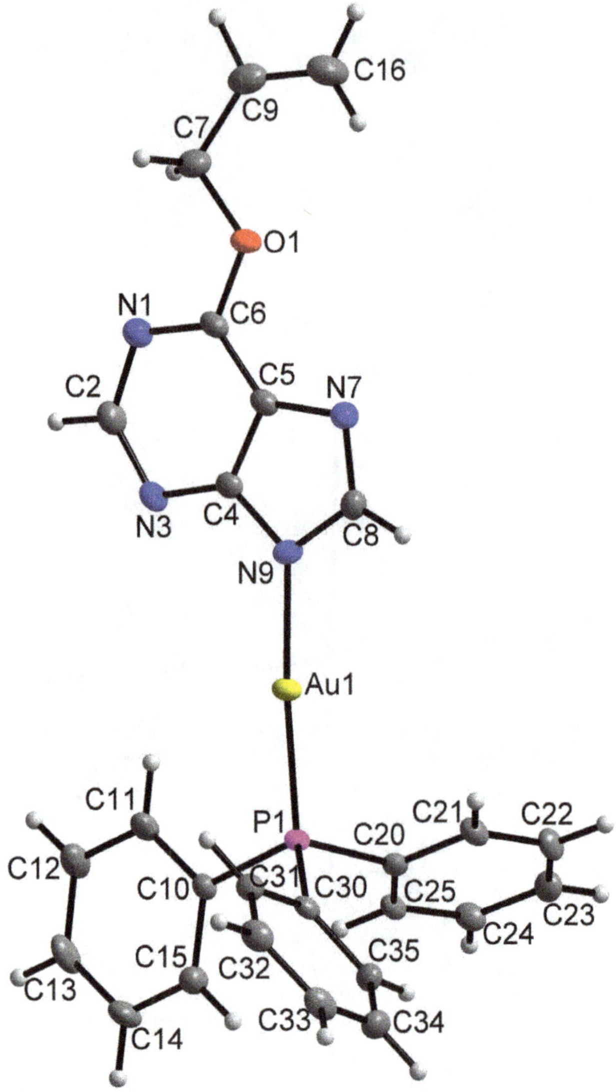

Figure 4. Molecular structure of [Au(L$_3$)(PPh$_3$)] (3). The molecular structure of **3** showing the atom numbering scheme. Non-hydrogen atoms are displayed as ellipsoids at the 50% probability level.

[Au(L)(PPh$_3$)] complexes, in which HL stands for 6-benzylaminopurine derivatives [15,16]. Concretely, the reactions of the acetone solutions of [AuCl(PPh$_3$)] (1 mmol in 10 mL) were mixed with the corresponding hypoxanthine derivative (HL$_n$; 1 mmol in 20 mL), and subsequently, 1 mL of 1 M NaOH was added into the reaction mixture. The mixture was stirred for 3 h, after which precipitated NaCl was filtered off. The colourless filtrate was evaporated to dryness and the residue was collected. Recrystallization was carried out from acetone. In the case when the residue was of gel-like consistency, 20 mL of diethyl ether was added and the suspension was sonicated to obtain a powder product. Crystals of complexes **1** and **3**, suitable for single crystal X-ray analysis, were prepared by a slow diffusion of *n*-hexane into a saturated solution of the appropriate complex in toluene. The purity and composition of the obtained gold(I) complexes **1**–**9** were established based on the methods of elemental analysis, electrospray-ionization mass spectrometry (ESI-MS), ^{1}H and ^{13}C NMR, and FT-IR spectroscopies, and thermal analysis (TG/DTA) (characterization data are given in File S1). The molecular and crystal structures were determined by single crystal X-ray analysis for complexes **1** and **3**.

Physical Measurements

Elemental analyses (C, H, N) were carried out on a Flash 2000 CHNO-S Analyser (Thermo Scientific, USA). FT-IR spectra were measured on a Nexus 670 FT-IR spectrometer (ThermoNicolet, USA) by the ATR technique in the 200–4000 cm^{-1} range. ^{1}H, ^{13}C and ^{31}P NMR spectra were measured in DMF-d_7 on a Varian 400 MHz NMR spectrometer at 300 K using tetramethylsilane (SiMe$_4$) (for ^{1}H and ^{13}C spectra) and 85% H_3PO_4 (for ^{31}P) as an internal reference standard. Mass spectra of methanol solutions of complexes were recorded on an LCQ Fleet Ion-Trap mass spectrometer using the positive mode electrospray ionization (Thermo Scientific, USA). Thermogravimetric (TG) and differential thermal (DTA) analyses were performed on a thermal analyser Exstar TG/DTA 6200 (Seiko Instruments Inc., Japan) in dynamic air conditions (50 mL min^{-1}) between room temperature (ca 25°C) and 950°C (gradient 2.5°C min^{-1}). Single crystal X-ray analyses were performed on an Xcalibur2 diffractometer equipped with a CCD detector Sapphire2 (Oxford Diffraction Ltd., Oxford, UK) using MoKα radiation (monochromator Enhance, Oxford Diffraction Ltd.), and using the ω-scan technique at 120 K. Data collection, data reduction and cell parameter refinements were performed by the CRYSALIS software package [32]. The molecular structures were solved by direct methods and all non-hydrogen atoms were refined anisotropically on F^2 using the full-matrix least-squares procedure (*SHELX-97*) [33]. H-atoms were found in difference maps and refined by using the riding model with C−H = 0.95, 0.98 and 0.99 Å, with $U_{iso}(H) = 1.2U_{eq}(CH, CH_2)$ and $1.5U_{eq}(CH_3)$. The highest residual peaks of 2.623 e Å^{-3} and 1.792 e Å^{-3} were located 0.85 Å from Au1 (for complex **1**), and 0.88 Å from Au1 (for complex **3**), respectively. Molecular graphics were drawn and additional structural parameters were interpreted in *DIAMOND* [34] and *Mercury* [35].

Maintenance and Preparation of Macrophages

The human monocytic leukaemia cell line THP-1 (ECACC, Salisbury, UK) was used for the *in vitro* anti-inflammatory activity evaluation. The cells were cultivated at 37°C in the RPMI 1640 medium supplemented with 2 mM L-glutamine, 10% FBS, 100 U/mL of penicillin and 100 μg/mL of streptomycin in humidified atmosphere containing 5% CO_2. Stabilized cells (3rd–15th passage) were split into microtitration plates to get the concentration of 500 000 cells/mL and the differentiation to macrophages was induced by addition of phorbol myristate acetate (PMA) dissolved in DMSO at the final concentration of 50 ng/ml and the cells were incubated for 24 h. Unlike monocytes, differentiated macrophages tend to adhere to the bottom of the cultivation plates. For the subsequent 24 h, the cells were incubated with the fresh complete RPMI medium, i.e. containing antibiotics and FBS, without PMA. Then, the medium was aspirated, and the cells were washed with PBS and cultivated in the serum-free RPMI 1640 medium for next 24 h. These prepared macrophages were used for the detection of inflammatory response.

In Vitro Cytotoxicity Testing

Cytotoxicity in THP-1 cells was determined by the WST-1 assay. The THP-1 cells (floating monocytes, 500 000 cells/mL) were incubated in 100 μL of the serum-free RPMI 1640 medium and seeded into 96-well plates in triplicate at 37°C. Measurements were taken 24 h after the treatment with the tested compounds dissolved in 0.1% DMSO in the concentration range of 0.16–

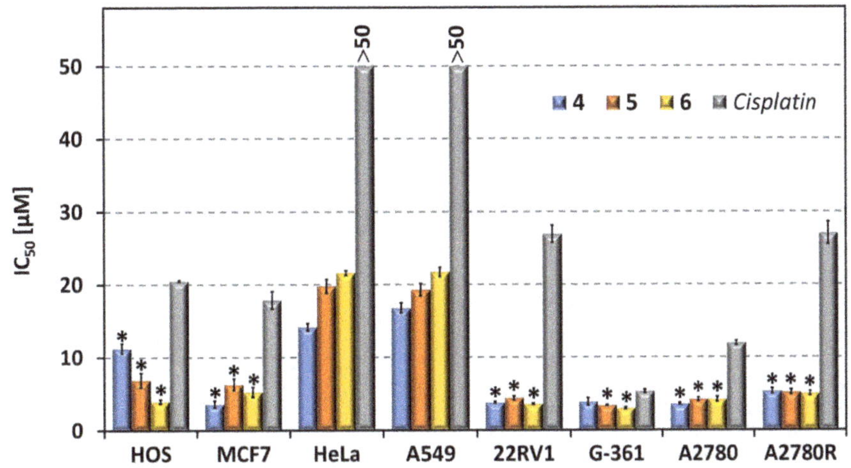

Figure 5. The results of *in vitro* cytotoxicity against selected cancer cell lines for complexes 4–6 and *cisplatin*. The cells were exposed to the employed complexes for 24 h. Measurements were performed in triplicate and each cytotoxicity experiment was repeated three times. The given IC_{50}±SE (µM) values represent an arithmetic mean. The asterisk (*) denotes significant difference (ANOVA, $p<0.05$) between **4–6** and *cisplatin*.

10 µM. Viability was determined by the WST-1 test according to the manufacturer's manual. The amount of created formazan (correlating with the number of metabolically active cells in the culture) was calculated as a percentage of the control cells, which were treated only with 0.1% DMSO and was set-up as 100%. The cytotoxic IC_{50} values of the tested compounds were calculated from the obtained data. The WST-1 assay was performed spectrophotometrically at 440 nm (FLUOstar Omega, BMG Labtech, Germany).

In vitro cytotoxicity of the presented compounds was further determined by the MTT assay in a wide range of human cancer cell lines, i.e. human breast adenocarcinoma (MCF7; ECACC no. 86012803), human osteosarcoma (HOS; ECACC no. 87070202), lung carcinoma (A549; ECACC no. 86012804), malignant melanoma (G-361; ECACC no. 88030401), cervix epitheloid carcinoma (HeLa; ECACC no. 93021013), ovarian carcinoma (A2780; ECACC no. 93112519), *cisplatin*-resistant ovarian carcinoma (A2780R; ECACC no. 93112517) and prostate carcinoma (22Rv1; ECACC no 105092802) cancer cell lines purchased from European Collection of Cell Cultures (ECACC). The cells were cultured according to the ECACC instructions. They were maintained at 37°C and 5% CO_2 in a humidified incubator. The cells were treated with the complexes **1**–**9**, free HL_{1-9} molecules, $HAuCl_4$, AuCl and *cisplatin* (applied up to 50 µM) for 24 h, using multi-well culture plates of 96 wells. In parallel, the cells were treated with vehicle (DMF; 0.1%, v/v) and Triton X-100 (1%, v/v) to evaluate the minimal (i.e. positive control), and maximal (i.e. negative control) cell damage, respectively. The MTT assay was performed spectrophotometrically at 540 nm (TECAN, Schoeller Instruments LLC, Prague, CZ).

Drug Treatment and Induction of Inflammatory Response

Differentiated macrophages were pretreated with 300 nM solutions of the complexes **1**–**9**, HL_{1-9}, AuCl, [AuCl(PPh_3)], PPh_3 and Auranofin dissolved in DMSO (the final DMSO concentration was 0.1%) and with 0.1% DMSO solution (vehicle) for 1 h; the given concentrations of the tested compounds lack the cytotoxic effect (cell viability >94%). The inflammatory response was triggered by addition of 1.0 µg/mL LPS dissolved in water to the pretreated macrophages, control cells were without the LPS treatment.

RNA Isolation and Gene Expression Evaluation

For the evaluation of the expression of TNF-α, IL-1β, and β-actin mRNA, the total RNA was isolated directly from the THP-1 cells in cultivation plates using a RealTime Ready Cell Lysis Kit, according to the manufacturer's instructions.

The gene expression was quantified by two-step reverse-transcription quantitative (real-time) PCR (RT-qPCR). The reverse transcription step was performed by Transcriptor Universal cDNA Master using cell lysate as a template. The reaction consists of 3 steps: (1) primer annealing, 29°C for 10 min; (2) reverse transcription, 55°C for 10 min; and (3) transcriptase inactivation, 85°C for 5 min. FastStart Universal Probe Master and Gene Expression assays were used for qPCR. These assays contain specific primers and TaqMan probes that bind to an exon-exon junction to avoid DNA contamination. The parameters for the qPCR work were adjusted according to the manufacturer's recommendations as follows: 50°C for 2 min, then 95°C for 10 min, followed by 40 cycles at 95°C for 15 s and 60°C for 1 min. The results were normalized to the amount of ROX reference dye, and the change in gene expression was determined by the $\Delta\Delta C_T$ method. Transcription of the control cells was set as 1 and other experimental groups were multiples of this value.

Evaluation of Cytokine Secretion by ELISA

Macrophages, which were pretreated with the tested compounds for 1 h, were incubated with LPS for next 24 h. After this period, the medium was collected and the concentration of TNF-α and IL-1β was measured by an Instant ELISA kit according to the manufactures' manual.

Determination of IκB Degradation by Western Blot

Macrophage-like THP-1 cells were pretreated with the tested compounds and stimulated by LPS as described above. Thirty minutes after the addition of LPS, the medium was aspirated and cells were washed by cold PBS. Subsequently, the cells were collected using the lysis buffer [50 mM Tris-HCl pH 7.5, 1 mM EGTA, 1 mM EDTA, 1 mM sodium orthovanadate, 50 mM sodium fluoride, 5 mM sodium pyrophosphate, 270 mM sucrose,

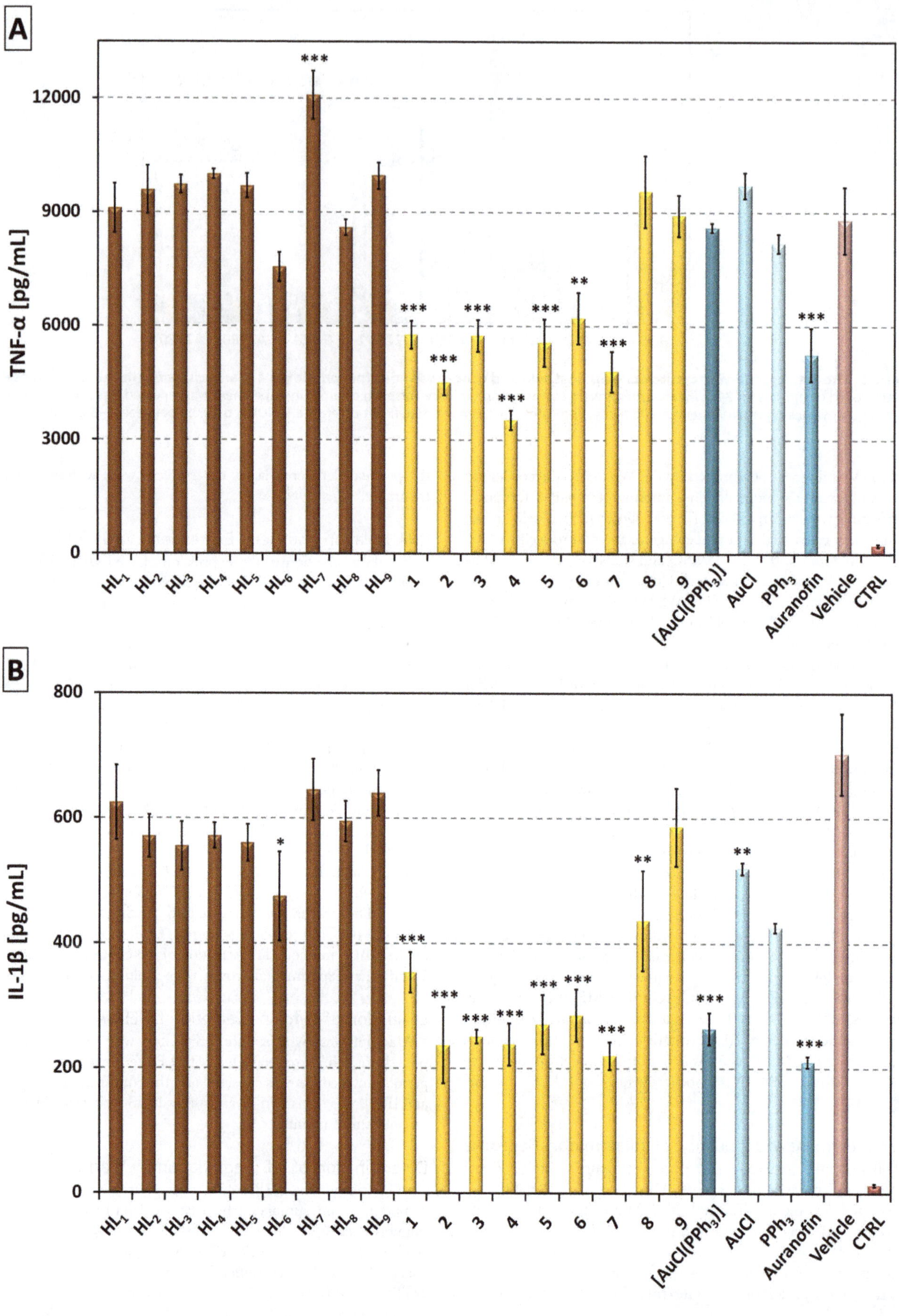
A
TNF-α [pg/mL]
12000
9000
6000
3000
0
HL1 HL2 HL3 HL4 HL5 HL6 HL7 HL8 HL9 1 2 3 4 5 6 7 8 9 [AuCl(PPh3)] AuCl PPh3 Auranofin Vehicle CTRL
B
IL-1β [pg/mL]
800
600
400
200
0
HL1 HL2 HL3 HL4 HL5 HL6 HL7 HL8 HL9 1 2 3 4 5 6 7 8 9 [AuCl(PPh3)] AuCl PPh3 Auranofin Vehicle CTRL

Figure 6. Effects of the Au(I) complexes 1–9, reference drug Auranofin, [AuCl(PPh_3)], AuCl, PPh_3 and HL_{1-9} on LPS-induced TNF-α (A) and IL-1β (B) secretion. The cells were pretreated with the tested compounds (300 nM) or the vehicle (0.1% DMSO) only. After 1 h of the incubation, the inflammatory response was induced by LPS [except for the control cells (CTRL)]. The secretion was determined 24 h after the LPS addition. The results are expressed as means±SE of three independent experiments. Significant difference in comparison to: *vehicle-treated cells ($p<0.05$), **vehicle-treated cells ($p<0.01$), ***vehicle-treated cells ($p<0.001$).

0.1% (v/v) Triton X-100, and cOmplete Protease Inhibitor Cocktail (Roche, Germany)] and scraper. The lysis of cells was facilitated by short (ca. 30 s) incubation in the ultrasonic water bath. The protein concentration was determined according to Bradford's method. For protein separation, 30 µg of protein was loaded onto 12% polyacrylamide gel. Then, they were electrophoretically transferred on the PVDF membranes, which were subsequently blocked by 5% BSA dissolved in TBST buffer [150 mM NaCl, 10 mM Tris base pH 7.5, 0.1% (v/v) Tween-20]. The membranes were incubated with the primary anti-IκB-α antibody at the concentration of 1:500, or with the primary anti-β-actin at the concentration of 1:5000 at 4°C for 16 h. After washing, the secondary anti-mouse IgG antibody diluted 1:2000 was applied on the membranes and incubated for 1 h at laboratory temperature (~22°C). The amount of the bound secondary antibody was detected colorimetrically by an Opti-4CN kit according to the manufacturer's manual.

Statistical Evaluation

The cytotoxicity data were expressed as the percentage of viability, when 100% represent the treatment with vehicle (DMF or DMSO). The experiments were conducted in triplicate using cells from different passages. The IC_{50} values were calculated from viability curves. The results are presented as arithmetic mean ± standard error of the mean (SE). The significance of the differences between the results was evaluated by the ANOVA analysis with $p<0.05$ considered to be significant (QC Expert 3.2, Statistical software, TriloByte Ltd., Pardubice, CZ).

The statistically significant differences between individual groups during anti-inflammatory activity testing were assessed by the one-way ANOVA test, followed by Tukey's *post-hoc* test for multiple comparisons. GraphPad Prism 5.02 (GraphPad Software Inc., San Diego, CA, USA) was used for the analysis.

Interactions with L-Cysteine and Reduced Glutathione Analyzed by Mass Spectrometry

The interaction experiments between the selected representative complexes **1** and **6**, bearing the same ethoxy-substitution on the C6 atom, but differing in the substituents in the C2 position, and the mixture of physiological levels of cysteine and glutathione were performed on a Thermo Scientific LTQ Fleet Ion-Trap mass spectrometer, using the positive ionization mode. The reaction system contained the physiological concentrations of L-cysteine (290 µM) and reduced glutathione (6 µM) [36] and the tested complex (20 µM) in the methanol:water (1:1, v/v) mixture. The reference system was comprised of the solution of complex (20 µM) in the methanol:water (1:1, v/v) mixture. The flow injection analysis (FIA) method was used to introduce the reaction system (5 µL spikes) into the mass spectrometer, while pure acetonitrile was used as a mobile phase. The ESI-source was set up as follows: source voltage was 4.5 kV, the vaporizer temperature was 160°C, the capillary temperature was 275°C, the sheath gas flow rate was 30 L/min, and auxiliary gas flow rate was 10 L/min. The system was calibrated according to the manufacturer specifications and no further tuning was needed.

Results and Discussion

General Properties of the Au(I) complexes

This work reports on the preparation, thorough characterization, and *in vitro* cytotoxic and anti-inflammatory activities of a series of gold(I)-triphenylphosphine complexes [Au(L_{1-9})(PPh_3)] involving mono- or disubstituted derivatives of hypoxanthine

Table 2. *In vitro* cytotoxicity of complexes 1–9 and *cisplatin* against MCF7 and HOS cancer cell lines.

	Cell Line		
Compound	**MCF7**	**HOS**	**THP-1**
1	15.22±0.78	19.20±0.71	1.17±0.04
2	27.10±0.21	30.02±2.13	1.03±0.04
3	12.40±1.07	15.60±1.10	1.87±0.09
4	3.66±0.48	11.30±0.67	2.15±0.19
5	6.30±0.80	6.56±0.97	1.89±0.11
6	5.23±0.68	3.96±0.29	1.94±0.12
7	>50	>50	1.97±0.14
8	>25	18.80±0.70	5.28±0.21
9	>25	16.80±0.27	>10
cisplatin	17.90±1.17	20.50±0.10	-
Auranofin	1.10±0.30[a]	n.d.	0.88±0.04

The results of the *in vitro* cytotoxic activity testing of **1–9** and *cisplatin* against human breast adenocarcinoma (MCF7) and osteosarcoma (HOS): cells were treated with the tested compounds for 24 h; measurements were performed in triplicate, and cytotoxicity experiment was repeated in three different cell passages; data are expressed as IC_{50}±SE (µM).
[a]adopted from Ref. [42]; n.d. – not determined.

Table 3. *In vitro* cytotoxicity of complexes 4–6 and *cisplatin* against a panel of cancer cell lines.

	Cell Line					
Compound	**A549**	**G-361**	**HeLa**	**A2780**	**A2780R**	**22Rv1**
4	16.8±0.7	3.9±0.5	14.2±0.5	3.6±0.1	4.3±0.2	3.8±0.1
5	19.3±0.8	3.4±0.1	19.8±0.9	4.2±0.2	4.8±0.6	4.4±0.3
6	21.7±0.4	3.0±0.1	21.6±0.3	4.2±0.3	5.1±0.4	3.6±0.1
cisplatin	>50	5.3±0.2	>50	12.0±0.3	27.0±1.5	26.9±1.2

The results of the *in vitro* cytotoxic activity testing of **4–6** and *cisplatin* against the human cancer cell lines. Cells were treated with the tested compounds for 24 h; measurements were performed in triplicate, and cytotoxicity experiments were repeated in three different cell passages; data are expressed as IC_{50}±SE (μM).

(HL_{1-9}). The complexes were synthesized by a modification of a previously published method [15,16], i.e. by a reaction of the precursor complex [AuCl(PPh_3)] with an equimolar amount of the corresponding organic molecule HL_{1-9} in acetone with the addition of 1 M NaOH. The prepared complexes **1–9** are very well soluble in acetone, alcoholic solvents, toluene, DMSO and DMF, and partially soluble in water at laboratory temperature. The complexes were prepared non-solvated, as evidenced by the results of simultaneous TG/DTA analysis (see Figure S3 in File S1). The complexes were further characterized as chemical individuals by elemental analysis, ^{1}H, ^{13}C and ^{31}P NMR spectroscopy, FT-IR spectroscopy and ESI–MS. Single crystals suitable for X-ray analysis were prepared in the cases of **1** and **3**, thus providing information about the molecular and crystal structures of the complexes (discussed in detail below).

^{1}H and ^{13}C NMR spectra were measured for all the presented complexes. The obtained results were very beneficial for the confirmation of the purity and composition of **1–9**. The observed signals unambiguously proved the presence of both hypoxanthine and phosphine derivatives in the structures of the Au(I) complexes as well as gave information about the coordination mode of these ligands. The most conclusive evidence concerning the identification of the donor atom of HL_{1-9} was obtained from the ^{13}C NMR spectra by comparing the chemical shifts in the uncoordinated and coordinated hypoxanthine derivative. The resulting differences, calculated as coordination shifts; $\Delta\delta = \delta_{complex} - \delta_{ligand}$, ppm; Table 1), showed that the greatest changes occurred for the signals corresponding to the carbons C4 and C8, shifted by 2.02–4.82 ppm, and 3.57–6.89 ppm, respectively. This observation indirectly pointed to N9 as the coordination site, as the two mentioned carbons lie in the direct vicinity to this nitrogen. The set of the most intensive signals at around 130 ppm, characteristic of all the spectra of **1–9**, was assigned to the carbon atoms of triphenylphosphine. Accordingly, the ^{1}H NMR spectra of all the nine Au(I) complexes showed very strong multiplet signals at around 7.70 ppm with the relative integral intensity well corresponding to the calculated value of 15 hydrogens of PPh_3. Additionally, the C8 H signal of the corresponding HL_{1-9} ligand was shifted by 0.08–0.27 ppm upfield in the spectra of the complexes with respect to the spectra of the uncoordinated HL_{1-9}, corresponding with the results following from ^{13}C NMR spectroscopy about N9 being the site of coordination to gold. What should be also pointed out is the absence of the signal assignable to the proton N9 H in the spectra of **1–9**, which well agrees with the presence of deprotonated hypoxanthine-based ligands in the studied complexes symbolized as L_{1-9}. All the ^{31}P NMR spectra of the complexes were characteristic of the presence of one singlet at 31.67–33.13 ppm (see Figure S5 in File S1), which is significantly shifted as compared to the signal of free PPh_3 (–5.96 ppm), which confirms the coordination of PPh_3 to gold(I) atom through phosphorus, thus forming the Au–P bond. In summary, the presence and chemical shift of all the detected signals in ^{1}H, ^{13}C and ^{31}P NMR spectra, as well as the relative intensity of the peaks in the proton spectra, indicate that the gold(I) atom in **1–9** is coordinated by one deprotonated hypoxanthine-derived compound (L_{1-9}) binding via N9 and one PPh_3 molecule. These conclusions are in good agreement with the results following from single crystal X-ray analysis of complexes **1** and **3** discussed below.

Mass spectra measured in the positive ionization mode also indirectly confirmed the composition of the presented complexes, as all the spectra of **1–9** contained the $[M+H]^+$ molecular peaks. The presence of the hypoxanthine-based derivatives was demonstrated by the observed peaks corresponding to the adducts of $[HL_n+Na/K]^+$ (for details of ESI+MS characterization, see File S1).

Further properties of the presented Au(I) complexes were studied by FT-IR spectroscopy. The courses of the spectra of **1–9** in the mid-IR region were qualitatively very similar to those of the uncoordinated HL_{1-9}. The very intensive peaks at 1600–1578 cm^{-1} could be assigned to the $\nu(C{\cdots}N)_{ring}$ stretching vibrations characteristic of heterocyclic molecules with nitrogen ring atoms. Further assigned characteristic vibrations could be found at 3057–3048 cm^{-1} for $\nu(C\text{-}H)_{ar}$, 2986–2889 cm^{-1} for $\nu(C\text{-}H)_{aliph}$, and also 1480–1436 cm^{-1} for $\nu(C{\cdots}C)_{ring}$. The typical vibrations of the ether functional group found in the *O*6-substituted hypoxanthine derivatives were detected at 1339–1272 cm^{-1} for the aromatic C6–O stretch and at 1118–1087 cm^{-1} for the O–C10 stretch. The medium to strong intensity bands found between 800–700 cm^{-1}, and at ca. 690 cm^{-1} can be attributed to the out-of-plane C–H bending vibrations, and ring bending, respectively, determining the presence of an aromatic ring in all the complexes **1–9** [37,38]. In the far spectra of the Au(I) complexes, new bands were identified as compared with the spectra of free HL_{1-9}. These maxima at 506–492 cm^{-1}, and 329–321 cm^{-1} could be assigned to ν(Au–N), and ν(Au–P) stretching vibrations, respectively, although it should be noted that triphenylphosphine alone has intensive vibrations in this region of IR spectra, so these bands could be overlapped [15,16,37,39].

Molecular and Crystal Structures of [Au(L_1)(PPh_3)](1) and [Au(L_3)(PPh_3)] (3)

The crystallization method of slow *n*-hexane diffusion into the saturated toluene solution of the complexes allowed the preparation of single crystals suitable for X-ray analysis of two complexes, [Au(L_1)(PPh_3)](**1**) and [Au(L_3)(PPh_3)] (**3**), where HL_1 = 6-ethoxy-9*H*-purine and HL_3 = 6-allyloxy-9*H*-purine. The molecular struc-

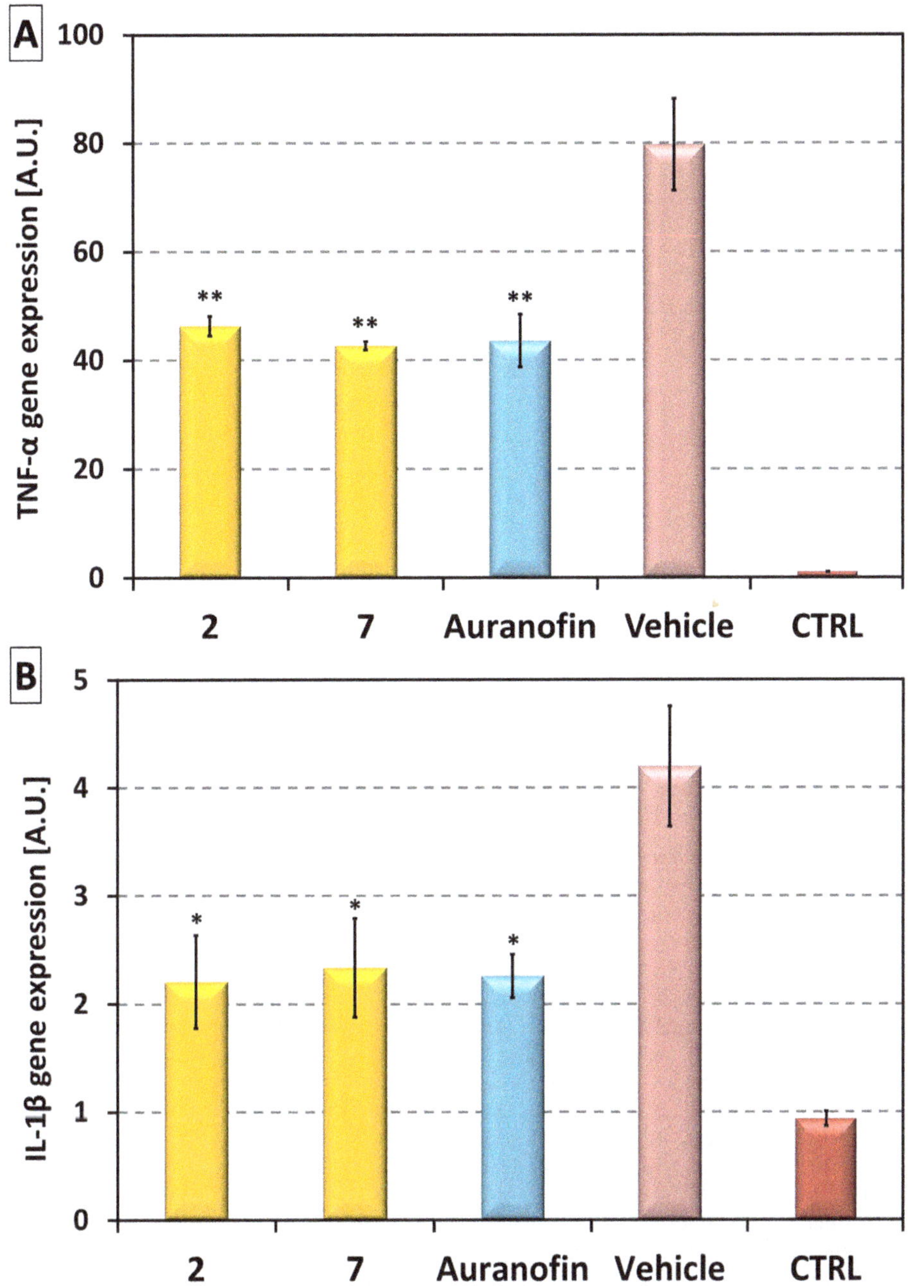

Figure 7. Effects of the Au(I) complexes 2 and 7, and reference drug Auranofin on gene expression of TNF-α (A) and IL-1β (B). THP-1 macrophages were pretreated with complexes **2**, **7** and Auranofin at the concentration of 300 nM or the vehicle (0.1% DMSO) only. After 1 h of the incubation, the inflammatory response was induced by LPS [except for the control cells (CTRL)]. After 2 h, the level of TNF-α and IL-1β mRNA was evaluated by RT-qPCR. The amount of cytokine mRNA was normalised to β-actin mRNA. The results are expressed as means±SE of three independent experiments. A.U. =arbitrary unit. Significant difference in comparison to: *vehicle-treated cells ($p<0.05$), **vehicle-treated cells ($p<0.01$).

tures are depicted in Figure 3, and 4, respectively. Crystal data and structure refinement parameters (Table S1 in File S1), selected bond lengths and angles (Table S2 in File S1), as well as non-covalent interaction parameters (Tables S3 and S4 in File S1) are given in File S1.

In both complexes **1** and **3**, the central gold(I) atom is two-coordinated in the distorted linear arrangement of the {NP} donor set formed by one *N*-donor deprotonated hypoxanthine derivative and the electroneutral molecule of triphenylphosphine bonded via phosphorus. Comparing the coordination bonds in **1** and **3**, both bond lengths are mutually comparable between the complexes, as they were found to be 2.046(3), and 2.042(3) Å for Au–N; and 2.2344(9), and 2.2356(8) Å for Au–P, respectively. On the other hand, it is evident that the Au–P bonds are significantly longer than the Au–N bonds, which is most likely connected with the bulky phenyl moieties surrounding the phosphorus donor atom in PPh_3. This bond distance difference is not uncommon in similar complexes. The search in the Cambridge Structural Database (CSD ver. 5.35, February 2014 update) [40] within the deposited 113 mononuclear compounds involving the N-Au-PPh_3 motif with

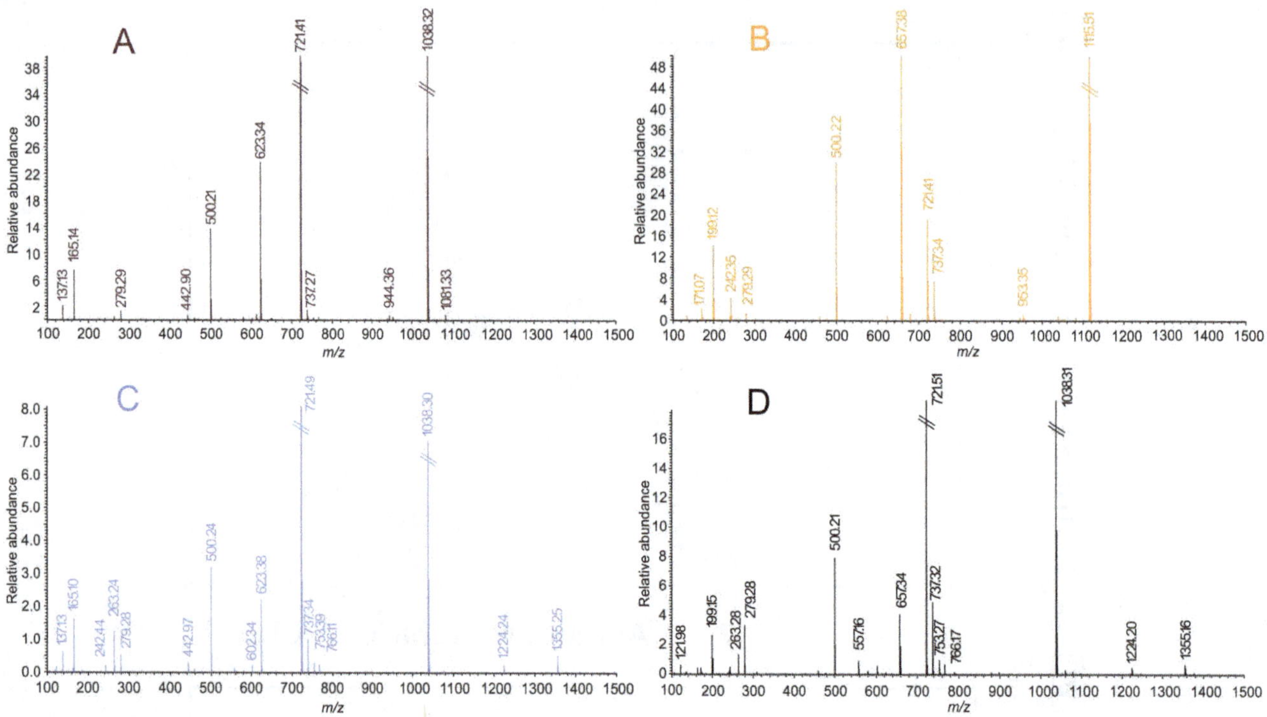

Figure 8. The results of the ESI-MS study of complex 1 (A) and 6 (B) solutions and interacting systems involving the mixture of physiological levels of cysteine and reduced glutathione and complex 1 (C) or complex 6 (D).

the central gold atom in the linear geometry proved that the Au–N and Au–P bond lengths in **1** and **3** fall within the interval of such bond lengths found in the above specified set of compounds, i.e. 1.971–2.134 Å, and 2.22–2.278 Å, respectively. The distortion of the linear geometry is well demonstrated on the dimensions of the N9–Au1–P1 angles, which are equal to 172.73(10)° in **1** and 175.65(8)° in **3**. These values also clearly reveal that the distortion from the ideal angle of 180° is significantly higher in complex **1** than in **3**. This difference could most likely be connected with a somewhat different array of non-covalent contacts found in the complexes. In general, the crystal structures of both complexes **1** and **3** are characterised by absence of strong non-covalent contacts, such as typical hydrogen bonds. The crystal structures of both the complexes are stabilized by C–H···C, C–H···N and C–H···O non-covalent contacts. For more details, see Supplementary Information, Tables S3 and S4 in File S1, Figures S1 and S2 in File S1.

In Vitro Cytotoxicity

For the evaluation of *in vitro* cytotoxicity, the presented complexes were tested by the MTT assay and the results were compared with the clinically applied metallodrug *cisplatin*, used as the reference standard, as well as with the starting compounds, i.e. hypoxanthine derivatives HL_{1-9}, and gold-containing inorganic compounds AuCl or $HAuCl_4$ (applied in the concentration range of 0.01–50.0 μM, unless their solubility was found to be lower). The first phase of testing involved screening of all the prepared complexes **1**–**9** against two human cancer cell lines, breast adenocarcinoma (MCF7) and osteosarcoma (HOS). The starting compounds were found inactive up to 50 μM or to the limiting concentration of their solubility against these cells. Then, this testing showed a varied effect of the tested complexes on the viability of the selected cancer cell lines. Complex **7** showed to be inactive up to the tested concentration range on both cell lines (IC_{50}>50 μM). Complexes **8** and **9** were found to be cytotoxic inactive against the MCF7 cells in the used concentration ranges given by their solubility, therefore their cytotoxicity can be evaluated as >25 μM. Complex **2** was moderately active on both cell lines, however, the IC_{50} values, i.e. 27.1±0.2 μM (MCF7) and 30.0±2.1 μM (HOS), were higher than those for *cisplatin* (in the case of MCF7, significantly higher, ANOVA, $p<0.05$). This pointed to the fact that the *n*-butyl group as the R1 substituent showed to be the least beneficial for the resulting cytotoxic activity against these cell lines within the tested series of compounds (*n*-Bu present in **2** and **7**). The best results were observed for the complexes **4**–**6**, all of which possessed significantly better cytotoxicity than *cisplatin* (ANOVA, $p<0.05$) against both cell lines, concretely the IC_{50} values were found to be 2–5-times lower. The most promising data were found for complex **4** against the MCF7 cell line, i.e. IC_{50} = 3.7±0.5 μM (17.9±1.2 μM for *cisplatin*), and for complex **6** against HOS cells, i.e. 4.0±0.3 μM as compared with 20.5±0.1 μM for *cisplatin* (Table 2).

Before using the THP-1 cell line for testing of the anti-phlogistic effect, cytotoxicity of complexes **1**–**9** and uncoordinated hypoxanthine derivatives HL_{1-9} was also tested on this cell line (Table 2). The IC_{50} values for **1**–**7** were between 1.03–2.15 μM, which are significantly lower than for the MCF7 and HOS cell lines. Interestingly, **8** has the IC_{50} only 5.3±0.2 μM and **9** does not even have any cytotoxic effect up to the concentration of 10 μM, whereas their structural analogues without chlorine at C2 (**3** and **4**) have the IC_{50} values equal to 1.87±0.09 μM, and 2.15±0.19 μM, respectively. In all the cases, cytotoxicity was lower (i.e. the IC_{50} values were higher; 1.03–5.28 μM) than for commercially used drug Auranofin (IC_{50} = 0.88±0.04 μM). Recently, the gold(I) complexes with the general composition $[Au(PPh_3)(Y)]$, where Y represents an *S*-coordinated thioamide ligand, showing remarkable cytotoxicity towards leiomyosarcoma cells with the IC_{50} values in the comparable range as **1**–**7** (0.7–2.1 μM) have been reported [41]. Complexes **1**–**8** additionally demonstrate the hormesis effect (higher viability; in this case up to 168%) around the concentration of 0.3 μM.

Based on the promising results for complexes **4**–**6** against all the three above mentioned cell lines, further testing was performed for these representatives on a panel of human cancer cell lines involving lung carcinoma (A549), malignant melanoma (G361), cervix epitheloid carcinoma (HeLa), ovarian carcinoma (A2780), ovarian carcinoma resistant to *cisplatin* (A2780R) and prostate carcinoma (22Rv1). The testing again revealed that the starting compounds (HL_n and AuCl, $HAuCl_4$) were not toxic in the tested concentration range, only a weak antiproliferative effect was observed for $HAuCl_4$ on the G361 cell line (38.1±0.8 μM). The IC_{50} values determined for **4**–**6** showed that viability of all the employed cell lines was reduced by the tested complexes comparably or better than by the metallodrug *cisplatin* (Table 3, Figure 5). Complexes **5** and **6** were significantly more *in vitro* antitumour active (ANOVA, $p<0.05$) against all the cell lines as compared with *cisplatin*, which is valid also for complex **4** with the exception of the G361 cells, against which its activity was found comparable with *cisplatin* (3.9±0.5 μM, and 5.3±0.2 μM, respectively). Focusing on individual cell lines, the lowest antiproliferative effect of **4**–**6** was observed for A549 and HeLa, which in the testing did not respond to the treatment by *cisplatin* up to 50 μM. The IC_{50} values for the tested Au(I) complexes showed moderate activity in the micromolar range (≈15–20 μM). On the other hand, low micromolar IC_{50} values (≈3–5 μM) resulted from the cytotoxicity testing against all the other cancer cell lines, *i.e.* G361, 22Rv1, A2780 as well as A2780R. It should be also pointed out that complexes **4**–**6** showed to be ca. 3-times (A2780), 5-times (A2780R) and 7-times (22Rv1) more effective than *cisplatin*. Moreover, the evaluation of cytotoxicity of **4**–**6** on both A2780 cell lines sensitive and resistant to *cisplatin* allowed the calculation of the resistance factors (RF), *i.e.* the ratio of IC_{50}(A2780R)/IC_{50}(A2780). The RF values are equal to 1.19 (**4**), 1.14 (**5**), 1.21 (**6**) and 2.25 (*cisplatin*), which unambiguously shows that **4**–**6** are able to circumvent the acquired resistance of cancer cells to *cisplatin*. It can be additionally pointed out that the tested complexes are comparably active on both A2780 and A2780R cell lines, as there is no statistically significant difference in their cytotoxic activity against these cancer cells (ANOVA, $p<0.001$).

In Vitro Anti-Inflammatory Activity

To evaluate the anti-inflammatory effect of the presented complexes *in vitro*, their ability to diminish the production of pro-inflammatory cytokines TNF-α and IL-1β in LPS-stimulated macrophages derived from the THP-1 cell line was determined. The results of this study showed that complexes **1**–**7** significantly decreased secretion of TNF-α in the LSP-stimulated cells, while complexes **8** and **9** exhibited no effect, as the extent of their influence on TNF-α secretion was comparable to the vehicle alone (0.1% DMSO) (Figure 6A). It is interesting to note, that the comparison of complexes **1**–**4** and their analogues **6**–**9** differing only in the substitution at C2 (hydrogen, and chlorine, respectively) showed that in all the cases, the complexes **1**–**4** were more effective in the TNF-α level attenuation. Moreover, all the active complexes (**1**–**7**) had comparable activity as the commercial reference drug Auranofin, but importantly they possessed a lower cytotoxic effect in the employed THP-1 cell line. To elucidate the role of each constituent part of the complexes (*N*-donor ligand, PPh_3 or gold(I) species) in diminishing TNF-α secretion, free hypoxanthine derivatives (HL_{1-9}), [AuCl(PPh_3)], PPh_3, and AuCl were also tested. It was found that none of these starting materials showed the anticipated effect. Moreover, the compound HL_7 significantly increased the production of TNF-α. These results indicated that in order to show the anti-inflammatory effect, the corresponding ligand has to be bonded into the Au(I)-complex. This observation is in agreement with the previous studies, where no anti-phlogistic effect was observed for free and uncoordinated purine-derived compounds applied as ligands in Au(III)-complexes [28].

The extent of the influence of complexes **1**–**9** on IL-1β secretion was very similar as for TNF-α (Figure 6B), but it should be noted that IL-1β production was affected slightly more than TNF-α. The same observation was also made in previous studies [15,43], which showed that the tested gold(I) complexes preferentially inhibit IL-1β production as compared to TNF-α. The results proved that similarly to TNF-α, compounds **1**–**7** significantly decreased the level of IL-1β, whereas complex **9** showed again no effect. The only difference as compared to the above-described TNF-α production influence study was found for complex **8**, which was inactive in the case of TNF-α secretion, but it significantly reduced the production of IL-1β. However, its inhibitory activity was still lower as compared with the activity of **1**–**7**. Testing of the constituent parts of the complexes as well as of starting materials revealed the element necessary for diminishing the production of IL-1β. The free HL_n molecules were again found to be inactive, with the exception of HL_6 which reduced the level of the cytokine significantly as compared with the vehicle-treated cells ($p<0.05$). On the other hand, unlike in the case of TNF-α, AuCl significantly decreased the level of this pro-inflammatory cytokine ($p<0.01$) as well as the [AuCl(PPh_3)] complex, which even curtailed its level as effectively as complexes **1**–**9**. These results indicate that the presence of the {Au-PPh_3} moiety in the complexes is crucial for the reduction of IL-1β secretion, but the coordinated *N*-donor organic ligand can dramatically change the activity of such a complex as it is visible on the example of the complexes **8** and **9** with low or no anti-inflammatory activity.

To determine whether the production of the pro-inflammatory cytokines TNF-α and IL-1β is regulated by a post-translation or post-transcription mechanism in the presence of the Au(I) complexes, the level of the corresponding mRNA was determined. The obtained results showed that selected representative complexes **2** and **7** were able to decrease the transcription of these cytokines after the LPS stimulation (Figure 7). This finding indicates that the target site for the Au(I) complexes should be up-stream the transcription, which is in accordance with previous studies [15,44].

The transcription of the cytokines TNF-α and IL-1β is controlled by transcription factor NF-κB. This protein is kept in cytoplasm by its inhibitor IκB. After the activation of the signalling pathway, this inhibitor is degraded [45]. Gold-containing compounds are known for their ability to inhibit this signalling pathway [46]. The results from the herein presented study are in agreement with the suggested mechanism. Complexes **2** and **7**, as well as Auranofin, were able to attenuate the degradation of IκB nonsignificantly (Figure S4 in File S1). This blocking of the NF-κB signalling pathway leads to lower transcription of TNF-α and IL-1β genes and thus, decreases their secretion.

Interactions with a Mixture of Cysteine and Glutathione Analysed by ESI-MS

As soft Lewis acids, Au(I) species prefer the formation of strong coordination bonds with soft Lewis base ligands, i.e. thiolate or selenolate ions, or phosphine derivatives, while the latter ones form the most stable bonds. It is a known fact, that Au(I) complexes behave likewise, as they bind to sulfanyl-containing substances, such as amino acid cysteine (Cys) or small proteins, such as glutathione (GSH), and with high molecular weight proteins (*e.g.* albumin or globulins [47]), in the biologically relevant environments (*i.e.* blood or serum) by the ligand exchange mechanism. The complexes formed this way can be considered as transport intermediates. The exchange of *N*-ligands for *S*-ligands occurs relatively quickly (within 20 minutes when interacting with albumin and globulins in the blood [48]), while the *P*-ligand exchange proceeds much more slowly. It seems that in this mechanism the cooperative effects of adjacent thiolato or selenolato ligands in the neighbourhood of the interaction site play an important role. In connection with the above mentioned, the ligand exchange is interpreted as one of the molecular mechanisms of incorporation of gold into the active site of selenium-containing flavoreductases, such as thioredoxin reductase [49]. In the scope of our work, we strived to uncover the molecular behaviour of selected complexes **1** and **6** (applied in the concentration of 20 μM, which approximately corresponds to the highest therapeutic blood levels of gold during chrysotherapy [50]) in biologically relevant conditions using a mixture of cysteine (at the 290 μM concentration) and reduced glutathione (at the 6 μM concentration) [36].

Based on the results of the ESI-MS experiments, we confirmed that both complexes **1** and **6** react with the used sulfhydryl-containing substances in time-independent manner by the ligand-exchange mechanism based on the substitution of the *N*-ligand (L_n) by the cysteine or glutathione molecule. This mechanism was confirmed by the emergence of ions at 1224.24 *m/z*, corresponding to the $[(Au\text{-}PPh_3)_2\text{+}GSH]^+$ intermediate, and an ion at 1355.25 *m/z*, corresponding to the ionic species $[Cys\text{+}(Au\text{-}PPh_3)_2\text{+}PPh_3\text{+}CH_3OH\text{+}Na]^+$ (see Figure 8). Unlike our previous reports on the biological activities of Au(I) complexes [15,16], in this interaction experiments we observed both the intermediates involving cysteine and glutathione molecules. This might indicate that the herein reported compounds are much more susceptible to the sulfur-containing molecules with several donor atoms, like glutathione.

In concordance with the above mentioned suggestion as well as in accordance with the previously reported behaviour of some Au(I) complexes in water-containing solutions [16], the mass spectra of the reacting systems involving sulfur-containing molecules and also the reference solutions of complexes revealed a considerable instability of the complexes demonstrated by the appearance of the intensive ion at 721.41 *m/z*, corresponding to the $[Au(PPh_3)_2]^+$ intermediate, and other ionic species involving the residue $Au\text{-}PPh_3$ (i.e. $[M\text{+}(Au\text{-}PPh_3)]^+$; 1081.33 *m/z* for complex **1**, and 1115.51 *m/z* for complex **6**), the free HL_n molecules ($[HL_1\text{+}H]^+$ at 165.10 *m/z* and ($[HL_6\text{+}H]^+$ at 199.12 *m/z*), or the free triphenylphosphine residue (i.e. $[PPh_3\text{+}H]^+$ at 263.24 *m/z* and $[Au\text{+}(PPh_3)_3\text{+}CH_3OH\text{+}Na]^+$ at 1038.30 *m/z*).

Conclusions

A series of gold(I) complexes of the general composition $[Au(L_n)(PPh_3)]$ (**1**–**9**), involving a combination of *N*-donor (HL_n) and *P*-donor triphenylphosphine ligands, was prepared and thoroughly characterized. The *in vitro* cytotoxicity results against a panel of nine human cancer cell lines (MCF7, HOS, A549, HeLa, A2780, A2780R, 22Rv1, G-361 and THP-1) revealed the complexes as more anticancer active than *cisplatin*, with the best $IC_{50} \approx 1\text{–}5$ μM. Moreover, the calculated resistance factors, i.e. the ratio of the IC_{50} values found for the *cisplatin* resistant and sensitive cell lines (A2780R)/IC_{50}(A2780) showed that the complexes are able to circumvent the acquired resistance of cancer cells to *cisplatin*, as the resistance factor values are equal to 1.19 (**4**), 1.14 (**5**), 1.21 (**6**) as compared to the value of 2.25 for *cisplatin*. Further, the complexes **1**–**9** were evaluated for their *in vitro* anti-inflammatory activity on the model of the LPS-activated THP-1 monocytes. It was found out that the complexes **1**–**7** exhibited the ability to influence the cell-cycle of THP-1 cells resulting in the hormetic effect, and they were also able to significantly attenuate the production of pro-inflammatory cytokines TNF-α and IL-1β at comparable levels as gold(I)-based reference drug Auranofin, but with lower toxicity than this metallodrug. Based on the results of the ESI-MS experiments may be concluded that representative complexes **1** and **6** react with the sulfur-containing substances (cysteine and reduced glutathione) in time-independent manner by the ligand-exchange mechanism based on the substitution of the *N*-ligand (L_n) by the cysteine or glutathione molecule.

Supporting Information

File S1 Supporting Information. The results of elemental analysis, FTIR, ^1H and ^{13}C NMR, and ESI–MS experiments for **1**–**9**. **Table S1.** Crystal data and structure refinements for [Au(L1)(PPh3)] (**1**) and [Au(L3)(PPh3)] (**3**). **Table S2.** Selected bond lengths and angles in complexes **1** and **3. Figure S1.** Parts of the crystal structure of complex $[Au(L_1)(PPh_3)]$ (**1**). **Table S3.** Selected non-covalent contacts and their parameters for **1. Figure S2.** Parts of the crystal structure of complex $[Au(L_3)(PPh_3)]$ (**3**). **Table S4.** Selected non-covalent contacts and their parameters for **3**. **Figure S3.** TG/DTA curves of the complexes **1** and **4**. **Figure S4.** Effects of the Au(I) complexes, and Auranofin on the LPS-induced degradation of IκB-α. **Figure S5.** ^{31}P NMR spectrum of complex **6**. (DOCX) CCDC Nos. 1010556 and 1010557 contain the supplementary crystallographic data for **1**, and **3**, respectively. These data can be obtained free of charge via http://www.ccdc.cam.ac.uk/conts/retrieving.html, or from the Cambridge Crystallographic Data Centre, 12 Union Road, Cambridge CB2 1EZ, UK; email: deposit@ccdc.cam.ac.uk.

Acknowledgments

The authors are grateful to Ms. Kateřina Kubešová for help with the cytotoxicity testing.

Author Contributions

Conceived and designed the experiments: RK J. Hosek JV ZD ZT. Performed the experiments: RK J. Hosek JV J. Hutyra ZD ZT. Analyzed the data: RK J. Hosek JV ZD ZT. Contributed to the writing of the manuscript: RK J. Hosek JV ZD ZT.

References

1. Berners-Price SJ (2011) Gold- Based Therapeutic Agents: A New Perspective. In: Bioinorganic Medicinal Chemistry. Alessio E, (Ed.). Weinheim: Wiley-VCH, Germany, 197–222.
2. Ho SI, Tiekink ERT (2005) Gold-Based Metallotherapeutics: Use and Potential. In: Metallotherapeutic Drugs and Metal-based Diagnostic Agents: The Use of Metals in Medicine. Gielen M, Tiekink ERT (Eds.). London: John Wiley and Sons, Ltd., England.
3. Shaw III CF (1999) Gold-Based Therapeutic Agents. Chem Rev 99: 2589–2600.
4. Berners-Price SJ, Filipovska A (2011) Gold compounds as therapeutic agents for human diseases. Metallomics 3: 863–873.

5. Sigler JW, Bluhm GB, Duncan H, Sharp JT, Ensign DC, et al. (1974) Gold Salts in the Treatment of Rheumatoid Arthritis: A Double-Blind Study. Ann Intern Med 80: 21−26.
6. Williams HJ, Ward JR, Reading JC, Brooks RH, Clegg DO, et al. (1992) Comparison of Auranofin, methotreaxate, and the combination of both in the treatment of rheumatoid arthritis. A controlled clinical trial. Arthritis Rheum 35: 259−269.
7. Kean WF, Hart L, Buchanan WW (1997) Auranofin. Br J Rheumatol 36: 560–572.
8. Madeira JM, Gibson DL, Kean WF, Klegeris A (2012) The biological activity of auranofin: implications for novel treatment of diseases. Inflammopharmacol 20: 297–306.
9. Rau R (2005) Have traditional DMARDs had their day? Effectiveness of parenteral gold compared to biologic agents. Clin Rheumatol 24: 189–202.
10. Ott I (2009) On the medicinal chemistry of gold complexes as anticancer drugs. Coord Chem Rev 253: 1670–1681.
11. Barreiro E, Casas JS, Couce MD, Sanchez-Gonzalez A, Sordo J, et al. (2008) Synthesis, structure and cytotoxicity of triphenylphosphinegold(I) sulfanylpropenoates. J Inorg Biochem 102: 184–192.
12. Ott I, Qian X, Xu Y, Kubutat D, Will J, et al (2009) A gold(I) phosphine complex containing naphthalimide ligand functions as a TrxR inhibiting antiproliferative agent and angiogenesis inhibitor. J Med Chem 52, 763–770.
13. Gallassi R, Burini A, Ricci S, Pellei M, Rigobello MP, et al. (2012) Synthesis and characterization of azolate gold(I) phosphane complexes as thioredoxin reductase inhibiting antitumor agents. Dalton Trans 41: 5307–5318.
14. Abbehausen C, Peterson EJ, de Paiva RE, Corbi PP, Formiqa AL, et al. (2013) Gold(I)-phosphine-N-heterocycles: biological activity and specific (ligand) interactions on the C-terminal HIVNCp7 zinc finger. Inorg Chem 52: 11280–11287.
15. Trávníček Z, Štarha P, Vančo J, Šilha T, Hošek J, et al. (2012) Anti-inflammatory Active Gold(I) Complexes Involving 6-substituted Purine Derivatives. J Med Chem 55: 4568–4579.
16. Hošek J, Vančo J, Štarha P, Paráková L, Trávníček Z (2013) Effect of 2-Chloro-Substitution of Adenine Moiety in Mixed-Ligand Gold(I) Triphenylphosphine Complexes on Anti-Inflammatory Activity: The Discrepancy between the In Vivo and In Vitro Models. PLoS ONE 8(11): e82441.
17. Craig S, Gao L, Lee I, Gray T, Berdis AJ (2012) Gold-Containing Indoles as Anticancer Agents That Potentiate the Cytotoxic Effects of Ionizing Radiation. J Med Chem 55: 2437–2451.
18. Gandin V, Fernandes AP, Rigobello MP, Dani B, Sorrentino F, et al. (2010) Cancer cell death induced by phosphine gold(I) compounds targeting thioredoxin reductase. Biochem Pharmacol 79: 90–101.
19. Gibson AE, Arris CE, Bentley J, Boyle FT, Curtin NJ, et al. (2002) Probing the ATP Ribose-Binding Domain of Cyclin-Dependent Kinases 1 and 2 with O6-Substituted Guanine Derivatives. J Med Chem 45: 3381–3393.
20. Arris CE, Boyle FT, Calvert AH, Curtin NJ, Endicott JA, et al. (2000) Identification of Novel Purine and Pyrimidine Cyclin-Dependent Kinase Inhibitors with Distinct Molecular Interactions and Tumor Cell Growth Inhibition Profiles. J Med Chem 43: 2797–2804.
21. Griffin RJ, Arris CE, Bleasdale C, Boyle FT, Calvert AH, et al. (2000) Resistance-Modifying Agents. 8. Inhibition of O6-Alkylguanine-DNA Alkyltransferase by O6-Alkenyl-, O6-Cycloalkenyl-, and O6-(2-Oxoalkyl)guanines and Potentiation of Temozolomide Cytotoxicity in Vitro by O6-(1-Cyclopentenylmethyl)guanine. J Med Chem 43: 4071–4083.
22. Schirrmacher R, Schirrmacher E, Mühlhausen U, Kaina B, Wängler B (2005) Synthetic Strategies Towards O^6-Substituted Guanine Derivatives and their Application in Medicine. Curr Org Synth 2: 215–230.
23. Štarha J, Hošek J, Vančo J, Dvořák Z, Suchý Jr P, et al. (2014) Pharmacological and Molecular Effects of Platinum(II) Complexes Involving 7-Azaindole Derivatives. PLoS ONE 9: e90341.
24. Vrzal R, Štarha P, Dvořák Z, Trávníček Z (2010) Evaluation of in vitro cytotoxicity and hepatotoxicity of platinum(II) and palladium(II) oxalato complexes with adenine derivatives as carrier ligands. J Inorg Biochem 104: 1130–1132.
25. Buchtík R, Trávníček Z, Vančo J (2012) In vitro cytotoxicity, DNA cleavage and SOD-mimic activity of copper(II) mixed-ligand quinolinonato complexes. J Inorg Biochem 116: 163–171.
26. Trávníček Z, Vančo J, Hošek J, Buchtík R, Dvořák Z (2012) Cellular responses induced by Cu(II) quinolinonato complexes in human tumor and hepatic cells. Chem Centr J 6: 160.
27. Trávníček Z, Matiková-Maľarová M, Novotná R, Vančo J, Štěpánková K, et al. (2011) In vitro and in vivo biological activity screening of Ru(III) complexes involving 6-benzylaminopurine derivatives with higher pro-apoptotic activity than NAMI-A. J Inorg Biochem 105: 937–948.
28. Křikavová R, Hošek J, Suchý P, Vančo J, Trávníček Z (2014) Diverse in vitro and in vivo anti-inflammatory effects of trichlorido-gold(III) complexes with N6-benzyladenine derivatives. J Inorg Biochem 134: 92–99.
29. Vančo J, Marek J, Trávníček Z, Račanská E, Muselík J, et al. (2008) Synthesis, structural characterization, antiradical and antidiabetic activities of copper(II) and zinc(II) Schiff base complexes derived from salicylaldehyde and beta-alanine. J Inorg Biochem 102: 595–605.
30. Mann FG, Wells AF, Purdie D (1937) The constitution of complex metallic salts. Part VI. The constitution of the phosphine and arsine derivatives of silver and aurous halides. The configuration of the coordinated argentous and aurous complex. J Chem Soc: 1828–1836.
31. Bruce MI, Nicholson BK, Shawkataly bin O, Shapley JR, Henly T (1989) Synthesis of gold-containing mixed-metal cluster complexes. Inorg Syn 26: 324–328.
32. Oxford Diffraction, CrysAlis RED and CrysAlis CCD Software (Ver. 1.171.33.52), Oxford Diffraction Ltd., Abingdon, Oxfordshire, UK.
33. Sheldrick GM (2008) Short History of SHELX. Acta Crystallogr, Sect A 64: 112–122.
34. Brandenburg K (2011) DIAMOND, Release 3.2i, Crystal Impact GbR, Bonn, Germany.
35. Macrae CF, Bruno IJ, Chisholm JA, Edgington PR, McCabe P, et al. (2008) Mercury CSD 2.0 - new features for the visualization and investigation of crystal structures. J Appl Cryst 41: 466–470.
36. Salemi G, Gueli MC, D'Amelio M, Saia V, Mangiapane P, et al. (2009) Blood levels of homocysteine, cysteine, glutathione, folic acid, and vitamin B12 in the acute phase of atherothrombotic stroke. Neurol Sci 30: 361–364.
37. Nakamoto K (1997) Infrared Spectra of Inorganic and Coordination Compounds, Part B, Applications in Coordination, Organometallic, and Bioinorganic Chemistry. Wiley, New York, USA.
38. Smith BC (1999) Infrared Spectral Interpretation: A Systematic Approach. CRC Press LLC, Florida, USA.
39. Faggianhi R, Howard-Locck HE, Lock CJL, Turner MA (1987) The reaction of chloro(triphenylphosphine)gold(I) with 1-methylthymine. Can J Chem 65: 1568–1575.
40. Allen FH (2002) The Cambridge Structural Database: a quarter of a million crystal structures and rising. Acta Crystallogr Sect B Struct Sci 58: 380–388.
41. Kouroulis KN, Hadjikakou SK, Kourkoumelis N, Kubicki M, Male L, et al. (2009) Synthesis, structural characterization and in vitro cytotoxicity of new Au(III) and Au(I) complexes with thioamides. Dalton Trans 47: 10446–10456.
42. Ott I, Schmidt K, Kircher B, Schumacher P, Wiglenda T, et al. (2005) Antitumor-Active Cobalt−Alkyne Complexes Derived from Acetylsalicylic Acid: Studies on the Mode of Drug Action. J Med Chem: 48 622–629.
43. Seitz M, Valbracht J, Quach J, Lotz M (2003) Gold sodium thiomalate and chloroquine inhibit cytokine production in monocytic THP-1 cells through distinct transcriptional and posttranslational mechanisms. J Clin Immunol 23: 477–484.
44. Han S, Kim K, Kim H, Kwon J, Lee YH, et al. (2008) Auranofin inhibits overproduction of pro-inflammatory cytokines, cyclooxygenase expression and PGE(2) production in macrophages. Arch Pharmacal Res 31: 67–74.
45. Hayden MS, Ghosh S (2008) Shared principles in NF-kappa B signaling. Cell 132: 344–362.
46. Jeon KI, Jeong JY, Jue DM (2000) Thiol-reactive metal compounds inhibit NF-kappa B activation by blocking I kappa B kinase. J Immunol 164: 5981–5989.
47. Shaw CF, Coffer MT, Klingbeil J, Mirabelli CK (1988) Application of phosphorus-31 NMR chemical shift: gold affinity correlation to hemoglobin-gold binding and the first inter-protein gold transfer reaction. J Am Chem Soc 110: 729–734.
48. Iqbal MS, Taqi SG, Arif M, Wasim M, Sher M (2009) In vitro distribution of gold in serum proteins after incubation of sodium aurothiomalate and auranofin with human blood and its pharmacological significance. Biol Trace Elem Res 130: 204–209.
49. Saccoccia F, Angelucci F, Boumis G, Brunori M, Miele AE, et al. (2012) On the mechanism and rate of gold incorporation into thiol-dependent flavoreductases. J Inorg Biochem 108: 105–111.
50. Lewis D, Capell HA, McNeil CJ, Iqbal MS, Brown DH, et al. (1983) Gold levels produced by treatment with auranofin and sodium aurothiomalate. Ann Rheum Dis 42: 566–570.

6

The Sensitivity of Cancer Cells to Pheophorbide a-Based Photodynamic Therapy Is Enhanced by *NRF2* Silencing

Bo-hyun Choi, In-geun Ryoo, Han Chang Kang, Mi-Kyoung Kwak*

College of pharmacy, The Catholic University of Korea, Bucheon, Gyeonggi-do, Republic of Korea

Abstract

Photodynamic therapy (PDT) has emerged as an effective treatment for various solid tumors. The transcription factor NRF2 is known to protect against oxidative and electrophilic stress; however, its constitutive activity in cancer confers resistance to anti-cancer drugs. In the present study, we investigated NRF2 signaling as a potential molecular determinant of pheophorbide a (Pba)-based PDT by using *NRF2*-knockdown breast carcinoma MDA-MB-231 cells. Cells with stable *NRF2* knockdown showed enhanced cytotoxicity and apoptotic/necrotic cell death following PDT along with increased levels of singlet oxygen and reactive oxygen species (ROS). A confocal microscopic visualization of fluorogenic Pba demonstrated that *NRF2*-knockdown cells accumulate more Pba than control cells. A subsequent analysis of the expression of membrane drug transporters showed that the basal expression of *BCRP* is NRF2-dependent. Among measured drug transporters, the basal expression of breast cancer resistance protein (BCRP; ABCG2) was only diminished by *NRF2*-knockdown. Furthermore, after incubation with the BCRP specific inhibitor, differential cellular Pba accumulation and ROS in two cell lines were abolished. In addition, *NRF2*-knockdown cells express low level of peroxiredoxin 3 compared to the control, which implies that diminished mitochondrial ROS defense system can be contributing to PDT sensitization. The role of the NRF2-BCRP pathway in Pba-PDT response was further confirmed in colon carcinoma HT29 cells. Specifically, *NRF2* knockdown resulted in enhanced cell death and increased singlet oxygen and ROS levels following PDT through the diminished expression of BCRP. Similarly, PDT-induced ROS generation was substantially increased by treatment with *NRF2* shRNA in breast carcinoma MCF-7 cells, colon carcinoma HCT116 cells, renal carcinoma A498 cells, and glioblastoma A172 cells. Taken together, these results indicate that the manipulation of NRF2 can enhance Pba-PDT sensitivity in multiple cancer cells.

Editor: Michael Hamblin, MGH, MMS, United States of America

Funding: This research was supported by the National Research Foundation (NRF) funded by the Ministry of Science, ICT and Future Planning (NRF-2013R1A2A2A01015497). The funders had no role in study design, data collection and analysis, decision to publish, or preparation of the manuscript.

Competing Interests: The authors have declared that no competing interests exist.

* Email: mkwak@catholic.ac.k

Introduction

Photodynamic therapy (PDT) has emerged as an efficient treatment for several solid tumors [1–3]. PDT requires three elements: i) a photosensitizer that can be selectively targeted to tumor tissues, ii) an appropriate light source that emits low-energy and tissue-penetrating light, and iii) molecular oxygen [4]. The first step of PDT is activation of a photosensitizer by light. When the activated photosensitizer in its excited state returns to its ground state, it transfers its energy to oxygen and generates singlet oxygen ($^1O_2$), a highly reactive and short-lived reactive oxygen species (ROS), as a type II reaction. At the same time, the activated photosensitizer can react directly with cellular components and transfers a hydrogen atom forming radicals, which eventually produces oxidation products through the reaction with oxygen (type I reaction) [5]. Singlet oxygen and ROS are highly oxidizing molecules; therefore PDT-treated cells undergo cell death through both necrosis and apoptosis [6]. In addition to its direct effect on tumor cells, PDT affects the tumor's microenvironment by destroying its microvasculature and by enhancing inflammatory responses and tumor-specific immune responses [4,7,8].

Pheophorbide a (Pba) is a product of chlorophyll breakdown, which is isolated from silkworm excreta [9] and Chinese medicinal herb *Scutellaria barbarta* [10]. Pba absorbs light at longer wavelengths than the first-generation photosensitizer photofrin. The maximum wavelength Pba is 666 nm, whereas that of photofrin is 630 nm [11]. Because tissue penetration is enhanced by longer wavelengths, Pba has been considered as a photosensitizer for the treatment of large tumors in the peritoneal cavity [12]. Similar to photofrin, Pba induces apoptosis and necrosis in pancreatic carcinoma, leukemia, and hepatocellular carcinoma cells [13–15]. In uterine carcinoma cells, the underlying mechanism of apoptosis is Pba accumulation in the mitochondria, which leads to the generation of ROS and release of cytochrome c [16,17]. Similarly, Pba causes mitochondria-dependent apoptosis in breast carcinoma MCF-7 cells [18]. Several *in vivo* animal studies have supported the efficacy of Pba-PDT in preventing tumorigenesis. For instance, a liposomal preparation of Pba-PDT delayed tumor growth in a colon carcinoma HT29 xenograft [19]. Intravenous administration of 0.3 mg/kg Pba followed by light irradiation significantly inhibited tumor growth in nude mice harboring a human hepatoma xenograft [11].

One factor determining the efficacy of PDT is the expression of ATP-binding cassette (ABC) transporters in the target tissue. These transporters control the intracellular accumulation of foreign chemicals by actively transporting them out of the cell [20]. The breast cancer resistance protein (BCRP or ABCG2) is an ABC transporter that was originally identified in doxorubicin-resistant breast cancer cells [21]. Overexpression of BCRP in tumors confers resistance to chemotherapy [22]. In addition to anti-cancer drugs, BCRP has been shown to transport porphyrin-type photosensitizers. Specifically, HEK cells overexpressing BCRP were resistant to Pba-induced cytotoxicity [23]. At the same time, *bcrp*-knockout mice were highly susceptible to dietary Pba-induced skin phototoxicity [24].

The transcription factor NF-E2-related factor 2 (NRF2) is a member of the cap'n'collar family of basic leucine-zipper (CNC-bZIP) transcription factors [25]. NRF2 activity is primarily regulated by the cytoplasmic protein Kelch-like ECH-associated protein 1 (KEAP1) [26,27]. Through binding to the Neh2 domain of NRF2, KEAP1 mediates ubiquitinylation and subsequent proteasomal degradation of NRF2. Under conditions of oxidative and electrophilic stress, NRF2 is liberated from KEAP1 and translocates into the nucleus, resulting in the transcription of multiple target genes that encode detoxifying enzymes, antioxidant proteins, stress-response proteins, and drug transporters [28–30]. Because its target genes have cytoprotective effects, NRF2 is considered as a critical player in the defense system against oxidative and electrophilic stress [31]. Accordingly, several studies have shown that genetic deletion of *nrf2* is associated with increased susceptibility to tissue damage and injury resulting from environmental and endogenous stressors [28,31,32]. On the other hand, increasing evidence suggests that cancer cells exploit the NRF2 system for survival by adapting to the stressful tumor microenvironment [33]. NRF2 signaling is constitutively activated in several tumor types and cultured cancer cell lines, which is associated with increased tumor growth and resistance to chemotherapeutic agents. In cancer cells, NRF2 signaling is up-regulated after exposure to chemotherapeutic drugs, which confers acquired resistance to chemotherapy [34–36]. Similarly, PDT with hypericin in human bladder carcinoma cells resulted in elevated expression of nuclear NRF2 protein and heme oxygenase-1 (HO-1) through $p38^{MAPK}$ and PI3K pathways [37]. Treatment of HepG2 cells with a non-toxic concentration of Pba followed by photo activation for 90 min resulted in increased expression of BCRP and heme oxygenase-1 (HO-1) in a NRF2-dependent manner [38].

In the present study, we investigated NRF2 as a novel molecular determinant of PDT efficacy. Because NRF2 regulates the expression of ROS-counteracting components and several drugs transporters, we hypothesized that manipulating NRF2 expression would enhance the efficacy of PDT. To test this hypothesis, we established stable *NRF2*-knockdown cell lines using human breast carcinoma MDA-MB-231 cells and colon carcinoma HT29 cells, and measured PDT sensitivity. Our results showed that *NRF2* knockdown enhances PDT-induced cell death by increasing the production of ROS. As an underlying mechanism, BCRP expression was repressed by *NRF2* knockdown, leading to increased cellular accumulation of Pba and increased production of singlet oxygen.

Materials and Methods

Materials

Pba was from Santa Cruz Biotechnology (Santa Cruz, CA, USA). NRF2 antibody was obtained from Abcam (Cambridge, MA, USA). Antibodies recognizing AKR1C1 and BCRP were purchased from Abnova (Taipei City, Taiwan) and Cell Signaling Technology (Beverly, MA, USA), respectively. PRDX3 and β-tubulin antibodies were obtained from Santa Cruz Biotechnology. Ko143, 3-(4,5-dimethylthiazol-2-yl)-2,5-diphenyltetrazolium bromide (MTT), and puromycin were obtained from Sigma-Aldrich (Saint Louis, MO, USA). 5(6)-Carboxy-2′,7′-dichlorofluorescein diacetate (DCFDA), trans-1-(2′methoxyvinyl) pyrene, and Mito-Green were purchased from Life Technologies (Carlsbad, CA, USA). The lentiviral system containing a pre-designed human *NRF2* shRNA and nonspecific scrambled RNA (scRNA) was bought from Sigma-Aldrich.

Cell culture

The human breast cancer cell line MDA-MB-231 and MCF-7, colon cancer cell line HT29 and HCT116, and human renal carcinoma A498 were obtained from American Type Culture Collection (Rockville, MD, USA). The human glioblastoma cell line A172 was purchased from Korean Cell Line Bank (Seoul, South Korea). MDA-MB-231, MCF7, A498, A172, and HCT116 were maintained in a medium containing Dulbecco's Modified Eagle Medium and Nutrient Mixture F-12 (Hyclone, Utah, USA) in the ratio of 1:1 supplemented with 10% fetal bovine serum (Hyclone) and penicillin/streptomycin (WelGene Inc., Daegu, South Korea). HT29 was maintained in RPMI-1640 medium (Hyclone) with 10% FBS and penicillin/streptomycin. The cells were grown at 37°C in a humidified 5% CO_2 atmosphere.

Production of lentiviral particles containing *NRF2* shRNA expression plasmid

Lentiviral particles with shRNA were produced in HEK 293T cells following the transfection of cells with *NRF2* shRNA expression plasmid and the packaging mix (Sigma-Aldrich) as described previously [36]. Briefly, HEK 293T cells were seeded in 60 mm plates at a density of 7×10^5 cells per well. The next day, medium was replaced by OptiMEM (Life Technologies) and subsequently, 1.5 μg pLKO.1-NRF2 shRNA, which contains the human *NRF2*-specific shRNA (5′-CCGGGCTCCTACTGT-GATGTGAAATCTCGAGATTTCACATCACAGTAGGA-3′), and the packaging mix were transfected into cells using Lipofectamine 2000 (Life Technologies). The pLKO.1-scRNA plasmid was used as a nonspecific control RNA. On the second day, after the removal of transfection complex, the complete medium was added into each well. Media containing lentiviral particles were harvested after 4 days.

Establishment of *NRF* knockdown cell line

MDA-MB-231 cells in 6-well plate were incubated with lentiviral particles containing either scRNA or NRF2 shRNA expression plasmid. After a 48 h-incubation, cells were recovered in the complete medium and the puromycin (1 μg/ml) selection was followed for up to 4 weeks. The *NRF2* knockdown HT29 cell line was established as previously reported [39].

Transient knockdown of NRF2

MCF-7, HCT116, A172 and A498 cells were seeded in 6-well plates at a density of 1×10^5 cells/well and grown for overnight. Next day, the cells were incubated with cholesterol for 15 min and then, the lentiviral particle containing scRNA or shNRF2 were added to each well. After 48 h incubation, viral particle-containing media were removed and cells were recovered in the fresh medium for overnight.

PDT and MTT analysis

MDA-MB-231 and HT29 were seeded at a density of 7×10^3 cells/well in 96-well plates and incubated for 20 h. The cells were treated with Pba (0–2.5 μg/ml) for 6 h and then irradiated with 0.3 (HT29) or 0.6 J/cm^2 (MDA-MB-231) laser in the absence of Pba. For the laser irradiation, the 670 nm LED Hybrid Lamp system (Quantum Spectra Life, Barneveld, WI) was used. The cells were recovered in complete medium for 18 h and incubated with MTT for 4 h. After removal of the MTT solution, 100 μl of dimethyl sulfoxide (DMSO) was added to each well and the absorbance was measured at 570 nm using a Spectro-star Nano microplate reader (BMG Labtechnologies, Offenburg, Germany).

Cytotoxicity measurement

Cytotoxicity by PDT was assessed using CytoTox-Fluor assay system (Promega, Madison, WI, USA). After PDT, cells were maintained for 24 h and then 50 μl bis-AAF-R110 substrate was added to each well. Substrate containing solution was incubated for a further 2 h with orbital shaking at 37°C. Intensities of fluorescence were measured using a SpectraMax M5 (Molecular Devices, Sunnyvale, CA) at the 485 nm Ex/520 nm Em.

Total RNA extraction and real-time PCR analysis

Total RNAs were isolated from cells using a Trizol reagent (Life Technologies). For the synthesis of cDNAs, reverse transcriptase (RT) reactions were performed by incubating 200 ng of total RNA with a reaction mixture containing 0.5 μg/μl oligo dT_{12-18} and 200 U/μl Moloney Murine Leukemia Virus RT (Life Technologies). For the real-time polymerase-chain reaction (PCR) analysis, Roche LightCycler (Mannheim, Germany) was used with the Takara SYBR Premix ExTaq system (Otsu, Japan). Primers were synthesized by Bioneer (Daejeon, South Korea) and the primer sequences for the human genes are: *NRF2*, 5′-ATAGCT-GAGCCCAGTATC-3′ and 5′-CATGCACGTGAGTGCTCT-3′; *HO-1*, 5′-GCTGCTGACCCATGACACCAAGG-3′ and 5′-AAGGACCCATCGGAGAAGCG-GAG-3′; aldo-keto reductase 1C1 (*AKR1C1*), 5′-CGAGAAGAACCATGGGTGGA-3′ and 5′-GGCCACAAA-GGACTGGGTCC-3′; NAD(P) quinone oxidoreductase-1 (*NQO1*), 5′- CAGTGGTTTGGAGTCCCTGCC-3′ and 5′-TCCCCGTGGATCCCTTGCAG-3′; the catalytic subunits of γ-glutamate cysteine ligase (*GCLC*), 5′-TGAAGGGA-CACCAGGACAGCC-3′ and 5′-GCAGTGTGAACCCAGGA-CAGC-3′; epoxide hydrolase-1 (*EPHX1*), 5′-GCCTGCACTT-GAACATGGCT-3′ and 5′-ATGTGCATGTAGCCGCTCTC-3′; superoxide dismutase 1 (*SOD1*), 5′-GATTCCATGTTCAT-GAGTTT-3′ and 5′-AGGATAACAGATGAGTTAAG-3′; *SOD 2*, 5′-AACCTCACATCAACGCGCAGAT-3′and 5′-TCAGTG-CAGGCTGAAGAGCTAT-3′; catalase (*CAT*), 5′- GTGCATG-CAGGACAATCAGG-3′ and 5′-GAATGCCCGCACCTGAG-TAA-3′; peroxiredoxin 3 (*PRDX3*), 5′- GCCGTTGTCAATG-GAGAGTTC-3′ and 5′-GCAAGATGGCTAAAGTGGGAA-3′; *PRDX5*, 5′- GGTGGCCTGTCTGAGTGTTA-3′ and 5′- ACC-ACCATGGAGAACCTCTTG-3′; glutathione peroxidase 1 (*GP X1*), 5′-TTCCCGTGCAACCAGTTTG-3′ and 5′-TTCACCT-CGCACTTCTCGAA-3′; *GPX4*, 5′-TCACCAAGTTCCTCA-TCGACA-3′ and 5′- GCCACACACTTGTGGAGCTA-3′; glutathione reductase (*GSR*), 5′-ACCCCGATGTATCACGCAG-TTA-3′ and 5′-TGTCAAAGTCTGCCTTCGTTGC-3′; glutaredoxin 2 (*GLRX2*), 5′-GTATTGCTCTCCATCCTCCTCG-3′ and 5′- CTGGGAGCCTTTATGAGCGT-3′. thioredoxin-2 (*TX N2*), 5′-CACACCACTGTGCGTGGAAA-3′ and 5′-ACTGTA-ACACCCAACCCAGC-3′; breast cancer resistance protein (*BC RP/ABCG2*), 5′- CACAACCATTGCATCTTGGCTG-3′ and 5′- TGAGAGATCGATGCCCTGCTTT-3′; multidrug resistance protein 1 (*MDR1/ABCB1*), 5′-CTATGCTGGATGTT-TCCGGT-3′ and 5′-TCTTCACCTGGCTCAGT-3′; multidrug resistance-associated protein 1 (*MRP1/ABCC1*), 5′-AGCTTTA-TGCCTGGGAGCTGGC-3′ and 5′-CGGCAAATGTG- CA-CAAGGCCAC-3′; *MRP2/ABCC2*, 5′-GCTGCCACACTTCA-GGCTCT-3′ and 5′-GGCAGCCAGCAGTGAAAAGC-3′; *MR P3/ABCC3*, 5′-ATACGCTCGCCACAGT-CCTT-3′ and 5′-GCTGGCCATGATGACCACAA-3′; *MRP4/ABCC4*, 5′-CTT-G- GATCGCAA-TACCCTTG-3′ and 5′-GACACCTCTCT-TCTGCTTTG-3′; *MRP5/ABCC5*, 5′-CAGAGACCGTGAA-GATTCCA-3′ and 5′-TTTGGAAGTAGTCCGGATGG-3′; *M RP6/ABCC6*, 5′-TGTGTGGCTCACCACGATG-3′ and 5′-C-ATAGGTAG- GTGGACAG-GTGG-3′; organic cation transporter novel 1 (*OCTN1;* SLC22A4), 5′-GCTGTATGTCTT-CACTGCTG-3′ and 5′-GGTGAGGATTCCAATCAGGA-3′; *OCTN2* (*SLC22A5*), 5′-ATTGTTGTGCCTTCCACTATC-3′ and 5′-GGTCATCCACAGCATTATGG-3′; multidrug and toxin extrusion transporter 2 (*MATE2*; *SLC47A2*), 5′-TTCATTC-CAGGACTTCCGGTG-3′ and 5′-AGGTGTGAGTGAGATG-GATGG-3′; hypoxanthine phosphoribosyltransferase-1 (HPRT1), 5′-TGGCGTCGTGATTAGTGATG-3′ and 5′-GCTACAATG-TG-ATGGCCTCC-3′.

Measurement of singlet oxygen

The cells were seeded in a cover glass dish (SPL Life science, Gyeonggi-do, South Korea) and cultured for overnight. After the Pba-laser irradiation, the cells were washed with PBS and incubated with 50 μM trans-1-(2′methoxyvinyl) pyrene (Life Technologies) for 30 min. For the nuclei staining, Hoechst 33342 (H342) was added to the above dishes and incubated for 10 min. Green fluorescence from singlet oxygen was detected immediately using a LSM 710 confocal microscope (Carl Zeiss, Jena, Germany) and intensities were quantified using a ZEN2011 software (Carl Zeiss).

Measurement of intracellular ROS

Cellular ROS levels were examined using a cell-permeable fluorogenic probe, carboxy-H_2DCFDA. The cells were seeded in a cover glass bottom dish (SPL Life science) and further incubated for overnight. After the Pba-laser therapy, cells were washed with PBS and incubated with 30 μM of carboxy-H_2DCFDA for 30 min at 37°C. For the nuclei staining, H342 was incubated for 10 min. Then confocal images were obtained and green fluorescent intensities were quantified using a LSM 710 confocal microscope and ZEN2011 software.

Measurement of Pba accumulation

Pba is a fluorogenic substance; therefore the level of intracellular accumulation of Pba was determined by measuring red fluorescence in the cell. MDA-MB-231 and HT29 on cover glass slides were incubated with Pba for 6 h. Then, Pba was removed and PBS washes were followed. Intensities of Pba red fluorescence were quantified in confocal images using ZEN2011 software. As an alternative way for quantification, cells were seeded in 96-well plates (BD Biosciences) and incubated with Pba for 6 h. After the cell wash, Pba red fluorescence was detected using a CellInsight Personal Cell Imager (Thermo Fisher Scientific, Waltham, MA, USA) and intensities were quantified by CellInsight software (Thermo Fisher Scientific).

Fluorometric determination of intracellular Pba

Cells in 96-well plates were incubated with Pba for 6 h and then were lysed using 1% SDS after PBS wash. DMSO was added to

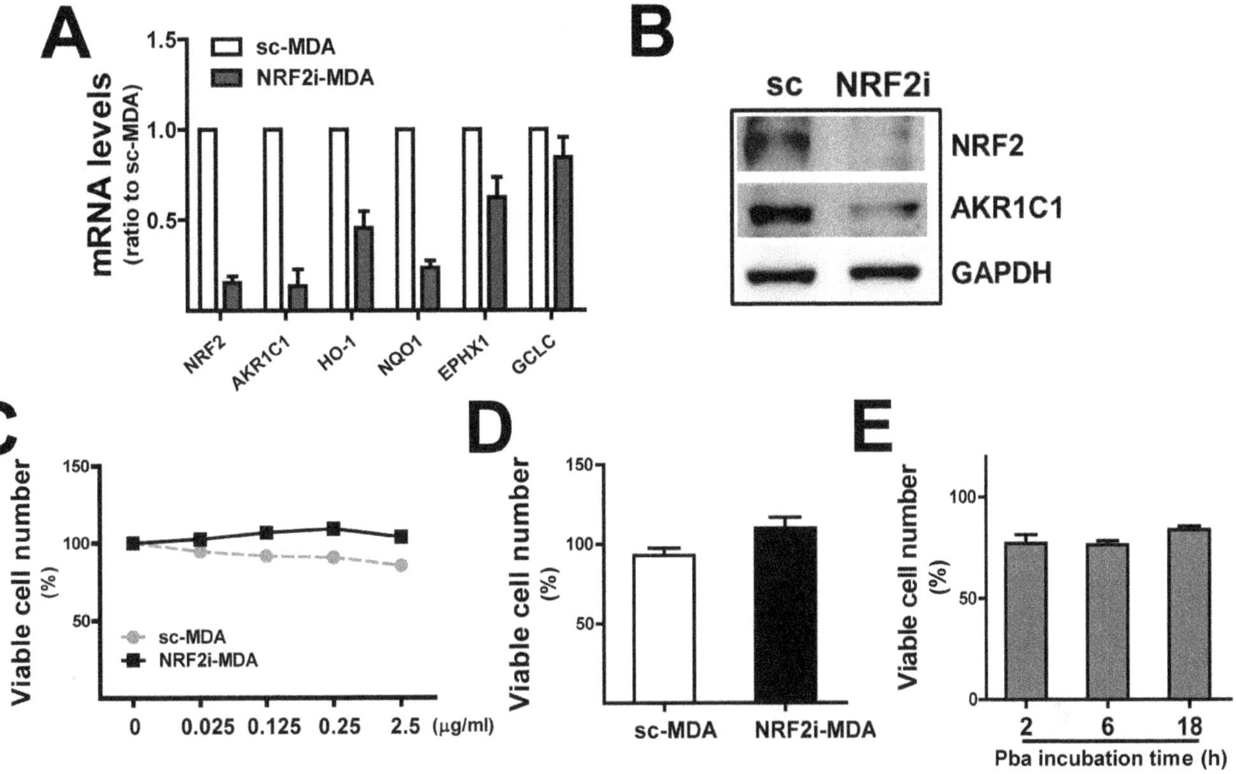

Figure 1. Effect of Pba and laser irradiation on MDA-MB-231. (A) Transcript levels of *NRF2*, *AKR1C1*, and *HO-1* were measured in the control (sc-MDA) and *NRF2*-knockdown cells (NRF2i-MDA) using relative quantification of real-time PCR. HPRT1 was used as a housekeeping control gene. Data represent ratios with respect to sc-MDA and are reported as mean ± standard deviations (SDs) of 3 experiments. (B) Protein levels of NRF2 and AKR1C1 were determined by Western blot analysis in the sc control and NRF2i-MDA cells. (C) The sc-MDA and NRF2i-MDA cells were incubated with Pba (0–2.5 μg/mL) for 6 h, and viable cells were quantified using an MTT assay after an 18 h recovery. (D) Cells were irradiated by a laser in the absence of Pba, and viable cells were quantified using an MTT assay after an 18 h recovery. (E) The sc-MDA was incubated with Pba for 2, 6, or 18 h and viable cell number was determined after laser irradiation. The data represent percentages with respect to the vehicle group for each cell line and are reported as the mean ±SD of 8 wells.

cell lysates to dissolve cellular Pba and fluorescence intensity was measured using a SpectraMax M5 at the 415 nm Ex/673 nm Em.

Western blot analysis

Cells were lysed with RIPA buffer (50 mM Tris [pH 7.4], 150 mM NaCl, 1 mM EDTA, and 1% nonyl phenoxypolyethoxylethanol 40) containing a protease inhibitor cocktail (Sigma-Aldrich). For BCRP protein extraction, 0.1% SDS was added to RIPA buffer. The protein concentration was determined using a DC protein assay kit (Bio-Rad, Hercules, CA, USA). The protein samples were separated by electrophoresis on 12% SDS-polyacrylamide gels and transferred to nitrocellulose membranes (Whatman, Dassel, Germany). Then, the membrane was blocked with 5% skim milk or 3% bovine serum albumin for 1 h and incubated with antibodies. The chemiluminescence images were captured using a Fujifilm LAS-4000 mini imager (Fujifilm, Tokyo, Japan) and intensities were quantified with corresponding software.

Flow cytometry

The NRFi-MDA cells were seeded in 60 cm^2 dishes at a density of 1×10^5 cells/well and cultured overnight. After the Pba-laser irradiation, the cells were trypsinized and spun down at 15,000 rpm for 10 min at 4°C. Then, 2×10^5 cells were transferred to 1.5 ml tube for centrifugation at 8,000 *g* for 5 min at 4°C. Then, 5 μl of fluorochrome conjugated Annexin V (BioLegend, San Diego, CA, USA) and 10 μl of propidium iodide (PI, BioLegend) solution were added into each tube and incubated with gentle vortex. The cells were incubated for 15 min at room temperature in the dark and then, 400 ul of Annexin V binding buffer (BioLegend) was added to each tube. Stained cells were analyzed using a Becton-Dickinson FACS Canto (SanJose, CA, USA) with and data were analyzed with FACSDiva software (BD).

Statistical analysis

Statistical significance was determined by a Student paired t-test followed or a one-way analysis of variance (one-way ANOVA) followed by the Student Newman–Keuls test for multiple comparisons using GraphPad Prism software (La Jolla CA, USA).

Results

Pba cytotoxicity is enhanced by *NRF2* knockdown in MDA-MB-231 breast cancer cells

In order to investigate the involvement of NRF2 in the efficacy of Pba-PDT for breast cancer, we established an *NRF2*-knockdown breast carcinoma cell line in MDA- MB-231 cells. Stable cell lines expressing nonspecific scrambled RNA (sc-MDA) or *NRF2*-specific shRNA (NRF2i-MDA) were attained from puromycin selection for 4 weeks. The expression levels of NRF2 and its target genes were evaluated in these cell lines. NRF2i-MDA cells showed an 85% reduction in *NRF2* mRNA and substantial decreases in expression of the NRF2 targets *AKR1C1*

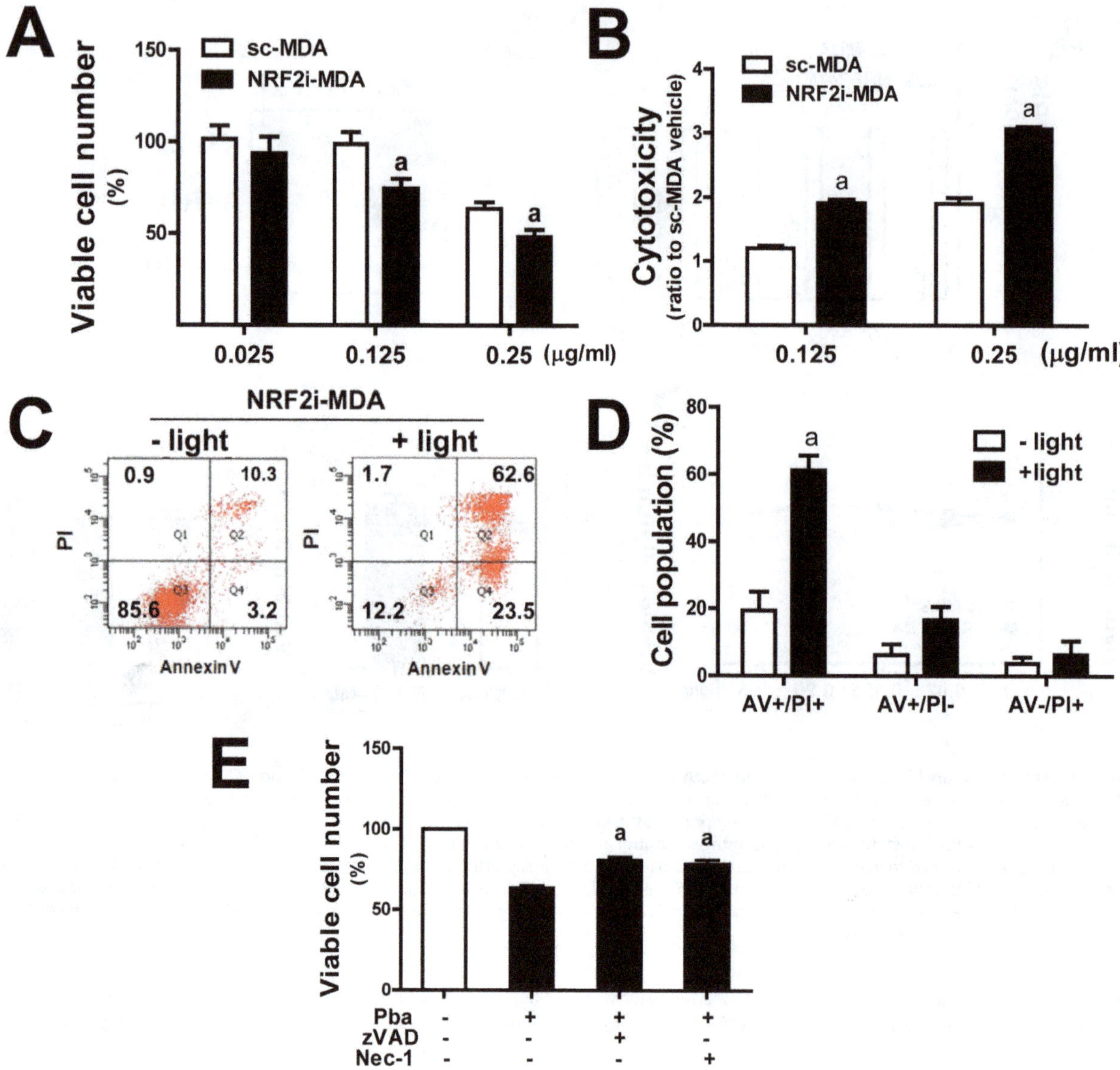

Figure 2. Effect of *NRF2* knockdown on Pba-laser treatment-induced cytotoxicity in MDA-MB-231. (A) The sc control and NRF2i-MDA cells were pre-incubated with Pba (0–2.5 μg/mL) for 6 h and were then irradiated by 0.6 J/cm^2 laser. Then MTT analysis was performed following an 18 h recovery. The data represent percentages with respect to the vehicle group for each cell line and are reported as the mean ±SD of 8 wells. [a]$P<0.05$ as compared with the sc-MDA control at each concentration of Pba. (B) PDT-induced cytotoxicity was assessed by measuring dead cell protease activity in a cell cultured medium. Cells were incubated with Pba (0.125 and 0.25 μg/mL) for 6 h followed by laser irradiation, and incubated for 18 h. Dead cell derived protease activity was determined using fluorogenic substrate AAF-R110. The data represent relative cytotoxicity with respect to the vehicle group for each cell line and are reported as the mean ±SD of 8 wells. [a]$P<0.05$ as compared with each sc-MDA control. (C) A flow cytometric analysis of apoptotic and necrotic cells was performed in NRF2i-MDA cells after Pba-laser treatment. The cells were incubated with PI and Annexin V, and cell populations were assessed. (D) The bar graph represents cell population in Annexin V (AV)+/PI+, AV+/PI-, or AV-/PI+ phase from three separate experiments. [a]$P<0.05$ as compared with no laser control. (E) NRF2i-MDA cells were co-incubated with Z-VAD-FMK (10 μM) or necrostatin (Nec-1, 50 μM) and Pba (0.125 μg/mL) for 6 h; then, cells were washed with PBS and irradiated with a laser. After 18 h incubation, viable cells were quantified using an MTT assay. The data are percentages with respect to the control (no PDT and vehicle treatment) and are reported as the mean ±SD of 8 wells. [a]$P<0.05$ as compared with the control.

and *HO-1* (Fig. 1A). Western blot analysis showed that proteins levels of NRF2 and AKR1C are substantially diminished in knockdown cells (Fig. 1B). These confirm the successful inhibition of NRF2 signaling in established stable cell line. Next, we examined the sensitivity of *NRF2*-knockdown MDA-MB-231 cells to the Pba and laser combination therapy. Without laser irradiation, incubation of sc-MDA and NRF2i-MDA cells with Pba (0.025–2.5 μg/mL, 24 h) did not significantly affect cell viability (Fig. 1C). Similarly, laser irradiation without Pba incubation did not affect cell viability (Fig. 1D). To assess PDT sensitivity, cells were irradiated with a 0.6-J/cm^2 laser after incubation with Pba and MTT analysis was performed following 18 h recovery. Initially, PDT effect was evaluated with varied incubation times of Pba. The incubation of Pba (0.125 μg/mL) for 2, 6, and 18 h showed similar cytotoxicity in the sc control cells (Fig. 1E). Based on this result, the 6 h-incubation of Pba was maintained in this study.

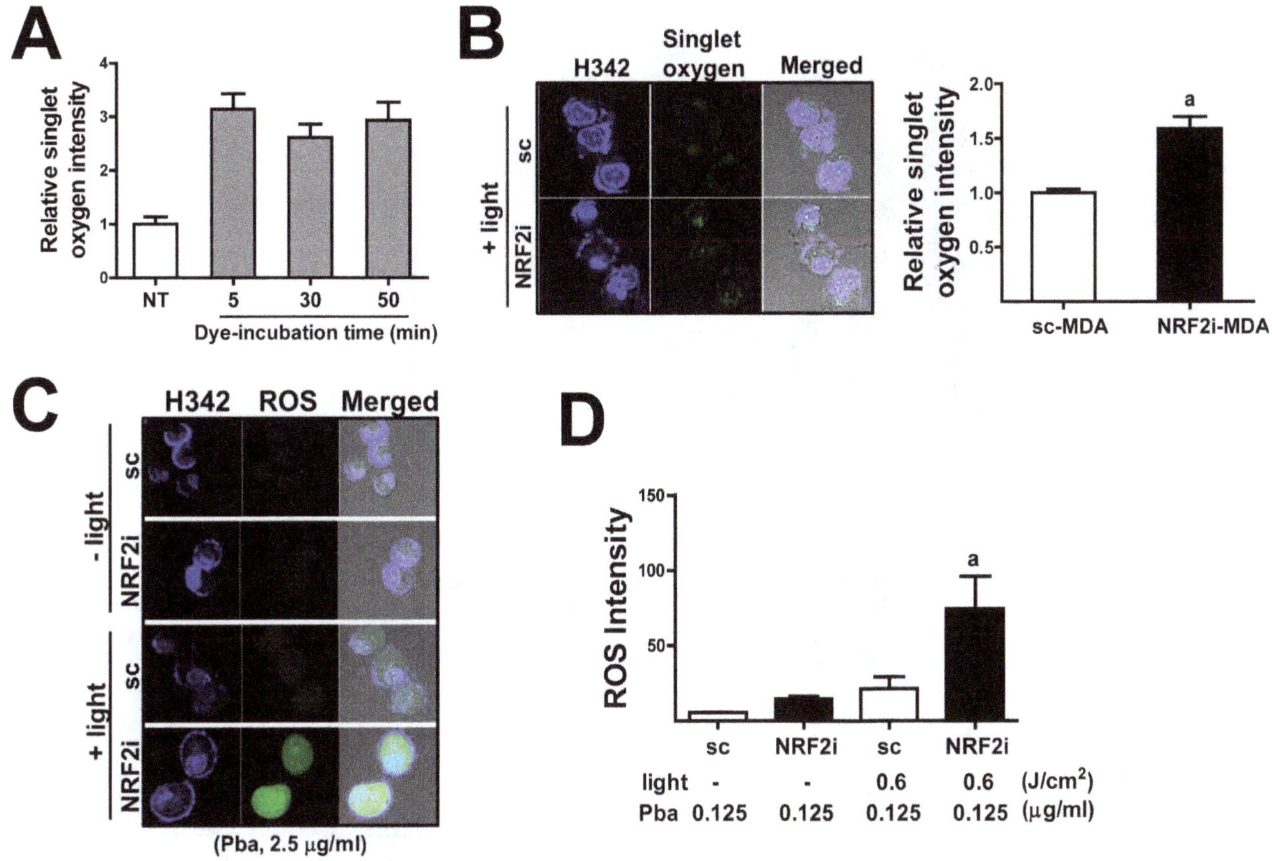

Figure 3. Singlet oxygen and ROS are elevated in *NRF2*-knockdown MDA-MB-231 cells. (A) The sc control cells were incubated with Pba for 6 h and irradiated by a 0.6 J/cm^2 laser. Right after PDT, a singlet oxygen sensitive trans-1-(2′methoxyvinyl) pyrene was added and cells were further incubated for 5, 30, or 50 min in the presence of trans-1-(2′methoxyvinyl) pyrene. Then confocal observation was performed to detect fluorogenic dye formation, which was formed by the reaction with singlet oxygen. (B) The sc and NRF2i cells were incubated with trans-1-(2′methoxyvinyl) pyrene for 30 min following PDT. Then confocal microscopic detection of singlet oxygen-derived fluorogenic pyrene was carried out. Green fluorescence from singlet oxygen reacted pyrene was quantified using a ZEN 2011 software. The data represent ratios with respect to sc-MDA cells and are reported as the mean ±SD of 3 experiments. [a]$P<0.05$ as compared with the sc-MDA control. Hoechst 33342 (H342) presents nuclear staining. ×100 magnification (C–D) The sc- and NRF2i-MDA cells were incubated with 2.5 μg/mL (C) or 0.125 μg/mL Pba (D) for 6 h and irradiated by a 0.6 J/cm^2 laser. Then, cells were incubated with DCFHA for 30 min, and ROS-derived green fluorescence was detected using a confocal microscope. The data represent ratios with respect to sc-MDA control cells treated with Pba only and are reported as the mean ±SD of 3 experiments. [a]$P<0.05$ as compared with sc-MDA with Pba and laser irradiation. ×100 magnification.

In MTT analysis, the NRF2-MDA cells were relatively more sensitive to Pba-based PDT: viable cell number after PDT was lower in the NRF2i-MDA cells than that in the control cells (Fig. 2A). Similarly, when dead cell-derived peptidase activity was measured in the medium using a CytoTox substrate *NRF2* knockdown cells showed a significantly high cytotoxicity compared to the sc control (Fig. 2B).

PDT induces cell death through apoptotic and necrotic pathways [6,40]. Next, in order to identify the mechanism of cell death involved in PDT-treated *NRF2* knockdown breast cancer cells, FACS analysis with Annexin V and PI double staining was performed. NRF2i-MDA cells were treated with PDT; immediately thereafter, cells were trypsinized and stained with Annexin V (early apoptosis marker) and PI (late apoptosis and necrosis marker). After Pba-laser combination treatment, the majority cell population shifted to the apoptotic-necrotic phase (Fig. 2C). Quantification of experimental repeats showed that 16.7% of cells were in the early apoptotic phase (Annexin V+/PI-) and 61.3% of cells were in the late apoptotic/necrotic phase (Annexin V+/PI+). Only 15.7% of cells were in the non-apoptotic and non-necrotic phase (Fig. 2D). These clearly show that PDT induces cell death involving the process of apoptosis and necrosis. As a confirmation, when cells were co-incubated with a caspase pan-inhibitor Z-VAD-FMK (10 μM) and PDT (Pba 0.125 μg/mL) percentage of viable cell number increased from 63% to 80.1% (Fig. 2E). In addition, the incubation with necrostatin (50 μM), a potent inhibitor of programed necrotic cell death, elevated viable cell number to 78.2%. Taken together, obtained results indicate that *NRF2* knockdown sensitized breast cancer MDA-MB-231 cells to Pba-based PDT, resulting in enhanced cell death.

PDT-stimulated ROS generation is elevated in *NRF2* knockdown MDA cells

Pba-laser combination therapy releases singlet oxygen within the cell, and the resulting ROS is a major contributor to PDT's cytotoxicity [5]. Therefore, we monitored PDT-derived singlet oxygen levels in both cell lines. Cells pre-treated with Pba (2.5 μg/mL for 6 h) were irradiated by a 0.6-J/cm^2 laser, and the levels of singlet oxygen were determined using trans-1-(2′methoxyvinyl) pyrene, a fluorescent dye, which is specific to singlet oxygen.

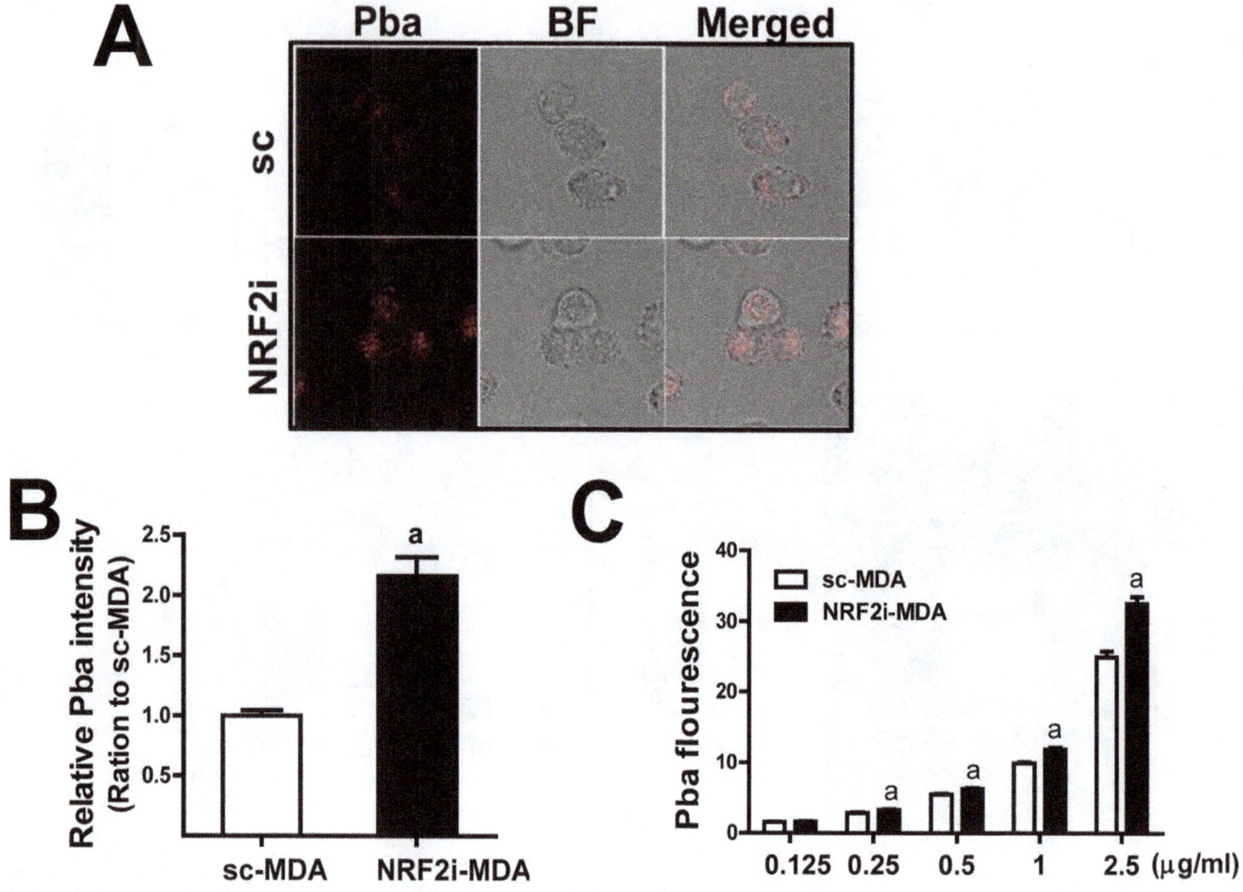

Figure 4. *NRF2* knockdown increases cellular accumulation of Pba. (A) The cells were incubated with Pba (2.5 μg/mL) for 6 h and then washed with PBS. Intracellular accumulation of Pba was monitored by confocal microscopy. BF, bright field; ×100 magnification (B) Intracellular accumulation of Pba (2.5 μg/mL, 6 h) was quantified using a Cell Insight system. The data are ratios with respect to the sc-MDA control and are reported as the mean ± standard error (SE) of 6 experiments. (C) Intracellular accumulation of Pba (0.25 and 0.5 μg/mL, 6 h) was assessed by fluorometric measurement in cell lysates. The data represent ratios with respect to each no PDT control are reported as the mean ±SD of 3 experiments. [a]$P<0.05$ as compared with sc-MDA with PDT.

Compared to treatment with Pba only or laser irradiation only, the trans-1-(2′methoxyvinyl) pyrene-based method showed that Pba-laser combination group displays an enhanced fluorescent signal within the cell (data not shown), confirming the increase in singlet oxygen upon PDT. In our initial assessment, the incubation of trans-1-(2′methoxyvinyl) pyrene for 5 min, 30 min and 50 min showed similar increase levels of singlet oxygen-derived fluorogenic pyrene intensity (Fig. 3A). This confirms that singlet oxygen-derived pyrene fluorescence can be reliably detectable during these incubations times; therefore a confocal determination was done after 30 min incubation of trans-1-(2′methoxyvinyl) pyrene in our study. The comparative measurement of singlet oxygen demonstrated that *NRF2*-knockdown MDA-MB-231 cells generate higher levels of singlet oxygen than the control cells (Fig. 3B). The fluorescent signals were distributed within the cytoplasm as well as the nucleus, and the total fluorescence intensity was 1.5-fold higher in the knockdown cells than that in the control cells. Accordingly, the total level of ROS, which was monitored using DCFDA, was substantially elevated after treatment with the Pba-laser combination in both cell lines; however, the increase was greater in the NRF2i-MDA cells. Specifically, after treatment with 2.5 μg/mL Pba and laser irradiation, the increase in ROS was 4.6-fold higher in the *NRF2*-knockdown cell line than in the control cell line (Fig. 3C). Similarly, after treatment with the low concentration of Pba (0.125 μg/mL) and laser irradiation, the increase in ROS was 3.5-fold higher in NRF2i-MDA cells (Fig. 3D). These results suggested that elevation in singlet oxygen and ROS enhances the sensitivity of *NRF2*-knockdown breast cancer cells to PDT.

Increased accumulation of Pba in *NRF2* knockdown breast cancer cells is resulted from diminished BCRP expression

The level of PDT-derived singlet oxygen was higher in NRF2i-MDA cells than in control cells (Fig. 3B), suggesting differential cellular level of Pba in *NRF2*-knockdown cells. Using the fluorescent property of Pba, we used confocal microscopy to monitor cellular levels of Pba (2.5 μg/ml) after a 6 h-incubation. The Pba-derived red fluorescence signal was greater in NRF2i-MDA cells than in control cells (Fig. 4A). Compared to control cells, NRF2i-MDA cells showed 2.2-fold greater Pba-derived fluorescent intensity when quantified using a Cell Insight System (Fig. 4B). The fluorometric measurement of Pba in cell lysates also showed similar results: cellular level of Pba is higher in knockdown cells throughout Pba concentrations (Fig. 4C).

These results demonstrated that NRF2 affects cellular accumulation of Pba and that differential expression of transporters may

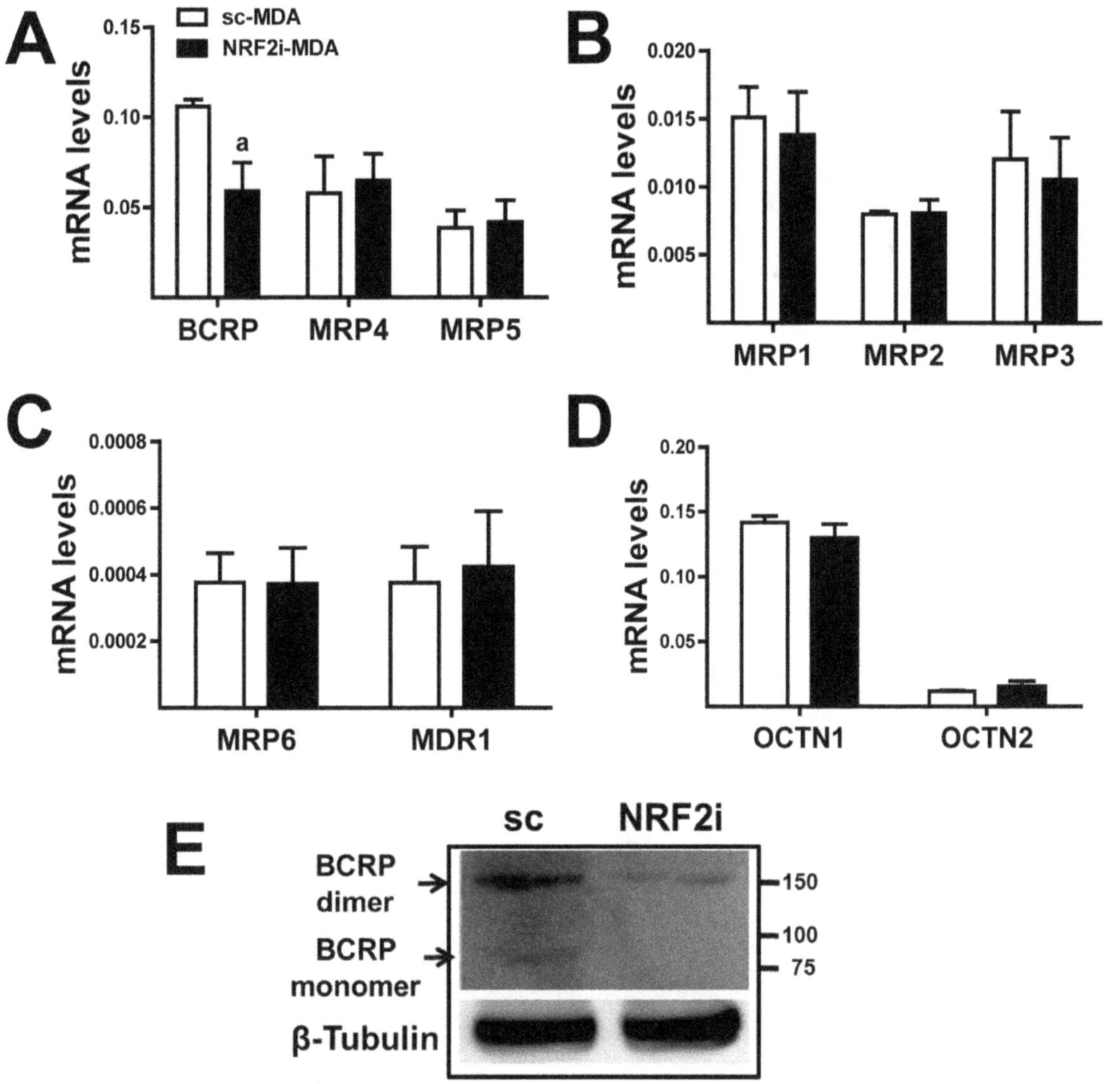

Figure 5. Increased Pba accumulation in *NRF2* knockdown cells is resulted from BCRP decrease. (A–C) Relative quantification of mRNA levels of ABC transporters (BCRP, MRP1-6, and MDR1) was performed in sc-DMA and NRF2i-MDA cells using real-time PCR. (D) Transcript levels of SLC transporters (OCTN1 and OCTN2) were determined using real-time PCR. The data are ratios with respect to the sc-MDA control for each gene and are reported as the mean ±SD of 3 experiments. (E) BCRP protein levels (dimer, 150 kDa; monomer, 75 kDa) in sc-MDA and NRF2i-MDA cells were determined using immunoblot analysis.

be associated with enhanced accumulation. Next, we measured mRNA levels of several ATP-binding cassette (ABC) transporters (*BCRP*, *MRP1-6*, and *MDR1*) and solute carrier (SLC) transporters (*OCTN1* and *OCTN2*) in order to identify the mechanisms underlying Pba accumulation in NRF2-MDA cells. Among these transporters, the transcript level of *BCRP* was significantly lower in NRF2i-MAD cells than that in control cells, whereas the levels of other transporters were not altered by *NRF2* knockdown (Fig. 5A–5D). The reduced level of BCRP in *NRF2* knockdown cells was confirmed by western-blot analysis: NRF2i-MDA cells displayed significantly reduced levels of the BCRP monomers and dimers (Fig. 5E). These data indicated that the basal expression of BCRP is controlled by NRF2 in MDA-MB-231 cells and that enhanced Pba accumulation in *NRF2*-knockdown cells can be associated with reduced expression of BCRP.

BCRP inhibitor treatment increases Pba accumulation, PDT-induced ROS increase and cytotoxicity

In order to strengthen the relationship between BRCP and PDT sensitivity, we incubated cells with a potent BCRP inhibitor, Ko143, and monitored PDT-derived ROS. The differential increase in ROS after PDT treatment between sc-MDA and NRF2i-MDA cells disappeared when they were co-incubated with 0.5 μM Ko143. Specifically, ROS generation in sc-MDA cells increased to the same level as that in NRF2i-MDA cells (Fig. 6A). Similarly, differential cellular levels of Pba in the sc control and NRF2 knockdown cells were abolished by the Ko143 incubation (Fig. 6B). In addition, viable cell number was significantly decreased by BCRP inhibitor (Fig. 6C). These results further support the role of NRF2-BCRP in Pba-PDT response. It is notable that the effects of Ko143 on Pba accumulation and cell viability are not identical. Upon Ko143 incubation, there was no statistical difference in cellular Pba levels in both cell lines,

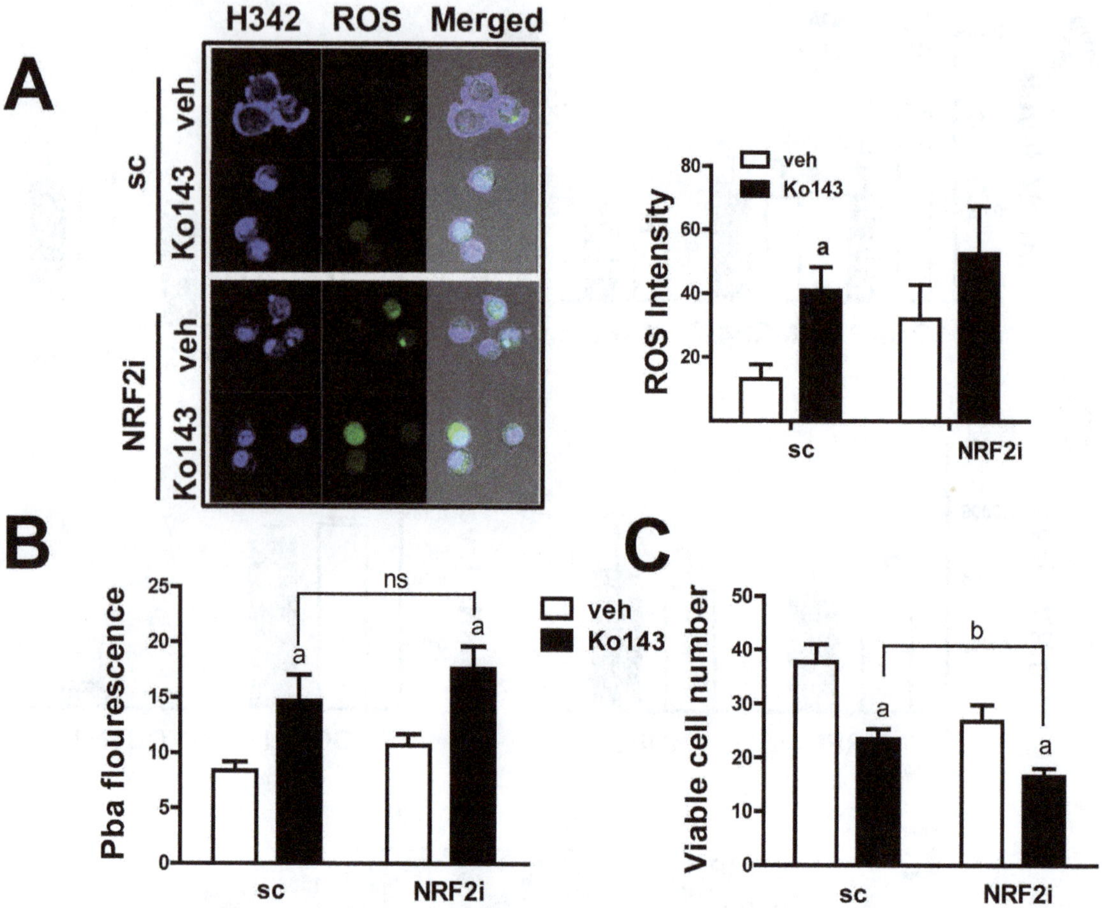

Figure 6. BCRP inhibitor treatment reverses Pba accumulation and PDT cytotoxicity in NRF2 knockdown cells. (A) The sc- and NRF2i-MDA cells were pre-incubated with the BCRP inhibitor Ko143 (0.5 μM) for 1 h followed by incubation with Pba (0.25 μg/mL) for 6 h. Then, the cells were irradiated with a 0.6 J/cm^2 laser, and ROS levels were quantified by DCFDA staining. The data are ratios with respect to the sc-MDA control without Ko146 pre-incubation and are reported as the mean ±SD of 3 experiments. (B–C) After PDT in the presence of Ko143, cellular level of Pba (B) and cell viability (C) were assessed. Cellular Pba level was determined by fluorometeric measurement of Pba in cell lysates. Cell viability was measured using MTT analysis. The data are reported as the mean ±SD of 8–10 wells. $^aP<0.05$ as compared with no Ko143 group of each cell line. $^bP<0.05$ as compared with the vehicle-treated sc (B) or Ko143-treated sc control group (C).

implying the critical role of BCRP in Pba accumulation; however the viability of knockdown cells was still low compared to the sc control. These suggest the role of additional NRF2 factors in PDT response determination.

The mitochondrial antioxidant peroxiredoxin 3 (PRDX3) is reduced in *NRF2* knockdown MDA-MB-231 cells

In an attempt to identify additional NRF2 factors participating PDT sensitization, the levels of mitochondrial ROS counteracting enzymes were examined. Particularly, it has been reported that PDT-induced cell death is associated with the accumulation of Pba in the mitochondria [17]. When cellular Pba localization was monitored in MDA-MB-231 cells after Pba incubation, Pba-derived red fluorescence and mitochondria-specific green fluorescence were largely co-localized (Fig. 7A). These data support the Pba accumulated in the mitochondria of MDA-MB-231 cells; therefore, the mitochondrial antioxidant system can be an additional determinant of PDT sensitivity. Among the 11 mitochondrial antioxidant genes we measured, only *PRDX3* was significantly down-regulated (~50%) by *NRF2* knockdown as compared to the control (Fig. 7B and 7C). The transcript levels of other genes, including superoxide dismutase 1/2 (SOD1/2), catalase (CAT), thioredoxin 2 (TXN2), glutaredoxin 1/4 (GLRX1/4), and PRDX5, were not affected by *NRF2* knockdown. The decrease of PRDX3 was confirmed in Western blot analysis (Fig. 7D). These results suggested that the basal expression of *PRDX3* is dependent on NRF2 and that decreased expression of this major mitochondrial ROS defense gene can participate in enhanced PDT response of knockdown cells.

PDT sensitivity is enhanced by *NRF2* knockdown in colon cancer HT29 cells

In order to confirm the role of NRF2-BCRP signaling in regulating the sensitivity to PDT, we examined the effect of *NRF2* knockdown on PDT response in the colon carcinoma HT29 cell line. The stable *NRF2*-knockdown cell line (NRF2i-HT) showed a substantial reduction in *NRF2*, *AKR1C1*, and *HO-1* mRNA (data not shown). MTT analysis following Pba and laser irradiation (0.3 J/cm^2) showed that *NRF2*-knockdown HT29 cells were more sensitive to PDT-induced cytotoxicity (Fig. 8A). Furthermore, the levels of singlet oxygen and ROS were higher in NRF2i-HT cells than in control cells (Fig. 8B and 8C). Finally, similar to MDA-MB-231 cells, there was greater intracellular Pba accumulation and lower expression of *BCRP* in NRF2i-HT cells (Fig. 8D and

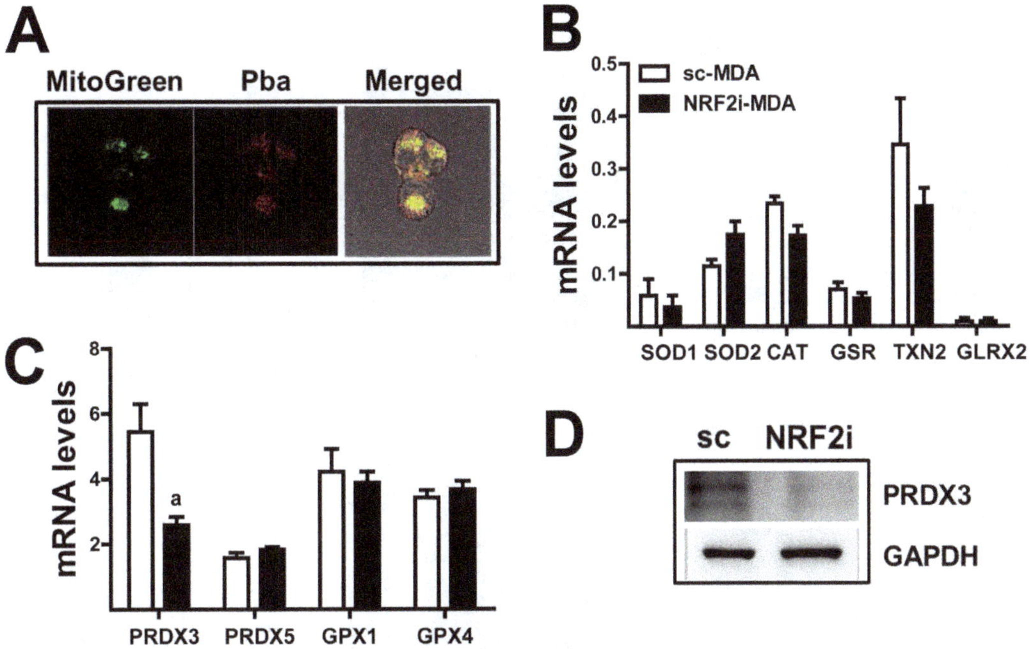

Figure 7. The mitochondrial ROS-counteracting protein PRDX3 is decreased in NRF2i-DMA cells. (A) The sc-MDA cells were incubated with 2.5 μg/mL Pba for 6 h and then washed with PBS. The cells were incubated with MitoGreen (0.5 μM) for 15 min, and a confocal microscopic observation was performed. Green fluorescence indicates mitochondria, red fluorescence indicates cellular Pba, and yellow color indicates co-localization of mitochondria and Pba. ×100 magnification (B–C) Transcript levels of ROS-scavenging genes were measured using real-time PCR analysis for relative quantification. The data are reported as the mean ±SD of 3–4 experiments. [a]$P<0.05$ as compared with the sc-MDA control for each gene. (D) Protein level of PRDX3 in the sc- and NRF2i- MDA was assessed using Western blot analysis.

8E). Taken together, these results indicated that NRF2 inhibition in colon cancer cells reduced *BCRP* expression and thereby enhanced PDT sensitivity.

Combination of lentiviral shRNA delivery and PDT in other types of cancer

Next, we examined the efficacy of *NRF2* siRNA delivery in PDT sensitization of 4 additional types of cancer cells: human breast carcinoma cell line MCF7, colon carcinoma cell line HCT116, renal carcinoma cell line A498, and glioblastoma cell line A172. These cells were incubated for 48 h with the *NRF2* shRNA-containing lentiviral particle and then subjected to PDT. Subsequently, cellular ROS level was assessed as a marker of PDT efficacy. The level of knockdown was not as high as in the stable cell line. Nevertheless, lentiviral delivery of shRNA significantly reduced the level of *NRF2* mRNA in each cell line: 44% reduction in HCT116, 35% reduction in MCF7, 22% reduction in A498, and 38% reduction in A172 (Fig. 9A–9D). Under conditions of *NRF2* depletion, PDT-induced ROS was substantially increased in all cell types. These data confirmed the beneficial effects of *NRF2* siRNA for sensitizing cancer cells to PDT.

Discussion

The activation of NRF2 using pharmacological interventions or genetic approaches can prevent oxidative stress-associated diseases, such as inflammatory diseases and cancer [27,28,31]. Whereas, a constitutive increase in NRF2 expression can promote cancer cell survival in the stressful tumor environment and in the presence of chemotherapeutic agents [33,41,42]. In the present study, we investigated NRF2 as a potential molecular determinant of the efficacy of Pba-based PDT in human breast carcinoma MDA-MB-231 cells and colon carcinoma HT29 cells. Stable knockdown of *NRF2* in both cancer cell lines enhanced cell death and substantially increased ROS levels following Pba-PDT as compared to the respective control cell lines. In particular, the level of singlet oxygen, which is a direct product of Pba photoactivation, was significantly higher in *NRF2*-knockdown cancer cells than in control cells, suggesting differential levels of cellular Pba between these cell lines. Indeed, confocal microscopic observation of fluorogenic Pba showed significantly higher cellular accumulation of Pba in knockdown cells as compared to control cells. A subsequent analysis of the expression of membrane drug transporters revealed that the basal expression of *BCRP* is NRF2-dependent. Among the measured ABC transporters and SLC transporters, only BCRP was down-regulated by *NRF2* knockdown. Accordingly, treatment with a BCRP-specific inhibitor enhanced PDT sensitivity in control cells but not knockdown cells. These results indicate that the inhibition of *NRF2* in cancer cells could enhance sensitivity to Pba-PDT by decreasing *BCRP* expression. In addition to photosensitizer accumulation, *NRF2* knockdown affected the expression of mitochondrial ROS-counteracting proteins. Among the examined ROS-scavenging proteins, including SOD1/2, CAT, GPX1/4, PRDX3/5, and TXN2, the transcript level of *PRDX3*, which is a major ROS scavenger in the mitochondria, was down-regulated by *NRF2* knockdown in MDA-MB-231 cells. Finally, we demonstrated that PDT-induced ROS was substantially elevated by the delivery of shRNA to other types of human cancer cell lines, including breast carcinoma MCF-7, colon carcinoma HCT116, renal carcinoma A498, and glioblastoma A172 cells. These results confirm that NRF2 is a molecular determinant of Pba-PDT sensitivity in various types of cancer cells.

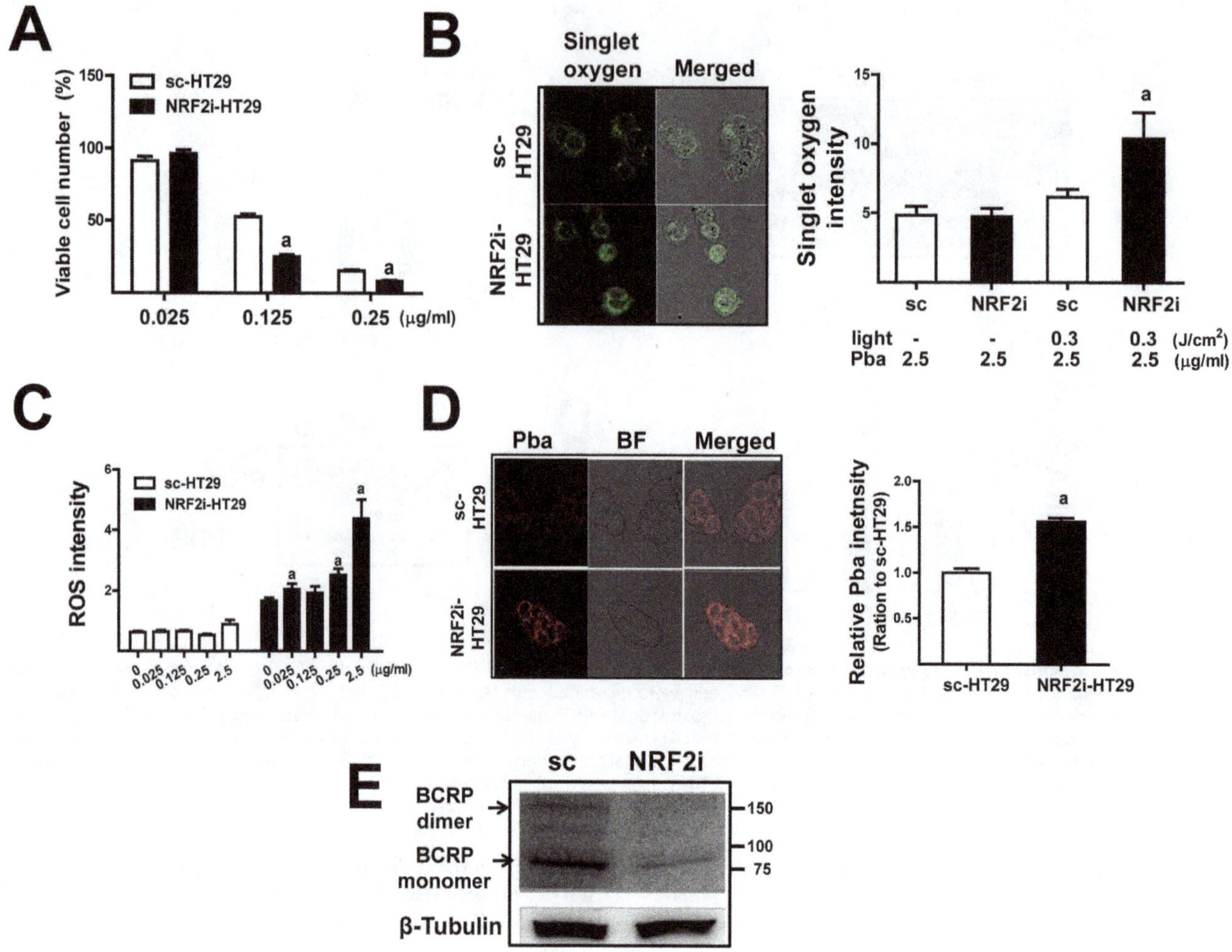

Figure 8. NRF2-BCRP inhibition enhances PDT sensitivity in colon cancer HT29 cells. (A) The HT29 cell lines with stable expression of nonspecific scRNA (sc-HT) and *NRF2* shRNA (NRF2i-HT) were incubated with Pba (0.025–2.5 μg/mL) for 6 h and then irradiated by a 0.3 J/cm^2 laser. After 18 h incubation in complete medium, viable cells were quantified using an MTT assay. The data are ratios with respect to the vehicle-treated sc-HT cells and are reported as the mean ±SD of 8 wells. [a]*P*<0.05 as compared with each sc-HT PDT group. (B) Singlet oxygen levels were quantified in PDT-treated sc- and NRF2i-HT cells using a specific fluorescent dye. The data are reported as the mean ±SD of 3 experiments. [a]*P*<0.05 as compared with the sc-HT PDT group. ×100 magnification (C) Levels of ROS in PDT-treated cells were quantified using a Cell Insight Personal Cell Imager. [a]*P*< 0.05 as compared with the no PDT group of each cell line. (D) The cells were incubated with Pba (2.5 μg/mL) for 6 h, and cellular Pba accumulation was monitored using a confocal microscopy. Pba accumulation was quantified using a Cell Insight system. The data are ratios with respect to the sc-HT control and are reported as the mean ±SE of 6 samples. BF, bright field; ×100 magnification (E) BCRP levels in sc-HT and NRF2i-HT cells were assessed by immunoblot analysis.

BCRP, an ABC transporter, exists in the plasma membrane as a homodimer, which is formed through disulfide bonds between extracellular cysteine residues of the BCRP molecule [43]. BCRP is overexpressed in many types of cancer and is strongly associated with chemoresistance by mediating the efflux of a wide range of anti-cancer agents, such as anthracyclines and methotrexate [21,44,45]. Chlorophyll-derived dietary phototoxins are known substrates of BCRP in animals. Using *bcrp*-deficient mice, Jonker et al. demonstrated that Pba-induced skin phototoxicity was increased in the absence of BCRP [24]. Later, Robey et al. provided direct evidence that Pba is a specific substrate of BCRP [23]. Among cancer cell lines expressing high levels of multidrug resistance-associated protein-1, P-glycoproteins, or BCRP, Pba transport was only detected in cells expressing BCRP and this transport was inhibited by a BCRP-specific inhibitor. Furthermore, other type of protoporphyrins, such as the clinical photosensitizer photochlor and verteporfin, are also known as BCRP substrates [46]. In a retrospective examination of BCRP levels in clinical samples, BCRP expression was significantly associated with the efficacy of photofrin-PDT in patients with early lung cancer [47]. Therefore, BCRP inhibition may be an effective method for enhancing PDT efficacy. Indeed, treatment of cells with imatinib mesylate, a BCRP inhibiting tyrosine kinase inhibitor, increased levels of the photosensitizer within tumors and enhanced the efficacy of PDT in mice [46]. These data implicated the role of BCRP in regulating the efficacy of PDT.

Drug transporters are transcriptionally regulated: the aryl hydrocarbon receptor (AhR), pregnane X receptor (PXR), and constitutive androstane receptor (CAR) are involved in their regulation [48,49]. Additionally, several research groups have reported the association of NRF2 in regulating the expression of drug transporters. Previously, Hayashi et al. reported that *Mrp-1* expression is up-regulated by treatment with diethyl maleate, which activates NRF2, and that the basal expression of Mrp-1 was

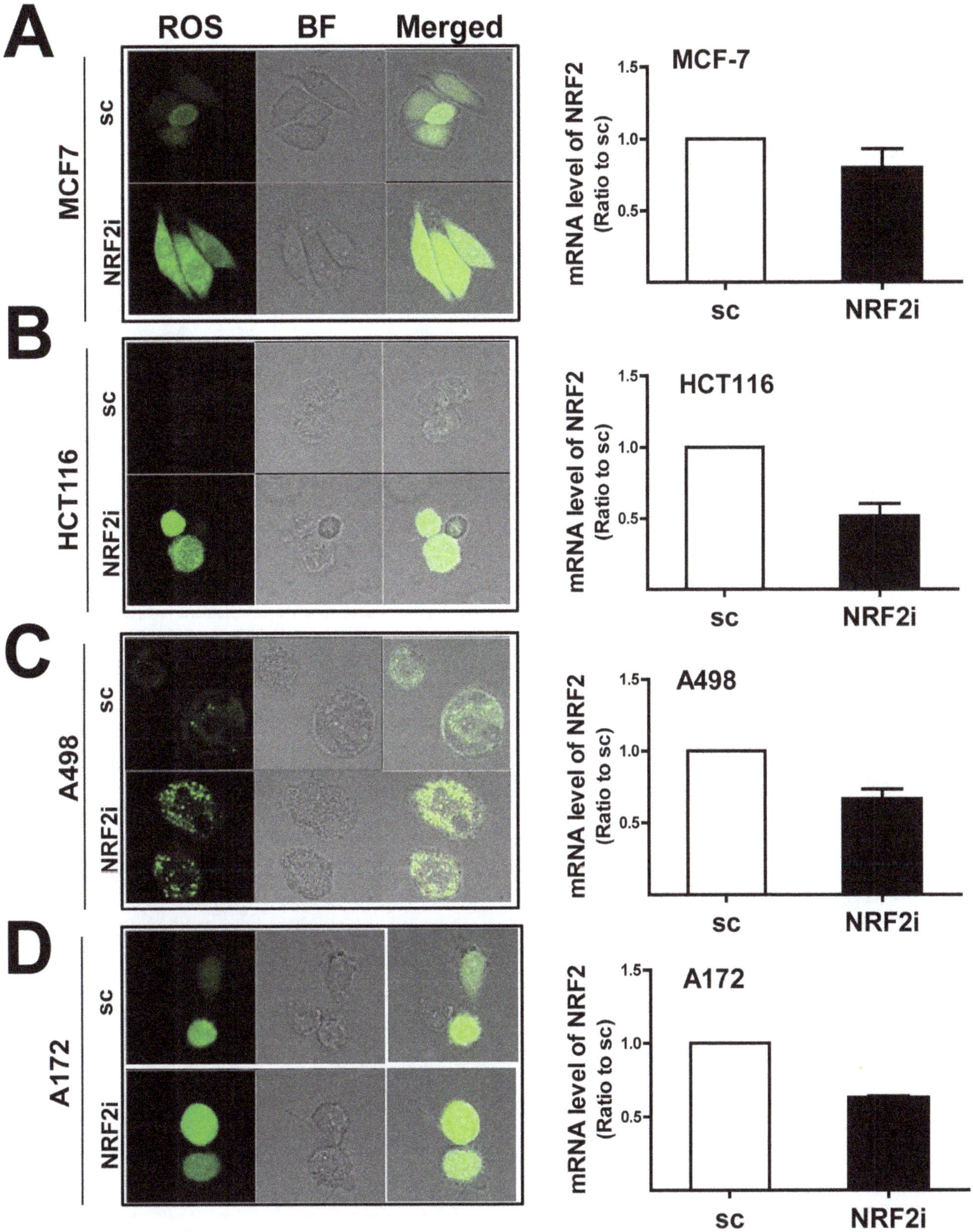

Figure 9. The combination of *NRF2* shRNA delivery and Pba PDT elevates ROS levels in additional cancer cell lines. The breast carcinoma MCF7 cell line (A), colon carcinoma HCT116 cell line (B), renal carcinoma A498 cell line (C), and glioblastoma A172 cell line (D) were transiently incubated with lentiviral particles containing *NRF2* shRNA. Cells were treated with PDT, and the levels of cellular ROS were monitored with DCFDA staining. Transcript levels of NRF2 were measured using relative quantification of real-time PCR in each cell line. BF, bright field; ×100 magnification.

lower in *nrf2*-deficient embryonic fibroblasts than that in wild-type cells [50]. Maher et al. demonstrated that the administration of NRF2 activators in mice increased the expression of Mrp2-6 in the liver [51]. Later, BCRP expression was reportedly up-regulated upon treatment with *tert*-butylhydroquinone through NRF2 in HepG2 cells [52]. In our study, NRF2 affected basal expression of BCRP. Specifically, the mRNA level and protein levels of both the BCRP monomer (70 kDa) and homodimer (140 kDa) were significantly decreased by *NRF2*-knockdown. In contrast, the levels of *MRP1-6*, *MDR1*, and *OCTN1-2* were unaffected by *NRF2*-knockdown, indicating that basal expression of BCRP is highly dependent on NRF2. Based on this specific link between NRF2 and BCRP in cancer cells, together with the effect on mitochondrial antioxidant genes, NRF2 can be a novel molecular target for enhancing the efficacy of Pha-PDT. This principle was validated in other cancer cell types, including HT29, HCT116, MCF-7, A498, and A172 cell lines.

The cellular mechanism underlying PDT phototoxicity involves apoptosis and necrosis [6]. As a mitochondria-dependent pathway, it was shown that PDT-ROS induces inner mitochondrial membrane permeabilization and subsequent cytochrome c release, which leads to apoptotic cell death [40,53]. In a confocal microscopic determination, we observed that cellular Pba is primarily co-localized with the mitochondrial dye, and this implies that mitochondria-mediated apoptosis can be involved in PDT cytotoxicity in MDA-MB cells. However, the treatment with pan-caspase inhibitor could not completely block PDT-mediated cell death. This indicates that PDT-induced cell death is developed by a complex mechanism. Another mechanism underlying PDT phototoxicity is necrosis. Although necrosis is a passive mechanism, necroptosis or programmed necrosis has recently emerged as a novel mechanism of cell death [54,55]. Oxidative stress has been proposed as a stimulator of necroptotic cell death [56]. Mouse embryonic fibroblasts with the deletion of *RIPK* gene, an essential component in necroptotic response, were resistant to hydrogen peroxide-induced cell death [57]. Treatment of mouse hippocampal cells with necroptosis-specific inhibitor necrostatin-1 prevented GSH depletion-induced cytotoxicity [58]. In our study, most of PDT-exposed *NRF2* knockdown cells were Annexin+/PI- and Annexin+/PI+ populations, which represent the early apoptotic and necrotic/late apoptotic cells, respectively. Accordantly, PDT-induced knockdown cell death affected by pharmacological inhibitors of apoptosis and necroptosis. The co-incubation of NRF2i cells with either Z-VAD-FMK (pan-caspase inhibitor) or necrostatin-1 attenuated PDT-induced cell death with a similar degree. These results indicate that Pba-PDT can induce cell death through both apoptotic and necroptotic mechanisms.

The role of NRF2 in cancer has received increasing attention, because constitutive activation of NRF2 has been identified in many human cancers [33,41]. Several different mechanisms have been proposed for the constitutive activation of NRF2 [42]. First, somatic mutations on *KEAP1* or *NRF2* have been reported to cause of gain-of-function NRF2 in cancer cell lines and tumor tissues. Second, reduced *KEAP1* expression due to promoter hypermethylation has been observed. Third, the *NRF2* transcription can be increased by signaling through oncogenes, such as *c-Myc* and *K-Ras*. Fourth, accumulation of p21 or p62 can disrupt the binding of KEAP1 to NRF2. Fifth, certain cancer metabolites, such as fumarate, can modify KEAP1 protein, causing it to activate NRF2. Although the underlying mechanisms may differ, the ultimate activation of NRF2's target genes, including detoxifying enzymes, antioxidant proteins, and drug transporters, confers cancer resistance to anti-cancer drugs. Therefore, the inhibition of *NRF2* expression using interfering RNA could restore chemosensitivity in various cancer cells [59,60]. Thus the potential role of NRF2 in PDT response can be hypothesized. It has been demonstrated that the expression of *HO-1*, a target gene of NRF2, is involved in the protection against photofrin-PDT toxicity and that HO-1 inhibitors potentiate the anti-tumor effect of PDT [37]. Another group reported that PDT with Pba, delta-aminolevulinic acid, and protoporphyrin IX increased the expression of *BCRP* and *HO-1* expression [38]. In that study, the authors raised the possibility that individual differences in PDT response can be associated with activation of BCRP and HO-1 in tumors. Together with these findings, our results provide clear evidence that NRF2 inhibition sensitizes cancer cells to Pba-based PDT through the modulation of BCRP expression.

Collectively, our results suggest that NRF2 is a molecular determinant of the efficacy of PDT in various cancer cell types. Therefore, manipulation of NRF2 activity in tumors can be a novel strategy for enhancing the efficacy of PDT.

Author Contributions

Conceived and designed the experiments: MKK. Performed the experiments: BHC IGR. Analyzed the data: BHC MKK. Contributed reagents/materials/analysis tools: HCK. Wrote the paper: BHC MKK.

References

1. Dolmans DE, Fukumura D, Jain RK (2003) Photodynamic therapy for cancer. Nat Rev Cancer 3: 380–387.
2. Hopper C (2000) Photodynamic therapy: a clinical reality in the treatment of cancer. Lancet Oncol 1: 212–219.
3. McBride G (2002) Studies expand potential uses of photodynamic therapy. J Natl Cancer Inst 94: 1740–1742.
4. Dougherty TJ, Gomer CJ, Henderson BW, Jori G, Kessel D, et al. (1998) Photodynamic therapy. J Natl Cancer Inst 90: 889–905.
5. Sharman WM, Allen CM, van Lier JE (2000) Role of activated oxygen species in photodynamic therapy. Methods Enzymol 319: 376–400.
6. Buytaert E, Dewaele M, Agostinis P (2007) Molecular effectors of multiple cell death pathways initiated by photodynamic therapy. Biochim Biophys Acta 1776: 86–107.
7. Castano AP, Mroz P, Hamblin MR (2006) Photodynamic therapy and anti-tumour immunity. Nat Rev Cancer 6: 535–545.
8. Nowis D, Makowski M, Stoklosa T, Legat M, Issat T, et al. (2005) Direct tumor damage mechanisms of photodynamic therapy. Acta Biochim Pol 52: 339–352.
9. Park YJ, Lee WY, Hahn BS, Han MJ, Yang WI, et al. (1989) Chlorophyll derivatives–a new photosensitizer for photodynamic therapy of cancer in mice. Yonsei Med J 30: 212–218.
10. Chan JY, Tang PM, Hon PM, Au SW, Tsui SK, et al. (2006) Pheophorbide a, a major antitumor component purified from Scutellaria barbata, induces apoptosis in human hepatocellular carcinoma cells. Planta Med 72: 28–33.
11. Li WT, Tsao HW, Chen YY, Cheng SW, Hsu YC (2007) A study on the photodynamic properties of chlorophyll derivatives using human hepatocellular carcinoma cells. Photochem Photobiol Sci 6: 1341–1348.
12. Xodo LE, Rapozzi V, Zacchigna M, Drioli S, Zorzet S (2012) The chlorophyll catabolite pheophorbide a as a photosensitizer for the photodynamic therapy. Curr Med Chem 19: 799–807.
13. Hajri A, Coffy S, Vallat F, Evrard S, Marescaux J, et al. (1999) Human pancreatic carcinoma cells are sensitive to photodynamic therapy in vitro and in vivo. Br J Surg 86: 899–906.
14. Hibasami H, Kyohkon M, Ohwaki S, Katsuzaki H, Imai K, et al. (2000) Pheophorbide a, a moiety of chlorophyll a, induces apoptosis in human lymphoid leukemia molt 4B cells. Int J Mol Med 6: 277–279.
15. Tang PM, Chan JY, Au SW, Kong SK, Tsui SK, et al. (2006) Pheophorbide a, an active compound isolated from Scutellaria barbata, possesses photodynamic activities by inducing apoptosis in human hepatocellular carcinoma. Cancer Biol Ther 5: 1111–1116.
16. Lee WY, Lim DS, Ko SH, Park YJ, Ryu KS, et al. (2004) Photoactivation of pheophorbide a induces a mitochondrial-mediated apoptosis in Jurkat leukaemia cells. J Photochem Photobiol B 75: 119–126.
17. Tang PM, Liu XZ, Zhang DM, Fong WP, Fung KP (2009) Pheophorbide a based photodynamic therapy induces apoptosis via mitochondrial-mediated pathway in human uterine carcinosarcoma. Cancer Biol Ther 8: 533–539.

18. Hoi SW, Wong HM, Chan JY, Yue GG, Tse GM, et al. (2012) Photodynamic therapy of Pheophorbide a inhibits the proliferation of human breast tumour via both caspase-dependent and -independent apoptotic pathways in in vitro and in vivo models. Phytother Res 26: 734–742.
19. Hajri A, Wack S, Meyer C, Smith MK, Leberquier C, et al. (2002) In vitro and in vivo efficacy of photofrin and pheophorbide a, a bacteriochlorin, in photodynamic therapy of colonic cancer cells. Photochem Photobiol 75: 140–148.
20. Wlcek K, Stieger B (2013) ATP-binding cassette transporters in liver. Biofactors.
21. Doyle LA, Yang W, Abruzzo LV, Krogmann T, Gao Y, et al. (1998) A multidrug resistance transporter from human MCF-7 breast cancer cells. Proc Natl Acad Sci U S A 95: 15665–15670.
22. Natarajan K, Xie Y, Baer MR, Ross DD (2012) Role of breast cancer resistance protein (BCRP/ABCG2) in cancer drug resistance. Biochem Pharmacol 83: 1084–1103.
23. Robey RW, Steadman K, Polgar O, Morisaki K, Blayney M, et al. (2004) Pheophorbide a is a specific probe for ABCG2 function and inhibition. Cancer Res 64: 1242–1246.
24. Jonker JW, Buitelaar M, Wagenaar E, Van Der Valk MA, Scheffer GL, et al. (2002) The breast cancer resistance protein protects against a major chlorophyll-derived dietary phototoxin and protoporphyria. Proc Natl Acad Sci U S A 99: 15649–15654.
25. Itoh K, Chiba T, Takahashi S, Ishii T, Igarashi K, et al. (1997) An Nrf2/small Maf heterodimer mediates the induction of phase II detoxifying enzyme genes through antioxidant response elements. Biochem Biophys Res Commun 236: 313–322.
26. Itoh K, Wakabayashi N, Katoh Y, Ishii T, Igarashi K, et al. (1999) Keap1 represses nuclear activation of antioxidant responsive elements by Nrf2 through binding to the amino-terminal Neh2 domain. Genes Dev 13: 76–86.
27. Kobayashi M, Yamamoto M (2005) Molecular mechanisms activating the Nrf2-Keap1 pathway of antioxidant gene regulation. Antioxid Redox Signal 7: 385–394.
28. Hayes JD, McMahon M, Chowdhry S, Dinkova-Kostova AT (2010) Cancer chemoprevention mechanisms mediated through the Keap1-Nrf2 pathway. Antioxid Redox Signal 13: 1713–1748.
29. Kwak MK, Wakabayashi N, Itoh K, Motohashi H, Yamamoto M, et al. (2003) Modulation of gene expression by cancer chemopreventive dithiolethiones through the Keap1-Nrf2 pathway. Identification of novel gene clusters for cell survival. J Biol Chem 278: 8135–8145.
30. Thimmulappa RK, Mai KH, Srisuma S, Kensler TW, Yamamoto M, et al. (2002) Identification of Nrf2-regulated genes induced by the chemopreventive agent sulforaphane by oligonucleotide microarray. Cancer Res 62: 5196–5203.
31. Kensler TW, Wakabayashi N, Biswal S (2007) Cell survival responses to environmental stresses via the Keap1-Nrf2-ARE pathway. Annu Rev Pharmacol Toxicol 47: 89–116.
32. Cho HY, Kleeberger SR (2010) Nrf2 protects against airway disorders. Toxicol Appl Pharmacol 244: 43–56.
33. Jaramillo MC, Zhang DD (2013) The emerging role of the Nrf2-Keap1 signaling pathway in cancer. Genes Dev 27: 2179–2191.
34. Chen CC, Chu CB, Liu KJ, Huang CY, Chang JY, et al. (2013) Gene expression profiling for analysis acquired oxaliplatin resistant factors in human gastric carcinoma TSGH-S3 cells: the role of IL-6 signaling and Nrf2/AKR1C axis identification. Biochem Pharmacol 86: 872–887.
35. Kim SK, Yang JW, Kim MR, Roh SH, Kim HG, et al. (2008) Increased expression of Nrf2/ARE-dependent anti-oxidant proteins in tamoxifen-resistant breast cancer cells. Free Radic Biol Med 45: 537–546.
36. Shim GS, Manandhar S, Shin DH, Kim TH, Kwak MK (2009) Acquisition of doxorubicin resistance in ovarian carcinoma cells accompanies activation of the NRF2 pathway. Free Radic Biol Med 47: 1619–1631.
37. Kocanova S, Buytaert E, Matroule JY, Piette J, Golab J, et al. (2007) Induction of heme-oxygenase 1 requires the p38MAPK and PI3K pathways and suppresses apoptotic cell death following hypericin-mediated photodynamic therapy. Apoptosis 12: 731–741.
38. Hagiya Y, Adachi T, Ogura S, An R, Tamura A, et al. (2008) Nrf2-dependent induction of human ABC transporter ABCG2 and heme oxygenase-1 in HepG2 cells by photoactivation of porphyrins: biochemical implications for cancer cell response to photodynamic therapy. J Exp Ther Oncol 7: 153–167.
39. Kim TH, Hur EG, Kang SJ, Kim JA, Thapa D, et al. (2011) NRF2 blockade suppresses colon tumor angiogenesis by inhibiting hypoxia-induced activation of HIF-1alpha. Cancer Res 71: 2260–2275.
40. Moor AC (2000) Signaling pathways in cell death and survival after photodynamic therapy. J Photochem Photobiol B 57: 1–13.
41. Hayes JD, McMahon M (2009) NRF2 and KEAP1 mutations: permanent activation of an adaptive response in cancer. Trends Biochem Sci 34: 176–188.
42. Mitsuishi Y, Motohashi H, Yamamoto M (2012) The Keap1-Nrf2 system in cancers: stress response and anabolic metabolism. Front Oncol 2: 200.
43. Lage H, Dietel M (2000) Effect of the breast-cancer resistance protein on atypical multidrug resistance. Lancet Oncol 1: 169–175.
44. Allen JD, Brinkhuis RF, Wijnholds J, Schinkel AH (1999) The mouse Bcrp1/Mxr/Abcp gene: amplification and overexpression in cell lines selected for resistance to topotecan, mitoxantrone, or doxorubicin. Cancer Res 59: 4237–4241.
45. Volk EL, Rohde K, Rhee M, McGuire JJ, Doyle LA, et al. (2000) Methotrexate cross-resistance in a mitoxantrone-selected multidrug-resistant MCF7 breast cancer cell line is attributable to enhanced energy-dependent drug efflux. Cancer Res 60: 3514–3521.
46. Liu W, Baer MR, Bowman MJ, Pera P, Zheng X, et al. (2007) The tyrosine kinase inhibitor imatinib mesylate enhances the efficacy of photodynamic therapy by inhibiting ABCG2. Clin Cancer Res 13: 2463–2470.
47. Usuda J, Tsunoda Y, Ichinose S, Ishizumi T, Ohtani K, et al. (2010) Breast cancer resistant protein (BCRP) is a molecular determinant of the outcome of photodynamic therapy (PDT) for centrally located early lung cancer. Lung Cancer 67: 198–204.
48. Klaassen CD, Slitt AL (2005) Regulation of hepatic transporters by xenobiotic receptors. Curr Drug Metab 6: 309–328.
49. Urquhart BL, Tirona RG, Kim RB (2007) Nuclear receptors and the regulation of drug-metabolizing enzymes and drug transporters: implications for interindividual variability in response to drugs. J Clin Pharmacol 47: 566–578.
50. Hayashi A, Suzuki H, Itoh K, Yamamoto M, Sugiyama Y (2003) Transcription factor Nrf2 is required for the constitutive and inducible expression of multidrug resistance-associated protein 1 in mouse embryo fibroblasts. Biochem Biophys Res Commun 310: 824–829.
51. Maher JM, Cheng X, Slitt AL, Dieter MZ, Klaassen CD (2005) Induction of the multidrug resistance-associated protein family of transporters by chemical activators of receptor-mediated pathways in mouse liver. Drug Metab Dispos 33: 956–962.
52. Adachi T, Nakagawa H, Chung I, Hagiya Y, Hoshijima K, et al. (2007) Nrf2-dependent and -independent induction of ABC transporters ABCC1, ABCC2, and ABCG2 in HepG2 cells under oxidative stress. J Exp Ther Oncol 6: 335–348.
53. Oleinick NL, Morris RL, Belichenko I (2002) The role of apoptosis in response to photodynamic therapy: what, where, why, and how. Photochem Photobiol Sci 1: 1–21.
54. Galluzzi L, Kepp O, Krautwald S, Kroemer G, Linkermann A (2014) Molecular mechanisms of regulated necrosis. Semin Cell Dev Biol.
55. Kaczmarek A, Vandenabeele P, Krysko DV (2013) Necroptosis: the release of damage-associated molecular patterns and its physiological relevance. Immunity 38: 209–223.
56. Vanlangenakker N, Vanden Berghe T, Vandenabeele P (2012) Many stimuli pull the necrotic trigger, an overview. Cell Death Differ 19: 75–86.
57. Shen HM, Lin Y, Choksi S, Tran J, Jin T, et al. (2004) Essential roles of receptor-interacting protein and TRAF2 in oxidative stress-induced cell death. Mol Cell Biol 24: 5914–5922.
58. Xu X, Chua CC, Kong J, Kostrzewa RM, Kumaraguru U, et al. (2007) Necrostatin-1 protects against glutamate-induced glutathione depletion and caspase-independent cell death in HT-22 cells. J Neurochem 103: 2004–2014.
59. Cho JM, Manandhar S, Lee HR, Park HM, Kwak MK (2008) Role of the Nrf2-antioxidant system in cytotoxicity mediated by anticancer cisplatin: implication to cancer cell resistance. Cancer Lett 260: 96–108.
60. Manandhar S, Choi BH, Jung KA, Ryoo IG, Song M, et al. (2012) NRF2 inhibition represses ErbB2 signaling in ovarian carcinoma cells: implications for tumor growth retardation and docetaxel sensitivity. Free Radic Biol Med 52: 1773–1785.

7

A Cell-Based High-Throughput Screen for Novel Chemical Inducers of Fetal Hemoglobin for Treatment of Hemoglobinopathies

Kenneth R. Peterson[1,2*], Flávia C. Costa[1¤a], Halyna Fedosyuk[1], Renee Y. Neades[1], Allen M. Chazelle[1], Lesya Zelenchuk[1¤b], Andrea H. Fonteles[1], Parmita Dalal[1], Anuradha Roy[3], Rathnam Chaguturu[3¤c], Biaoru Li[4], Betty S. Pace[4,5]

1 Department of Biochemistry and Molecular Biology, University of Kansas Medical Center, Kansas City, Kansas, United States of America, **2** Department of Anatomy and Cell Biology, University of Kansas Medical Center, Kansas City, Kansas, United States of America, **3** High Throughput Screening Laboratory, University of Kansas, Lawrence, Kansas, United States of America, **4** Department of Pediatrics, Georgia Regents University, Augusta, Georgia, United States of America, **5** Department of Molecular and Cell Biology, Georgia Regents University, Augusta, Georgia, United States of America

Abstract

Decades of research have established that the most effective treatment for sickle cell disease (SCD) is increased fetal hemoglobin (HbF). Identification of a drug specific for inducing γ-globin expression in pediatric and adult patients, with minimal off-target effects, continues to be an elusive goal. One hurdle has been an assay amenable to a high-throughput screen (HTS) of chemicals that displays a robust γ-globin off-on switch to identify potential lead compounds. Assay systems developed in our labs to understand the mechanisms underlying the γ- to β-globin gene expression switch during development has allowed us to generate a cell-based assay that was adapted for a HTS of 121,035 compounds. Using chemical inducer of dimerization (CID)-dependent bone marrow cells (BMCs) derived from human γ-globin promoter-firefly luciferase β-globin promoter-Renilla luciferase β-globin yeast artificial chromosome (γ-luc β-luc β-YAC) transgenic mice, we were able to identify 232 lead chemical compounds that induced γ-globin 2-fold or higher, with minimal or no β-globin induction, minimal cytotoxicity and that did not directly influence the luciferase enzyme. Secondary assays in CID-dependent wild-type β-YAC BMCs and human primary erythroid progenitor cells confirmed the induction profiles of seven of the 232 hits that were cherry-picked for further analysis.

Editor: Bridget Wagner, Broad Institute of Harvard and MIT, United States of America

Funding: This work was supported by Public Health Service National Institutes of Health (NIH.gov) grants HL069234 to BSP (subcontract to KRP), and HL067336, DK061804, and DK081290 to KRP. KU-HTSL is a KU Cancer Center Shared Resource, and is funded in part by National Intitutes of Health COBRE Grant 8 P30 GM103495 (B. Timmermann, PI) and the NCI Cancer Support Grant, 5 P30 CA168524 (R. Jensen, PI). The funders had no role in study design, data collection and analysis, decision to publish, or preparation of the manuscript.

Competing Interests: The authors have declared that no competing interests exist.

* Email: kpeterson@kumc.edu

¤a Current address: College of Biosciences, Kansas City University of Medicine and Biosciences, Kansas City, Missouri, United States of America
¤b Current address: The Kidney Institute, University of Kansas Medical Center, Kansas City, Kansas, United States of America
¤c Current address: SRI International, Harrisonburg, Virginia, United States of America

Introduction

Sickle cell disease (SCD) is the most common monogenetic disease diagnosed in the United States, affecting approximately 1 of 400 African-American infants [1]. The high morbidity rate of SCD patients is related to vascular complications that include multiple chronic organ damage affecting the brain, heart, lungs, kidneys, liver, eyes, skin, and skeleton. Vaso-occlusive crises result in acute and chronic severe pain, as well as acute chest syndrome, splenic sequestration, hemolytic anemia, stroke, acute and chronic multi-system organ damage, and shortened life expectancy [2], [3]. Understanding the molecular mechanisms underlying the human γ- to β-globin gene switch has long been recognized as important in the treatment of SCD, since a wealth of evidence has demonstrated that increased fetal hemoglobin (HbF) significantly ameliorates the clinical complications associated with this disease Individuals with defective adult β-globin genes, as is the case for SCD or β-thalassemia, are more-or-less phenotypically normal if they carry compensatory mutations that result in hereditary persistence of fetal hemoglobin (HPFH). Thus, a logical clinical goal for treatment of the β-hemoglobinopathies is to up-regulate γ-globin synthesis pharmacologically.

An increase in HbF parameters (% HbF and % F cells) prevents sickling *in vivo*. Hydroxyurea (HU), a ribonucleotide reductase inhibitor that arrests DNA synthesis, was shown to increase HbF production and improve the clinical symptoms of SCD [4], [5]. HU is currently the only FDA-approved drug to treat SCD, but the side effects and safety issues associated with long-term use are unknown [6]. Fetal hemoglobin synthesis can be stimulated by several other pharmacologic compounds including 5-azacytidine,

AraC, butyrate and other short chain fatty acids [7], [8], [9], [10], [11], [12], [13], [14]. However, therapies specific for SCD, that do not affect cell physiology globally, remain elusive.

High-throughput (HTS) technology has been used successfully in the past 20 years in the pharmaceutical industry for lead drug discovery [15], [16]. Development of the technology has been propelled by advancements in combinatorial chemistry, human genome sequencing, and automation of drug screens. It is an enabling technology and the number of researchers that have applied this powerful tool in biomedical research has increased. Successful examples include discoveries of novel inhibitors of protein arginine methyltransferase [17], metalloform-selective methionine aminopeptidase [18], and cystic fibrosis transmembrane conductance regulator [19].

Based on our previous data using wild-type CID-dependent β-YAC BMCs, we generated dual-luciferase β-YAC (dual-luc β-YAC) BMCs containing γ-globin promoter-firefly luciferase (γ-luc) and β-globin promoter-Renilla luciferase (β-luc) fusions from γ-luc β-luc β-YAC transgenic mice. The γ-luc gene fusion was not active unless a γ-globin inducing compound was applied, a true "off-on" switch similar to our wild-type CID-dependent β-YAC BMCs, whereas the β-luc gene fusion was active. These cells were adapted to a HTS platform to allow rapid identification of chemical scaffolds that produced firefly luciferase-positive cells (γ-globin), but did not further induce Renilla luciferase (β-globin). Out of 121,035 compounds tested, 233 lead compounds that induce γ-globin gene expression were identified in this cell-based HTS system.

Materials and Methods

Detailed Materials and Methods may be found in the accompanying Supplemental Materials and Methods file (File S1).

Generation of the dual-luc β-YAC construct, production of transgenic mice and derivation of CID-dependent BMCs

A firefly luciferase gene cassette was incorporated into the $^{A}\gamma$-globin gene (Figure 1A) of a 155 Kb β-YAC [20] and the resultant γ-luc β-YAC was modified by introduction of a Renilla luciferase gene cassette into the β-globin gene using homologous recombination in yeast [21] for both steps, essentially as described [22]. The resultant β-YAC was purified and microinjected into fertilized oocytes to produce transgenic mice [23]. CID-dependent BMCs were established from these animals and maintained as previously [24].

Ethics Statement

The mouse work was carried out in strict accordance with the recommendations in the Guide for the Care and Use of Laboratory Animals of the National Institutes of Health. The protocol was approved by the Institutional Animal Care and Use Committee of the University of Kansas Medical Center (ACUP Number: 2012–2060). All efforts were made to minimize suffering.

High-throughput screening assay

For HTS experiments, the dual luc β-YAC BMCs were seeded into 384-well plates (Greiner Bio-One, Monroe, NC) at a density of 10,000 cells/30 µl/well by Wellmate bulk dispenser (Thermo-Scientific Inc., Waltham, MA) in complete media containing the CID, CL-COB-II-293 (synthesized by the University of Kansas COBRE CCET Core C Synthesis Lab, commonly called AP20187). The CID-dependent dual luc β-YAC BMCs were responsive to known γ-globin inducers including valproic acid, sodium butyrate, valeric acid and hydroxyurea (data not shown). Sodium butyrate (2 mM) was selected as the positive control for screening, as a consistent 5–6 fold increase in firefly luciferase activity was obtained in four independent experiments with four different passage numbers. Since both the cell viability and luciferase induction was unaffected at DMSO concentrations below 0.5%, the compound libraries were screened at 10 µM concentration in 0.35% DMSO. Compounds were transferred acoustically using a Labcyte Echo 550 dispenser (Labcyte Inc., Sunnyvale, CA). Based on previous optimizations, 10,000 cells/well in IMDM containing CL-COB-II-293 (100 nM) were added to the wells of 384-well assay plates. The negative (n = 16, DMSO) and positive (n = 16, sodium butyrate, 2 mM) controls were added to the first two columns of each plate to assure uniformity across plates and screening batches. The cells were exposed to compounds for 24 hours at 37°C, 5% CO_2 in a 95% humidified incubator. After 24 hours incubation, Steady Glo luciferase detection reagent (Promega, Madison, WI) was used for cell lysis and generation of a luminescent signal, proportional to γ-globin promoter driven firefly luciferase reporter expression. The luminescence intensities were read 30 minutes later on a Tecan Safire2 microplate reader (Tecan, Männedorf, Switzerland). The luminescence values were used for calculating fold-induction of luciferase over DMSO treated controls. The controls were used to calculate a Z′ factor value for each plate, a measure of screening assay quality.

Compound libraries. For this study, the optimized cell-based assay utilized the following six compound collections: 1) MicroSource Spectrum (2,000 compounds containing FDA approved drugs, bioactive, natural products, MicroSource Discovery Systems, Gaylordsville, CT, www.msdiscovery.com), 2) Prestwick Chemical Library (1,120 compounds, Prestwick Chemical, ILLKIRCH France), 3) The University of Kansas Center of Excellence in Chemical Methodologies & Library Development (KU-CMLD, 1,920 compounds with novel diverse scaffolds), 4) ChemBridge Library (43,736 drug-like diverse chemical structures, ChemBridge Corporation, San Diego, CA, www.chembridge.com), 5) ChemDiv Library (56,232 compounds, diversity set from ChemDiv Inc., San Diego, CA), and 6) Orthogonally Compressed Library [(OCL), collection of 16,000 compounds from The Lankenau Institute for Medical Research (LIMR), Chemical Genomics Center (LCGC) Inc., Wynnwood, PA).

Data analysis. The active compounds from the primary screen were cherry-picked from mother plates and retested for firefly luciferase induction in an eight concentration dose-response assay (two fold dilution starting at 30 µM). The fold-induction values from dose-response curves were used for preliminary scaffold analysis and clustering using the Tripos Selector program and analyzed using the Jarvis Patrick routine, using default parameters [The Tripos Associates (Cetara), St. Louis, MO]. From each preliminary cluster, the largest conserved substructure present in at least half of the cluster members was identified.

Secondary screening. Some of the primary screen active compounds were repurchased and tested for activity in cell-based assays using the primary screening reporter cells in a ten concentration dose-response. Both firefly luciferase induction (γ-globin promoter activation using the One-Glo luciferase detection system; Promega, Madison, WI), and Renilla luciferase induction (β-globin induction the using Renilla-Glo Luciferase detection system; Promega, Madison, WI), were measured for specificity of compound activity. The cytotoxicity of the compounds was measured after 24 hours in the same cells using Cell-Titer Glo reagent (Promega, Madison, WI). The compounds were also tested

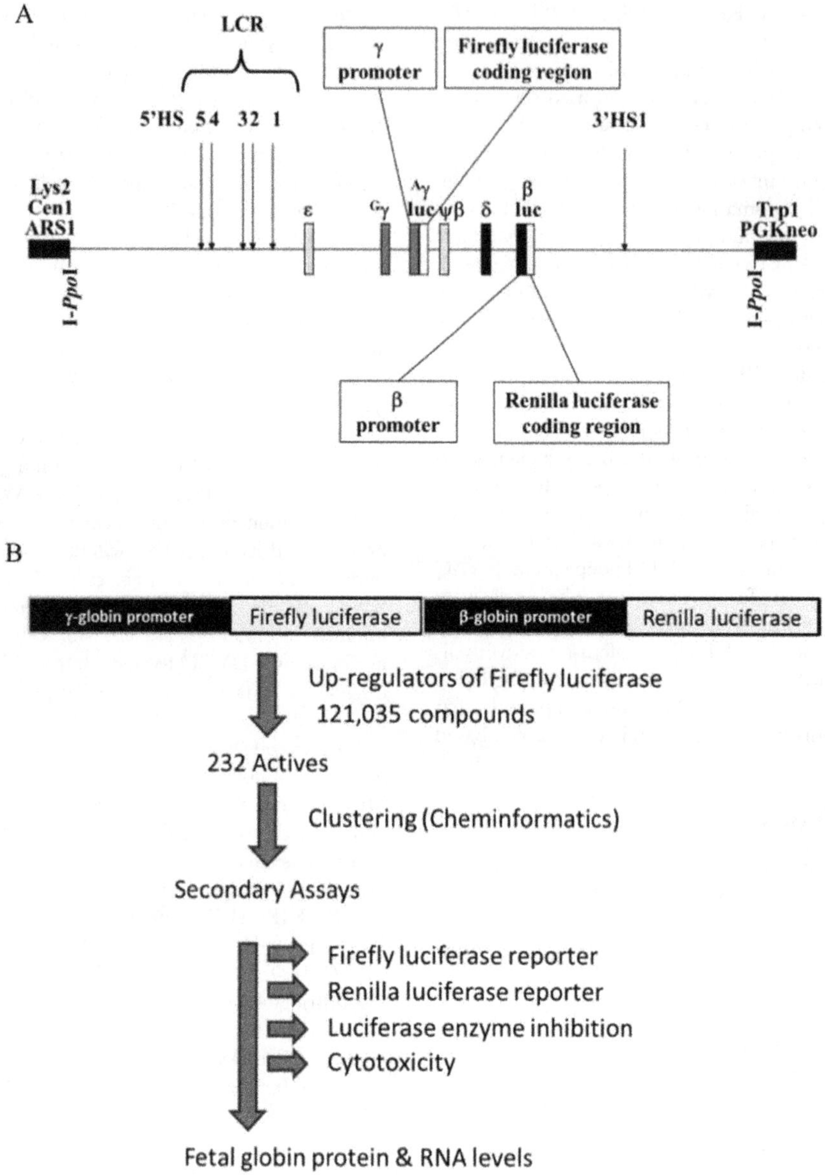

Figure 1. Schematic diagrams of the β-YAC construct and HTS work flow. Panel A) γ-luc β-luc β-YAC construct used to generate transgenic mice and derivative CID-dependent murine BMCs. This β-YAC was assembled as described in Materials and Methods and was derived from the *Ppo*-155 β-YAC [22]. The β-YAC is indicated as a line with the β-like globin genes or β-like globin promoter-luciferase fusions shown as boxes with the names of the genes above them. More detailed information regarding the components of the two luc fusions are indicated above and below the β-YAC illustration. Boxes at the left and right ends are modified pYAC4 vector [42] sequences. The LCR 5'HSs, 3'HS1 and YAC/yeast gene components are indicated above the line. LYS2, yeast lysine synthesis gene; ARS1, autonomous replicating sequence (yeast origin of replication); CEN1, yeast centromere; TRP1, yeast tryptophan synthesis gene; PGKneo, mammalian G418-resistance cassette. Engineered restriction enzyme sites utilized YAC structural determinations are shown below the line. **Panel B) High-throughput screening work flow and secondary assays.** The process flow of the high-throughput screen for identification of active compounds up-regulating fetal γ-globin gene expression is shown. The assay utilized immortalized multi-potential cells derived from the bone marrow of transgenic mice stably expressing a dual luciferase construct with firefly luciferase under control of the fetal $^{A}\gamma$-globin promoter and Renilla luciferase under the control of the adult β-globin promoter. The screening parameters were optimized in 384-well format and the cells were characterized for their ability to respond to at least 10 known inducers of fetal globin including hydroxyurea, sodium butyrate, valproic acid, and valeric acid. The assay was used to screen 120,035 compounds from the KU compound collection; 232 of which were found to up regulate firefly luciferase. The actives were clustered into 12 structural groups and fresh compounds were repurchased from various vendors. Three cell-based secondary assays were performed using the freshly available compounds: 1) up-regulation of firefly luciferase, 2) activity of Renilla luciferase, and 3) general cytotoxicity. The active compounds were also tested for inhibition of purified luciferase in an optimized biochemical assay. Profiling of the compounds revealed that of the 232 compounds tested, at least 124 compounds selectively up-regulated firefly luciferase but did not up-regulate Renilla luciferase. The 124 compounds which selectively up-regulated firefly luciferase activity also did not inhibit purified luciferase enzyme activity and were largely non-toxic to bone marrow progenitor cells.

Table 1. Primary screen.

Compound Source	No. of Compounds
Validation Library (Microsource, Prestwick and CMLD)	5,067
ChemBridge Library	43,736
ChemDiv Library	56,232
Orthogonally compressed library (LCGC)	16,000
Total No. of compounds	121,035

Actives: 232.
Overall hit rate: 0.19%.

in a biochemical screen for any inhibition to purified firefly luciferase enzyme (15 nM).

Verification assays for γ-globin transcription and HbF synthesis in murine CID-dependent wild-type β-YAC BMCs or human CD34$^+$ primary progenitor cells

Human erythroid progenitors were generated *in vitro* from adult CD34$^+$ stem cells (STEMCELL Technologies, Inc., Vancouver, Canada) using a 2-stage culture system that achieves terminal erythroid differentiation [25]. Standard, but variant, methods for quantitative reverse transcription-PCR (qRT-PCR) and flow-activated cell sorting (FACS) were employed for the two cell types as detailed in File S1. ELISA was used to measure HbF in CID-dependent wild-type β-YAC BMCs as described in the supplement.

Results

Cell-based assay system characteristics

We developed CID-dependent ^{A}γ-luc β-luc ββ-YAC BMCs from our transgenic mice as a powerful tool for screening activators of γ-globin [26]. This cell-based assay has a strong γ-globin gene expression off-on switch, a characteristic which is lacking in existing erythroid cell lines. A chimeric growth switch consisting of the thrombopoietin receptor (mpl) signaling domain fused to a FKBP12 ligand-binding domain is activated on addition of a CID. The CID, CL-COB-II-293 (AP20187), enforces dimerization by binding two FKBP12 ligand-binding domains on two neighboring molecules with 1:2 stoichiometry. Dimerization causes signaling from the mpl receptor sequences. The resultant multi-potential transgenic BMCs express exclusively human β-globin from the wild-type β-YAC transgene [26]. γ-globin synthesis is not detected in wild-type β-YAC BMCs, but expression can be reactivated in the presence of 5-azacytidine (5-Aza), butyric acid and other fatty acids, hydroxyurea, or hemin.

The 150 Kb dual luc β-YAC was synthesized as described in Materials and Methods; a schematic diagram is shown in Figure 1A. Mouse L cells, a non-erythroid control, lipofected with the dual luc β-YAC, constitutively expressed γ-luc and β-luc, similar to wild-type β-YAC L cell lines and induction with hemin/HMBA was not observed (data not shown) [27], [28]. MEL585 cells or GM979 cells similarly transfected trended towards establishing proper luciferase expression patterns appropriate to each cell line with extended time in culture, but displayed mixed responsiveness to terminal differentiation agents or inducers, similar to cell lines produced with the wild-type β-YAC (data not shown). However, both firefly and Renilla luciferase activities steadily declined in cell pools or clones, whether induced or not, after 28 weeks of culture.

Transgenic mice were also produced with this dual luc β-YAC. The hematopoietic tissues of staged conceptuses were assayed for γ-firefly luciferase and β-Renilla luciferase. Generally, the two gene fusions showed correct developmental regulation, with γ-luc predominating during primitive erythropoiesis in the yolk sac and β-luc during the later stages of definitive erythropoiesis in the fetal liver and in the adult bone marrow (data not shown). CID-dependent dual luc β-YAC BMCs displayed a β-like globin gene expression pattern that was identical to previously established CID-dependent wild-type β-YAC BMCs, however γ-firefly-luc or β-Renilla-luc transcription/enzyme activity were the parameters measured, rather than native γ- or β-globin transcript/protein levels. In the absence of any HbF activating compounds, these cells were γ-luc$^-$ β-luc$^+$ (data not shown). Using this cell-based assay, a HTS and secondary verification assays were performed as outlined in Figure 1B.

Primary HTS

Parameters for the HTS are described in Methods and outcomes are summarized in Tables 1 and 2. The screening assay was found to be robust with an acceptable dynamic range between the positive (sodium butyrate induction) and negative DMSO

Table 2. Reordered compounds.

Compound Source	No. of Compounds	Amount (mgs)
ChemBridge Library	171	2
ChemDiv Library	21	2
Orthogonally compressed library (LCGC)	40	2–5
Total No. of compounds	232	

100% DMSO: 50 or 100 mM.

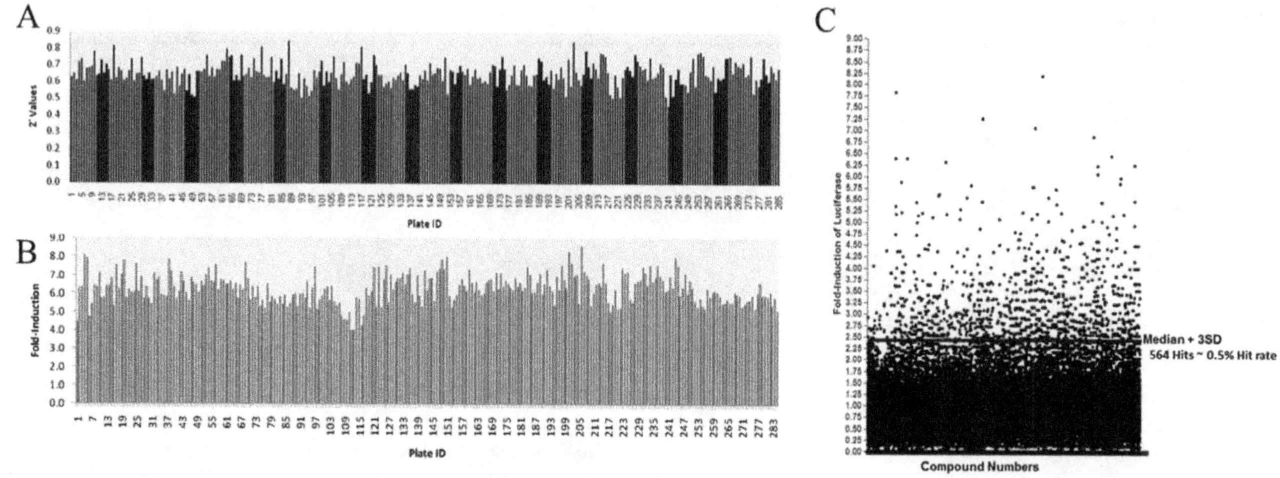

Figure 2. High-throughput screening for firefly luciferase inducers. Panel A) Distribution of Z′ scores. An average Z′ of 0.65±0.067 was obtained across all assay plates indicating suitability of the assay for high-throughput screening of 121,035 compounds. **Panel B**) Sodium butyrate-induced firefly luciferase expression. The treatment of cells with the positive control sodium butyrate resulted in an average increase in firefly luciferase expression by 6.3±0.77-fold across all 300 plates tested. **Panel C**) Scattergram of fold-induction of all 121,085 compounds tested using CID-dependent dual-luc β-YAC BMCs. 564 active compounds were identified that induced firefly luciferase greater than 3 standard deviations above the plate median.

vehicle baseline controls across all the plates screened. The good separation of controls, as well as low variability around the means of the controls, resulted in an average Z′ factor value of 0.65±0.06 (Figure 2A) [29]. An average 6.3±0.7-fold induction of firefly luciferase was obtained with treatment of cells with 2 mM sodium butyrate (Figure 2B). The majority of compounds screened did not induce firefly luciferase. As shown in the scattergram of fold-induction of all 121,035 compounds screened (Figure 2C), only 564 compounds induced luciferase to greater than or equal to that of the plate median+3SD, resulting in a hit rate of 0.49%. A maximum fold-activation of >8-fold was obtained with some compounds in the primary screen. The actives from the primary screen were cherry-picked from mother plates and retested for firefly luciferase induction in an eight concentration dose-response (two fold dilution starting at 30 μM). Of 564 compounds, 328 compounds were dose-responsive with 83 compounds inducing luciferase to greater than 2.5 fold. The compounds were subjected to cheminformatics analysis to define the structural groups and the range of activities within each group (data not shown). At least 12 distinct clusters were identified using the Tripos Selector program. From each preliminary cluster, the largest conserved substructure present in at least half of the cluster members was identified. These data will used to guide efforts to progress these compounds forward as potential therapeutics and assist in choosing additional compound banks to screen.

Secondary assays

In order to establish that the firefly induction activity was not due to breakdown products of library compounds, some of the active compounds were repurchased as fresh powders (>95% purity). Of the 121,035 compounds screened, 232 actives that met the criteria outlined above, were identified and repurchased for further testing and validation. The number of actives within the 232 hit set identified in the primary screen of the CID-dependent dual luc BMCs that had γ-firefly luciferase induction 2-fold or higher was 211, thus 90% of the originally identified actives were reconfirmed (Figure 3A). The activity of the repurchased compounds was tested in a 10 concentration dose-response in the following 3 cell-based assays using the same CID-dependent dual luc BMCs used in the primary screen: 1) γ-firefly luciferase induction assay, 2) β-Renilla luciferase induction, and 3) cytotoxicity assays (Figure 1B). In addition to the three cell-based assays, a biochemical screen was set up using purified firefly luciferase to identify compounds that directly inhibit luciferase enzyme activity. Luciferase enzyme binders/modulators have been implicated in stabilizing luciferase RNA and hence appear as false positives in luciferase-based screens [30]. Based on these four secondary assays, at least 124 compounds were found to specifically induce firefly luciferase between 2- to 11-fold (Figure 3A), did not induce β-globin promoter-Renilla luciferase, and were not cytotoxic to the dual reporter-expressing BMCs (data not shown). None of the 124 compounds inhibited purified firefly luciferase.

Some of these compounds were tested in physiologically relevant non-reporter assay systems [31]. Seven cherry-picked repurchased compounds showed fold-induction of firefly luciferase (Figure 3B). The corresponding induction of Renilla luciferase activity is also shown in Figure 3B. These compounds were also tested for their ability to inhibit firefly luciferase enzyme in a biochemical assay (Figure 3C). The cytotoxicity of these compounds in CID-dependent dual luc β-YAC BMCs is shown in Figure 3D. All compounds were found to specifically up-regulate firefly luciferase with no significant induction of the Renilla reporter. While most of the compounds were not cytotoxic, a few compounds were found to affect cell viability at higher concentrations. Compounds #1 and #157 appear to be less cytotoxic than the control (Figure 3D); however in subsequent assays described below these compounds did not have a stimulatory effect on cell proliferation. Thus, the increased γ-globin signal was not a consequence of increased cell number.

Most of the firefly luciferase inducers did not significantly inhibit the luciferase enzyme (IC50>100 μM). Table 3 shows the EC50 values for the molar concentrations of these compounds resulting in 50% stimulation of firefly luciferase expression and their corresponding IC50 values for the molar concentrations resulting in 50% loss of cell viability. The therapeutic index for each compound was calculated from the ratio of IC50 for cytotoxicity to

A

Fold-Induction	Number
11-11.99	2
9-9.99	1
7-7.99	1
6.0-6.99	3
5.0-5.99	10
4.0-4.99	32
3.0-3.99	73
2.0-2.99	82
1.5-1.99	11
1.0-1.49	17

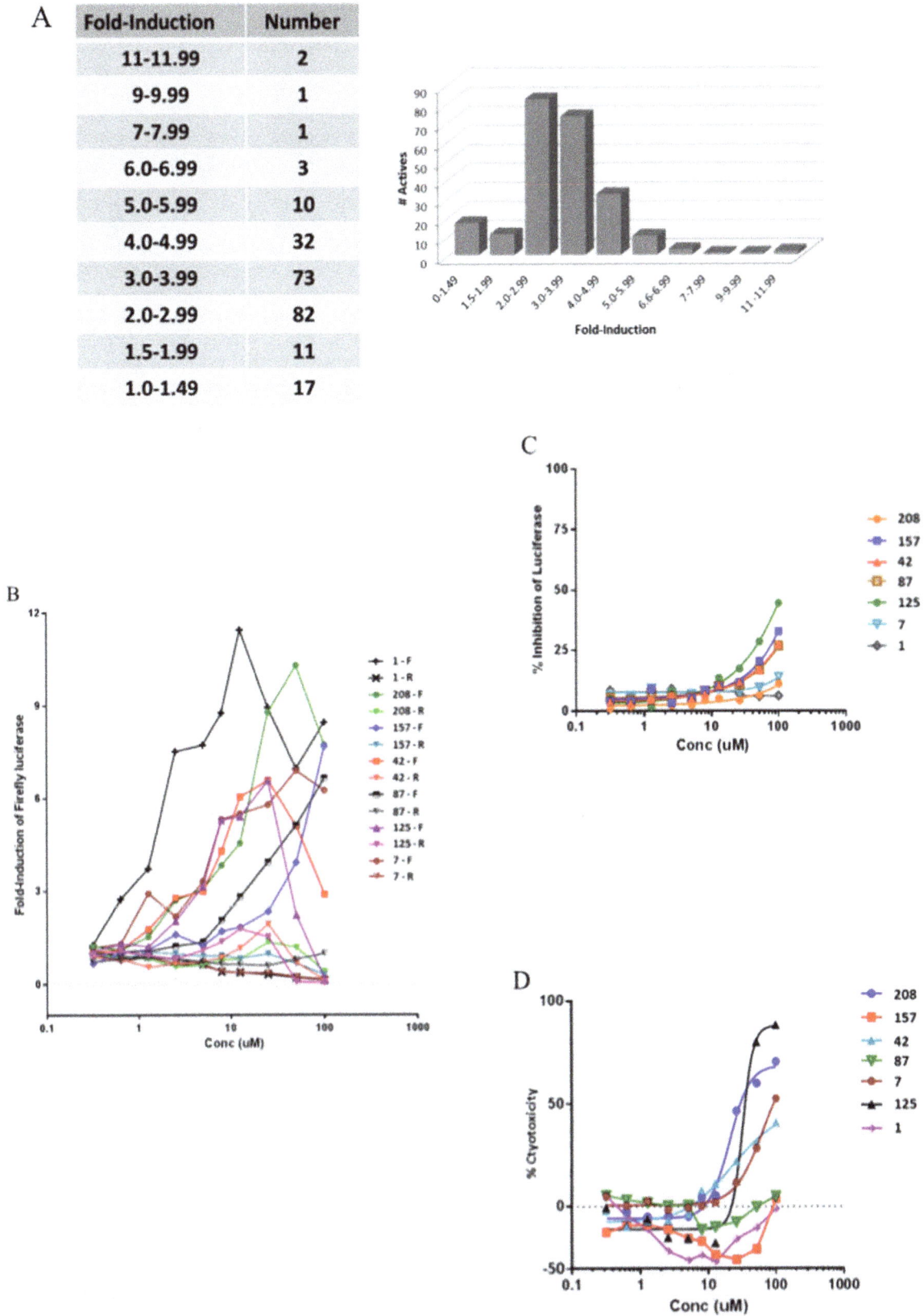

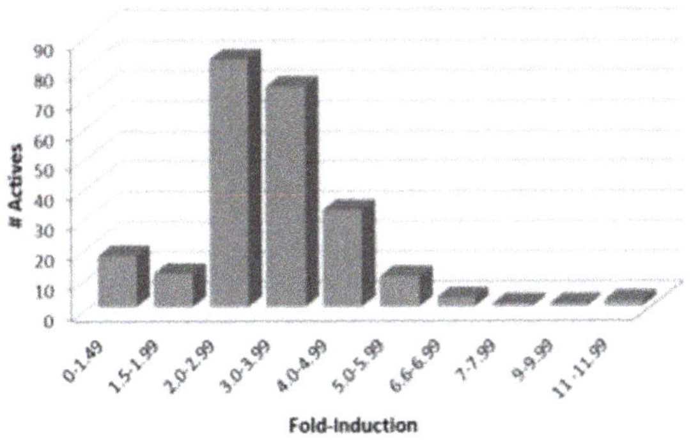

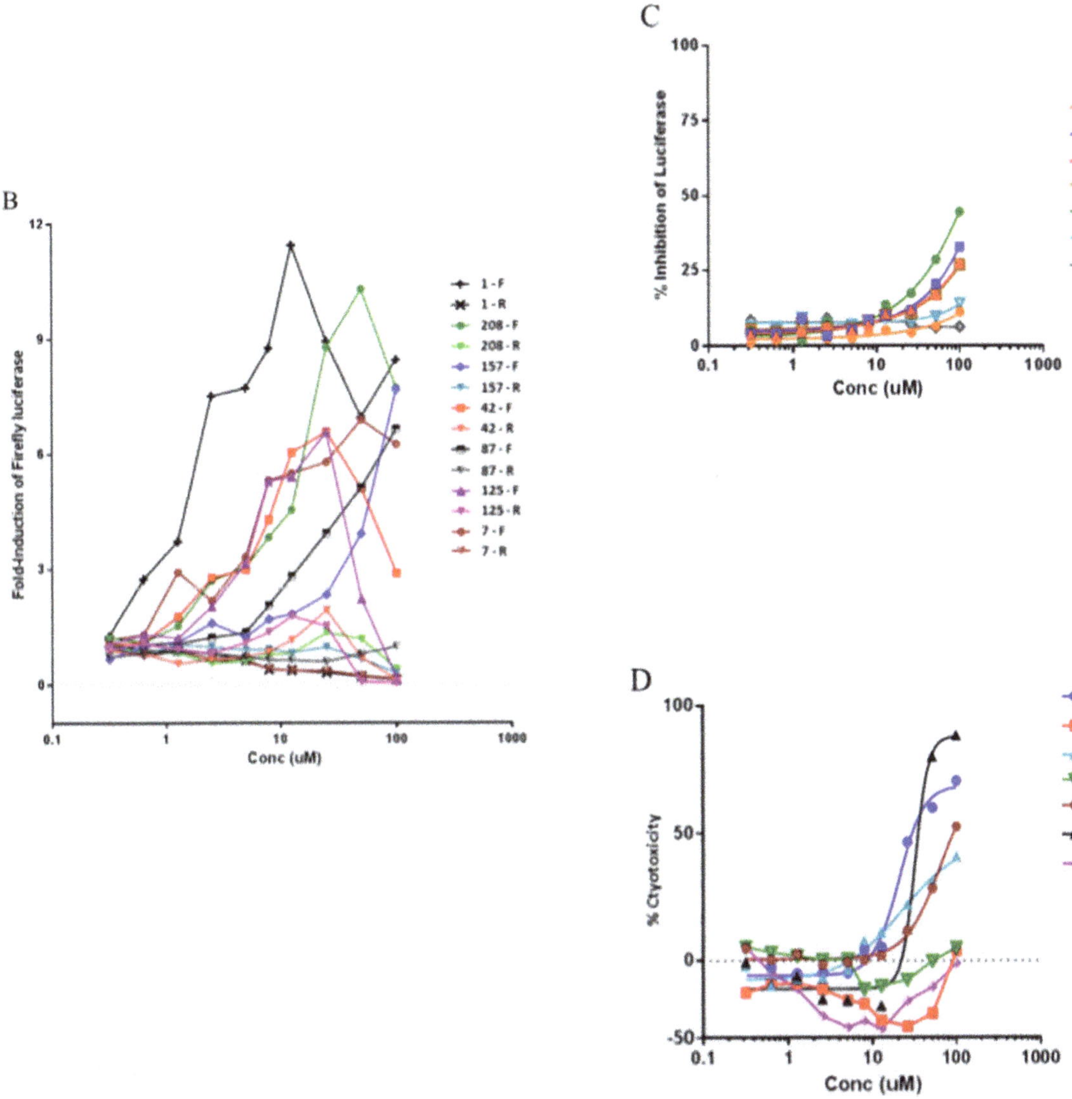

Figure 3. Reconfirmation and secondary assays of γ-globin inducer compounds. Panel A) Reconfirmation of γ-luc inducibility by 232 actives from primary HTS. Four secondary assays were employed including two reconfirmation assays for firefly luciferase induction and cytotoxicity, and two specificity assays for Renilla luciferase activity and luciferase enzyme modulators. All assays were a 10-point dose-response. A summary of firefly induction is shown in this figure. 211 of the 232 compounds had firefly induction of 2-fold or higher; a 90% reconfirmation rate.

Panels B-D) Performance of seven γ-firefly inducers in the initial four secondary assays - detailed 10-point dose-response data. Comparison of compound activity from dose-response data is shown for firefly and Renilla luciferase activity (**Panel B**), purified firefly luciferase enzyme inhibition (**Panel C**), and cytotoxicity (**Panel D**). Assays were performed as described in Materials and Methods.

EC50 for luciferase stimulation. A larger window indicates significant separation of stimulatory activity of the compound from its cytotoxic effects. As shown in Table 3, the therapeutic windows were found to be significant for a majority of the compounds tested. Compound 1 with EC50 ~1.4 μM and no detectable cytotoxicity exhibited the most favorable profile.

Fetal hemoglobin activation in CID-dependent wild-type β-YAC BMCs

The HTS and initial validation of hits measured luciferase activity from fusions to the γ- and β-globin gene promoters. Thus, an important first secondary assay was to demonstrate that our actives effectively induced native γ-globin mRNA and protein, as well as the formation of HbF. For this purpose we utilized CID-dependent BMCs derived from wild-type β-YAC transgenic mice [26]. Criteria for cherry-picking compounds for testing in secondary assays included those with the highest fold induction, coupled with lowest toxicity. These are the top seven compounds listed in the table from Figure 3A. Compound #1 was dropped from further consideration because cell survival proved to be lower than expected based on the HTS results.

To confirm the effectiveness of these compounds, human γ- and β-globin gene expression was measured by qPCR in RNA samples from wild-type β-YAC BMCs treated with the 6 remaining compounds (Figure 4). γ-globin expression increased 26.9-fold with compound #42 and 13.6-fold with compound #208. Compounds #7 and #87 also induced γ-globin expression (3.7- and 2.3-fold, respectively). Sodium butyrate (NaB) and DMSO treatment was performed in parallel as a positive control and solvent control, respectively; 9.9-fold induction of γ-globin expression was observed with NaB treatment. Two of the compounds did not increase γ-globin transcription (#125 and #157). No induction of adult β-globin was observed with any of the 7 compounds tested.

γ-globin (HbF)-expressing F cells were measured in parallel to confirm the induction of γ-globin expression at the protein level. Compound #208 showed 16% F cells and compound #42 had 14.1% F cells, compared to 15.9% F cells with NaB treatment and no change in F cells in DMSO only-treated and untreated samples (Figure 5A). These results are consistent with the induction of γ-globin observed at mRNA levels. Interestingly, compounds #7 and #87 showed higher induction of γ-globin at the protein level than mRNA, with 12.3% and 9.9% F cells (Figure 5A). The change in number of cells expressing γ-globin ranged from 14-46-fold (compounds #125 and #157 not included) compared to untreated cells, and in general, mirrored the % F cells measured (Figure 5B). Compound #42 was an exception with fewer cells expressing γ-globin compared to the number of F cells, whereas the opposite was true for compound # 87 and especially for compound #208. For compound # 208 this outcome might have been related to lower viability of cells following treatment (Figure 5C).

Based on the RT-qPCR and flow cytometry data for the six compounds assessed, #125 and #157 were dropped from further analyses based on lack of γ-globin transcript induction. Change in HbF was measured by ELISA following treatment with the remaining compounds in the wild-type β-YAC BMCs, as described in Materials and Methods. The pattern of expression of HbF by ELISA was similar to the mRNA expression results (Figure 5D). Treatment with compound #42 produced the greatest increase in HbF with the least variability, followed by compound #208 (with much greater variability), and then compound #7. The smallest response was seen with compound #87. The variation in response to #208 may be related to the much larger decrease in viability we observed with this compound (40%; Figure 5C)

Fetal hemoglobin activation in human primary erythroid progenitor cells

Our last set of studies was aimed at demonstrating the ability of the lead compounds to induce HbF expression in human erythroid progenitors generated in liquid cultures. CD34+ cells were cultured in a 2-stage system as described in Materials and Methods. Initial studies were performed to monitor terminal erythroid maturation and the γ- to β-globin switch in this system. Cells were harvested every 2–3 days and morphology was examined by Giemsa staining. We observed a steady progression of erythropoiesis with 19% reticulocytes and mature red blood cells by day 14 (Figure 6A). We next performed qRT-PCR to follow the γ- to β-globin switch, which was observed around day 10 in culture (Figure 6B). These data support the use of this system to test the ability of lead compounds to activate human γ-globin.

Table 3. EC50, IC50 and therapeutic index for seven cherry-picked compounds.

	Firefly Luciferase		Cytotoxicity	
Compound ID	**EC50 (μM)**	**Fold-induction**	**IC50 (μM)**	**Therapeutic Index**
1	1.4	8.6	>100	>100
7	5.9	6.5	87.6	15
42	9.8	5.2	>100	>100
87	49.3	9.6	>100	>100
125	5.7	7.0	35.0	6
157	30.0	9.5	>100	>100
208	14.3	10.1	24.3	2

>100: Less than 10% or no cytotoxicity up to 100 μM tested.

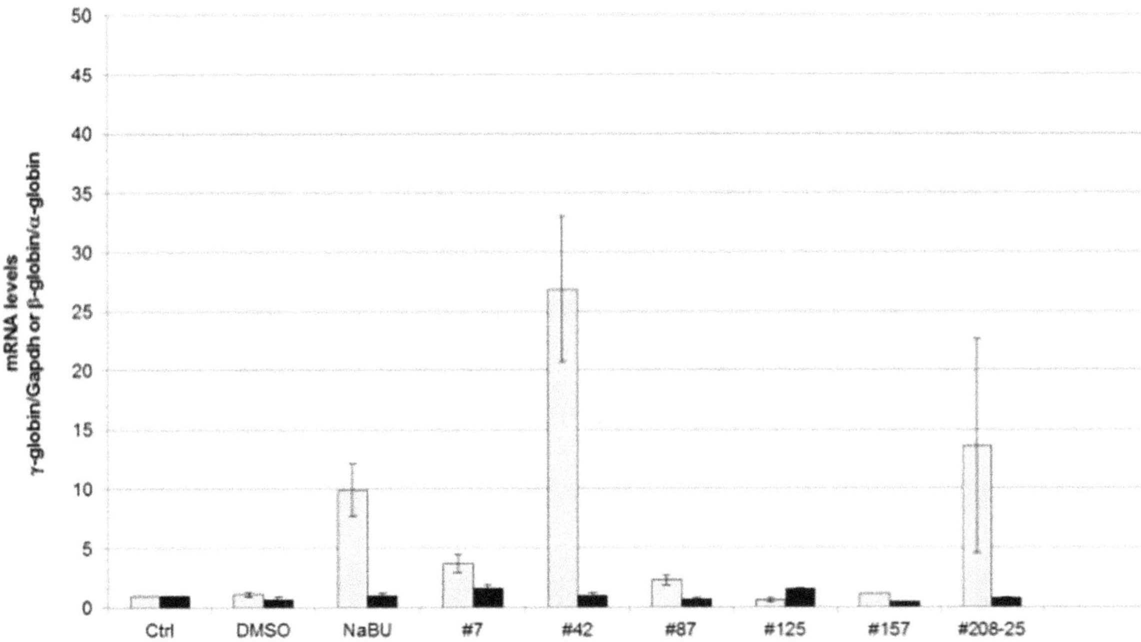

Figure 4. γ-globin and β-globin mRNA levels in compound-treated CID-dependent wild-type β-YAC mouse bone marrow cells. qRT-PCR was performed as described in Materials and Methods. Fold change in mRNA level is shown on the y-axis; sample names are shown on the x-axis. Ctrl, untreated cells; DMSO, cells treated with DMSO only; NaB, 2 mM sodium butyrate; #7, 50 μM; #42, 15 μM, #87; 100 μM; #125, 30 μM; #157, 100 μM; #208-25, 25 μM. Gray bars, γ-globin mRNA expression; black bars, β-globin mRNA expression. Data shown are the results of two-three separate experiments, with each sample duplicated within an experiment. P≤0.01 for NaB and compound # 42; P≤0.05 for compounds #42 and #208.

The various compounds were added on day 8 for 48 hours and cell viability, measured by trypan blue exclusion, remained greater than 97% throughout the culture period. Using qRT-PCR, the γ-globin to β-globin (γ/β) ratio was increased 1.8-fold for the positive control sodium butyrate when compared to DMSO (Figure 6C). In contrast, the γ/β ratio for lead compounds #7, #42, #87 and #208 was increased 2.8-, 2.9-, 1.6- and 2.2-fold, respectively.

FACS analysis was conducted to determine if the lead compounds induce HbF synthesis in erythroid progenitors by measuring the % HbF-positive cells (Figure 7A). We observed a 7-fold increase in % HbF-positive cells after sodium butyrate treatment compared to a 2.7-5.1-fold increase mediated by the lead compounds (Figure 7B). DMSO alone did not change the levels of HbF-positive cells significantly. These data demonstrate the ability of the lead compounds #7, #42, #87 and #208 to act as HbF-inducers in human primary erythroid cells.

Discussion

Proteins with potential therapeutic value must meet the criteria implied or predicted for druggable targets based on evolutionary relationships, 3D-structural properties, features derived from amino-acid sequence or properties of ligands known to bind the protein. Proteins with narrow specificity for regulating γ-globin gene expression constitute potential ideal druggable targets, but none have been identified. Alternate approaches utilized molecular modeling to identify new therapeutic candidates based on compounds previously shown to induce HbF, such as short-chain fatty acids and derivatives [32], a chemical genetic strategy in primary cells for HDAC1 and 2 inhibitors [33], an optical assay in which the color is proportional to the anti-sickling effect of the test compound [34] or a more naïve cell-based γ-globin expression reporter HTS assay [35]. This latter approach relied on phenotype (γ-globin induction, enhanced HbF expression) to identify useful agents, rather than searching for compounds or ligands that directly affect a target protein. The lack of fetal γ-globin-specific regulatory proteins that meet druggability criteria has made this approach the method of choice for identification of potential new therapeutic compounds to treat β-hemoglobinopathies. Research on γ-globin gene regulation may result in the discovery of fetal-specific activators or repressors that may be druggable. In the meantime, phenotypic selection for HbF chemical inducers using assays amenable to HTS of large compound libraries will allow exhaustive assessment of all available compound and drug libraries.

The reporter assay in the cell-based HTS mentioned above was not robust [34], but the cell-based system we developed provides a tightly-regulated γ-globin expression "off-on" switch with a readout that was adapted for HTS. Identification of pharmacologic agents capable of reactivating γ-globin gene expression has been complicated by the lack of suitable cell lines. Essentially, cell lines were not available that displayed a suitable "off-on" switch for γ-globin gene expression, including mouse human globin transgenic MEL cells, HFE-MEL switching hybrids, and human K562 or HEL cells. We rationalized that a better approach would be to use primary progenitors derived from β-YAC transgenic mouse bone marrow using a novel method to immortalize these cells [24], [26], [36]. A CID was used to specifically and reversibly control the growth of primary, multi-potential hematopoietic cell populations *in vitro* and establish cell culture. In CID-dependent wild-type β-YAC BMCs, β-globin is expressed, but γ-globin expression is not detectable. However, expression is inducible using a variety of drugs known to increase HbF. Endogenous mouse β^{maj}-globin and α-globin are also synthesized [26].

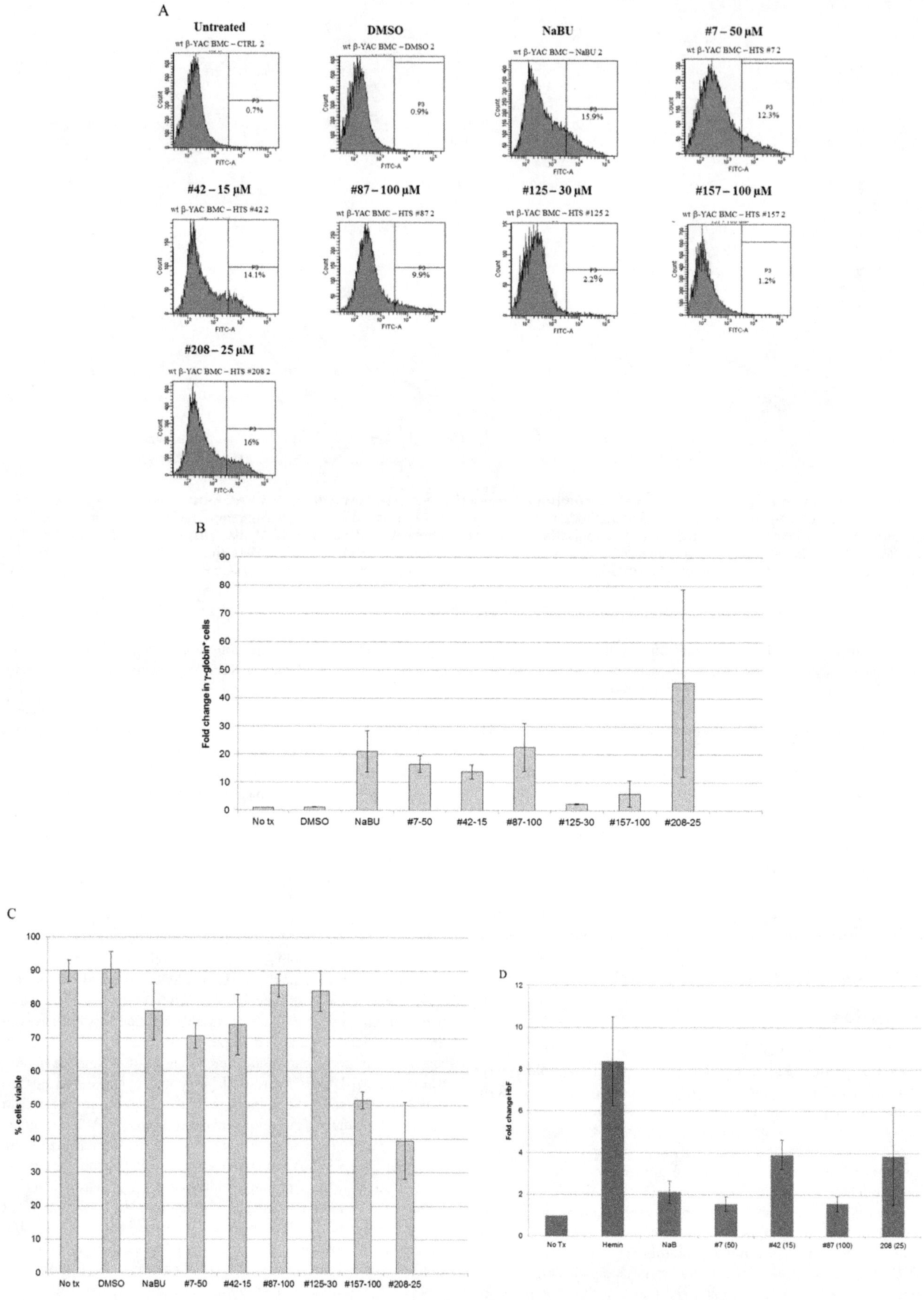
A
Untreated
DMSO
NaBU
#7 – 50 μM
0.7%
0.9%
15.9%
12.3%
#42 – 15 μM
#87 – 100 μM
#125 – 30 μM
#157 – 100 μM
14.1%
9.9%
2.2%
1.2%
#208 – 25 μM
16%
Count
FITC-A
B
Fold change in γ-globin+ cells
No tx
DMSO
NaBU
#7-50
#42-15
#87-100
#125-30
#157-100
#208-25
C
% cells viable
No tx
DMSO
NaBU
#7-50
#42-15
#87-100
#125-30
#157-100
#208-25
D
Fold change HbF
No Tx
Hemin
NaB
#7 (50)
#42 (15)
#87 (100)
208 (25)

Figure 5. Induction of HbF by lead compounds in CID-dependent mouse BMCs. Panel A) FACS analysis of HbF levels in compound-treated CID-dependent wild-type β-YAC mouse bone marrow cells. The protocol was carried out as described in Materials and Methods using anti-human HbF FITC-conjugated antibody. Samples are labeled as described in the legend to Figure 4, but compound concentration follows the compound number. Representative data from one experiment is shown here, but the experiment was replicated two to three times for each sample with similar results (summarized in Panels B and C). **Panels B-C) Summary of FACS analysis of HbF levels in compound-treated CID-dependent wild-type β-YAC mouse bone marrow cells. Panel B)** fold change in γ-globin (FITC)$^+$ cells. **Panel C)** percent viable cells. Bars show mean and standard error of the mean in control and compound-treated cells for each panel. **Panel D) HbF induction measured by ELISA in compound-treated CID-dependent wild-type β-YAC mouse bone marrow cells.** The assay was carried out as described in Materials and Methods. Fold induction of HbF is shown on the y-axis; cell treatment and concentration, where applicable, are shown on the x-axis. Data represent the mean and standard error of the mean from four experiments with duplicate samples within each experiment.

Addition of erythropoietin (Epo) and stem cell factor (SCF) modestly enhance globin gene expression; a cocktail of Epo, granulocyte monoctye-colony stimulating factor (GM-CSF) and interleukin-3 (IL-3) does not. BMCs derived from -117 Greek HPFH β-YAC transgenic mice [37] recapitulated the HPFH phenotype. A γ-globin-specific synthetic Zn finger activator protein (gg1-VP64) [38], [39] induced γ-globin synthesis in wild-type β-YAC BMCs, as does enforced expression of other fetal-specific transcriptional activators including FKLF and FGIF [26]. Differentiation into terminal erythrocytes is not required, since globin gene expression patterns are similar in both our BMC and erythroid cell populations.

CID-dependent bone marrow cells were established from $^{A}\gamma$-luc β-luc β-YAC transgenic mice. These cells were utilized to develop and benchmark a robust HTS assay to identify compounds that 1) induced γ-globin gene expression, 2) did not induce β-globin gene

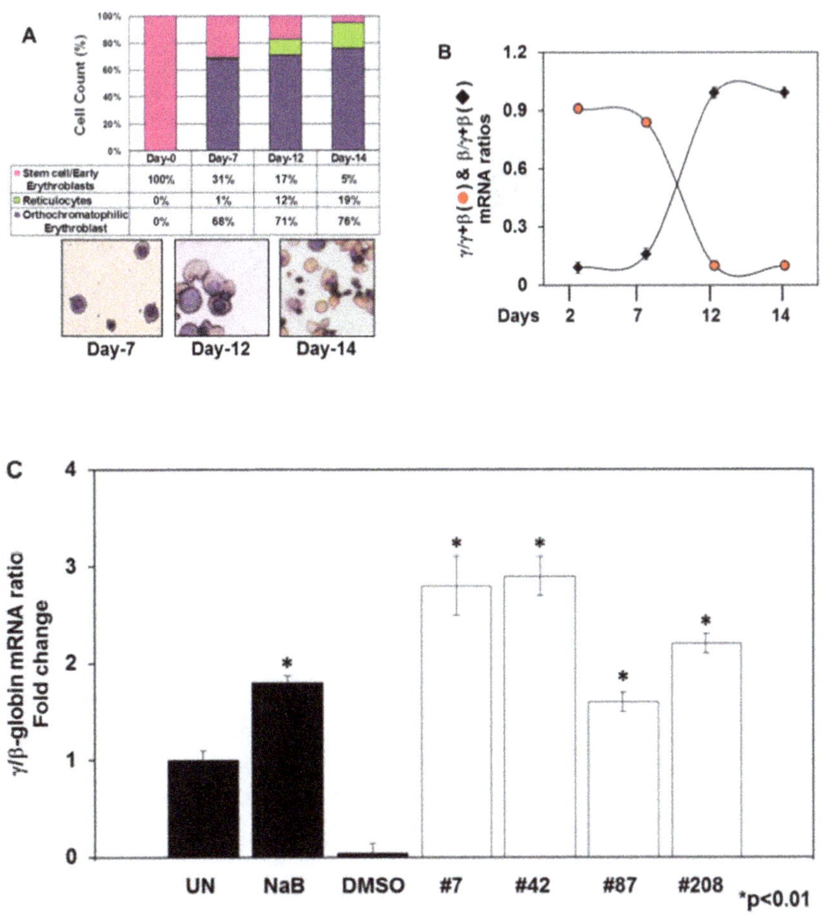

Figure 6. γ-globin expression is induced in compound-treated human primary erythroid progenitors. Human erythroid progenitors were generated from adult CD34$^+$ cells in liquid culture as described in Materials and Method). Cells were analyzed for morphology, globin gene expression and HbF induction after treatment with the lead compounds. **Panel A**) Erythroid cells were harvested on the days indicated for cell morphology determination by Geimsa staining. The percentage of different erythroid progenitors at each stage is shown as a function of days in culture. At least 500 cells were counted by light microscopy from duplicate slides. Representative cell morphology is shown in the images at 40× magnification. **Panel B**) qRT-PCR was performed as described in Materials and Methods. The levels of γ- and β-globin expression were normalized to GAPH; expression of each gene is shown as a fraction of the total globin (γ+β). Note the γ-to β-globin switch around day 10. **Panel C**) Fold change in γ-globin/β-globin mRNA ratio after normalization to GAPDH is shown on the y-axis. UN, untreated cells; DMSO, cells treated with DMSO only; NaB, 2 mM sodium butyrate; lead compounds: #7, 50 μM; #42, 15 μM, #87; 100 μM; #208, 25 μM. Data shown are the mean and standard error of the mean of three independent samples.

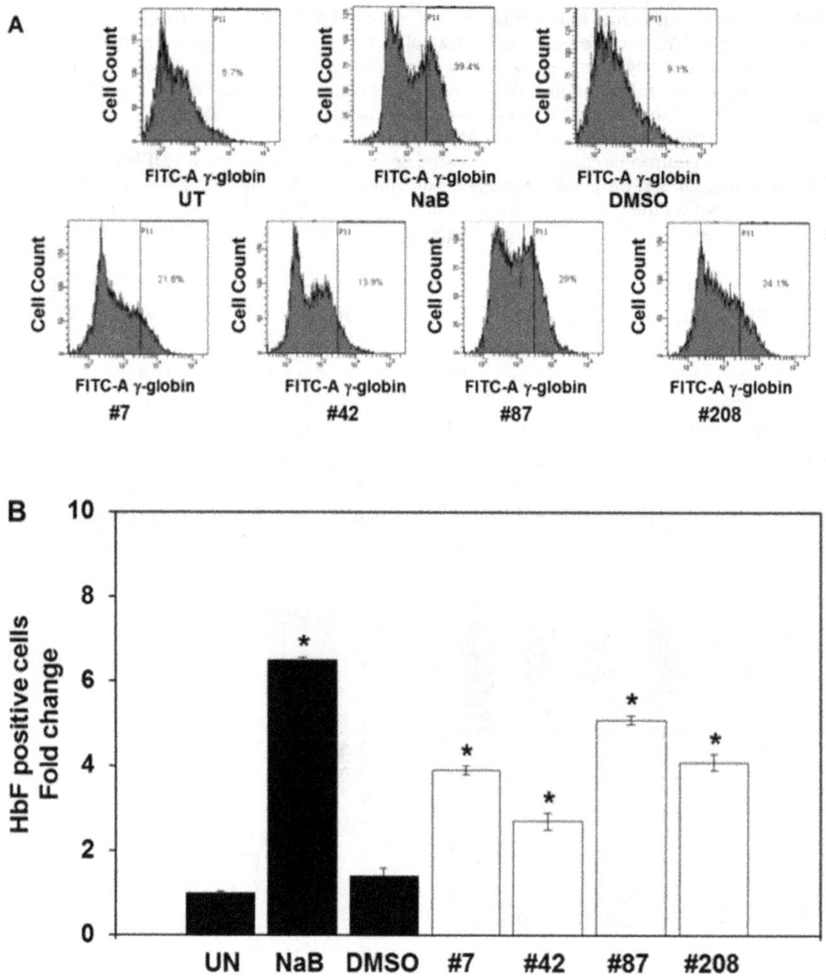

Figure 7. The lead compounds induce HbF expression in human primary erythroid cells. FACS analysis was performed with erythroid progenitors treated for 48 hours with each of the four lead chemical compounds. The protocol was carried out as described in Materials and Methods using anti-human HbF FITC-conjugated antibody. **Panel A**) Representative FACS tracings are shown; experiments were replicated three times for each compound with similar results. **Panel B**) Based on the FACS data the % HbF-positive cells (FITC-A) was calculated for the different treatment conditions. Shown in the graph is the fold change in HbF-positive cells. Data are shown as the mean and standard error of the mean in control and compound-treated cells for each sample. *; $P<0.01$.

expression, 3) were not cytotoxic and 4) did not directly affect luciferase enzymatic activity. The HTS surveyed 121,035 compounds from various libraries and yielded 232 hits that induced γ-luc 2- to 11-fold. Of these, 211 were reconfirmed for γ-luc induction, and 124 met the constraints of the four listed criteria following a 4-assay, 10 point dose-response secondary screen. Six of the top 124 actives were cherry-picked for further analysis and conformation in other cell-based systems.

Our first assessment was in wild-type β-YAC BMCs, where normal γ-globin transcript and protein levels could be measured in the multi-potential mouse BMC background, rather than luciferase activity. Using the optimum dose for each compound, four of the six compounds induced γ-globin transcription 2- to 26-fold and had increased F cells ranging from 9.9 to 16% in wild-type β-YAC BMCs. ELISA concurred with these data; an approximately 2- to 4-fold increase in HbF was observed; the same pattern of change seen in mRNA levels was reflected in protein levels.

Although different cell lines have been used extensively to screen chemical compound libraries for HbF inducers, these lines do not undergo hemoglobin switching. Thus, the output of these screens may yield false-positive hits that do not correlate with their ability to induce HbF in primary human erythroid progenitors. The dual luciferase reporter system established in primary mouse BMCs immortalized by the CID and used for the HTS described in this report more closely mimics human erythroid progenitors. Our studies in erythroid progenitors generated from adult human primary CD34$^+$ stem cells confirmed the validity of using the CID-dependent β-YAC BMCs for the HTS. In addition, the data demonstrated that this system recapitulated erythropoiesis and the γ to β-globin switch in a manner similar to that previously published using another liquid culture system [40], [41]. The advantage of the human progenitor terminal differentiation protocol is that we produce mature erythrocytes and mimic the γ- to β-globin switch similar to normal erythropoiesis *in vivo*, thereby adding further credibility to our hit identification. The fact that HbF was induced by lead compounds #7, #42, #87 and #208 to levels greater than sodium butyrate suggests that these agents are candidates for further drug development using medicinal chemistry approaches to treat β-hemoglobinopathies.

Acknowledgments

The HTS facility would like to thank Drs. Joseph Heppert, Roy Jensen, Barbara Timmermann and Scott Weir for their continued support of the KU HTSL and drug discovery research at KU.

Author Contributions

Conceived and designed the experiments: KRP FCC RYN AR RC BSP. Performed the experiments: KRP FCC HF RYN AMC LZ AHF PD AR BL BSP. Analyzed the data: KRP FCC HF RYN AMC PD AR RC BSP. Contributed reagents/materials/analysis tools: KRP RYN BL BSP. Contributed to the writing of the manuscript: KRP FCC RYN AR BSP.

References

1. Ashley-Koch A, Yang Q, Olney RS (2000) Sickle hemoglobin (HbS) allele and sickle cell disease: a HuGE review. Am J Epidemiol 151: 839–845.
2. Lancaster JR Jr (2003) Sickle cell disease: loss of the blood's WD40? Trends Pharmacol Sci 24: 389–391.
3. Vichinsky E (2002) New therapies in sickle cell disease. Lancet 360: 629–631.
4. Charache S (1997) Mechanism of action of hydroxyurea in the management of sickle cell anemia in adults. Semin Hematol 34(3 Suppl 3): 15–21.
5. Steinberg MH, Lu ZH, Barton FB, Terrin ML, Charache S, et al. (1997) Fetal hemoglobin in sickle cell anemia: determinants of response to hydroxyurea. Multicenter Study of Hydroxyurea. Blood 89: 1078–1088.
6. Davies SC, Gilmore A (2003) The role of hydroxyurea in the management of sickle cell disease. Blood Rev 17: 99–109.
7. DeSimone J, Heller P, Hall L, Zwiers D (1982) 5-azacytidine stimulates fetal hemoglobin synthesis (HbF) in anemic baboons. Proc Natl Acad Sci USA 79: 4428–4431.
8. Ley TJ, DeSimone J, Anagnou NP, Keller GH, Humphries RK, et al. (1982) 5-Azacytidine selectively increases γ-globin synthesis in a patient with β+ thalassemia. N Engl J Med 307: 1469–1475.
9. Letvin NL, Linch D, Beardsley GP, McIntyre KW, Nathan DG (1984) Augmentation of fetal-hemoglobin production in anemic monkeys by hydroxyurea. N Engl J Med 310: 869–873.
10. Papayannopoulou T, Torrealba de Ron A, Veith R, Knitter G, Stamatoyannopoulos G (1984) Arabinosylcytosine induces fetal hemoglobin in baboons by perturbing erythroid cell differentiation kinetics. Science 224: 617–619.
11. Perrine SP, Rudolph A, Faller DV, Roman C, Cohen RA, et al. (1988) Butyrate infusions in the ovine fetus delays the biologic clock for globin gene switching. Proc Natl Acad Sci USA 85: 8540–8542.
12. Constantoulakis P, Papayannopoulou T, Stamatoyannopoulos (1988) α-amino-N-butyric acid stimulates fetal hemoglobin in the adult. Blood 72: 1961–1967.
13. Liakopoulou E, Blau CA, Li Q, Josephson B, Wolf JA, et al. (1995) Stimulation of fetal hemoglobin production by short chain fatty acids. Blood 86: 3227–3235.
14. Little JA, Dempsey NJ, Tuchman M, Ginder GD (1995) Metabolic persistence of fetal hemoglobin. Blood 85: 1712–1718.
15. Hertzberg RP, Pope AJ (2000) High-throughput screening: new technology for the 21st century. Curr Opin Chem Biol 4: 445–451.
16. Fox S, Wang H, Sopchak L, Farr-Jones S (2002) High throughput screening 2002: moving toward increased success rates. J Biomol Screen 7: 313–316.
17. Cheng D, Yadav N, King RW, Swanson MS, Weinstein EJ, et al. (2004) Small molecule regulators of protein arginine methyltransferases. J Biol Chem 279: 23892–23899.
18. Ye QZ, Xie SX, Huang M, Huang WJ, Lu JP, et al. (2004) Metalloform-selective inhibitors of E. coli methionine aminopeptidase and X-ray structure of a Mn(II)-form enzyme complexed with an inhibitor. J Am Chem Soc 126: 13940–13941.
19. Ma T, Thiagarajah JR, Yang H, Sonawane ND, Folli C et al. (2002) Thiazolidinone CFTR inhibitor identified by high-throughput screening blocks cholera toxin-induced intestinal fluid secretion. J Clin Invest 110: 1651–1658.
20. Gaensler KM, Burmeister M, Brownstein BH, Taillon-Miller P, Myers RM (1991) Physical mapping of yeast artificial chromosomes containing sequences from the human β-globin gene region. Genomics 10: 976–984.
21. Rothstein RJ (1983) One-step gene disruption in yeast. Meth Enzymol 101: 202–210.
22. Peterson KR, Navas PA, Li Q, Stamatoyannopoulos G (1998) LCR-dependent gene expression in β-globin YAC transgenics: detailed structural studies validate functional analysis even in the presence of fragmented YACs. Hum Mol Genet 7: 2079–2088.
23. Peterson KR, Clegg CH, Huxley C, Josephson BM, Haugen HS, et al. (1993) Transgenic mice containing a 248-kb yeast artificial chromosome carrying the human β-globin locus display proper developmental control of human globin genes. Proc Natl Acad Sci USA 90: 7593–7597.
24. Blau CA, Peterson KR (2006) Establishment of cell lines that exhibit correct ontogenic stage-specific gene expression profiles from tissues of YAC transgenic mice using chemically induced growth signals. In: MacKenzie, A, editor. Methods in Molecular Biology, Vol. 349: YAC Protocols, 2nd ed. Totowa, NJ: Humana Press. pp. 163–173.
25. Hebiguchi M, Hirokawa M, Guo YM, Saito K, Wakui H, et al. (2008) Dynamics of human erythroblast enucleation. Int J Hematol 88: 498–507.
26. Blau CA, Barbas CF 3rd, Bomhoff A, Neades R, Yan J, et al. (2005) γ-globin gene expression in CID-dependent multi-potential cells established from β-YAC transgenic mice. J Biol Chem 280: 36642–36647.
27. Peterson KR, Zitnik G, Huxley C, Lowrey CH, Gnirke A, et al. (1993) Use of yeast artificial chromosomes (YACs) for studying control of gene expression: regulation of the genes of a human β-globin locus YAC following transfer to mouse erythroleukemia lines. Proc Natl Acad Sci USA 90: 11207–11211.
28. Vassilopoulos G, Navas PA, Skarpidi E, Peterson KR, Lowrey CH, et al. (1999) Correct function of the locus control region may require passage through a non-erythroid cellular environment. Blood 93: 703–712.
29. Zhang JH, Chung TD, Oldenburg KR (1999) A simple statistical parameter for use in evaluation and validation of high throughput screening assays. J Biomol Screen 4: 67–73.
30. Auld DS, Thorne N, Nguyen DT, Inglese J (2008) A specific mechanism for nonspecific activation in reporter-gene assays. ACS Chem Biol 3: 463–470.
31. Roy A, Taylor BJ, McDonald PR, Price AR, Chaguturu R (2009) Hit-to-probe-to-lead optimization strategies: a biological perspective to conquer the valley of death. In Seethala R, Zhang L, editors. Handbook of Drug Screening. Zug Switzerland: Informa Healthcare. pp. 21–55.
32. Boosalis MS, Castaneda SA, Trudel M, Mabaera R, White GL, et al. (2011) Novel therapeutic candidates, identified by molecular modeling, induce γ-globin expression in vivo. Blood Cells Mol Dis 47: 107–116.
33. Bradner JE, Mak R, Tanguturi SK, Mazitschek R, Haggarty SJ, et al. (2010) Chemical genetic strategy identifies histone deacetylase 1 (HDAC1) and HDAC2 as therapeutic targets in sickle cell disease. Proc Natl Acad Sci USA 107: 12617–12622.
34. Pais E, Cambridge JS, Johnson CS, Meiselman HJ, Fisher TC, et al. (2009) A novel high-throughput screening assay for sickle cell disease drug discovery. J Biomolec Screen 14: 330–336.
35. Haley JD, Smith DE, Schwedes J, Brennan R, Pearce C, et al. (2003) Identification and characterization of mechanistically distinct inducers of γ-globin transcription. Biochem Pharmacol 66: 1755–1768.
36. Jin L, Siritanaratkul N, Emery DW, Richard RE, Kaushansky K, et al. (1998) Targeted expansion of genetically modified bone marrow cells. Proc Natl Acad Sci USA 95: 8093–8097.
37. Peterson KR, Li Q, Clegg CH, Furukawa T, Navas PA, et al. (1995) Use of YACs in studies of mammalian development: Production of β-globin locus YAC mice carrying human globin developmental mutants. Proc Natl Acad Sci USA 92: 5655–5659.
38. Graslund T, Li X, Magnenat L, Popkov M, Barbas CF 3rd (2005) Exploring strategies for the design of artificial transcription factors. J Biol Chem 280: 3707–3714.
39. Tschulena U, Peterson KR, Gonzalez B, Fedosyuk H, Barbas CF 3rd (2009) Positive selection of DNA-protein interactions in mammalian cells through phenotypic coupling with retrovirus production. Nat Struct Mol Biol 16: 1195–1199.
40. Muralidhar SA, Ramakrishnan V, Kalra IS, Li W, Pace BS (2011) Histone deacetylase 9 activates γ-globin gene expression in primary erythroid cells. J Biol Chem 286: 2343–2353.
41. Kalra IS, Alam MM, Choudhary PK, Pace BS (2011) Krüppel-like factor 4 activates HBG gene expression in primary erythroid cells. Br J Haematol 154: 248–259.
42. Kuhn RM, Ludwig RA (1994) Complete sequence of the yeast artificial chromosome cloning vector pYAC4. Gene 141: 125–127.

8

Carbon Black Nanoparticles Promote Endothelial Activation and Lipid Accumulation in Macrophages Independently of Intracellular ROS Production

Yi Cao, Martin Roursgaard*, Pernille Høgh Danielsen, Peter Møller, Steffen Loft

Section of Environmental Health, Department of Public Health, University of Copenhagen, Copenhagen, Denmark

Abstract

Exposure to nanoparticles (NPs) may cause vascular effects including endothelial dysfunction and foam cell formation, with oxidative stress and inflammation as supposed central mechanisms. We investigated oxidative stress, endothelial dysfunction and lipid accumulation caused by nano-sized carbon black (CB) exposure in cultured human umbilical vein endothelial cells (HUVECs), THP-1 (monocytes) and THP-1 derived macrophages (THP-1a). The proliferation of HUVECs or co-cultures of HUVECs and THP-1 cells were unaffected by CB exposure, whereas there was increased cytotoxicity, assessed by the LDH and WST-1 assays, especially in THP-1 and THP-1a cells. The CB exposure decreased the glutathione (GSH) content in THP-1 and THP-1a cells, whereas GSH was increased in HUVECs. The reactive oxygen species (ROS) production was increased in all cell types after CB exposure. A reduction of the intracellular GSH concentration by buthionine sulfoximine (BSO) pre-treatment further increased the CB-induced ROS production in THP-1 cells and HUVECs. The expression of adhesion molecules ICAM-1 and VCAM-1, but not adhesion of THP-1 to HUVECs or culture dishes, was elevated by CB exposure, whereas these effects were unaffected by BSO pre-treatment. qRT-PCR showed increased *VCAM1* expression, but no change in *GCLM* and *HMOX1* expression in CB-exposed HUVECs. Pre-exposure to CB induced lipid accumulation in THP-1a cells, which was not affected by the presence of the antioxidant N-acetylcysteine. In addition, the concentrations of CB to induce lipid accumulation were lower than the concentrations to promote intracellular ROS production in THP-1a cells. In conclusion, exposure to nano-sized CB induced endothelial dysfunction and foam cell formation, which was not dependent on intracellular ROS production.

Editor: Clarissa Menezes Maya-Monteiro, Fundação Oswaldo Cruz, Brazil

Funding: This work was supported by the Centre for Pharmaceutical Nanoscience and Nanotoxicology financed by the Danish Strategic Research Council and by the Lundbeck Foundation Center for Biomembranes in Nanomedicine (CBN). The funders had no role in study design, data collection and analysis, decision to publish, or preparation of the manuscript.

Competing Interests: The authors have declared that no competing interests exist.

* Email: mwro@sund.ku.dk

Introduction

Exposure to nanoparticles (NPs) has been suggested to cause vascular health effects with oxidative stress and inflammation as central mechanisms [1]. The NP-mediated vascular effects include expression of endothelial cell adhesion molecules such as intercellular adhesion molecule 1 (ICAM-1) and vascular cell adhesion molecule 1 (VCAM-1), vasomotor dysfunction and accelerated progression of atherosclerosis [1]. The expression of ICAM-1 and VCAM-1 promotes the firm adhesion of monocytes onto the endothelium and the monocytes can subsequently differentiate into macrophages, migrate to the intima and transform to foam cells [2]. It has been shown that exposure of endothelial cells to NPs promotes the expression of ICAM-1 and VCAM-1 as well as adhesion of monocytes onto the endothelial cells [3,4]. Furthermore, it has also been shown that NP exposure induces intracellular lipid accumulation [5–7]. The process of endothelial activation might not require oxidative stress, as suggested by increased adhesion molecule expression by NP exposure in a manner not associated with generation of ROS [8,9]. In addition, it has been shown that addition of the antioxidant ascorbic acid to the cell culture medium did not alleviate particle-induced ICAM-1 and VCAM-1 expression on human umbilical vein endothelial cells (HUVECs) [10]. On the other hand, NP induced lipid accumulation in rat cells was inhibited by pre-treatment with the antioxidant N-acetylcysteine (NAC) [11].

We hypothesized that oxidatively stressed endothelial cells would be more readily activated and interact more strongly with monocytes or macrophages, and that oxidative stress could further promote the lipid accumulation in macrophages by exposure to NPs. To this end we investigated the effect of exposure to nano-sized carbon black (CB) on the activation of endothelial cells by ICAM-1 and VCAM-1 expression on HUVECs and adhesion of THP-1 monocytes onto HUVECs as well as lipid accumulation in THP-1 macrophages. We used nano-sized CB because it generates high levels of intracellular ROS [12]. In addition, we have previously shown that HUVECs express increased levels of ICAM-1 and VCAM-1 after exposure to nano-sized CB [9,10,13]. CB is widely used as black pigment in rubber, paints and inks as well as being a widely used type of particle in toxicological studies including studies on ROS production [14], endothelial-dependent vasomotor function [15] and atherosclerosis [16]. The intracellular ROS generation and GSH concentration were used as markers of oxidative stress, whereas the mRNA expression of adhesion molecule *VCAM-1* as well as the oxidative stress response genes in the NRF-2 signaling pathway, glutamate-cysteine ligase, modifier subunit (*GCLM*), the rate limiting enzyme in GSH synthesis, and heme oxygenase 1 (*HMOX1*), one of the essential enzymes in heme catabolism [17], was assessed in HUVECs by qRT-PCR.

Materials and Methods

Cell lines

The HUVECs and culture medium were purchased from Cell Applications (San Diego, CA, USA). The cells were cultured in Endothelial Cell Growth Medium Kit with 2% serum at 37°C in an incubator with 5% CO_2. The medium was changed 24–36 h after seeding and the cells were cultured until they were 90% confluent. The cells were used between passages 2–5 because they maintain their morphologic and phenotypic characteristics within these passages [9,13]. The THP-1 monocytes were obtained from the American Type Culture Collection (Manassas, VA, USA) and was cultured in RPMI with 10% serum as previously described [18]. The THP-1 cells were differentiated into adherent macrophages (denoted THP-1a) by treatment with 10 ng/ml phorbol 12-myristate 13-acetate (PMA, Sigma, St. Louis, MO, USA) overnight [19]. The THP-1a cells attach to the surface of the culture flasks, whereas THP-1 cells stay in suspension and were removed with the supernatant.

Particles

CB particles (Printex 90) were obtained from Evonik Industries, Frankfurt, Germany (primary particle size 14 nm; surface area 300 m^2/g). Printex 90 is an extensively studied model NP and has been characterized elsewhere [20,21]. The mean size of the particles suspended in media was 85±38 nm [13]. The uptake of CB in cells has been confirmed by transmission electron micrograph (TEM) [13]. A stock solution of CB was prepared by sonicating a 1 mg/ml suspension of particles in double distilled water (Sigma-Aldrich), using a Branson Sonifier S-450D (Branson Ultrasonics Corp., Danbury, CT, USA) equipped with a disrupter horn (Model number: 101-147-037) before each experiment. The suspension was sonicated for 8 min with alternating 10 s pulses and 10 s pauses at amplitude of 10% and continuously cooling on ice to avoid sample heating and evaporation [13]. After sonication, the suspension was diluted in cell culture medium and used only freshly. For all the experiments except real-time RT-PCR, cells were incubated with 200 µl CB solutions in 96-wells plates (growth area 0.32 cm^2). The concentrations of CB were 0, 2.5, 12.5, 25, and 100 µg/ml, which were equal to the concentrations of 0, 1.6, 7.8, 15.6, 62.5 µg/cm^2. Our previous studies showed increased levels of ICAM-1 and VCAM-1 in HUVECs after exposure to these concentrations of CB [9,10,13]. As we observed increased lipid accumulation in THP-1a cells by CB as low as 2.5 µg/ml (see in results section), we also included lower concentrations of CB of 0.25, 2.5, 25, 250, 2500 ng/ml, which were equal to the concentrations of 0.16, 1.6, 15.6, 156.3, 1562.5 ng/cm^2. For real-time RT-PCR, cells were incubated with 5 ml CB solutions in 6-wells plates.

Cytotoxicity

The cytotoxicity was measured with the WST-1 or lactate dehydrogenase (LDH) assays (Roche Diagnostics GmbH, Mannheim, Germany) according to the manufacturer's instructions. The WST-1 assay is regarded to reflect mitochondrial succinate dehydrogenase activity, although it should not be interpreted as a specific measurement for this enzyme. The LDH assay is considered to reflect leakage of this cytosolic enzyme through the cell membrane to the extracellular fluid.

Briefly, 5×10^4 THP-1, 5×10^4 THP-1a or 2×10^4 HUVECs were seeded in 96-wells plates and incubated with CB for 24 h. Then, the supernatant was collected for LDH assay and cells were rinsed once for WST-1 assay. The cells were incubated with 100 µl fresh medium containing 10% WST-1 reagent for 2 h and the absorbance was measured at 450 nm with 630 nm as reference by an ELISA reader (Labsystems, Multiskan Ascent). For LDH assay, 100 µl supernatant was incubated with 100 µl LDH reaction buffer provided in the kit for 1 h and the absorbance was measured at 490 nm with 630 nm as reference using an ELISA reader. We have previously shown that the CB particles do not interact with LDH enzyme activity [13,22].

Cell viability was further assessed in THP-1 cells by trypan blue exclusion. After exposure of 5×10^4 THP-1 cells to 100 µg/ml CB, 40 µl cell suspension was mixed with 40 µl 0.4% trypan blue. The non-colored viable cells and blue-stained non-viable cells were counted in a hemacytometer.

Cell proliferation assay

The proliferation of THP-1 cells and HUVECs was measured with the BrdU cell proliferation assay kit (Roche Diagnostics GmbH, Mannheim, Germany) according to the manufacturer's instructions. Briefly, 2×10^4 THP-1, 5×10^3 HUVECs or a mixture of THP-1 or THP-1a (1×10^4) with HUVECs (2.5×10^3) were exposed to CB suspension in the presence of BrdU for 24 h. After exposure, the medium were removed and cells were fixed for 30 min in fix solution, and then the BrdU-labelled DNA was bind to antibody for 90 min in antibody solution. After washing three times, the substrate solution was added to detect the immune complexes. The reaction was stopped with 50 µl 2 M HCl, and the absorbance was measured at 450 nm with 690 nm as reference. To confirm the proliferation results of THP-1 cell, 5×10^4/well of THP-1 cells were exposed to 100 µg/ml CB for 24 h, and the cell number was counted using a CASY Technology Cell counter (Scharfe System, Stuttgart, Germany). The proliferation of HUVECs was also measured after 24 h exposure to 10 ng/ml vascular endothelial growth factor (VEGF, Gibco, Camarillo, CA, USA) to assess the maximal proliferation capacity or 100 ng/ml tumor necrosis factor (TNF, Gibco, Carlsbad, CA, USA) because it is used as positive control for the expression of cell adhesion molecules (see below). Moreover, we assessed the proliferation of HUVECs after pre-treatment with the Ca^{2+} chelator BAPTA-AM (10 µM; Sigma, St. Louis, MO, USA) for 1 h before the 24 h exposure period because the VEGF-stimulated cell proliferation is mediated by increases in the intracellular Ca^{2+} concentration [23].

ROS measurement

The intracellular ROS production was measured with the fluorescent probe 2′,7′-dichlorofluorescein diacetate (DCFH-DA; Invitrogen A/S Taastrup, Denmark) [24]. A 10 mM DCFH-DA stock solution was made in methanol. 5×10^4 THP-1a cells or 2×10^4 HUVECs in a 96-wells plate were stained with 2 µM DCFH-DA in Hanks balanced salt solution (Sigma-Aldrich) at 37°C for 15 min and then rinsed twice in Hanks' balanced salt solution. The THP-1 suspension cells were incubated with probe as described above and then transferred to a 96 well plate as 5×10^4 cells/well. The cells were then incubated with CB in Hanks' balanced salt solution and the fluorescence was measured every 15 min for 3 h (λ_{ex} = 485 nm; λ_{em} = 538 nm) in a fluorescence spectrophotometer (Fluoroskan Ascent FL; Labsystems).

The accumulated ROS production over time was calculated as the area under the curve (AUC). The results are reported as fold increase compared with the control. The ROS production showed a bell-shaped concentration-effect relationship with a peak level at 12.5 μg/ml. This has also been observed in earlier investigations with CB and other types of particles with the same protocol [10,11,25,26]. We show the results from the cell cultures that were exposed to 25 or 100 μg/ml, although these results were not included in the statistical analysis.

As we observed increased lipid accumulation in THP-1a cells after 24 h exposure to lower concentrations of CB (see in results section), we also measured intracellular ROS production in THP-1a cells after exposure to lower concentrations of CB. Here 5×10^4 THP-1a cells were exposed to CB concentrations of 0.25, 2.5, 25, 250, 2500 ng/ml for 24 h, rinsed, and the ROS production was measured as indicated above.

We also detected the ROS production by fluorescence microscopy. After exposure, 2×10^4 HUVECs or 5×10^4 THP-1a on 8-well microscopy chamber slides (Ibidi, Munich, Germany) were stained with 25 μM DCFH-DA in medium for 30 min, rinsed twice with medium, and then examined by combined differential interference contrast (DIC) and fluorescence microscopy in a Leica AF6000 inverted widefield microscope with a 63 times dry objective with NA 0.7 (Leica Microsystems GmbH, Wetzlar, Germany).

Intracellular GSH concentration

The intracellular GSH concentration was measured with the fluorescent probe ThioGlo-1 (Covalent Technologies, Inc., Walnut Creek, CA, USA) [27]. A 2 mM ThioGlo-1 stock solution was made in DMSO. 5×10^4 THP-1, 5×10^4 THP-1a or 2×10^4 HUVECs seeded in 96-well plates was incubated with CB for 3 h or 24 h. After exposure, the cells were rinsed once with PBS, incubated with 10 μM ThioGlo-1 for approximately 5 min and then measured by fluorescence spectrophotometer ($\lambda_{ex} = 355$ nm; $\lambda_{em} = 460$ nm). A standard curve was made by incubating 10 μM ThioGlo-1 with GSH ranged from 16 to 0.125 μM (two fold dilution). The GSH concentration is expressed as nmol/10^6 cells, and is considered to be an observation of GSH equivalents.

BSO treatment

The intracellular GSH concentration was reduced by incubating the cells with 100 μM of BSO (Sigma-Aldrich, St. Louis, MO, USA) for 24 h. The cells were subsequently rinsed with PBS and exposed to CB or TNF.

THP-1 cell adhesion assay

The adhesion of THP-1 cells onto HUVCs was performed as previously described [3]. Briefly, 2×10^4 HUVECs in 96-well plates were co-cultured with 5×10^3 BrdU-labeled THP-1 cells, and exposed to CB or the positive controls TNF (100 ng/ml) and PMA (100 ng/ml) for 24 h. We assessed the CB-mediated interaction between THP-1 cells and BSO pre-treatment HUVECs in co-culture. Only the HUVECs were pre-treated with 100 μM of BSO for 24 h because there was increased CB-mediated ROS production in BSO pre-treated HUVECs, but not in THP-1 cells.

After exposure, the cells were rinsed twice with 100 μl PBS and the BrdU contents both in the co-culture and supernatant were determined according to manufacturer's instructions (Roche Diagnostics GmbH, Mannheim, Germany) as indicated in Cell proliferating assay section. The percentage of THP-1 cells remaining attached in the co-culture was calculated [3].

Measurement of ICAM-1 and VCAM-1

The surface expression of ICAM-1 and VCAM-1 was measured with a modified ELISA procedure [10,13,26]. The expression of cell adhesion molecules were investigated in cultures with 2×10^4 HUVECs, 1.8×10^4 HUVEC $+5\times10^3$ TPH-1a, 1×10^4 HUVECs $+2.5\times10^4$ THP-1a, or 5×10^4 THP-1a in 96-well plates. The cells were exposed to CB or TNF as positive control (100 ng/ml) for 24 h. Subsequently, the cells were incubated with anti-ICAM-1 or anti-VCAM-1 (both from R&D systems, Abingdon, UK) in a 1:500 dilution for 1 h at 37°C. After being rinsed for three times in 1% BSA medium, the cells were incubated with 1:25 000 diluted secondary antibody (anti-goat IgG peroxidase coupled antibody; Sigma, MI, USA) in PBS with 0.1% Tween 20 for 1 h on ice. After washing 5 times with ice-cold PBS/Tween 20 solution, the cells were incubated with a substrate solution containing 0.4 mg/ml o-phenylenediamine (OPD; Sigma, St. Louis, MO, USA) and 3.5 mM H_2O_2 in phosphate-citrate buffer (phosphate-citrate buffer tablets, Sigma) for 30 min in the dark. The absorbance was measured in at 450 nm.

We assessed the interference of particles with the assay by exposing HUVECs to 100 ng/ml TNF for 24 h to induce the expression of ICAM-1 and VCAM-1, followed by 30 min exposure to CB. This short CB exposure was expected to have little effect on ICAM-1 and VCAM-1 expression on HUVECs, whereas the adherent CB particles might affect the measurement in the ICAM-1 and VCAM-1 assays.

Lipid accumulation in THP-1a cells

The lipid accumulation in THP-1a was measured by the fluorescent probe Nile Red (Sigma, St. Louis, MO, USA). THP-1a cells (5×10^4 cells/well) in 96-well black plates were exposed to various concentrations of CB for 24 h, with or without the presence of 1 mM NAC. After washing, the cells were incubated with either medium containing 1% BSA (for control) or 0.5 mM free fatty acid (FFA; oleic/palmitic acid, 2:1; in medium with 1% BSA) for another 3 h. After one wash, the cells were stained in Hanks solution containing 0.5 μg/ml Nile red and 0.01% Pluronic F127 (Sigma-Aldrich, St. Louis, MO) for 15 min in the dark and subsequently rinsed twice. The fluorescence was measured in a fluorescence spectrophotometer ($\lambda_{ex} = 544$ nm, $\lambda_{em} = 590$ nm). There was a remarkable decrease in the Nile red signal at the concentration of 100 μg/ml; probably due to the interactions of CB with the probe. Therefore we show the results from the cell cultures that were exposed to 0 to 25 μg/ml CB.

The lipid accumulation was further assessed with fluorescence microscopy using the two different fluorescent probes Nile Red and Bodipy 493/503 (Molecular Probes, Eugene, OR). Briefly, 5×10^4 THP-1a cells were seeded on 8-well microscopy chamber slides and after exposure to particles (25 ng/ml or 2.5 μg/ml) and/or FFA, the cells washed with PBS and fixed with 4% paraformaldehyde for 30 min at room temperature. After another wash the fixed cells were stained 10 min with Nile Red (as described above) and Hoechst 33342 or Bodipy (1 μg/ml) and Hoechst 33342 followed by washing and addition of two drops of mounting media (Ibidi). The microscopy was done with a Leica AF6000 inverted wide field microscope with a 40 times dry objective with NA 0.7. Each sample was captured as a z-stack in 5 random areas including at least 50 cells, followed by 3D deconvolution and 3D projection using Leica LAS AF 2.6.0.7266. The resulting images were analyzed with ImageJ (1.47V) to obtain the area of lipid droplets per cell.

Gene expression of *GCLM*, *HMOX1* and *VCAM1* in HUVECs

The mRNA levels of *GCLM* (Gene ID: 601176), *HMOX1* (Gene ID: 141250) *and VCAM1* (Gene ID: 19225) were measured in HUVECs as previously described [25]. HUVECs (5×10^5 cells/well) were seeded in 0.1% gelatine pre-coated 6-well plates and exposed to 100 μg/ml of CB for 3 h. Total RNA was extracted using TRIzol reagent (Invitrogen A/S, Taastrup, Denmark) and treated with DNAse (Promega Biotech AB, Denmark). The cDNA synthesis was done with the High Capacity cDNA Reverse Transcription Kit based on the GeneAmp PCR system 2700. The quantitative RT-PCR reactions were carried out with TaqMan Gene Assays on ABI PRISM 7900HT. All kits were obtained from Applied Biosystems, Naerum, Denmark. We used 18S rRNA as reference gene (Eukaryotic 18S rRNA Endogenous Control, 4352930E, Applied Biosystems, Naerum, Denmark). The gene expression levels were reported as the ratio between the mRNA level of the target genes and the 18S rRNA reference gene using the comparative $2^{-\Delta Ct}$ method.

Statistics

The results were analyzed by full-factorial ANOVA with least statistical difference as post-hoc test or linear regression analysis using Statistica version 5.5 (StatSoft Inc., Tulsa, OK, USA). Tests for normal distribution of residuals were carried out with the Kolmogorov-Smirnov test. The distribution of residuals for the ROS production did not follow a normal distribution as assessed by the Kolmogorov-Smirnov test, whereas it was by the Shapiro-Wilk test. The results of BSO pretreatment for CB-mediated ROS production in cells were not normally distributed on normal scale, whereas a log-transformation produced residuals that were normally distributed without affecting the statistically significant differences between the groups. The residuals of the ANOVA analysis of the VCAM-1 expression did not follow a normal distribution on either normal or log-transformed scale. However, this was because of a low value for the positive control (TNF) in one experiment; removal of this result produced residuals that followed a normal distribution. For the assessment of the interaction of BSO pretreatment, the residuals of the VCAM-1 expression was not normally distributed, which was due to one high value in the BSO group that was exposed to 25 μg/ml of CB. Removal of this result from the regression analysis produced residuals with normal distribution, whereas it did not affect the statistical outcome of the test. P–values<0.05 were considered to be statistically significant.

Results

Cytotoxicity

The results from the WST-1 assay showed increased cytotoxicity in the three types of cells at 100 μg/ml ($P<0.05$), whereas the exposure to 12.5 and 25 μg/ml of CB also decreased the WST-1 formation THP-1 and THP-1a cells ($P<0.05$) (Figure 1A). The results from the LDH assay only showed increased membrane leakage at 100 μg/ml CB in THP-1 cells ($P<0.05$) (Figure 1B).

The viability of THP-1 cells after exposure for 24 h to CB was also measured by the trypan blue assay (Figure S1 in File S1). The viability of both the control and 100 μg/ml CB exposed THP-1 cells were over 90%, and there was no effect of CB exposure.

BrdU cell proliferation assay

Figure 2 shows that the proliferation rate of THP-1 cells, HUVECs or co-cultures of both cell types was not significantly affected by the 24 h exposure to CB. The cell proliferation rate was also unaltered after treatment with TNF (83±4%) or VEGF (95±6%), indicating that the HUVECs had maximal proliferation capacity. The effect of pre-treatment of HUVECs with the Ca^{2+} chelator BAPTA-AM, which interferes with the VEGF-mediated increase in intracellular Ca^{2+} concentration, decreased the cell proliferation in HUVECs that were incubated in the presence (26±3%) or absence of VEGF (22±4%).

To confirm the lack of effect on the THP-1 cells, their number was also counted after 24 h CB exposure (Figure S2 in File S1). The results showed that the exposure to 100 μg/ml of CB did not affect the number of THP-1 cells.

Intracellular GSH concentration

Figure 3 shows the GSH concentration in cells after exposure to CB. The concentration of GSH was unaltered in all cell types after 3 h exposure to CB (Figure 3A). The GSH concentration was decreased in the THP-1a cells after 24 h exposure to 12.5 ($P<0.05$), 25 ($P=0.056$) and 100 μg/ml CB ($P<0.05$). In the HUVECs, 24 h exposure to 25 or 100 μg/ml CB ($P<0.05$) increased the GSH content, whereas there was no difference in the GSH concentration in the CB exposed THP-1 cells. The experiments for the 3 and 24 h exposures were carried out on different days. Therefore, we have not statistically analyzed for differences in the absolute GSH values in the cells after 3 or 24 h incubation. The exposure to PMA, which was used to activate the THP-1 cells, did not affect the GSH concentration in THP-1 cells (data not shown).

Intracellular ROS production

The 3 h exposure to CB was associated with increased intracellular ROS production in all cell types (Figure 4A). In keeping with earlier findings, we observed bell-shaped concentration-response curves for the intracellular ROS production [10,13], and the results from 25 and 100 μg/ml were not included in the statistical analysis as these concentrations are speculated to interfere with the measurements [10,25]. The ROS production was increased at the concentrations of 2.5 and 12.5 μg/ml in the THP-1 ($P<0.05$), THP-1a cells ($P<0.05$) and HUVECs ($P<0.05$). The intracellular ROS generation was further directly observed by fluorescent microscopy to investigate the possible interaction between the particles and the measurement. It showed that the CB exposure induced ROS production in a concentration-dependent manner and there was no obvious decline in ROS signal in HUVECs or THP-1a cells after exposure to 100 μg/ml CB as compared with control or 12.5 μg/ml of CB (Figure S3 in File S1).

The exposure to 10 and 100 ng/ml PMA, which was used to activate the THP-1 cells, increased the ROS production in THP-1 cells by 1.36-fold (95% CI: 0.98–1.72) and 1.57-fold (95% CI: 1.13–1.88), respectively (data not shown).

In another set of experiments we pre-treated the cells with 100 μM of BSO to reduce the intracellular concentration of GSH. The pre-treatment with 100 μM of BSO resulted in a 30% (from 7.2 to 5.0 nmol/10^6 cells), 28% (from 4.7 to 3.4 nmol/10^6 cells) decrease and no effect (from 4.2–4.7 nmol/10^6 cells) on the level of GSH in HUVECs, THP-1a and THP-1 cells, respectively. This pre-treatment was associated with increased CB-induced ROS production in THP-1 cells exposed to 2.5 ($P<0.05$) or 12.5 μg/ml ($P<0.05$), whereas the BSO pre-treatment did not affect the CB-induced ROS production in THP-1a cells. The BSO pre-treated HUVECs also showed higher ROS production as compared with non-treated HUVECs after exposure to 2.5 ($P<0.05$) or 12.5 μg/ml ($P<0.05$) of CB (Figure 4B).

As we observed increased lipid accumulation in THP-1a cells after 24 h exposure to lower concentrations of CB (see result below), we also measured intracellular ROS production in THP-

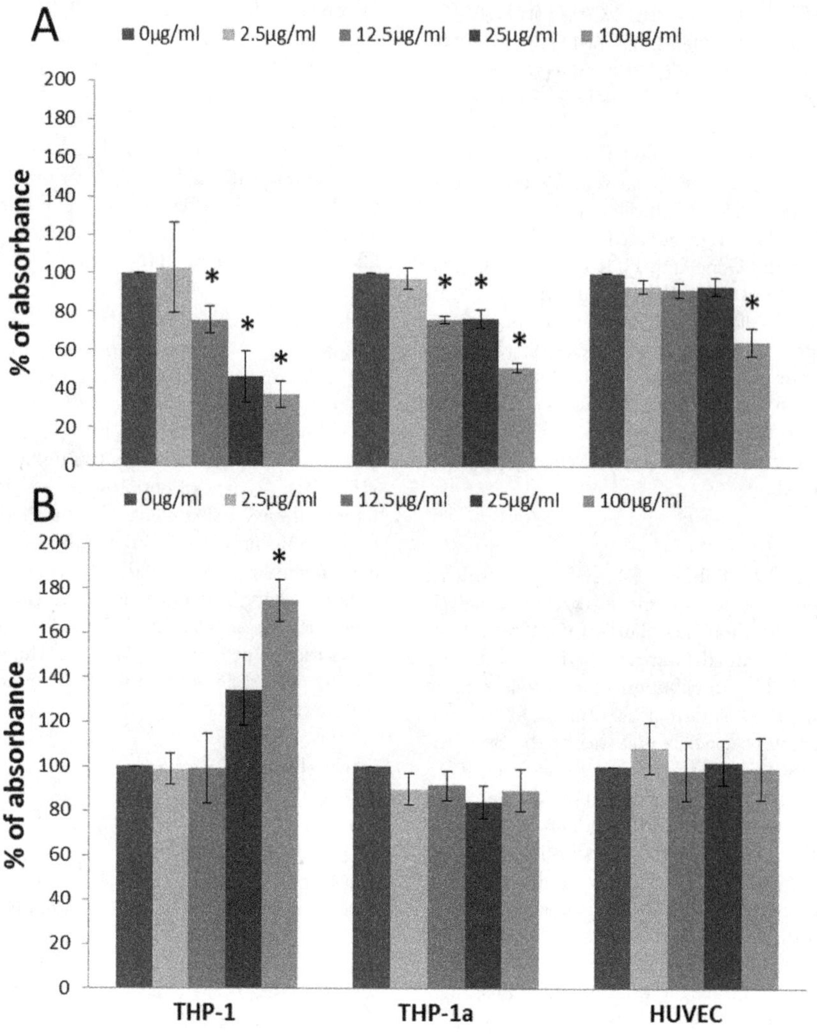

Figure 1. Cytotoxicity measured by the WST-1 assay (A) and LDH leakage (B) after 24 h CB exposure of THP-1, THP-1a and HUVECs. The data represent the percentage of absorbance compared with the unexposed control cells. Bars are means ±SEM of three independent experiments. *P<0.05 compared with unexposed cells.

1a cells after 24 h exposure to lower concentrations of CB to correlate intracellular ROS production with lipid accumulation (Figure 4C). 2500 ng/ml CB exposure significantly increased intracellular ROS production ($p<0.05$) by 1.29-fold (95% CI: 1.03–1.55 fold), whereas lower concentrations of CB did not significantly affect intracellular ROS production.

ICAM-1 and VCAM-1 surface expression

Figure 5 shows the ICAM-1 and VCAM-1 surface expression after 24 h of CB exposure in HUVECs and THP-1a monocultures and co-cultures of these. The ICAM-1 expression was significantly increased in 100 µg/ml CB- exposed HUVEC monocultures ($P<0.01$), the co-culture of 1.8×10^4 HUVEC $+5\times10^3$ THP-1a ($P<0.01$), and the TNF-exposed (positive control) ($P<0.001$) (Figure 5A). The VCAM-1 expression was only significantly increased after 100 µg/ml of CB or TNF-treatment in HUVEC monocultures ($P<0.01$) (Figure 5B).

Figure 5C shows the effect of BSO pre-treatment on the CB-mediated expression of ICAM-1 and VCAM-1 in HUVECs. The exposure to CB increased the expression of ICAM-1 ($P<0.01$) and VCAM-1 ($P<0.01$), whereas no difference in the slopes of the CB-mediated concentration-response relationships in HUVECs without or with BSO pre-treatment was observed ($P=0.91$ for ICAM-1 and $P=0.70$ for VCAM-1). The slopes ($\beta\pm$SE) were 0.16 ± 0.07 ($P<0.05$) and 0.15 ± 0.08 ($P=0.08$) for the CB-mediated ICAM-1 expression in HUVECs without or with BSO pre-treatment, respectively. For the CB-mediated VCAM-1 expression in HUVECs, the slopes were 0.18 ± 0.08 ($P<0.05$) and 0.14 ± 0.05 ($P<0.01$) without or with BSO pre-treatment, respectively. The reference control TNF also increased the expression of ICAM-1 ($P<0.001$) and VCAM-1 ($P<0.001$) in the HUVECs. The effect of TNF was not affected by pretreatment with BSO for ICAM-1 ($P=0.39$) and VCAM-1 ($P=0.15$).

The possible interaction effect of CB particles on the ICAM-1 and VCAM-1 assays is shown in Figure S4 in File S1. TNF exposure for 24 h increased the ICAM-1 and VCAM-1 expression approximately 3-fold on HUVECs, whereas a subsequent 30 min exposure to CB only caused a slight decrease in the antibody-based measurement of ICAM-1 and VCAM-1, indicating that no interaction between CB and the antibody-based detection of cell adhesion molecules is taking place.

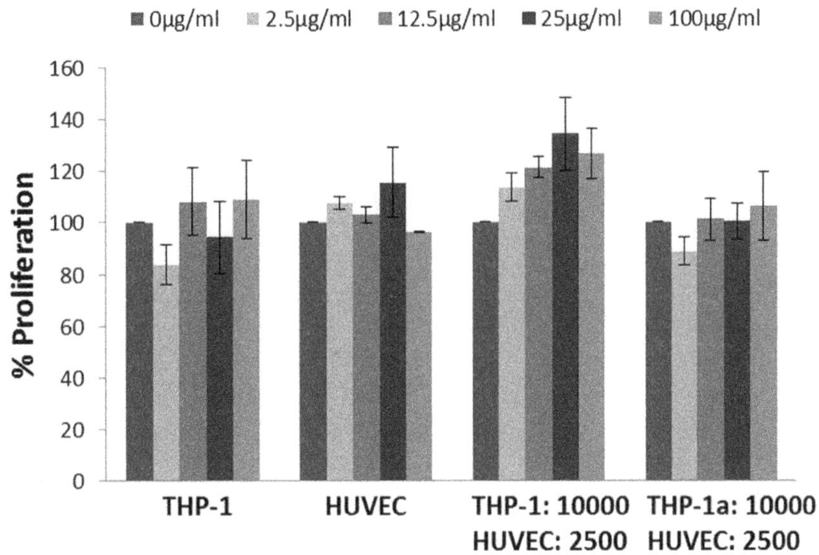

Figure 2. Cell proliferation of THP-1 and HUVECs in monocultures or co-culture after 24 h exposure to CB, measured by the BrdU assay. Data are expressed as percentage of absorbance compared with the unexposed cells. The bars are means ±SEM of at least three independent experiments with n = 3 for each. *P<0.05 compared with unexposed cells.

THP-1 adhesion

The CB exposure did not alter the level of adhesion of THP-1 cells to the mono-layer of HUVECs or culture dishes (Figure 6A). The positive control TNF was associated with increased adhesion of THP-1 cells onto HUVECs ($P<0.05$) and PMA (positive inducer of THP-1a macrophages) significantly increased THP-1 adhesion to both HUVECs ($P<0.05$) and culture dishes ($P<0.05$).

The pre-treatment of HUVECs with BSO was associated with decreased adhesion of THP-1 cells onto HUVECs in co-cultures that were not exposed to CB ($P<0.05$) and those that were exposed to TNF ($P<0.05$). Although we observed a similar tendency in co-cultures exposed to 25 µg/ml of CB ($P<0.05$), it was not a concentration-dependent effect (Figure 6B).

Lipid accumulation in THP-1a cells

The result of the lipid accumulation in THP-1a cells is shown in Figure 7. Pre-exposure to CB for 24 h increased lipid accumulation in THP-1a cells with a bell-shaped concentration-response curve. The CB exposure was associated with a significant increase in lipid accumulation at a concentration of 2.5 µg/ml ($p<0.05$). There was 30% (95% CI: 6.9%–60%) and 36% (95% CI: 11%–67%) higher lipid load in the cells that had been exposed to 2.5 µg/ml of CB and co-treated without or with FAA, respectively. In the cells that had been exposed to 2.5 µg/ml of CB and NAC, there was 82% (95% CI: 45%–123%) and 38% (95% CI: 10%–74%) higher lipid load in cells that were co-treated without or with FFA, respectively. The 3 h exposure to FFA was associated with a minor 11% (95% CI: 3.0%–20%) increase of the lipid level ($p<0.05$ for single-factor effect of FFA treatment) (Figure 7A). Pre-exposure to lower concentrations of CB ranging from 2500 ng/ml to 0.25 ng/ml for 24 h also increased lipid accumulation in THP-1a cells with or without further exposure to FFA ($p<0.05$ for 2500 ng/ml and $p<0.01$ for other concentrations) (Figure 7B).

Using fluorescence microscopy for further semi-quantitative determination of lipid accumulation, we observed increased lipid accumulation in THP-1a cells that were incubated with CB and/or FFA. Staining with Nile Red showed predominantly increased lipid content in cells exposed to CB and FFA (Figure 7C), whereas Bodipy 493/503 staining revealed increased lipid content in CB exposed cells without FFA treatment (Figure 7D). Although the lipid stains differ somewhat in regard to effect of FFA treatment, the collective interpretation from the fluorescence microscopy is that CB exposure is associated with increased lipid content in THP-1a cells.

Gene expressions

Because we observed increased ROS production at 3 h after the CB exposure and increased GSH content in HUVECs at 24 h, we measured the expression of *GCLM*, *HMOX1* and *VCAM1* after 3 h exposure to CB. The results showed that CB exposure did not alter the expressions of *GCLM* ($P = 0.75$) and *HMOX1* ($P = 0.97$) in HUVECs, whereas there was a concentration- dependent increase in *VCAM1* expression ($P<0.05$) (Figure 8).

Discussion

In this study we assessed the in vitro effects of CB exposure on oxidative stress, endothelial activation and foam cell formation which are important events in the early development of atherosclerosis [2]. The results showed that CB exposure increased the expression of ICAM-1 at protein level and VCAM-1 at both protein and gene level in HUVECs, whereas the adhesion of THP-1cells to HUVECs or culture dishes was unaffected by the exposure. In a previous study, we showed that exposure to particles from combustion of diesel or wood was associated with increased VCAM-1 expression, whereas only the wood smoke particles enhanced the adhesion of THP-1 cells onto HUVECs [3]. It is therefore possible that particle-induced monocyte adhesion onto endothelium depends on the activation of both types of cells. Nevertheless, CB exposure has been found to be associated with vasomotor dysfunction in aorta rings and altered pressure-diameter relationship in mesenteric artery segments from mice [13]. These effects correlated with the observations in HUVECs in mono-culture, including increased expression of cell adhesion molecules and ROS production. However, it can be argued that HUVECs mono-culture is a rather simple exposure

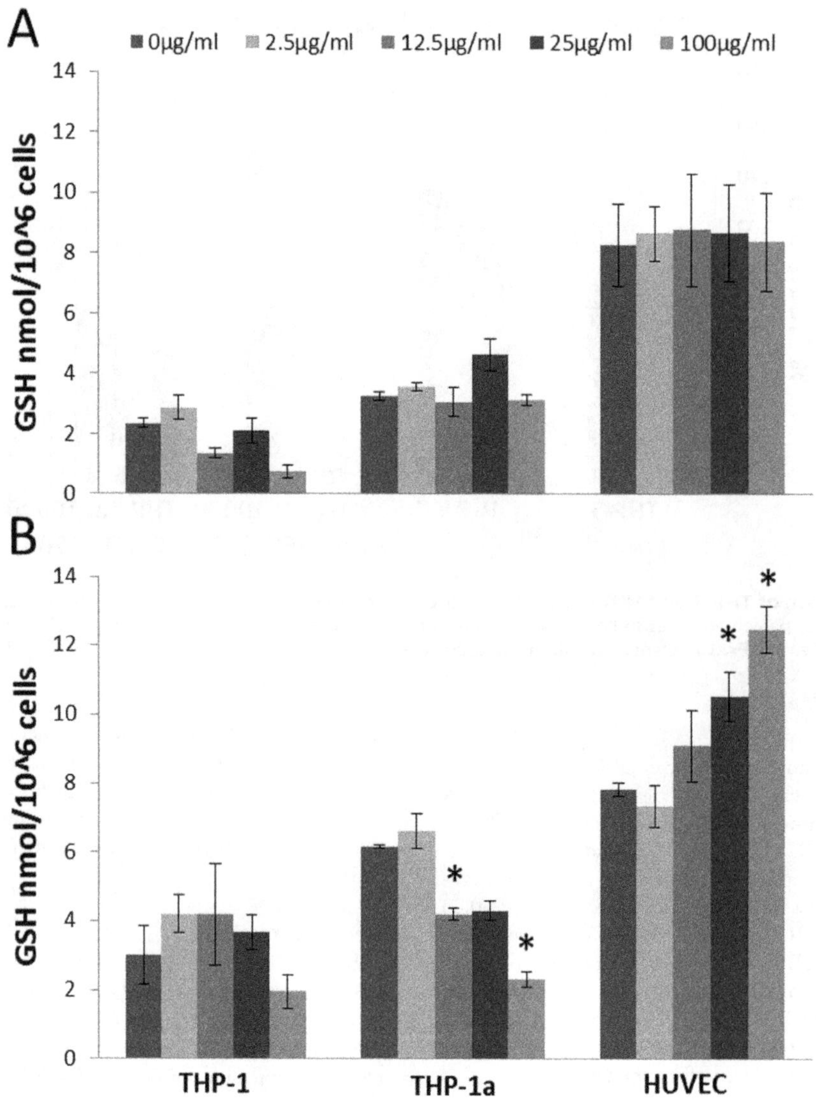

Figure 3. GSH concentration in HUVECs, THP-1 or THP-1a cells after 3 h (A) or 24 h (B) exposure to CB. Data are expressed as nmol/10^6 cells and bars are means ±SEM of three independent experiments. *P<0.05 compared with unexposed cells.

system and therefore co-culture was used here. This showed that the addition of THP-1a cells did not increase the CB-mediated expression of ICAM-1 and VCAM-1 on HUVECs. This is in accordance with earlier observations that THP-1 cells did not increase the expression of IL-1β, IL-6, IL-8 and TNF after exposure to CB [28]. Overall, the results indicate that CB possesses the ability to cause a modest activation of endothelial cells *in vitro*.

The CB exposure significantly increased the lipid accumulation in THP-1a cells, suggesting that CB exposure may promote the transformation of monocytes to foam cells, which is an important event in the atherogenesis [2]. This is consistent with previous studies showing that NP exposure could induce intracellular lipid accumulation [6,7,11] and it supports the observation that pulmonary exposure to CB accelerated progression of atherosclerosis [16]. However, the presence of the antioxidant NAC showed no effect on lipid accumulation induced by CB, and the concentrations of CB needed to induce lipid accumulation were apparently lower than the concentrations to promote intracellular ROS production in THP-1a cells, which indicated that CB induced lipid accumulation is independent of intracellular ROS production. This is in contrast to the effect of other NPs like cadmium telluride that can induce lipid droplet in an oxidant-dependent way [11].

We measured the intracellular ROS production by the DCHF assay that has been widely used in research on oxidative stress for years [29]. In keeping with earlier findings, we observed bell-shaped concentration-response curves for the intracellular ROS production in experiments were the cells loaded with DFCH before the exposure to CB [10,13,25]. This exposure condition enables the possibility to measure the intracellular ROS production in real-time, although the limitation is possible quenching of the signal by the particles in the cell culture medium. We have previously shown that addition of DCFH to HepG2 cells after the exposure to CB was associated with increased intracellular ROS production that did not show a bell-shaped concentration-response curve [30]. Those results showed essentially the same trend as the results in Figure S3 in File S1, albeit it was a different cell type.

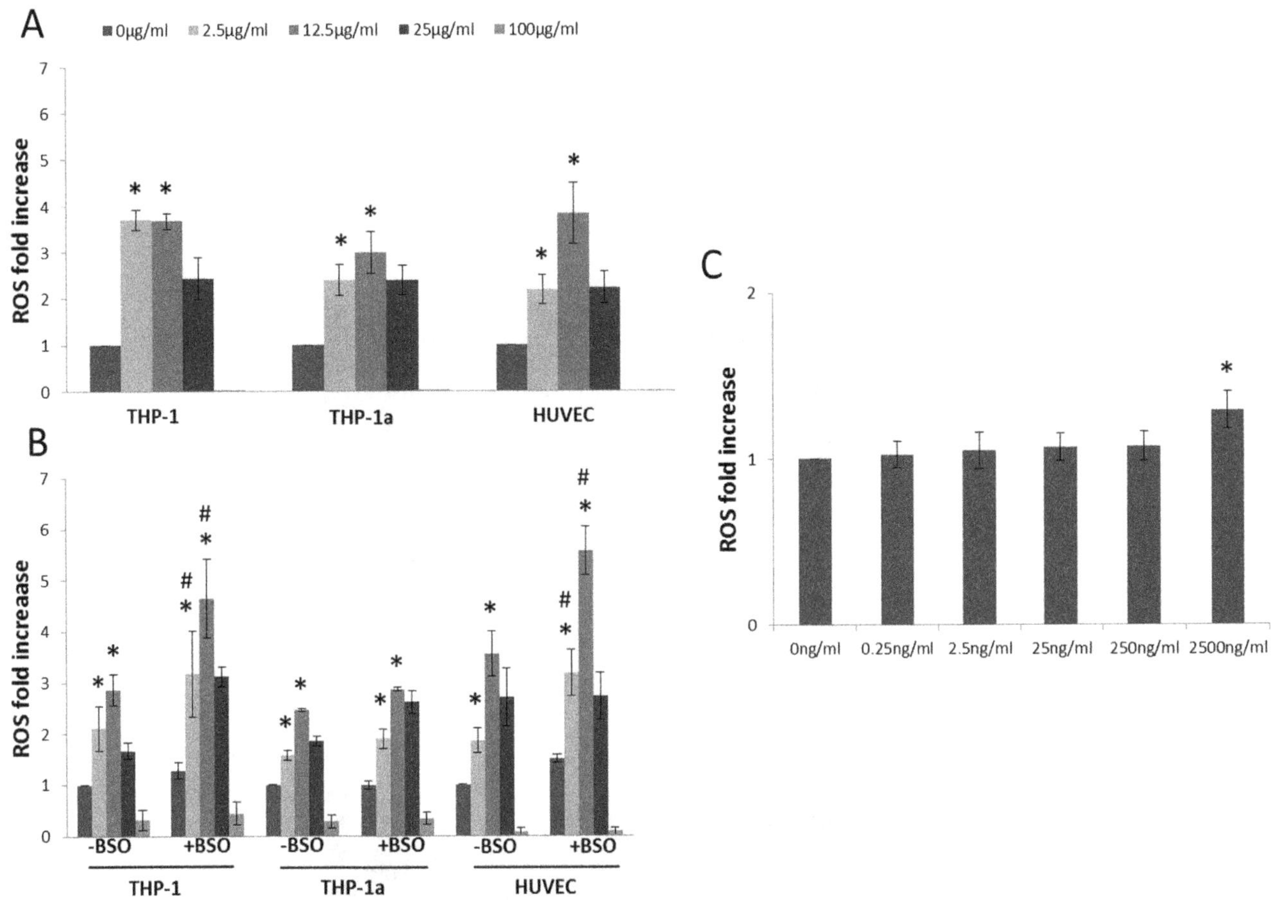

Figure 4. Intracellular ROS production during 3 h incubation with CB in HUVECs, THP-1 or THP-1a cells (A) or cells with or without BSO pre-treatment (B). C. Intracellular ROS production in THP-1a cells after 24 h exposure to lower concentrations of CB. Data are expressed as fold increase of ROS compared with unexposed control cells and bars are means ±SEM of 3–4 independent experiments. *P<0.05 compared with unexposed cells. #P<0.05 compared with BSO-untreated groups.

The collective interpretation of the Printex 90 exposure in our experiments is mediates the generation of intracellular ROS as measured by the DCFH assay. This is supported by studies on other types of probes for intracellular ROS production such as hydroethidium for detection of superoxide anion radicals [31].

It is generally acknowledged that the DCFH assay does not have specificity to particular types of ROS in the context of an intracellular environment. Interestingly some studies have shown that lysosomal permeabilization and subsequent increased release of iron to the cytosol is an important source of intracellular ROS as detected by the DCFH assay [32,33]. Studies in acellular conditions have also highlighted iron or heme-compounds as potent oxidants of DCFH [34,35]. It is therefore possible that the increased intracellular ROS production in CB-exposed cells arises as a consequence of "free" iron from compartments such as the lysosome or mitochondria. We have shown in several studies that CB in acellular conditions oxidizes DCFH [12,13]. In addition, the same type of CB generated ROS in acellular conditions be electron spin resonance [36], indicating the intrinsic ability of CB to generate ROS.

For all cell types there was CB-induced ROS production, whereas the intracellular GSH concentration remained unaffected during the same time period of 3 h CB exposure. To further explore the possible relationship between CB-induced endothelial activation and intracellular ROS level, we reduced the intracellular GSH concentration by BSO pretreatment prior to CB exposure. This increased the CB-induced ROS production especially in the THP-1 cells and HUVECs. The combined results from the BSO pre-treatment experiments indicate that the response is cell type specific, which might be related to the *de novo* synthesis of GSH and its interaction with other cellular components of the antioxidant defense system. We did not attempt to completely deplete the GSH because it might render the cells more susceptible to cytotoxicity by exposure to particles [37]. Too low GSH levels may also affect ROS-mediated redox signaling in macrophages, as seen in another study [38]. The BSO treatment did not affect CB-induced ICAM-1 and VCAM-1 surface expression or the THP-1 adhesion to HUVECs, which indicates that endothelial activation by CB exposure could be independent of oxidative stress. This is consistent with earlier observation where maintenance of ascorbate levels in HUVECs attenuated the CB-induced ROS production without affecting the expression of ICAM-1 and VCAM-1 [10]. Indeed, our results showed that depletion of GSH by BSO pre-treatment resulted in slightly reduced ICAM-1 and VCAM-1 expressions by TNF exposure and significantly reduced the TNF-mediated adhesion of THP-1 cells onto HUVECs. This is consistent with the observation that excessive BSO pre-treatment can lead to cellular adaptive response through the activation of the NRF-2 pathway and thus altered cell survival response [39]. However, the CB exposure for

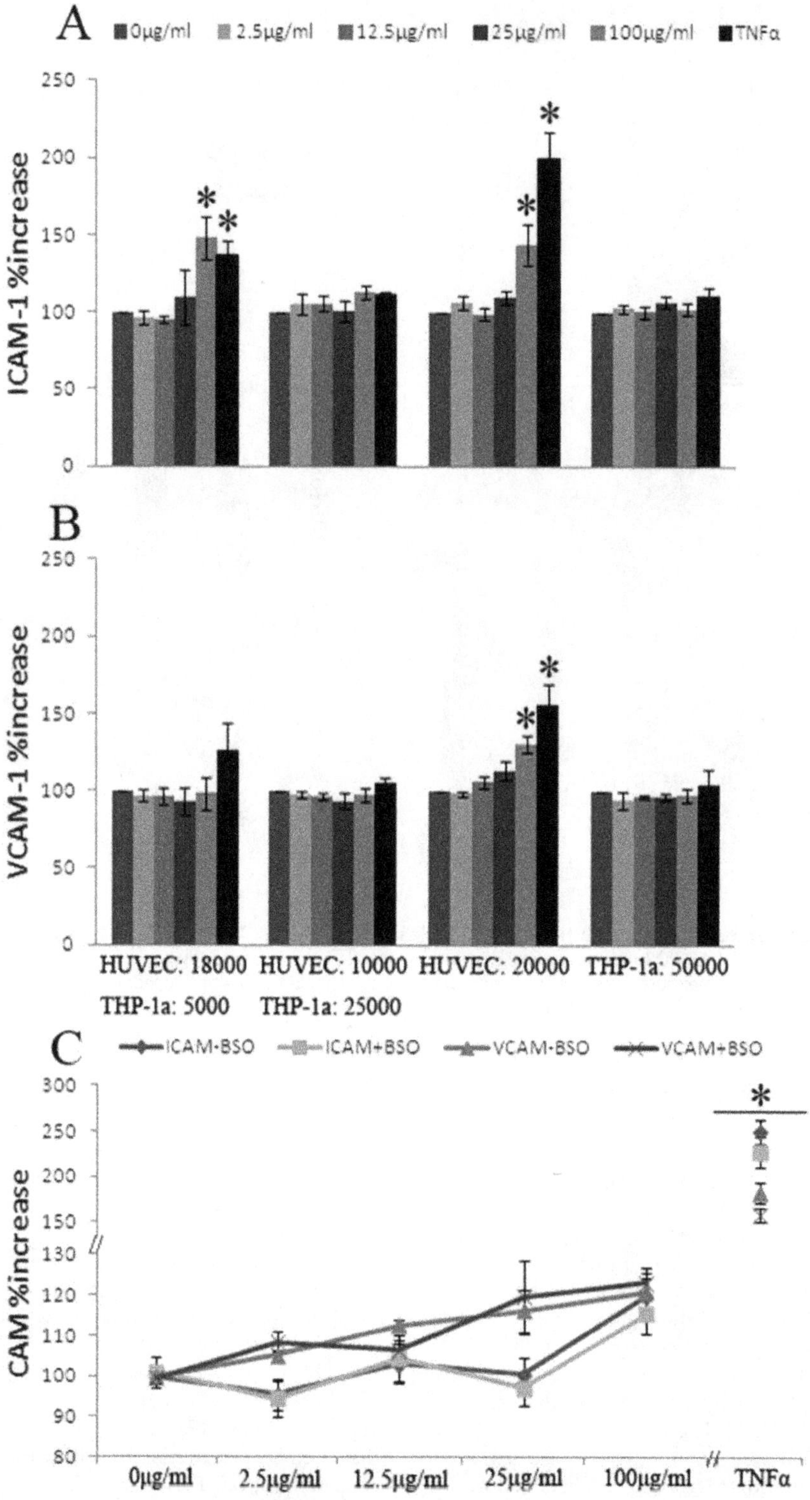

Figure 5. ICAM-1 and VCAM-1 surface expression after 24 h CB exposure in mono-cultures of HUVECs or THP-1a cells, co-cultures with 90% HUVECs and 10% THP-1a cells or 50% HUVECs and 50%THP-1a cells with number of seeded cells indicated (A and B) and effect of BSO pre-treatment on ICAM-1 and VCAM-1 surface expression in HUVECs (C). Data are expressed as percentage of absorbance of unexposed control cells and bars are means ±SEM of at least three independent experiments. *P<0.05 compared with unexposed cells.

3 h did not change the expressions of *GCLM* and *HMOX1*. Up regulation of *GCLM* with possibly increased synthesis capacity might be related to the elevated GSH levels found after CB exposure in HUVECs. However, the unaltered *HMOX1* expression is consistent with no sign of oxidative stress and even elevated GSH levels despite ROS formation detected by DCFH in

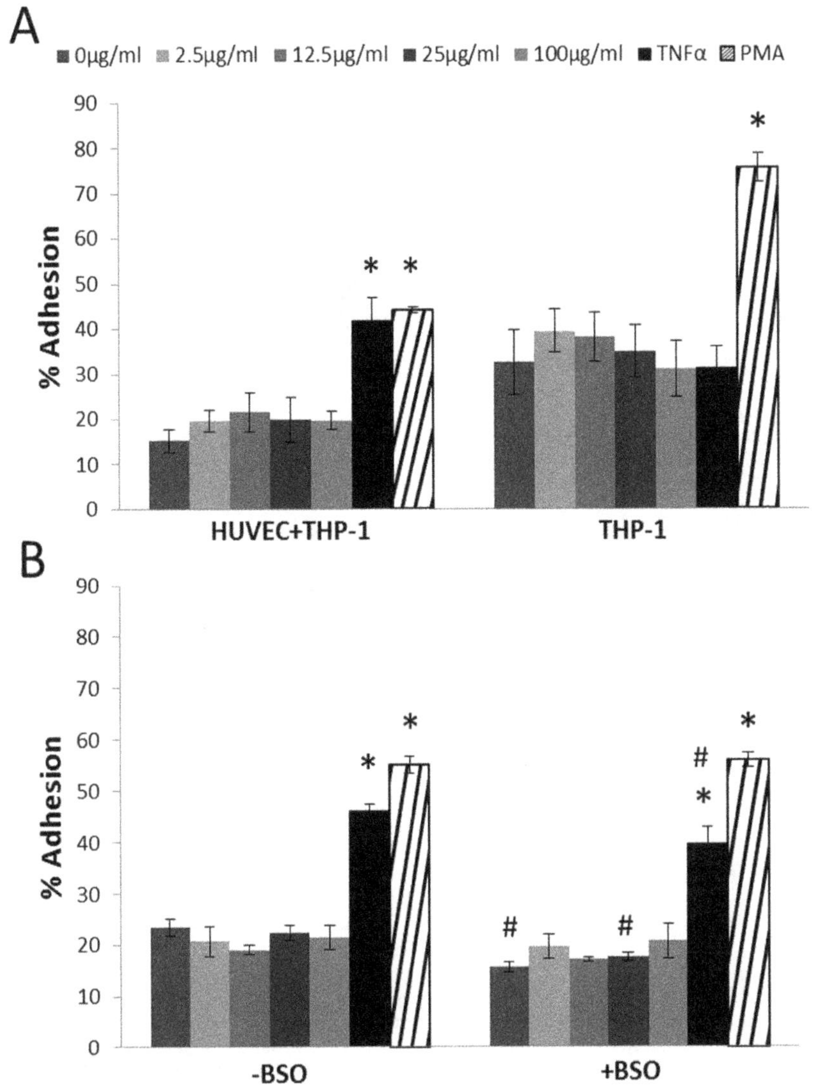

Figure 6. THP-1 adhesion to HUVEC cells or culture dishes assessed by BrdU labeling after 24 h CB exposure (A). In a separate experiment, HUVECs were exposed to 100 μM of BSO for 24 h before they were exposed to CB in co-culture with THP-1 cells (B). Data are expressed as percentage of adherent THP-1 cells compared with the total number of THP-1 cells (cell culture+supernatant) and bars are means ±SEM of three independent experiments *$P<0.05$ compared with unexposed cells, #$P<0.05$ compared with co-cultures where the HUVECs were not pre-treated with BSO.

HUVECs. In contrast, it has been shown that the *VCAM1* expression was sensitive to fluctuations in the redox state and mediators that are generated by inflammation [40], whereas the expression of VCAM-1 did not depend on the superoxide anion radical levels in vessel segments form mice [41]. Indeed, we observed an increased expression of *VCAM1* after the 3 h exposure to CB. This indicates that the gene expression of *VCAM-1* might be sensitive to intracellular generation of ROS without overt oxidative stress, or that the mRNA up regulation is unrelated to ROS formation like the enhanced expression of VCAM-1 on the plasma membrane of HUVECs induced by CB.

PMA was used to differentiate THP-1 cells to become adherent macrophage-like cells (THP-1a cells). It has been suggested that ROS have an initial signaling role for the differentiation of THP-1 cells to macrophages [19]. Here we also found that PMA treatment slightly increased ROS production in THP-1 cells, although this was much lower than the CB-induced ROS production. However, the slightly increased ROS production of THP-1a cells as compared with undifferentiated THP-1cells could also be related to higher phagocytosis activity in the former as also evidenced by higher mitochondrial activity and oxidative respiration [42]. The CB induced ROS production was not associated with enhanced adhesion of THP-1 cells to HUVECs or culture dishes.

We measured cell viability by several methods to determine concentrations with minimum cytotoxicity in order to be able to interpret the data related to atherosclerosis processes. The WST-1 and LDH assays are considered to be indicators of effect to mitochondria and cell membrane, respectively, whereas the proliferation ability can be regarded as an overall indicator of the cellular well-being in as much as the cells will not proliferate if they are damaged. The exposure to CB at high concentration was associated with cytotoxicity in THP-1 cells, without any effect on the proliferation in the same exposure period or decreased viability

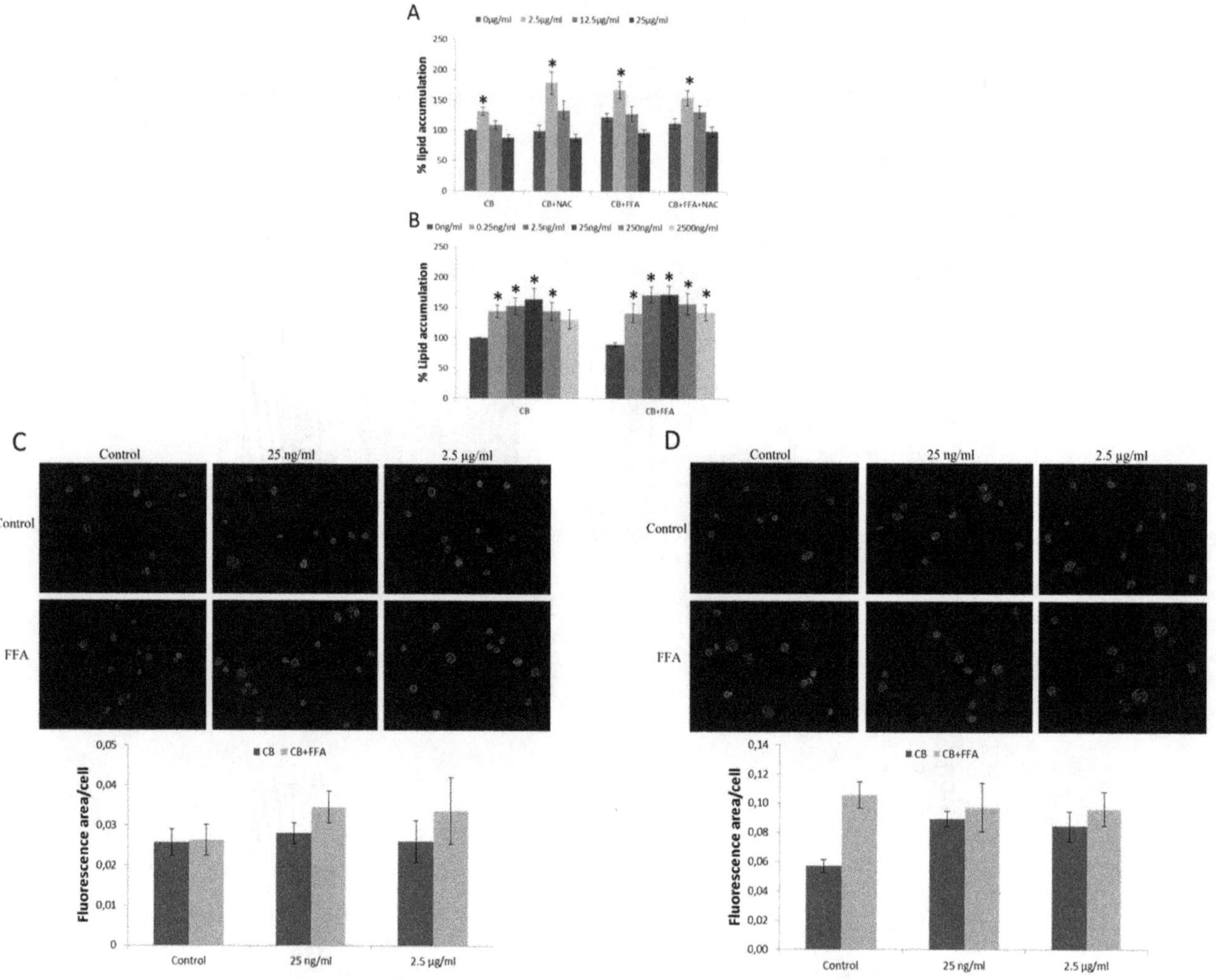

Figure 7. Accumulation of lipids in THP-1a cells after 24 h exposure to CB with or without the presence of NAC (A) or lower concentrations of CB (B) and subsequently treated with free fatty acids (FFA) for 3 h. Data are expressed as percentage increase of lipid accumulation compared with unexposed control cells and bars are means ±SEM of 4–10 independent experiments. *P<0.05 compared with unexposed cells. Semi-quantitative determination of lipid accumulation were performed by microscopy with Nile Red and Bodipy 493/503: C) Cells are stained with Nile Red (red) and Hoechst (blue), D) Cells are stained with Bodipy 493/503 (green) and Hoechst (blue) and representative images are shown in top, and calculation of the lipid fluorescence area per cell shown below calculated from 5 independent areas with SEM.

assessed by trypan blue exclusion. This is in agreement with earlier observations that the LDH release was increased in A549 lung epithelial cells after exposure to diesel exhaust particles, although it had little effect on the ability to proliferate and form colonies [43].

There were increased oxidative stress endpoints and lipid accumulation at the concentration of 2.5 µg/ml, whereas the expression of ICAM-1 and VCAM-1 was increased at 25 and 100 µg/ml. These are high but typical concentrations in particle toxicology. The relevance to the human exposure situation is difficult to assess firmly because studies on translocation usually use other types of particles, which can be traced systemically. In perspective, the dose was 1 mg/mouse by i.t. instillation in a study that showed increased level of atherosclerosis after exposure to CB [16]. This corresponds to 10 µg/ml in blood, assuming 1% translocation of the deposited dose in a blood volume of 1 ml in mice. It has further been estimated that a 24 h exposure to1 mg/m^3 of NPs with a diameter around 14–20 nm would correspond to an average exposure of 0.15 µg/cm^2 lung surface, which equals 0.24 µg/ml (240 ng/ml) in 96-wells plates [44]. This corresponds to a concentration of 2.4 ng/ml in blood, assuming the same 1% translocation to 1 ml blood. As the Occupational Exposure Limit

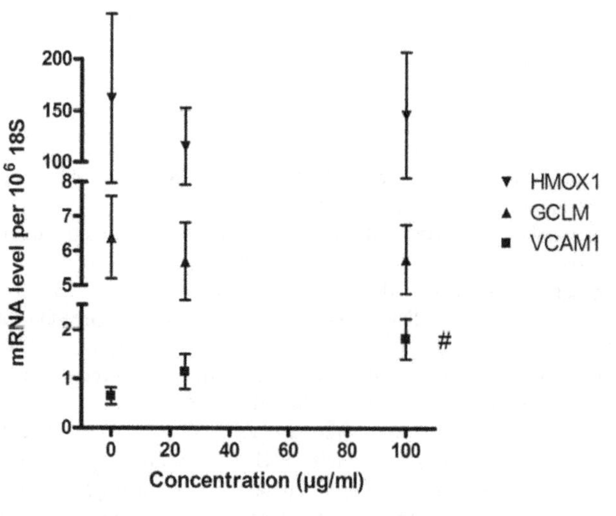

Figure 8. mRNA expression of *GCLM, HMOX1* and *VCAM1* in HUVECs after exposure to CB for 3 h. The symbols represent the mean and SEM of three independent experiments. #P<0.05 (linear regression analysis).

for carbon black is 3.5 mg/m^3, the exposure concentration levels used in this study were high and endothelial cells and monocytes will probably never be exposed to such concentrations *in vivo*. Nevertheless, the mechanistic effects have to be investigated both in realistic concentrations as well as under circumstances where effects are observable. On the other hand, we found an increase in the lipid accumulation by CB at concentrations ranging from 2.5 μg/ml to 0.25 ng/ml, which could be achieved *in vivo*. As in atherosclerosis, there are increased level of differentiated macrophages adherent to the endothelium [2], CB exposure could promote the lipid laden foam cell formation *in vivo*.

In conclusion, the results showed that exposure to nano-sized CB increased the expression of ICAM-1 and VCAM-1 on endothelial cells. This expression was not enhanced by BSO pretreatment, although BSO augmented the CB-mediated ROS generation. In addition, CB exposure increased the lipid accumulation in THP-1 macrophages, but the presence of antioxidants did not affect the lipid accumulation induced by CB. Further, very low concentrations of CB promoted lipid accumulation without obvious effect on intracellular ROS production. Our results suggest that CB induces endothelial adhesion molecule expression and foam cell formation independent of CB-induced ROS generation.

Supporting Information

File S1 Figure S1. Cytotoxicity of CB on THP-1 cells after 24 h exposure as measured by trypan blue assay. Figure S2. Cell number of THP-1 cells after 24 h CB. Figure S3. Representative micrographs showing the intracellular ROS production after 3 h incubation with CB in HUVECs or THP-1a cells. Figure S4. Interaction effect of a 30 min CB exposure on the ICAM-1 and VCAM-1 assays.

Author Contributions

Conceived and designed the experiments: YC MR PM SL. Performed the experiments: YC MR PD. Analyzed the data: YC MR PD PM SL. Contributed reagents/materials/analysis tools: PM SL. Wrote the paper: YC MR PD PM SL.

References

1. Moller P, Mikkelsen L, Vesterdal LK, Folkmann JK, Forchhammer L, et al. (2011) Hazard identification of particulate matter on vasomotor dysfunction and progression of atherosclerosis. Crit Rev Toxicol 41: 339–368.
2. Packard RRS, Libby P (2008) Inflammation in Atherosclerosis: From Vascular Biology to Biomarker Discovery and Risk Prediction. Clin Chem 54: 24–38.
3. Forchhammer L, Loft S, Roursgaard M, Cao Y, Riddervold IS, et al. (2012) Expression of adhesion molecules, monocyte interactions and oxidative stress in human endothelial cells exposed to wood smoke and diesel exhaust particulate matter. Toxicol Lett 209: 121–128.
4. Montiel-Davalos A, Ibarra-Sanchez MD, Ventura-Gallegos JL, Alfaro-Moreno E, Lopez-Marure R (2010) Oxidative stress and apoptosis are induced in human endothelial cells exposed to urban particulate matter. Toxicol in Vitro 24: 135–141.
5. Cao Y, Jacobsen NR, Danielsen PH, Lenz AG, Stoeger T, et al. (2014) Vascular Effects of Multiwalled Carbon Nanotubes in Dyslipidemic ApoE-/- Mice and Cultured Endothelial Cells. Toxicological Sciences 138: 104–116.
6. Przybytkowski E, Behrendt M, Dubois D, Maysinger D (2009) Nanoparticles can induce changes in the intracellular metabolism of lipids without compromising cellular viability. FEBS J 276: 6204–6217.
7. Tsukahara T, Haniu H (2011) Nanoparticle-mediated intracellular lipid accumulation during C2C12 cell differentiation. Biochem Biophys Res Commun 406: 558–563.
8. Gojova A, Guo B, Kota RS, Rutledge JC, Kennedy IM, et al. (2007) Induction of inflammation in vascular endothelial cells by metal oxide nanoparticles: Effect of particle composition. Environ Health Perspect 115: 403–409.
9. Mikkelsen L, Jensen KA, Koponen IK, Saber AT, Wallin H, et al. (2012) Cytotoxicity, oxidative stress and expression of adhesion molecules in human umbilical vein endothelial cells exposed to dust from paints with or without nanoparticles. Nanotoxicology 7: 117–134.
10. Frikke-Schmidt H, Roursgaard M, Lykkesfeldt J, Loft S, Nojgaard JK, et al. (2011) Effect of vitamin C and iron chelation on diesel exhaust particle and carbon black induced oxidative damage and cell adhesion molecule expression in human endothelial cells. Toxicol Lett 203: 181–189.
11. Khatchadourian A, Maysinger D (2009) Lipid Droplets: Their Role in Nanoparticle-Induced Oxidative Stress. Mol Pharm 6: 1125–1137.
12. Jacobsen NR, Pojana G, White P, Moller P, Cohn CA, et al. (2008) Genotoxicity, cytotoxicity, and reactive oxygen species induced by single-walled carbon nanotubes and C-60 fullerenes in the FE1-Muta (TM) mouse lung epithelial cells. Environ Mol Mutagen 49: 476–487.
13. Vesterdal LK, Mikkelsen L, Folkmann JK, Sheykhzade M, Cao Y, et al. (2012) Carbon black nanoparticles and vascular dysfunction in cultured endothelial cells and artery segments. Toxicol Lett 214: 19–26.
14. Moller P, Jacobsen NR, Folkmann JK, Danielsen PH, Mikkelsen L, et al. (2010) Role of oxidative damage in toxicity of particulates. Free Radic Res 44: 1–46.
15. Vesterdal L, Folkmann J, Jacobsen N, Sheykhzade M, Wallin H, et al. (2010) Pulmonary exposure to carbon black nanoparticles and vascular effects. Part Fibre Toxicol 7: 33.
16. Niwa Y, Hiura Y, Murayama T, Yokode M, Iwai N (2007) Nano-sized carbon black exposure exacerbates atherosclerosis in LDL-receptor knockout mice. Circ J 71: 1157–1161.
17. Kensler TW, Wakabayash N, Biswal S (2007) Cell survival responses to environmental stresses via the Keap1-Nrf2-ARE pathway. Annu Rev Pharmacol Toxicol 47: 89–116.
18. Danielsen PH, Loft S, Kocbach A, Schwarze PE, Moller P (2009) Oxidative damage to DNA and repair induced by Norwegian wood smoke particles in human A549 and THP-1 cell lines. Mutat Res 674: 116–122.
19. Traore K, Trush MA, George M, Spannhake EW, Anderson W, et al. (2005) Signal transduction of phorbol 12-myristate 13-acetate (PMA)-induced growth inhibition of human monocytic leukemia THP-1 cells is reactive oxygen dependent. Leuk Res 29: 863–879.
20. Bourdon J, Saber A, Jacobsen N, Jensen K, Madsen A, et al. (2012) Carbon black nanoparticle instillation induces sustained inflammation and genotoxicity in mouse lung and liver. Part Fibre Toxicol 9: 5.
21. Jackson P, Hougaard KS, Boisen AM, Jacobsen NR, Jensen KA, et al. (2012) Pulmonary exposure to carbon black by inhalation or instillation in pregnant mice: effects on liver DNA strand breaks in dams and offspring. Nanotoxicology 6: 486–500.
22. Jacobsen NR, Saber AT, White P, Moller P, Pojana G, et al. (2007) Increased mutant frequency by carbon black, but not quartz, in the lacZ and cII transgenes of muta mouse lung epithelial cells. Environ Mol Mutagen 48: 451–461.
23. McLaughlin AP, De Vries GW (2001) Role of PLCgamma and Ca(2+) in VEGF- and FGF-induced choroidal endothelial cell proliferation. Am J Physiol Cell Physiol 281: C1448–C1456.
24. Dikalov S, Griendling KK, Harrison DG (2007) Measurement of Reactive Oxygen Species in Cardiovascular Studies. Hypertension 49: 717–727.
25. Danielsen PH, Moller P, Jensen KA, Sharma AK, Wallin H, et al. (2011) Oxidative Stress, DNA Damage, and Inflammation Induced by Ambient Air and Wood Smoke Particulate Matter in Human A549 and THP-1 Cell Lines. Chem Res Toxicol 24: 168–184.
26. Hemmingsen JG, Moller P, Nojgaard JK, Roursgaard M, Loft S (2011) Oxidative Stress, Genotoxicity, And Vascular Cell Adhesion Molecule Expression in Cells Exposed to Particulate Matter from Combustion of Conventional Diesel and Methyl Ester Biodiesel Blends. Environ Sci Technol 45: 8545–8551.
27. Cao Y, Liang S, Zheng Y, Liu D, Zhang B, et al. (2011) Induction of GSNO reductase but not NOS in the lungs of mice exposed to glucan-spiked dust. Environ Toxicol 26: 279–286.
28. Murphy F, Schinwald A, Poland C, Donaldson K (2012) The mechanism of pleural inflammation by long carbon nanotubes: interaction of long fibres with macrophages stimulates them to amplify pro-inflammatory responses in mesothelial cells. Part Fibre Toxicol 9: 8.
29. Chen X, Zhong Z, Xu Z, Chen L, Wang Y (2010) 2′, 7′-Dichlorodihydrofluorescein as a fluorescent probe for reactive oxygen species measurement: Forty years of application and controversy. Free Radic Res 44: 587–604.
30. Vesterdal LK, Danielsen PH, Folkmann JK, Jespersen LF, Aguilar-Pelaez K, et al. (2013) Accumulation of lipids and oxidatively damaged DNA in hepatocytes exposed to particles. Toxicol Appl Pharmacol 10.
31. Hussain S, Thomassen L, Ferecatu I, Borot MC, Andreau K, et al. (2010) Carbon black and titanium dioxide nanoparticles elicit distinct apoptotic pathways in bronchial epithelial cells. Particle and Fibre Toxicology 7: 10.
32. Karlsson M, Kurz T, Brunk UT, Nilsson SE, Frennesson CI (2010) What does the commonly used DCF test for oxidative stress really show? Biochem J 428: 183–190.
33. Ohashi T, Mizutani A, Murakami A, Kojo S, Ishii T, et al. (2002) Rapid oxidation of dichlorodihydrofluorescin with heme and hemoproteins: formation of the fluorescein is independent of the generation of reactive oxygen species. FEBS Lett 511: 21–27.

34. LeBel CP, Ischiropoulos H, Bondy SC (1992) Evaluation of the probe 2′, 7′-dichlorofluorescin as an indicator of reactive oxygen species formation and oxidative stress. Chem Res Toxicol 5: 227–231.
35. Zhu H, Bannenberg GL, Moldeus P, Shertzer HG (1994) Oxidation pathways for the intracellular probe 2′, 7′-dichlorofluorescein. Arch Toxicol 68: 582–587.
36. Peebles BC, Dutta PK, Waldman WJ, Villamena FA, Nash K, et al. (2011) Physicochemical and toxicological properties of commercial carbon blacks modified by reaction with ozone. Environ Sci Technol 45: 10668–10675.
37. Anderson CP, Reynolds CP (2002) Synergistic cytotoxicity of buthionine sulfoximine (BSO) and intensive melphalan (L-PAM) for neuroblastoma cell lines established at relapse after myeloablative therapy. Bone Marrow Transplantation 30: 135–140.
38. Forman HJ, Fukuto JM, Torres M (2004) Redox signaling: thiol chemistry defines which reactive oxygen and nitrogen species can act as second messengers. Am J Physiol Cell Physiol 287: C246–C256.
39. Speciale A, Anwar S, Ricciardi E, Chirafisi J, Saija A, et al. (2011) Cellular adaptive response to glutathione depletion modulates endothelial dysfunction triggered by TNF-alpha. Toxicol Lett 207: 291–297.
40. Cook-Mills JM, Marchese ME, Abdala-Valencia H (2011) Vascular Cell Adhesion Molecule-1 Expression and Signaling During Disease: Regulation by Reactive Oxygen Species and Antioxidants. Antioxid Redox Signal 15: 1607–1638.
41. Willett NJ, Kundu K, Knight SF, Dikalov S, Murthy N, et al. (2011) Redox Signaling in an In Vivo Murine Model of Low Magnitude Oscillatory Wall Shear Stress. Antioxid Redox Signal 15: 1369–1378.
42. Jantzen K, Roursgaard M, Desler C, Loft S, Rasmussen LJ, et al. (2012) Oxidative damage to DNA by diesel exhaust particle exposure in co-cultures of human lung epithelial cells and macrophages. Mutagenesis 27: 693–701.
43. Danielsen P, Loft S, Moller P (2008) DNA damage and cytotoxicity in type II lung epithelial (A549) cell cultures after exposure to diesel exhaust and urban street particles. Part Fibre Toxicol 5: 6.
44. Gangwal S, Brown JS, Wang A, Houck KA, Dix DJ, et al. (2011) Informing Selection of Nanomaterial Concentrations for ToxCast in Vitro Testing Based on Occupational Exposure Potential. Environ Health Perspect 119: 1539–1546.

9

Functional Bioassays for Immune Monitoring of High-Risk Neuroblastoma Patients Treated with ch14.18/CHO Anti-GD_2 Antibody

Nikolai Siebert, Diana Seidel, Christin Eger, Madlen Jüttner, Holger N. Lode*

Department of Pediatric Oncology and Hematology, University Medicine Greifswald, Greifswald, Germany

Abstract

Effective treatment of high-risk neuroblastoma (NB) remains a major challenge in pediatric oncology. Human/mouse chimeric monoclonal anti-GD_2 antibody (mAb) ch14.18 is emerging as a treatment option to improve outcome. After establishing a production process in Chinese hamster ovary (CHO) cells, ch14.18/CHO was made available in Europe for clinical trials. Here, we describe validated functional bioassays for the purpose of immune monitoring of these trials and demonstrate GD_2-specific immune effector functions of ch14.18/CHO in treated patients. Two calcein-based bioassays for complement-dependent- (CDC) and antibody-dependent cellular cytotoxicity (ADCC) were set up based on patient serum and immune cells tested against NB cells. For this purpose, we identified LA-N-1 NB cells as best suited within a panel of cell lines. Assay conditions were first established using serum and cells of healthy donors. We found an effector-to-target (E:T) cell ratio of 20:1 for PBMC preparations as best suited for GD_2-specific ADCC analysis. A simplified method of effector cell preparation by lysis of erythrocytes was evaluated revealing equivalent results at an E:T ratio of 40:1. Optimal results for CDC were found with a serum dilution at 1:8. For validation, both within-assay and inter-assay precision were determined and coefficients of variation (CV) were below 20%. Sample quality following storage at room temperature (RT) showed that sodium-heparin-anticoagulated blood and serum are stable for 48 h and 96 h, respectively. Application of these bioassays to blood samples of three selected high-risk NB patients treated with ch14.18/CHO (100 mg/m^2) revealed GD_2-specific increases in CDC (4.5–9.4 fold) and ADCC (4.6–6.0 fold) on day 8 compared to baseline, indicating assay applicability for the monitoring of multicenter clinical trials requiring sample shipment at RT for central lab analysis.

Editor: Pierre Busson, Gustave Roussy, France

Funding: Financial support was provided by the Hector-Stiftung, Germany, University Medicine Greifswald, Germany. Further financial support was provided by Apeiron Biologics, Vienna, Austria. The funders had no role in study design, data collection and analysis, decision to publish, or preparation of the manuscript.

* Email: lode@uni-greifswald.de

Introduction

Monoclonal antibodies targeting disialoganglioside GD_2 emerge as an important treatment option for NB, a dismal pediatric malignancy characterized by high expression of GD_2 on tumor cells [1,2]. Ganglioside GD_2 is a glycolipid antigen devoid of an intracellular signal transduction domain. Therefore the mechanism of action of anti-GD_2 monoclonal Ab mostly rely on immune effector functions mediated by mAbs, which are more and more recognized as the key features of this class of cancer therapeutics [3]. These features include the activation of CDC and ADCC.

CDC is induced through binding of a serine protease complex C1 to the Fc domains of two or more mAbs binding to antigens expressed on tumor cells. This classical complement pathway results in an activation cascade resulting in the membrane attack complex disrupting the target cell. ADCC is a result of Fc-gamma receptor (FcγR) mediated interaction with effector immune cells such as natural killer (NK) cells, macrophages and granulocytes [3]. The binding of FcγR to Fc domain induces both release of granzymes and perforin from effector cells leading to a target cell lysis and Fc-dependent tumor cell phagocytosis.

The clinical development of anti-GD_2 monoclonal antibodies for NB patients originated from the discovery of two distinct murine anti-GD_2 antibodies designated 3F8 [4] and 14.18 [5], respectively. High-risk NB patients were successfully treated within clinical trials with both antibodies mostly conducted by cooperating academic groups of pediatric oncologists. In a more multi center and international approach, the human/mouse chimeric version of 14.18 (ch14.18) has demonstrated activity and efficacy as a monotherapy [6,7] and in combination with cytokines [8]. In Europe, ch14.18 antibody was made available for clinical trials following the recloning of the antibody genes into CHO cells which was designated as ch14.18/CHO. This is important, as ch14.18/CHO revealed superior activity in mediating ADCC compared to ch14.18 antibody produced in other cell lines [9]. Subsequently, a validated industrial production process was established. This development was initiated by SIOPEN, a group of international clinical leaders in the field of neuroblastoma and funded by charities throughout Europe. Four European clinical trials with different treatment schedules of ch14.18/CHO are being conducted to investigate the influence of a combined immunotherapy of ch14.18/CHO, interleukin-2 (IL-2) and 13-cis-retinoid acid on the outcome of patients with high-risk NB in the absence or presence of haploidentical blood stem cell transplantation. The first trial established the safety profile of ch14.18/CHO in children with high risk NB [10]. The European phase III clinical trial (HR-NBL 1.5/ESIOP, Eudra CT: 2006-001489-17) and the trial in the context of haploidentical stem cell transplantation (Eudra CT: 2009-015936-14) are based on a short term infusion of 20 mg/m^2/d ch14.18 over 8 h on five subsequent days. To reduce side effects including neuropathic pain, a Phase I/II clinical trial was initiated based on the same cumulative dose of ch14.18/CHO (100 mg/m^2/cycle) infused over a longer time period (ten days) (Eudra CT: 2009-018077-3). Within these trial protocols, a set of immune monitoring assays including the detection of ch14.18/CHO serum levels [11] and human anti-ch14.18/CHO immune responses [12], are implemented with the aim to identify immune biomarkers correlating with clinical response to ch14.18/CHO therapy. For a comprehensive assessment, validated bioassays to determine effector functions of ch14.18/CHO namely patient specific ADCC and CDC are of critical importance.

For analysis of patient-specific CDC and ADCC, we established and validated two non-radioactive and non-toxic cytotoxicity assays based on release of acetomethoxy derivate of calcein (calcein-AM), which is a membrane-permeable live-cell labeling dye. With these assays, we demonstrate GD_2 specific CDC and ADCC activity in ch14.18/CHO treated patients and demonstrated feasibility in the context of multicenter clinical trials.

Materials and Methods

Ethic statement

Participants were informed about the testing procedure and gave written informed consent. The study complies with the Declaration of Helsinki and was approved by the ethics committee of the University Medicine of Greifswald, Germany. *De novo* cell line establishment (HGW-1, HGW-2, HGW-3 and HGW-5 cell line) complies with the written informed consent from the donor, parents and legal guardians.

Tissue culture

Human GD_2-positive NB cell line LA-N-1 [13] and human melanoma cell line M21 (kindly provided by Prof. R. A. Reisfeld) [14] were cultured in RPMI supplemented with 4.5 g/l glucose, 2 mM stable glutamine (PAA, Pasching, Austria), 10% FCS and 100 U/ml penicillin and 0.1 mg/ml streptomycin (1x P/S; PAA, Pasching, Austria). Human GD_2-positive NB cell lines CHLA-20 [15], HGW-1, HGW-2, HGW-3 and HGW-5 were cultured in IMDM supplemented with 4 mM stable glutamine, 20% FCS, 1x ITS (BD Biosciences, Heidelberg, Germany) and 1x P/S. Human GD_2-negative NB cell line SK-N-SH [16] was cultured in DMEM supplemented with 4.5 g/l glucose, 2 mM stable glutamine, 10% FCS and 1x P/S. Hybridoma cells producing ganglidiomab were cultured in DMEM supplemented with 4.5 g/l glucose, 2 mM stable glutamine, 10% FCS, 1x P/S, 1x nonessential amino acids (PAA, Pasching, Austria) and 50 µM β-mercaptoethanol (Sigma Aldrich, Steinheim, Germany).

In order to establish new NB cell lines, tumor tissues and bone marrow samples from NB patients were used. Tumor tissue was first minced followed by homogenisation using 70 µM cell strainer (BD Biosciences, Heidelberg, Germany) and bone marrow samples were treated for 10 min with cold erythrocyte lysis buffer (0.15 M ammonium chloride, 10 mM potassium bicarbonate, 0.1 mM ethylenediaminetetraacetic acid, pH 7.4). After two wash steps (1x PBS, 5 min, 300×g, RT) cell pellets were resuspended in 10 ml 1x PBS and layered over 10 ml of Lymphocyte Separation Medium (PAA, Pasching, Austria). After centrifugation (30 min, 300×g, RT without brake) the upper layer was discarded, a layer of primary cells was carefully transferred into a new tube and the remaining Lymphocyte Separation Medium was washed off with 1x PBS supplemented with 0.5% BSA (Sigma Aldrich, Steinheim, Germany) and 2 mM EDTA (Sigma Aldrich, Steinheim, Germany) (pH 7.4, 10 ml, 5 min, 300×g, RT, brake on). Thereafter, the supernatant was carefully removed and the cell pellet was resuspended with 10 ml 1x PBS/0.5% BSA/2 mM EDTA buffer (pH 7.4) followed by cell counting and evaluation of cell viability. Finally, 1×10^7 vital cells were used for isolation of GD_2-positive cell subset with MACS technique (Miltenyi Biotec, Teterow, Germany).

For this purpose 1×10^7 primary cells were resuspended in 200 µl 1x PBS/0.5% BSA/2 mM EDTA buffer (pH 7.4) and then incubated on ice with 20 µl FcR-blocking reagent (Miltenyi Biotec, Teterow, Germany) for 5 min. Thereafter, the murine anti-GD_2 Ab 14G2a (1.0 µg) was added followed by incubation for 10 min on ice. After washing with 1x PBS/0.5% BSA/2 mM EDTA buffer (15 ml, pH 7.4, 5 min, 300×g, +4°C) cell pellet was resuspended in 100 µl 1x PBS/0.5% BSA/2 mM EDTA buffer and 20 µl magnetic microbeads conjugated with anti-mouse IgG (Miltenyi Biotec, Teterow, Germany) were added followed by incubation on ice for 15 min. Next, the cells were washed again by adding 15 ml 1x PBS/0.5% BSA/2 mM EDTA buffer (pH 7.4) and centrifuged at 300×g for 5 min at +4°C. 1 ml of 1x PBS/0.5% BSA/2 mM EDTA buffer was used to resuspend the cell pellet and magnetic separation of GD_2-positive cells was proceeded in MACS-separator (Miltenyi Biotec, Teterow, Germany) by applying the cell suspension onto the LS-separation column (Miltenyi Biotec, Teterow, Germany). The column was washed three times (3 ml, 1x PBS/0.5% BSA/2 mM EDTA buffer, pH 7.4) and then removed from the MACS-separator and placed into a collection tube. Cell fraction containing magnetically labeled GD_2-positive cells were immediately flushed out by firmly applying the plunger supplied with the column (Miltenyi Biotec, Teterow, Germany). Finally, primary cells were washed with 1x PBS (pH 7.4, 5 min, 300×g, RT) and the cell pellet was resuspended in culture medium as described above.

Genetic characterization of *de novo* neuroblastoma cell lines

To determine DNA profiles of newly established cell lines, short tandem repeats (STR) analysis was done (Eurofins MWG Operon, Ebersberg, Germany). Evaluation of genetic aberrations of each newly established cell line was performed by high resolution SNP array analysis using the Affymetrix ultra HD SNP array (CytoScan HD Array). The combination of copy number with the allele information, i.e. zygosity status, enables the detection of loss of heterozygosity with copy losses as well as copy neutral allelic changes.

Analysis of neuroblastoma surface markers by flow cytometry

For analysis of GD_2 and CD56 surface expression, 1×10^6 cells were stained with 1.0 µg ch14.18/CHO and 0.05 µg anti-CD56-APC (clone HCD56, BioLegend, Fell, Germany) in a total volume of 100 µl for 20 min, on ice, in the dark. The chimeric anti-CD20 antibody rituximab (Roche, Mannheim, Germany) and APC-labeled mouse IgG1 (clone MOPC-21, BioLegend, Fell, Germany) were used as negative controls for ch14.18 and anti-CD56, respectively. Cells were washed once with 1 ml wash buffer (1x PBS, 1% BSA, 0.1% NaN_3, 0.1% EDTA, pH 7.4) (300×g, 5 min, RT). Supernatant was discarded and cells were incubated with 0.017 µg of PE-labeled anti-human IgG antibody (clone HP6017, BioLegend, Fell, Germany) in a total volume of 100 µl for 20 min, on ice, in the dark. Cells were washed once and resuspended in 500 µl wash buffer for flow cytometric analysis. To exclude dead cells from analysis, 4 µl of a 0.1 mg/ml DAPI solution (Sigma-Aldrich, Steinheim, Germany) were added 5 min prior to acquisition. For each sample 20,000 live cells were analyzed. Sample acquisition was performed at a BD FACS CANTOII using FACSDiva software (BD Biosciences, Heidelberg, Germany) and data was analyzed using FlowJo 7.6.1 software (Treestar, Ashland, OR, USA). For comparison of GD_2 expression on *de novo* NB cell lines, the ratio of mean fluorescence intensity (MFI) relative to isotype control was calculated according to the formula: geometric fluorescence mean of GD_2 stained sample/ geometric fluorescence mean of isotype control.

Tyrosine hydroxylase and MDR1 gene expression analysis by RT-PCR

Total RNA was isolated from $\leq 1\times10^7$ cells using the RNA isolation Kit (QIAGEN GmbH, Hilden, Germany) according to the manufacturer's instructions. RNA concentration was determined spectrophotometrically (BioPhotometer plus, Eppendorf, Hamburg, Germany) and 1.0 µg of total RNA was used for cDNA synthesis using qScript cDNA Synthesis Kit (Quanta BioSciences, Gaithersburg, MD, USA) according to the manufacturer's protocol.

Analysis of human TH (hTH) mRNA expression was performed using gene-specific primers designed with online primer design tool Primer3 and used for PCR. For the detection of hTH mRNA, the forward primer sequence used was 5′-GGC CCA AGG TCC CCT GGT TC-3′ and the reverse primer sequence was 5′-ACA GCA GGC CGG CCA CAG GC-3′. HTH was amplified by 25 cycles consisting of 95°C (30 s) for denaturation, 62°C (30 s) for primer-specific annealing, and 72°C (30 s) for elongation. The PCR product size was 405 bp. PCR without cDNA template (no template control) served as a negative control and GAPDH as a housekeeping gene (forward primer: 5′-GAG TCA ACG GAT TTG GTC GT-3′ and reverse primer: 5′-TTG ATT TTG GAG GGA TCT CG-3′, product size: 238 bp).

To evaluate expression of MDR1 gene, specific primers were designed as described above. Following primer sequences were used for PCR: 5′-GCT CCT GAC TAT GCC AAA GC-3′ (forward primer) and 5′-TCT TCA CCT CCA GGC TCA GT-3′ (reverse primer). MDR1 PCR product (202 bp) was amplified by 25 cycles consisting of 95°C (15 s) for denaturation, 61°C (15 s) for primer-specific annealing, and 72°C (15 s) for elongation. Negative control and GAPDH as an internal control (forward primer: 5′-GAG TCA ACG GAT TTG GTC GT-3′ and reverse primer: 5′-TGT GGT CAT GAG TCC TTC CA-3′, product size: 512 bp) were used as described above. After separation by electrophoresis on 2% agarose gel, PCR products were visualized by ethidium bromide (ImageJ Program). Expression of MDR1 gene product was analyzed relative to the internal control GAPDH.

Isolation of ganglidiomab from hybridoma supernatants

Ganglidiomab anti-idiotype (anti-Id) Ab was isolated from hybridoma cells as previously described [17]. Briefly, the concentration of ganglidiomab in hybridoma supernatants was determined by ELISA using ch14.18/CHO as a capture mAb [17]. Hybridoma supernatants containing 50 µg/ml of ganglidiomab were filtered and ganglidiomab was concentrated followed by binding to protein G as previously described. After wash steps ganglidiomab was eluted and quantified with ELISA using ch14.18/CHO as a capture mAb [17]. The final product contained 500 µg/ml of ganglidiomab and was used for further assay developments.

Serum preparation

Blood was collected using BD Vacutainer plastic serum tubes (BD Biosciences, Heidelberg, Germany). Serum was prepared from clotted blood samples by centrifugation for 10 min at 1,700×g, RT and stored in aliquots at −80°C. Serum used for ADCC assays was heat inactivated at 56° for 30 min. Serum as a source for complements in CDC assays was used without further manipulation.

Isolation of effector cells

Isolation of peripheral blood mononuclear cells (PBMCs). Blood was collected using BD Vacutainer plastic sodium-heparin tubes (BD Biosciences, Heidelberg, Germany) 6 ml of blood were carefully layered over 6 ml of Lymphocyte Separation Medium (PAA, Pasching, Austria). After centrifugation (30 min, 300×g, RT without brake) following four layers were defined: a) a clear upper layer (diluted plasma and platelets), b) a fluffy white layer of PBMCs, c) a clear Lymphocyte Separation Medium layer and d) a lowest substantial pellet of red blood cells containing granulocytes. After the upper layer was discarded, a layer of PBMCs was carefully transferred into a new tube and the remaining Lymphocyte Separation Medium was washed off twice with 1x PBS (10 ml, 5 min, 300×g, RT, brake on). Thereafter, the supernatant was carefully removed and the cell pellet was resuspended with 10 ml 1x PBS followed by counting of PBMCs. To determine relative amounts of lymphocytes, granulocytes and monocytes in PBMCs, cells (2×10^5) were resuspended in 2 ml 1x PBS and attached to glass slides using cytospin centrifugation (10 min, 200×g, RT). Cytospins were stained using the panoptic method of Pappenheim following the manufacturer's guidelines and a differential leucocyte count was performed by light microscopy. The lowest layer containing erythrocytes and granulocytes was used for further isolation of granulocytes.

Isolation of granulocytes. The lowest layer obtained during the isolation of PMBCs as described above was resuspended in 4 ml of cold erythrocyte lysis buffer (0,15 M ammonium chloride, 10 mM potassium bicarbonate, 0.1 mM ethylenediaminetetraacetic acid, pH 7.4) and incubated for 10 min on ice. Further, cell suspension was centrifuged for 5 min at 300×g (+4°C). Thereafter, the supernatant was carefully removed and the cell pellet was resuspended in 15 ml 1x PBS and centrifuged (5 min, 300×g, + 4°C). Then, granulocytes were resuspended in 10 ml 1x PBS and counted. The relative amount of granulocytes was determined by light microscopy following cytospin as described above.

Isolation of leukocytes. Leukocytes were isolated from 6 ml of sodium-heparin blood not older than 24 hours using cold erythrocyte lysis buffer. Briefly, 6 ml of whole blood was gently mixed with 12 ml of cold erythrocyte lysis buffer, incubated for 10 min on ice and centrifuged for 5 min at 300×g (+4°C). Thereafter, cell pellet was resuspended in 15 ml 1x PBS and centrifuged again (5 min, 300×g, +4°C). Finally, leukocytes were resuspended in 10 ml 1x PBS and counted.

Calcein-AM cytotoxicity assay. In order to evaluate patient-specific ch14.18/CHO-mediated CDC as well as ADCC, two calcein-AM-based release assays were established. For ADCC,

Table 1. Genetic aberrations of *de novo* neuroblastoma cell lines.

	MYCN amplification	NMYC copy number	1p deletion	11q gain	17q gain
HGW-1	+	36	−	+	+
HGW-2	N.D.	N.D.	N.D.	N.D.	N.D.
HGW-3	+	14	+	−	+
HGW-5	+	25	+	−	+

Genetic aberrations of *de novo* neuroblastoma cell lines were evaluated using high resolution SNP array analysis. N.D; not done.

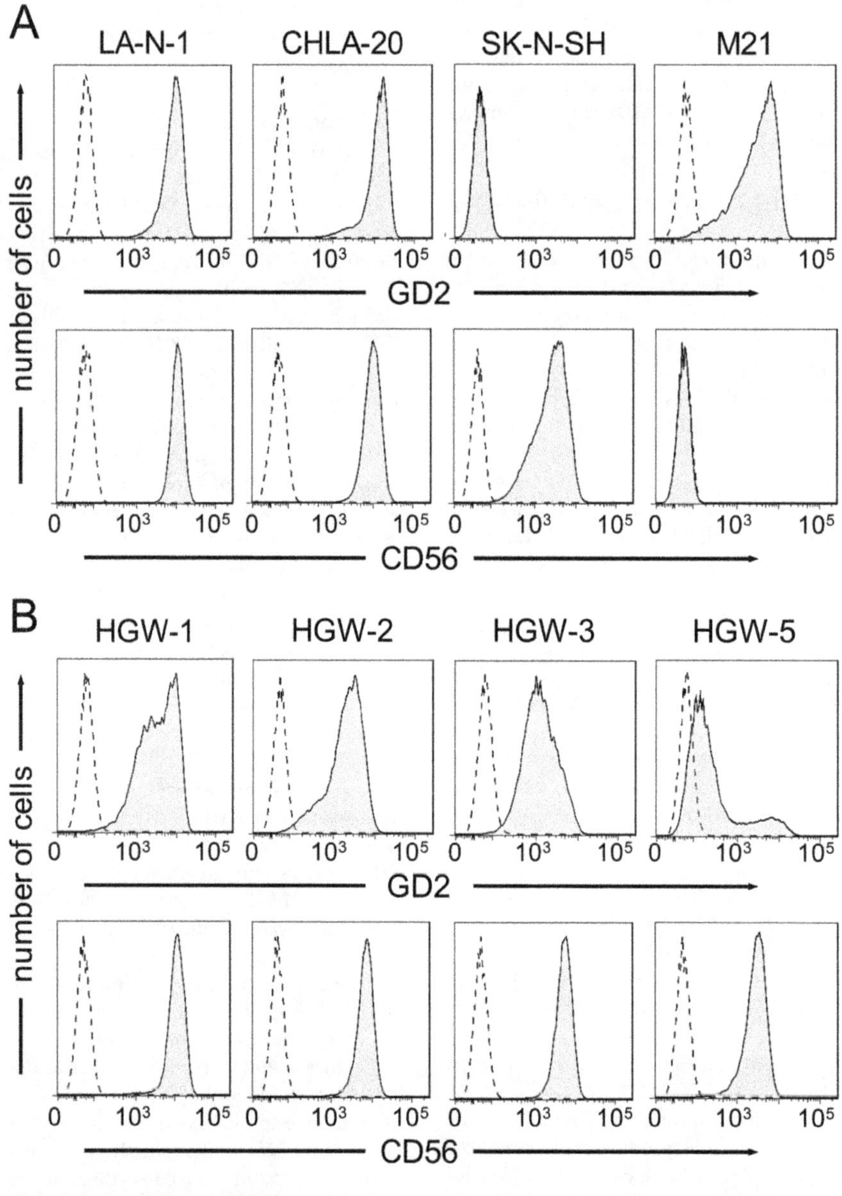

Figure 1. Flow cytometric analysis of GD_2 and CD56 expression. NB cells were stained with 1.0 μg ch14.18/CHO and 0.05 μg anti-CD56-APC, followed by incubation with 0.017 μg of PE-labeled anti-human IgG secondary antibody. Chimeric anti-CD20 antibody and APC-labeled mouse IgG1 were utilized as isotype controls, respectively. (**A**) Expression of GD_2 (upper panel, black filled curve) and CD56 (lower panel, black filled curve) on NB cell lines LA-N-1, CHLA-20, SK-N-SH and the melanoma cell line M21. Respective isotype controls are indicated in both panels as black dashed curves. Results are presented as representative histograms. (**B**) Selected histograms of GD_2 (upper panel, black filled curve) and CD56 (lower panel, black filled curve) expression on *de novo* NB cell lines HGW-1, HGW-2, HGW-3 and HGW-5. Respective isotype controls are shown as black dashed curves in both panels.

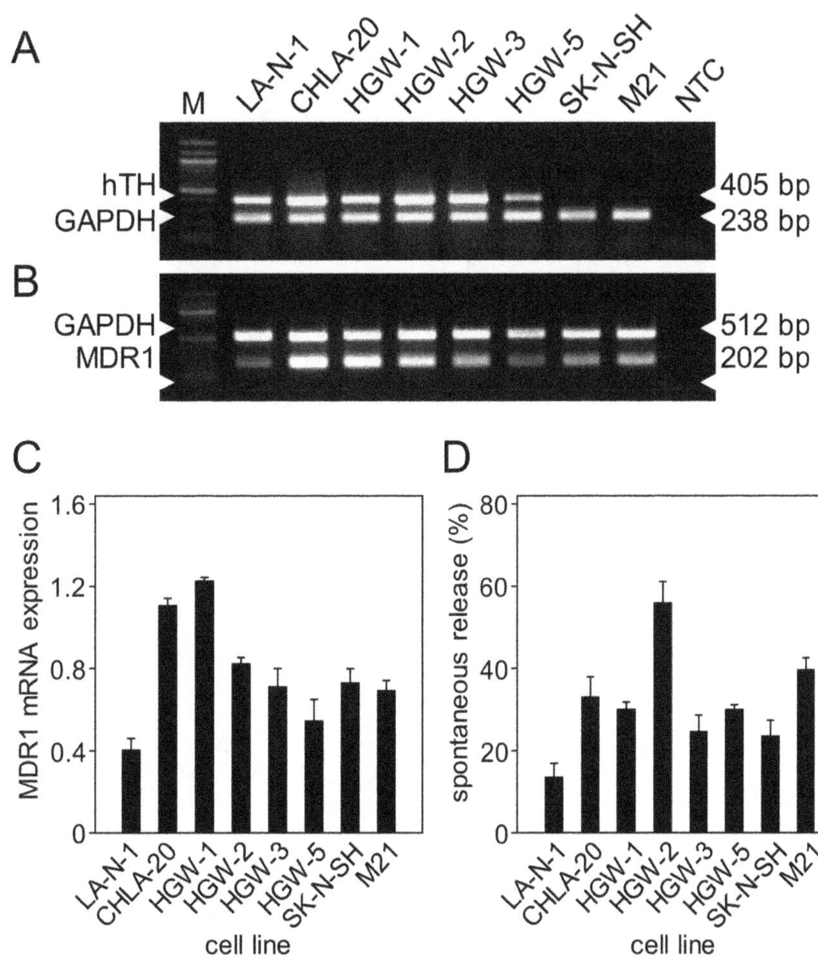

Figure 2. RT-PCR analysis of human tyrosine hydroxylase and MDR1 mRNA expression and level of spontaneous release of calcein from NB cell lines. RNA of human NB cell lines LA-N-1, CHLA-20, HGW-1, HGW-2, HGW-3 and HGW-5 was used for RT-PCR analysis of hTH (**A**) and MDR1 (**B**) gene expression (PCR-product sizes 405 bp and 202 bp, respectively). Expression of GAPDH mRNA served as internal control. (**C**) Densitometric analysis of MDR1 mRNA expression relative to GAPDH. Values are given as means ± SE of three independent experiments. HTH-negative NB cell line SK-N-SH and melanoma cell line M21 served as negative controls for hTH mRNA RT-PCR analysis. NTC, no template control. (**D**) Levels of spontaneous release of calcein from NB cells examined after 4 h incubation of calcein-labeled cells with 12.5% heat inactivated serum.

NB target cells labeled with membrane-permeable fluorescent dye calcein-AM were incubated with effector cells and serum of treated patients. For CDC, patient serum was incubated with calcein-AM-labeled target cells without effector cells.

Since high spontaneous release of calcein from labeled target cells is an obstacle for calculation of CDC, the level of spontaneous release was analyzed in a panel of GD_2-positive NB cell lines (LA-N-1, CHLA-20, HGW-1, HGW-2, HGW-3 and HGW-5) and GD_2-positive melanoma cell line M21. GD_2-negative NB cell line SK-N-SH served as a negative control. 0.6×10^6 cells were harvested, counted and washed twice with 10 ml 1x PBS (5 min, 300×g, RT). Cell pellet was then resuspended in 1 ml of respective culture medium and incubated with 10 µM calcein-AM (Sigma Aldrich, Steinheim, Germany) for 30 min at 37°C shaking at 100x rpm under CO_2-free atmosphere (dark). After two wash steps in serum-free medium, supernatants were collected for background calculation. For spontaneous release determination, 5×10^3 of calcein-AM labeled target cells were added to each well of a 96-well plate (PAA, Pasching, Austria) and incubated with 12.5% heat-inactivated serum of a healthy donor (30 min, 56°C) for 4 h at 37°C, in the dark. To achieve final volume of 200 µl/well, serum-free cell culture medium (RPMI) was added. For maximum release, target cells were disrupted using ultrasonic homogenizer (30 s, RT). Then, supernatants (50 µl) of each well were transferred to a black 96-well plate for determination of fluorescence at 495 nm excitation and 515 nm emission wavelengths by Synergy HT multimode microplate reader (BioTek Germany, Bad Friedrichshall, Germany). Experiments were analyzed in triplicates using six replicate wells for spontaneous release (target cells only). Spontaneous release in percent was calculated according to the formula: (spontaneous release - background)/(maximum release - background)×100%.

Assay conditions for complement-dependent cytotoxicity. In order to determine an optimal dilution factor, serum of a healthy donor was serially diluted to investigate the impact of different serum concentrations on CDC activity. Nine serum concentrations were analyzed: 100%, 50%, 25%, 12.5%, 6.2%, 3.1%, 1.6%, 0.8% and 0.4%. 0.6×10^6 LA-N-1 cells were labeled with calcein-AM as previously described followed by incubation for 4 h (+37°C, dark) with two defined concentrations of anti-GD_2 mAb ch14.18/CHO (1.0 and 0.1 µg/ml) prepared using serum of a healthy donor. Additionally, to prove CDC

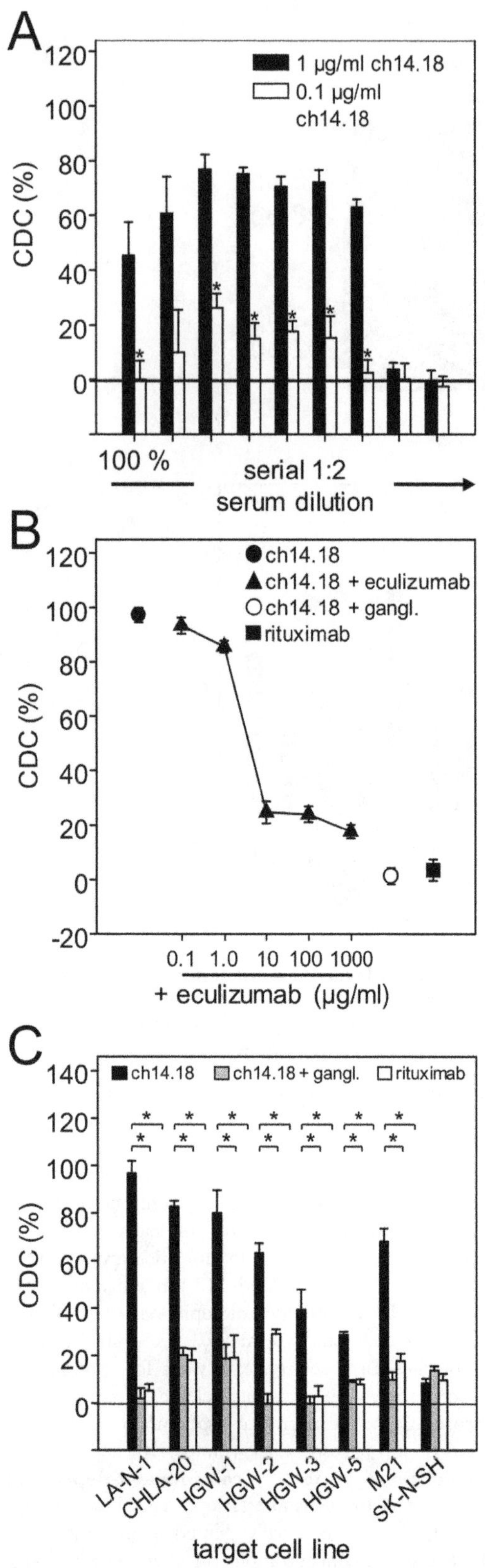

Figure 3. Assessment of variables for the complement-dependent cytotoxicity bioassay. (**A**) Analysis of CDC mediated by different serum concentrations (100%, 50%, 25%, 12.5%, 6.3%, 3.1%, 1.6%, 0.8%, 0.4%) using NB cell line LA-N-1 as a target cell line and two defined concentrations of anti-GD_2 Ab ch14.18/CHO (1.0 µg/ml (black column) and 0.1 µg/ml (white column). (**B**) Concentration-dependent inhibition of CDC mediated by 1.0 µg/ml ch14.18/CHO (closed circle) by complement inhibitor eculizumab (closed triangles). Pre-incubation with excess of anti-Id Ab ganglidiomab (5.0 µg/ml; open circle) was performed to show GD_2-specific target cell lysis. Rituximab (1.0 µg/ml; closed square) served as a negative control. (**C**) Evaluation of CDC mediated by different NB cell lines, 12.5% serum and anti-GD_2 Ab ch14.18/CHO (1 µg/ml; black column). Ganglidiomab (5.0 µg/ml; grey columns) and rituximab (1.0 µg/ml; white columns) served as controls. Data are shown as mean values ± SE of three independent experiments performed at least in triplicates. *t*-test; $^*P < 0.05$.

specificity of the target cell lysis, a humanized mAb eculizumab (trade name Soliris; Alexion Europe SAS, Paris, France) selectively inhibiting the cleavage of complement protein C5 to C5a and C5b by the C5 convertase was used. GD_2-specific CDC of NB cells LA-N-1 was induced by 1.0 µg/ml ch14.18 prepared in serum of a healthy donor (12.5% end concentration). To inhibit ch14.18-mediated CDC, samples were pre-incubated with 1:10 serial dilutions of 1.0 mg/ml eculizumab prepared in 1x PBS (final concentration: 1000, 100, 10, 1, 0.1 and 0.01 µg/ml). Samples pre-incubated with excess of GD_2-mimicking anti-idiotype (anti-Id) Ab ganglidiomab (5.0 µg/ml) were included to show GD_2-specific target cell lysis. MAb rituximab (1.0 µg/ml) was used as a negative control. CDC was calculated according to the formula: (test release - spontaneous release)/(maximum release - spontaneous release)×100%.

To establish a suitable target cell line for calcein-AM-based cytotoxicity assay, selected GD_2-positive NB cell lines LA-N-1, CHLA-20, HGW-1, HGW-2, HGW-3 and HGW-5 as well as a GD_2-positive melanoma cell line M21 were used. GD_2-negative NB cell line SK-N-SH served as a negative control. CDC was performed using 12.5% diluted serum of a healthy donor and 1.0 µg/ml ch14.18/CHO. Rituximab served as a negative control. Additionally, samples pre-incubated with excess ganglidiomab (5.0 µg/ml) were included to show GD_2-specific target cell lysis. 0.5×10^3 calcein-labeled cells/well of each target cell line were used and CDC was evaluated as described above.

To show inter-individual variations in CDC activity, serum samples collected from four healthy donors (D1, D2, D3 and D4) were used. CDC was performed using NB cell line LA-N-1 as a target cell line, 1:8 diluted donor-specific serum (12.5% final concentration) and 1:10 serial dilutions of 1.0 µg/ml ch14.18/CHO (1,000, 100, 10, 1.0, 0.1 and 0.01 ng/ml).

To analyze CDC-mediated by different anti-GD_2 mAb (murine 14G2a, chimeric human/murine ch14.18/CHO and IL-2 conjugated humanized hu14.18-IL-2) were used. Serial 1:2 dilutions of each Ab (final concentration of 1.0, 0.5, 0.25, 0.12, 0.06 and 0.03 µg/ml) were added to calcein-labeled LA-N-1 target cells and incubated with 12.5% serum of a healthy donor for 4 h at 37°C, in the dark. Two anti-GD_2 Ab lacking binding sites for complement proteins (ch14.18-delta-CH2 and hu14.18 containing mutated Fc part) as well as anti-CD20 mAb rituximab served as negative controls. Moreover, to show GD_2-dependent specificity of CDC, additional controls containing respective anti-GD_2 Ab were pre-incubated with excess of GD_2-mimicking anti-Id Ab ganglidiomab (5.0 µg/ml). CDC was evaluated as previously described.

Antibody-dependent cell-mediated cytotoxicity. A systematic analysis of the source of the effector cells and the effector to target (E:T) cell ratio was performed using 10 µg/ml of anti-GD_2 Ab ch14.18/CHO and LA-N-1 NB cell line as described above. Three effector cell populations (leukocytes, PBMCs and granulocytes) of a healthy donor (D1) were analyzed at different E:T ratios (80:1, 40:1 20:1, 10:1, 5:1, 2.5:1 and 1.25:1). Additionally, ADCC-mediated by activated effector cells was analyzed. Therefore, effector cells were cultivated for 64 h in

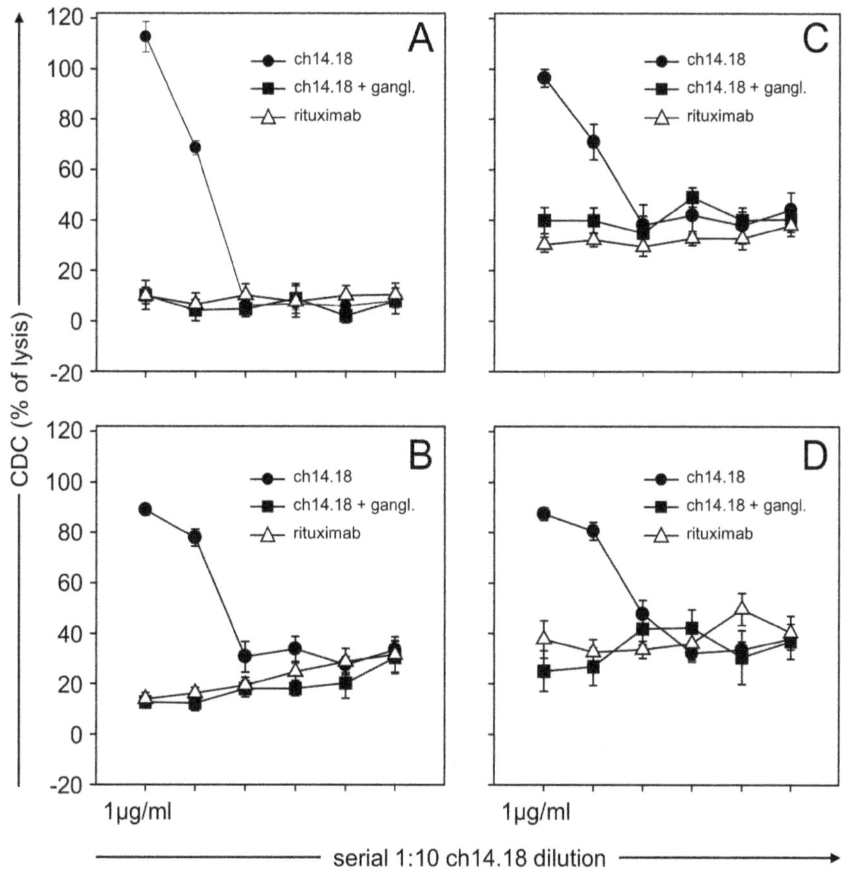

Figure 4. Evaluation of donor-specific CDC. Serum samples (12.5% final concentration) of four healthy donors D1 (**A**), D2 (**B**), D3 (**C**) and D4 (**D**) were analyzed using calcein-AM-based cytotoxicity assay as described in section "Materials and Methods". Serial dilutions of 1.0 µg/ml ch14.18/CHO were used for CDC (closed circles). Rituximab served as a negative control (1 µg/ml; open triangles). To show GD_2-specific target cell lysis, samples were pre-incubated with excess of GD_2-mimicking anti-Id Ab ganglidiomab (5 µg/ml; closed squares). Data are shown as mean values ± SE of three independent experiments performed at least in triplicates.

RPMI culture medium supplemented with IL-2 (1000 IE/ml; Novartis, Nürnberg, Germany), 4.5 g/l glucose, 2 mM stable glutamine, 10% FCS and 1x P/S. After pre-incubation of labeled target cells (5×10^3/well) with ch14.18/CHO for 30 min at +37°C (dark), effector cells were added for further 4 h (+37°C, dark). Rituximab served as a negative control. GD_2-specific ADCC of NB cells was demonstrated by pre-incubation of ch14.18/CHO with excess of anti-Id Ab ganglidiomab (50 µg/ml). To achieve a final volume of 200 µl/well, LA-N-1 cell culture medium was used. Finally, fluorescence levels of supernatants (50 µl) were measured as described above. Experiments were analyzed in triplicates using six replicate wells for spontaneous (target cells only) and three replicates for maximum release. ADCC was calculated according to the formula: (test release - spontaneous release)/(maximum release - spontaneous release)×100%.

To investigate the sensitivity, a concentration range of ch14.18/CHO mAb inducing measurable ADCC, serial Ab dilutions were prepared (10,000, 1,000, 100, 10, 1, 0.1 and 0.01 ng/ml). ADCC evaluation was performed using LA-N-1 as a target cell line and activated leukocytes of a healthy donor (D1) as effector cells at E:T ratio of 40:1 as described above. Rituximab and ganglidiomab containing controls were included as described above.

Assay validation and run acceptance analysis. To show reproducibility, accuracy and precision of the established cytotoxicity assay, both within-assay and inter-assay precision analysis were determined according to international guidelines for bioanalytical method validation [18]. For both data validation and run acceptance analysis, we included in each analytical run a quality control containing a known concentration of ch14.18/CHO mAb (1.0 µg/ml) prepared in serum of a healthy donor (D1).

Within-assay precision was determined with ten triplicated samples containing 1.0 µg/ml ch14.18/CHO in serum of a healthy donor. The within-assay precision value was calculated as follows: (standard deviation (SD) of replicates divided by mean of replicates)×100%. To confirm consistency of measurements over time, the inter-assay precision was calculated. For this, ten triplicated samples containing a defined concentration of ch14.18/CHO (1.0 µg/ml) prepared in serum of a healthy donor were analyzed by different operators on different days. The inter-assay precision was calculated according to the formula: (SD of replicates divided by mean of replicates)×100%.

For validation of cytotoxicity analysis, we developed a set of tailored QCs containing defined concentrations of ch14.18/CHO (1.0 µg/ml) prepared in serum of a healthy donor. For each serum batch the level of cytotoxicity was first determined in at least six independent measurements by different operators on different days. Then, we calculated the CV for these assays and plotted the results over time. Only the serum batch spiked with ch14.18/

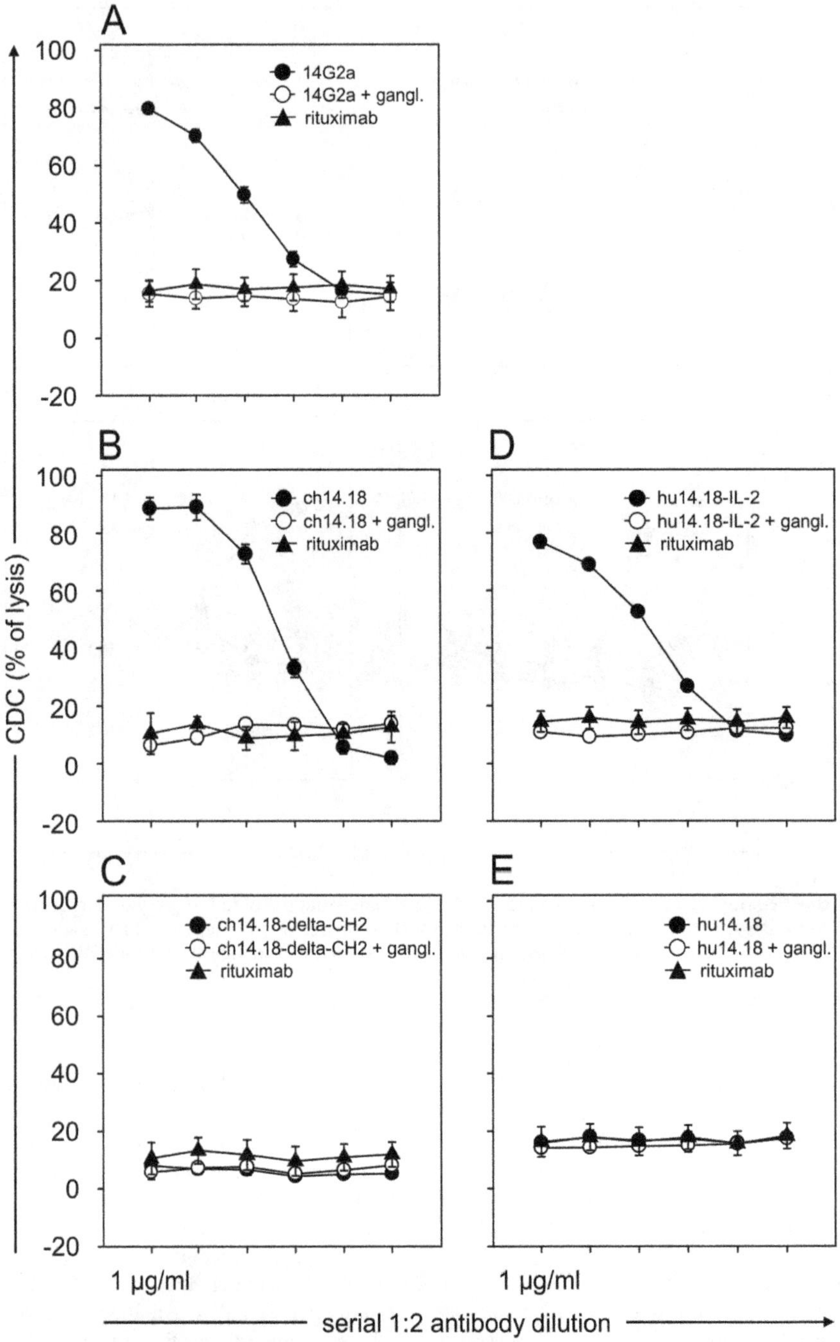

Figure 5. Evaluation of CDC-mediated by different anti-GD_2 Ab. Serial dilutions (final concentration of 1.0, 0.5, 0.25, 0.12, 0.06 and 0.03 µg/ml) of murine 14G2a (**A**, closed circles), chimeric human/murine ch14.18/CHO (**B**, closed circles), and IL-2 conjugated humanized hu14.18-IL-2 (**D**, closed circles) were used for CDC. Complement fixation deficient mutants chimeric ch14.18-delta-CH2 (**C**, closed circles) and humanized hu14.18 (**E**, closed circles) as well as rituximab (closed triangles) served as negative controls. To show GD_2-dependent specificity of CDC induced, additional controls containing respective anti-GD_2 Ab were pre-incubated with excess of GD_2-mimicking anti-Id Ab ganglidiomab (5 µg/ml; open circles). Data are shown as mean values ± SE of three independent experiments performed at least in triplicates.

CHO showing CV under 20% was used as QC and included in each analytical run for run acceptance analysis.

To accept or reject analytical runs, QCs were included in each run. Deviation of the QC results from their nominal value was calculated as absolute value (modulus) using the formula: | 100% - (MEAN/nominal value)×100% |, according to international guidelines for bioanalytical method validation [18]. If the differences between the QC and its respective nominal values exceeded 20%, the run was rejected and the data were not included in the data analysis. Only runs including QC deviating from the nominal within 20% were accepted.

Evaluation of CDC and ADCC in neuroblastoma patients. The established cytotoxicity assay was applied to serum and sodium-heparin blood samples collected from three

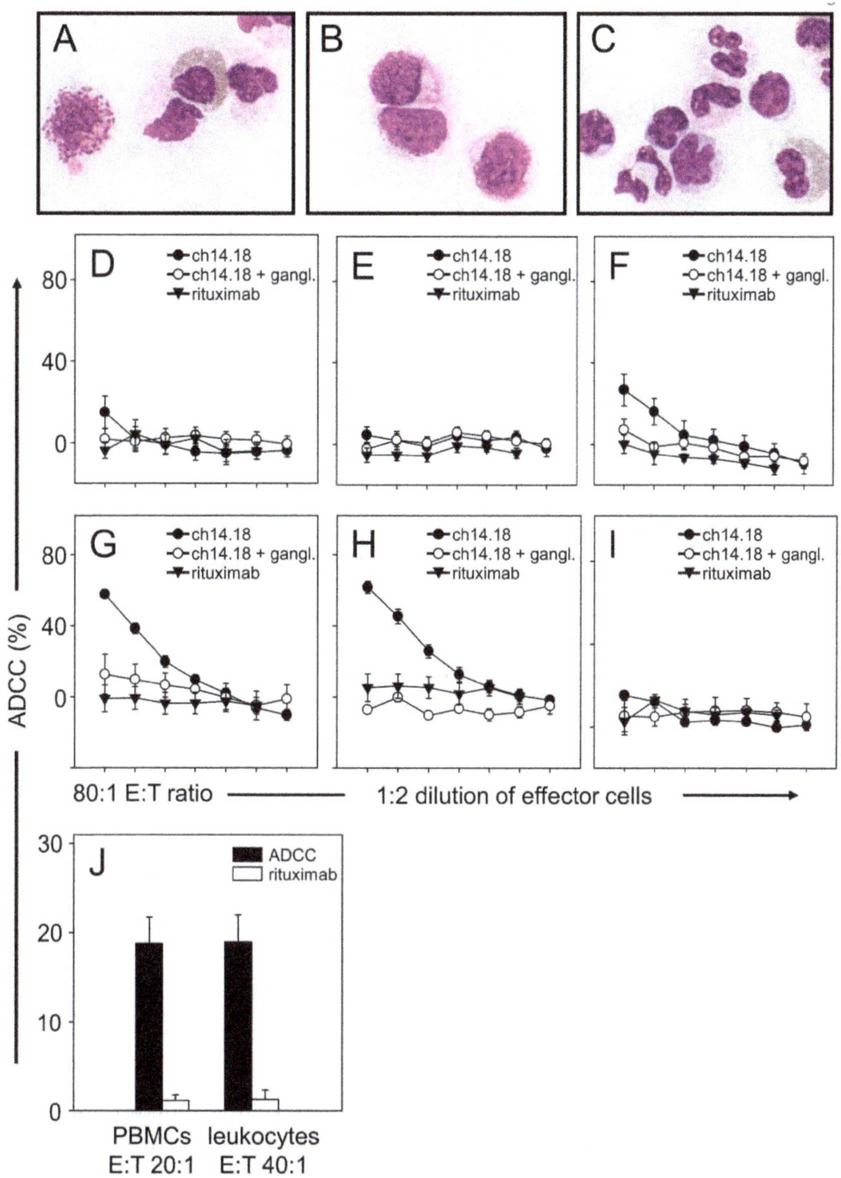

Figure 6. Evaluation of ADCC-mediated by different effector cell subsets. Three populations of freshly isolated effector cells of a healthy donor were compared for ADCC: leukocytes (**A**), PBMCs (**B**) and granulocyte rich fraction (**C**). ADCC were performed using calcein-AM-based cytotoxicity assay as described in Materials and Methods. Effector cells were incubated with 10 µg/ml ch14.18/CHO (closed circles) and calcein-labeled target cells LA-N-1 at different E:T ratios (80:1, 40:1, 20:1, 10:1, 5:1, 2.5:1 and 1.25:1) and ADCC mediated by leukocytes (**D**), PBMCs (**E**) and effector cells of granulocytes rich fraction (**F**) were examined. In order to simulate the use of IL-2 in combination with ch14.18/CHO in clinical trials, effector cells were incubated for 64 h in cell culture medium supplemented with 1,000 IU/ml IL-2. ADCC mediated by IL-2 treated leukocytes (**G**), IL-2 treated PBMCs (**H**) and IL-2 treated cells of granulocyte rich fraction (**I**) were calculated as described in Materials and Method. Rituximab served as a negative control (closed triangles). GD_2-specific ADCC of NB cells was demonstrated by pre-incubation of ch14.18/CHO with excess of anti-Id Ab ganglidiomab (open circles). Data are shown as mean values ± SE of three independent experiments performed at least in triplicates. (**J**) Comparison of ADCC mediated by leukocytes at E:T ratio of 40:1 and PBMCs at E:T ratio 20:1 isolated from the same blood sample of five selected NB patients treated with a combination of IL-2 and ch14.18/CHO (black columns). Rituximab served as a negative control (white columns).

selected NB patients (patient 1, patient 2, patient 3) treated in a European anti-GD_2 immunotherapy study with ch14.18/CHO in combination with IL-2. Patients received 6×10^6 IU/m^2 s.c. IL-2 (day 1–5; 8–12) and ten day long-term infusion (LTI) of 100 mg/m^2 ch14.18/CHO (day 8–17). CDC and ADCC were determined at two time points: prior to start of treatment (day 1) and on day 15 as described above.

Stability of CDC and effector cell viability. To evaluate the impact of shipping condition on CDC, viability and cell count of effector cells, we analyzed both serum and whole blood samples of a healthy donor (D1) stored under different conditions or subjected to five freeze-thaw cycles. The serum samples were prepared as described above. For evaluation of repeated freezing and thawing or storing at RT (up to 96 h), serum samples aliquots containing two defined ch14.18/CHO concentrations (1 and 0.1 µg/ml) were used. For evaluation of leukocyte viability and cell count, whole blood samples were collected in either BD Vacutainer plastic K2EDTA- (BD Biosciences, Heidelberg,

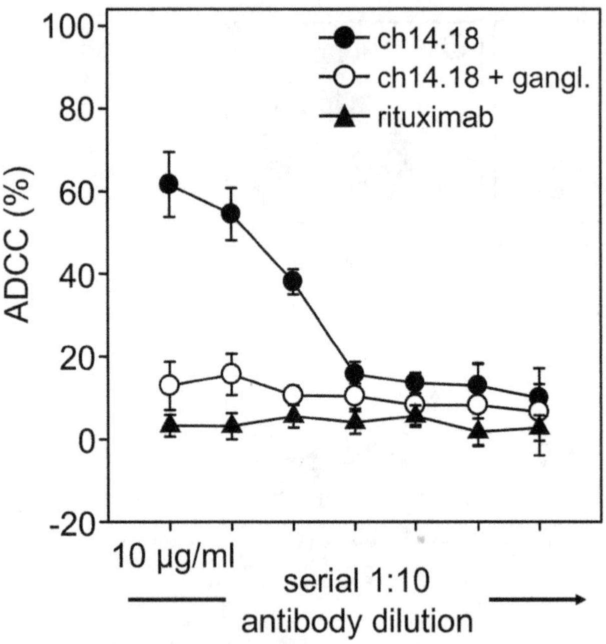

Figure 7. Determination of ADCC sensitivity. Different concentrations of anti-GD_2 mAb ch14.18/CHO (10,000, 1,000, 100, 10, 1, 0.1 and 0.01 ng/ml, closed circles) were used to investigate a concentration range of Ab inducing a detectable ADCC. Activated leukocytes of a healthy donor were incubated with calcein-labeled LA-N-1 cells at E:T ratio of 40:1. Rituximab (closed triangles) and anti-Id Ab ganglidiomab (open circles) containing controls were included as described in Materials and Methods. Data are shown as mean values ± SE of three Independent experiments performed at least in triplicates.

Germany) or BD Vacutainer plastic sodium-heparin-containing tubes (BD Biosciences, Heidelberg, Germany) and stored at RT for up to 72 h. CDC was evaluated using the established cytotoxicity assay. Rituximab containing samples and Ab-free sera were used as negative controls. Viability of leukocytes was evaluated using trypan blue test and a cell count with automated cell counter (EMD Millipore Corporation, Billerica, MA, USA).

Statistics. After testing for normality and equal variance across groups, differences between groups were assessed with the Students *t*-test. A P level of < 0.05 was considered significant. All data are given as means ± SD or means ± SEM. Analysis was performed using the software SigmaStat (Jandel, San Rafael, CA).

Results

Target cell line selection to establish CDC and ADCC bioassays

The selection of a suitable target cell line to set up immune bioassays for the monitoring of clinical trials was done with a panel of seven NB cell lines. The panel consisted of three cell lines propagated for many years (LA-N-1, CHLA-20, and SK-N-SH) and of four lines newly established from patients with relapsed NB. This was accomplished by isolation of GD_2-positive cells from primary tumor tissue or bone marrow by MACS and culture in IMDM-based medium as described in Materials and Methods. Newly established cell lines were named HGW-1 (bone marrow originated), HGW-2 (primary tumor originated), HGW-3 (primary tumor originated) and HGW-5 (bone marrow originated). HGW-1,2 and 5 cell lines were MYCN amplified and positive for 17 q gain (Table 1). HGW-3 and HGW-5 cells also showed the typical deletion of chromosome 1p. HGW-1 showed gain of 11q in contrast to the other lines (Table 1). Analysis of HGW-2 is pending. Finally, cell line DNA profiles determined with STR analysis clearly showed the *de novo* nature of each cell line.

Further characterization of these new HGW cell lines were done in comparison to NB cell lines LA-N-1, CHLA-20 and SK-N-SH as well as a melanoma cell line M21.

Since GD_2 is the target antigen of ch14.18, its expression on the target cell line is crucial to set up CDC and ADCC bioassays. The GD_2 expression analysis was complemented with CD56 since both surface molecules are typical features of NB cells.

NB origin of newly established cell lines HGW-1, HGW-2, HGW-3 and HGW-5 was confirmed by detection ob both CD56 and GD_2 NB expression markers (Fig. 1B). All *de novo* cell lines showed homogeneous expression of CD56 and heterogeneous expression of GD_2 (Fig. 1B). To compare GD_2 expression profiles, MFI ratios were used. The highest MFI ratio was found on HGW-1 (63.4). HGW-2 and -3 displayed MFI ratios of 46.9 and 22.9, respectively. The lowest MFI ratio was calculated for HGW-5 (5.0). Interestingly, GD_2 expression analysis of HGW-5 revealed two distinct subpopulations. About 84% of cells had a GD_2^{dim} phenotype (MFI ratio 3.0) and the smaller subpopulation of about 16% had a GD_2^{bright} expression pattern (MFI ratio 80.5; Fig. 1B). In contrast, HGW-3 cell line which consists of two morphologically distinctive cell populations (adherent and suspension cells) did not show differences in GD_2 expression profiles.

The NB cell lines LA-N-1 and CHLA-20 used as controls revealed high expression of both NB marker GD_2 and CD56 (Fig. 1A). In contrast, SK-N-SH showed high expression of CD56 but lacked expression of GD_2 (Fig. 1A), therefore, SK-N-SH was excluded from consideration as a target cell line for the bioassays. As expected, a melanoma cell line M21 did not show CD56 expression but a high expression of GD_2 (Fig. 1A).

In order to further characterize the newly established HGW cell lines, we also investigated expression of hTH, the first step enzyme of catecholamine biosynthesis, which is a typical feature of NB cells. Expression of hTH mRNA was found in all newly established NB cell lines HGW-1, HGW-2, HGW-3 and HGW-5 as well as in NB cell lines LA-N-1 and CHLA-20 (Fig. 2A) in contrast to the melanoma cell line M21 used as a negative control. The NB cell line SK-N-SH was surprisingly hTH negative further supporting the decision to exclude this cell line from further consideration.

The analysis of MDR1 gene expression was used as further selection criterion since calcein is an MDR1 substrate. Therefore, high MDR1 expression results in active transport of calcein into the extracellular space which accounts for a high background in calcein release assays [19]. The weakest mRNA expression of MDR1 was found in LA-N-1. (Fig. 2B–C). CHLA-20 and HGW-1 showed about three-fold and SK-N-SH, M21, HGW-2 and -3 about two-fold higher levels of MDR1 mRNA expression compared to LA-N-1 (Fig. 2B–C). These findings correlate with spontaneous release data for cell lines analyzed revealing the lowest level of spontaneous release in LA-N-1 cells (Fig. 2D).

Assessment of variables for the complement-dependent cytotoxicity bioassay

The optimal serum dilution used for the CDC bioassay with patient samples was evaluated by using a serial 1:2.dilution (undiluted, 1:2, 1:4, 1:8, 1:16, 1:32, 1:64, 1:128, 1:256) of serum of a healthy donor in the presence and absence of two distinct concentrations of anti-GD_2 Ab ch14.18/CHO, i.e. 1.0 and 0.1 µg/ml, respectively. Interestingly, we found a bell-shaped curve of ch14.18-mediated CDC activity with decreasing serum concentrations at both ch14.18 concentration levels (Fig. 3A).

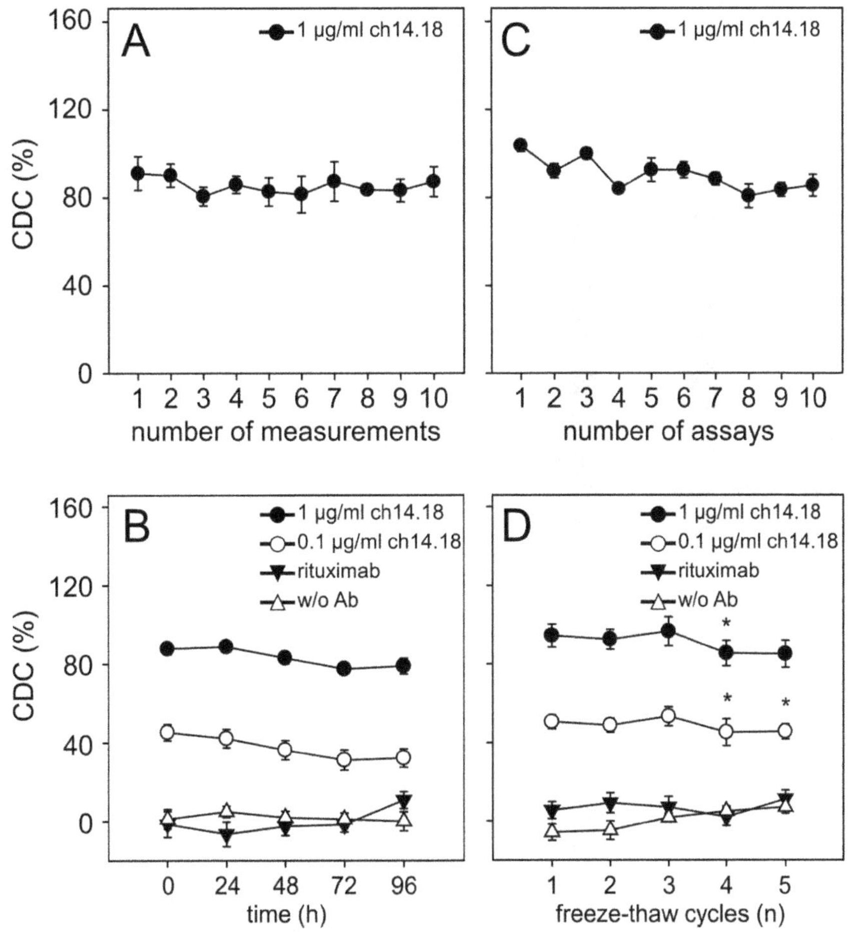

Figure 8. Within-assay precision, inter-assay precision and sample stability. For reliable and reproducible evaluation of cytotoxicity, within-assay and inter-assay precision analyses were performed (**A** and **C**). Both parameters were calculated according to the formula: SD/mean×100% and found to be under 20%. To determine within-assay precision (**A**), triplicated serum samples of a healthy donor (12.5% final concentration) with defined ch14.18/CHO concentrations (1.0 µg/ml) and calcein-labeled LA-N-1 target cells were analyzed. The cytotoxicity analysis was repeated ten times on the same plate. Results are presented as mean CDC of triplicates ± SD for ten data sets. Inter-assay precision (**C**) was determined on different days by different operators. Ten independent measurements of serum samples containing 1.0 µg/ml ch14.18/CHO and calcein-labeled LA-N-1 target cells were performed. The analyzed cytotoxicity levels are given as mean values ± SD for ten independent assays. To determine stability of CDC (**B** and **D**), two ch14.18/CHO concentrations 1.0 µg/ml (closed circles) and 0.1 µg/ml (open circles) prepared in 12.5% serum of a healthy donor were analyzed with established cytotoxicity assay. Samples were subjected to either storage at room temperature for up to 96 h (**B**) or to five freeze-thaw cycles (**D**). Rituximab containing (closed triangles) and Ab-free controls (open triangles) were included as described in Materials and Methods. Data are shown as mean CDC values ± SE of two independent experiments performed at least in triplicates.

Table 2. Effect of anticoagulants on leukocyte count and viability.

Leukocyte viability (%)				
storing time (h)	0	24	48	72
EDTA-blood	98.5±0.5	88.5±3.5	80.0±6.0	80. 0±6.0
Na-heparin-blood	99.0±0.0	96.5±2.5	95.5±2.5	91.0±5.0
Leukocyte count (1×10^9 cells/l)				
storing time (h)	0	24	48	72
EDTA-blood	2.00±0.00	1.00±0.22	0.71±0.29	0.53±0.21
Na-heparin-blood	2.00±0.00	1.84±0.08	1.68±0.43	1.33±0.53

Leukocytes were isolated from sodium-heparin- and EDTA whole blood samples followed by analysis of cell viability and count. Values are represented as mean ± SE of two independent experiments.

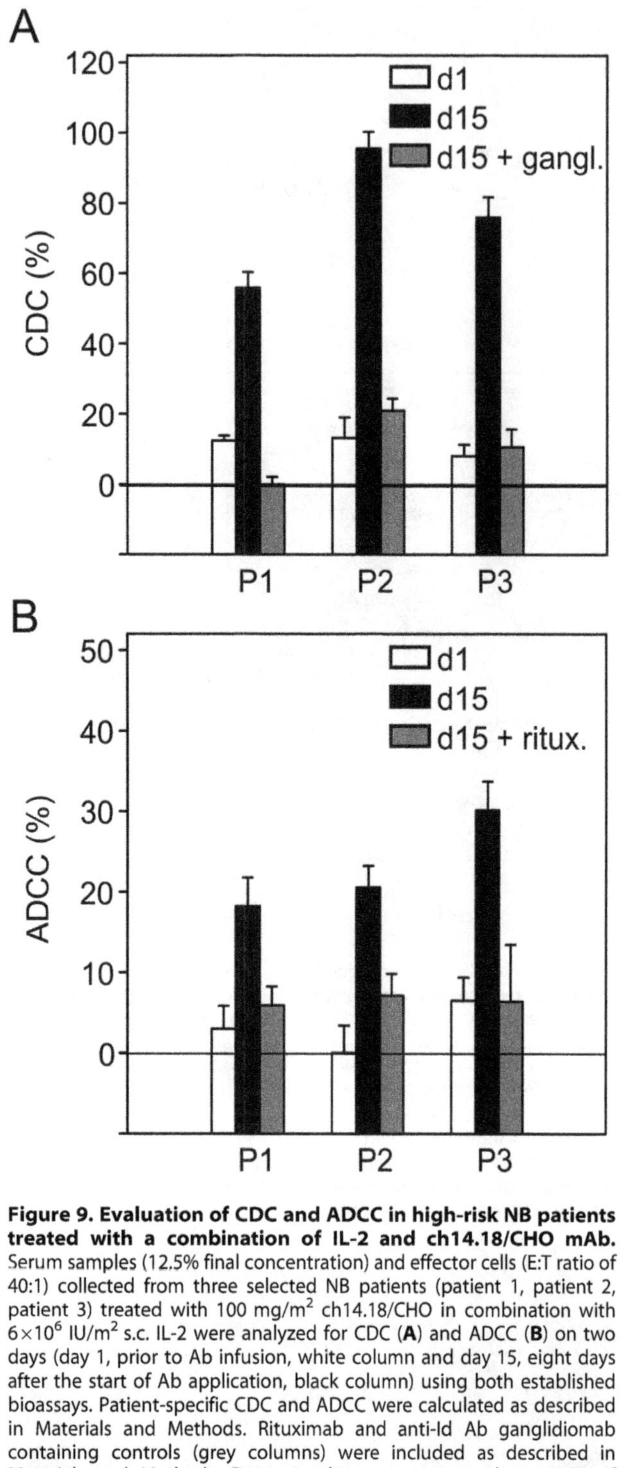

Figure 9. Evaluation of CDC and ADCC in high-risk NB patients treated with a combination of IL-2 and ch14.18/CHO mAb. Serum samples (12.5% final concentration) and effector cells (E:T ratio of 40:1) collected from three selected NB patients (patient 1, patient 2, patient 3) treated with 100 mg/m^2 ch14.18/CHO in combination with 6×10^6 IU/m^2 s.c. IL-2 were analyzed for CDC (**A**) and ADCC (**B**) on two days (day 1, prior to Ab infusion, white column and day 15, eight days after the start of Ab application, black column) using both established bioassays. Patient-specific CDC and ADCC were calculated as described in Materials and Methods. Rituximab and anti-Id Ab ganglidiomab containing controls (grey columns) were included as described in Materials and Methods. Data are shown as mean values ± SE of independent experiments performed at least in triplicates. *t*-test; *$P<0.05$.

CDC-mediated by 1.0 µg/ml ch14.18/CHO (Fig. 3A, black columns) revealed a maximum of about 80% target cell lysis in a serum dilution range from 1:4 to 1:64. In contrast, addition of undiluted or 1:2, 1:128 and 1:256 diluted serum resulted in lower CDC activity levels (45%, 65%, 4% and 4%, respectively). A similar pattern was observed with 0.1 µg/ml ch14.18/CHO. At this antibody concentration, CDC-mediated a maximum of about 30% target cell lysis at serum dilution of 1:4, 1:8, 1:16 and 1:32 (Fig. 3A, white columns). Again, the undiluted as well as 1:128 and 1:256 diluted sera (final concentrations: 3.1% and 1.6%, respectively) could not induce measurable CDC-mediated target cell lysis, and CDC-mediated by 1:2 diluted serum was found to be only at 14%.

In summary, the highest CDC-mediated target cell lysis was observed by both concentrations of ch14.18/CHO (1.0 and 0.1 µg/ml) to be between 1:4 and 1:32. Based on these data we defined the serum dilution at 1:8 as the standard procedure to evaluate CDC in treated patients.

To further confirm that the cytotoxic activity observed in these experiments is mediated by the complement system, we added the complement inhibitor eculizumab (trade name Soliris) to our system (Fig. 3B, closed triangles). Ch14.18 (1.0 µg/ml) prepared in serum of a healthy donor (D1) (12.5% final concentration) induced a LA-N-1 target cell lysis of 100%. Co-incubation with a serial dilution of 1.0 mg/ml eculizumab inhibited the cytotoxic activity in a concentration-dependent manner resulting in almost complete abrogation of ch14.18-mediated target cell lysis (Fig. 3B, closed triangles). These findings prove the complement-mediated cytotoxic effect. GD_2 specificity was also demonstrated by pre-incubation of ch14.18 with excess of anti-Id Ab ganglidiomab (Fig. 3B, open circle) or by replacing ch14.18 with similar concentration of mAb rituximab used as a negative control (Fig. 3B, closed square).

In order to make a final decision on the target NB cell line to be used for the bioassays, we analyzed CDC against our panel of cell lines with 12.5% serum (1:8 dilution) as a source of complement and 1.0 µg/ml ch14.18/CHO (Fig. 3C). The highest level of ch14.18/CHO-mediated CDC was observed using LA-N-1 (97%) NB cells compared to all other cell lines analyzed in particular HGW-5. These differences in GD_2-specific lysis correlate with GD_2 expression profiles of NB cell lines analyzed with flow cytometry (Fig. 1B). GD_2 negative SK-N-SH cells were used as a negative control. Importantly, pre-incubation with excess of anti-Id ganglidiomab resulted in complete abrogation of CDC in that cell line. Interestingly, for some cell lines, we found antibody-independent target cell lysis in samples incubated with 1.0 µg/ml non-specific rituximab or excess of anti-Id ganglidiomab (CHLA-20, HGW-1, HGW-5 and M21), indicating the activation of Ab-independent alternative complement activation pathways. In summary, LA-N-1 showed the highest sensitivity and specificity for GD_2-specific CDC-mediated by ch14.18/CHO which was therefore selected as the designated cell line to establish the bioassays.

The impact of the source of complement on ch14.18/CHO-mediated CDC against LA-N-1 NB target cells was analyzed using sera of four healthy donors (D1–4) (Fig. 4) and compared to that of rituximab used as a negative control. The cytotoxic activity mediated by 1.0 µg/ml ch14.18/CHO did not reveal significant inter-individual variations with a maximum activity between 90–100%. GD_2 specificity was demonstrated by a complete inhibition of CDC-mediated cytotoxicity to the level of the negative control (rituximab) after pre-incubation of serum samples with 5.0 µg/ml anti-Id Ab ganglidiomab. Interestingly, different inter-individual levels of ch14.18/CHO-independent anti-tumor cytotoxicity could be observed in serum samples of the selected donors in a range of 10% to 40%, indicating the presence of natural CDC activity against LA-N-1 as a result of complement activation mediated by the non-classical pathway [20]. Ch14.18/CHO concentrations below 10 ng/ml did not mediate detectable CDC in all donor sera analyzed. Based on these data we used for further experiments serum of a donor D1 lacking Ab-independent cytotoxicity (Fig. 4A).

CDC-mediated by different anti-GD_2 mAb constructs including 14G2a, ch14.18/CHO, hu14.18-IL-2 was compared to complement fixation deficient mutants hu14.18 K322 [21] and ch14.18-delta-CH2 against LA-N-1 NB target cells using serum of a healthy donor D1 described above (Fig. 5). The level of a concentration-dependent CDC activity observed was highest with ch14.18/CHO followed by 14G2a and hu14.18-IL2 (Fig. 1B and D) compared to rituximab negative controls. The activity was GD_2-specific since pre-incubation of samples with 5.0 µg/ml anti-Id ganglidiomab completely inhibited target cell lysis (Fig. 5). As expected, no detectable CDC could be observed with anti-GD_2 antibody constructs which lack complement binding sites (ch14.18-delta-CH2 and hu14.18 K322) (Fig. 5C and E). In summary, the CDC assay revealed consistent GD_2-specific results related to the presence and absence of a complement fixation moiety within the anti-GD_2 construct, with the highest level for ch14.18/CHO.

Antibody-dependent cell-mediated cytotoxicity bioassay

The analysis of ADCC was also performed using LA-N-1 NB target cells labeled with calcein as described in Materials and Methods. Assay conditions related to effector cell preparation and determination of an optimal effector-to-target cell ratio were done with blood samples of a healthy donor D1 in the presence of 10 µg/ml ch14.18/CHO compared to rituximab and to samples incubated with ch14.18/CHO and anti-Id used as negative controls (Fig. 6A–I) as well as patients treated with ch14.18/CHO (Fig. 6J), respectively.

For the analysis of ch14.18/CHO-mediated ADCC, three distinct sources of effector cells were systematically evaluated. The first source consisted of a leukocyte preparation following red blood cell lysis of anti-coagulated blood (Fig. 6C). The second and third source was prepared from blood samples centrifuged in a blood separation media as described in Materials and Methods. Lymphocyte rich PBMCs were collected from the fluffy white layer (Fig. 6B) and a granulocyte rich cell fraction was collected from the lowest layer followed by lysis of erythrocytes as described above (Fig. 6A). Additionally, amounts of lymphocytes, granulocytes and monocytes were determined in both PBMC and granulocyte cell fractions showing about 80% lymphocytes, 10% granulocytes and 10% monocytes and 25% lymphocytes, 72% granulocytes and 3% monocytes in PBMC and granulocyte rich fraction, respectively.

The initial evaluation included such effector cells prepared from a healthy donor D1 either used immediately after isolation (0 h; Fig. 6D–F) or after incubation in medium containing 1,000 IU/ml IL-2 for 64 h (Fig. 6G–I). The IL-2 incubation was done in order to simulate the use of IL-2 in combination with ch14.18/CHO in clinical trials.

Of the fresh isolated effector cell preparations used immediately after isolation, only the granulocyte rich cell fraction mediated a significant ADCC reaction at an E:T ratio of 80:1. This effect was GD_2-specific since anti-Id ganglidiomab completely inhibited ch14.18-mediated ADCC (Fig. 6F). In contrast, both freshly isolated leukocytes and lymphocyte rich PBMCs did not show significant cytotoxic activity against LA-N-1 NB target cells at any E:T ratio (Fig. 6D–E). This sharply contrasts to the response observed following IL-2 incubation (Fig. 6G–H). A strong increase of ADCC-mediated by leukocytes and lymphocyte rich PBMCs (Fig. 6G–H) but not by the granulocyte rich fraction was observed (Fig. 6I). All responses were GD_2-specific and correlated with the E:T ratio. In conclusion, leukocytes prepared by red blood cell lysis of anti-coagulated blood and the lymphocyte rich PBMC preparations revealed equivocal ADCC responses at an E:T ratio of 20:1 and 40:1.

In order to confirm these results, we isolated leukocytes and lymphocyte rich PBMC preparations from the same blood sample obtained from five NB patients treated with a combination of IL-2 and ch14.18/CHO (Fig. 6J). Again, both effector cell preparations revealed inter-exchangeable results when used at an E:T ratio of 20:1 (PBMCs) and 40:1 (leukocytes) in contrast to rituximab controls, respectively, which in conclusion are both appropriate for immune monitoring.

The sensitivity of the ADCC reaction was determined using leukocytes prepared by red blood cell lysis of anticoagulated blood of a healthy donor (D1) cultivated in medium containing 1,000 IU/ml IL-2 for 64 hours at an E:T ratio of 40:1 in the presence of varying concentrations of ch14.18/CHO (Fig. 7). A concentration-dependent ADCC was observed with a limit of detection at 10 ng/ml ch14.18/CHO. Again, the response was GD_2-specific, since pre-incubation with anti-Id ganglidiomab inhibited the cytotoxic activity to the level of background responses observed with rituximab used as a negative control.

Validation of bioassays, quality controls, run acceptance criteria and sample stability

The within-assay precision and the inter-assay variation were assessed according to international consensus recommendations for the bioanalytical method validation [18]. We defined values of CV for both within- and inter-assay variation up to 20% as acceptable. For within-assay precision, CDC of ten samples containing 1.0 µg/ml ch14.18/CHO prepared in serum of a healthy donor (D1) was performed and CDC data were used for calculation of CV (Fig. 8A). Each sample was analyzed in duplicates on the same plate. Analysis revealed a CV of 9% indicating reproducible performance of the assay. The inter-assay CV was determined in triplicates by changing the operators on ten different days. This analysis revealed a CV of 12% (Fig. 8C) clearly showing that results obtained are operator-independent and consistent over time.

To accept or reject experimental runs, QCs containing a known concentration of ch14.18/CHO (1.0 µg/ml) in serum of a healthy donor (D1) were included in each analysis. The deviation coefficients were calculated using QC results obtained after each analysis and the respective QC nominal value. The differences did not exceed 20% allowing analysis acceptance.

In order to test sample stability and subsequent use in the bioassays described after distinct storage conditions, we used healthy donor serum (D1) containing two defined concentrations of ch14.18/CHO (1.0 and 0.1 µg/ml). Neither storage at RT for up to 96 hours (Fig. 8B) nor up to three repeated freeze thaw cycles (Fig. 8D) revealed significant changes in the level of CDC-mediated by ch14.18/CHO. Next, we analyzed leukocyte count and viability in blood samples using two anticoagulants, EDTA and sodium-heparin, respectively (Table 2). In general, sodium-heparin anticoagulated whole blood revealed longer stability compared to EDTA anti-coagulated blood with acceptable quality for up to 48 h storage at RT. Blood stored at RT for 72 h negatively affected both leukocyte count and viability independent on anticoagulants. These data were confirmed by ADCC analysis using effector cells prepared from samples stored as described above.

We also evaluated the impact of storage conditions on the granulocyte rich effector cell fractions. We prepared them from blood samples after 2 and 4 hours of storing at RT and included granulocyte rich fractions freshly isolated, but cultured for 64 h as described in Materials and Methods (data not shown). We could observe a reduction in granulocyte count by only 17% and 21% at 2 and 4 hour time points, respectively. Interestingly, the cell viability of granulocytes rich fractions was 99% at both time points. The cell count of granulocytes was reduced by 60% after 64 h of culture with nearly 100% viability consistent with the known fragility of this cell population. This finding is in line with a reduction of the cytotoxic efficacy by 50% compared to fresh isolated granulocytes at the 64 h time point. Therefore, analysis of granulocyte mediated ADCC clearly requires fresh blood samples and timely processing.

In summary, sodium-heparin anti-coagulated blood and serum can be stored together at RT for up to 48 h allowing for a timely transfer of the samples from clinical study sites for central lab analysis of CDC and ADCC using the described bioassays.

Evaluation of CDC and ADCC bioassays in neuroblastoma patients

Serum samples and anti-coagulated blood (heparin) were collected from three selected NB patients (patient 1, patient 2, patient 3) treated within a Phase I/II clinical trial where patients are treated with a cumulative dose of ch14.18/CHO (100 mg/ m^2/cycle) infused over a time period of ten days (Eudra CT: 2009-018077-3). The collected samples were taken at base line before start of immunotherapy and on day 8 after start of antibody infusion. The collected serum samples were used after heat-inactivation for ADCC- and untreated for CDC-assays containing a patient-specific level of ch14.18/CHO Ab as a result from the treatment (i.e. without exogenous addition of ch14.18/CHO). The serum levels of ch14.18/CHO were determined as previously described [11] (P1: 13.30±0.08 μg/ml, P2: 15.14±0.24 μg/ml, P3: 11.39±0.24 μg/ml).

The effector cells were also used without further *ex vivo* stimulation at an E:T ratio of 40:1.

ADCC and CDC analyzed with these blood and serum samples resulted in a significant increase of CDC (Fig. 9A) and ADCC (Fig. 9B) in all treated patients. When serum samples were replaced with rituximab or pre-incubated with excess of anti-Id Ab ganglidiomab, only background cytotoxicity was observed in both bioassays. In summary, the ADCC and CDC methodology described here indicate GD_2-specific cytotoxic activity in blood and serum samples obtained from patients treated with ch14.18.

Discussion

Ab are important therapeutics for the treatment of malignant disease and many mechanisms have been proposed to explain the clinical anti-tumor activity of mAb targeting a tumor associated antigen. Some Ab act through their ability to disrupt signaling pathways involved in the maintenance of their malignant phenotype such as blockade of ligands binding to growth factor receptors (e.g.cetuximab; EGFR) [22]. However, the ability of Ab to initiate a tumor-specific immune response has been less well recognized. Several studies have established the importance of ADCC-mediated through Fc-Fcγ receptor interaction as well as CDC for the *in vivo* anti-tumor effects of mAb. This was demonstrated in mice which lack Fcγ receptor expression or which are deficient in C1q, a critical component of the complement system. In both types of mouse strains the anti-tumoral activity of anti-CD20 Ab was diminished compared to wild-type strains [23,24].

The initiation of a tumor-specific immune response is also an important mechanism of action related to passive immunotherapies based on application of anti-GD_2 mAb. This intervention emerges as an established concept for the treatment of NB, a challenging malignancy in pediatric oncology [25]. The target of this strategy is ganglioside GD_2, a glycolipid expressed on the cell surface of malignant cells of neuroectodermal origin devoid of an intracellular signaling domain. Therefore, the evaluation of tumor-specific anti-NB immune responses mediated by ADCC and CDC should capture the core components of the clinical activity observed with this class of anti-tumor Ab.

Here, we describe two rapid non-radioactive and non-toxic ADCC and CDC assays allowing for analysis of samples collected from NB patients treated with anti-GD_2 Ab ch14.18/CHO for the purpose of immune monitoring of ongoing clinical trials. Importantly, we demonstrated increased GD_2 specific CDC and ADCC in three selected high-risk NB patients treated with ch14.18/CHO indicating expected effector functions of ch14.18/ CHO in treated patients.

Among non-radioactive agents that can be used for such cytotoxicity assays, calcein-AM is one of the most prominent fluorescent dyes [26] used for labeling of target cells. Here, expression of multidrug transporter P-glycoprotein (MDR-1) is a hindering factor extruding calcein from target cells independently of CDC or ADCC. To avoid this problem, we selected LA-N-1 cells from a panel of NB cell lines. LA-N-1 showed low P-glycoprotein expression levels and subsequently low background signals after calcein labeling. Moreover, the most homogeneous and strongest GD_2 expression and the highest level of GD_2-specific lysis in contrast to all other NB cell lines of the available panel resulted in the decision to establish CDC and ADCC bioassays with LA-N-1 target cells. We also aimed to optimize the bioassays to reduce both preparation time required for effector cell isolation as well as sample volume, which is particularly important in a pediatric population. To this end, a minimum of 100 μl of serum and a blood sample containing 200,000 leukocytes are sufficient which can be isolated within 10 min from small blood volume of less than 500 μl.

A second challenge to overcome is the fact that European NB trials are generally multi-center in nature and require sample transfer to a central laboratory for analysis. Therefore, the impact of shipping conditions is of great importance. According to our present data, serum samples could be stored at RT for four days and subjected three times to repeated thawing and freezing without significant influence on CDC. For the analysis of ADCC, blood needs to be anticoagulated. Although EDTA is the most commonly used anticoagulant, it is known that it affects both erythrocytes and leukocytes, causing membrane damage [27]. Here, we compared the impact of two anti-coagulants, EDTA and sodium-heparin, on leukocyte count and viability and count in blood samples stored at RT for 72 h. We could not observe any significant changes in cell-viability and -count of effector cells in sodium-heparin-anticoagulated blood for up to 48 h at RT in contrast to EDTA-anticoagulated blood samples. In contrast, the analysis of granulocyte rich effector cell fractions revealed a reduction of granulocyte counts and anti-tumor cytotoxic activity during storage of blood samples. Therefore, the evaluation of granulocyte-mediated ADCC as a biomarker requires timely processing and analysis, which is unsuitable for central lab testing in a multicenter setup of a clinical trial. In summary, serum and in sodium-heparin-anticoagulated blood samples can be shipped within 48 h for central laboratory bioassay analysis. We analyzed CDC and ADCC in three selected high-risk NB patients participating in this trial and could observe a significant increase of both anti-tumor CDC and ADCC after Ab administration indicating beneficial effects of this immunotherapy.

In order to permit a valid interpretation of data from functional assays employed for quantitative determination of cytotoxicity in biological samples, reproducible and reliable data must be generated operator independent in a laboratory performing such analyses [28]. To validate the established assay and to show its reproducibility, accuracy and precision, both within-assay and inter-assay precision analysis were determined and QC were included in each analytical run according to the international guidelines for bioanalytical method validation [18]. We found CV of both within-assay and inter-assay to be under 20% indicating operator-independent and reproducible performance over time.

Recently, a concept of a personalized medicine in NB treatment becomes more important [29]. In line with the fact that the extraordinary diversity of the clinical course in NB patients is reflected by a substantial genetic variation [29], we observed inter-individual differences in a basic Ab-independent cytotoxicity in NB patients as well as about 40% inter-individual differences in healthy donors anylzed. By using the bioassays described here in combination with pharmacokinetic [11] and human anti-chimeric response analysis [12], we aim to monitor patients currently treated in clinical trials with ch14.18/CHO in order to work towards the establishment of a set of biomarkers potentially predictive of response.

Taken together, we reported two validated non-toxic and non-radioactive *in vitro* assays for rapid analysis of patient-specific CDC and ADCC in small volume samples collected from NB patients treated with anti-GD_2 Ab. These two assays allow reliable analysis within 48 h after sample collection for standard laboratory purposes and large-scale applications in clinical trials and are therefore a suitable tool for immune monitoring also in the multicenter setting.

Acknowledgments

We would like to acknowledge the cooperating group of pediatric oncologists of the SIOPEN-R-NET for the production of ch14.18/CHO antibody carried out by Polymun Scientific, Vienna, Austria which was financed by charities throughout Europe and Dr. Peter Ambros for SNP array analysis of *de novo* NB cell lines. We also thank Theodor Koepp and Manuela Brueser (University Medicine Greifswald, Pediatric Hematology and Oncology, Greifswald, Germany) for excellent technical assistance.

Author Contributions

Conceived and designed the experiments: NS HNL. Performed the experiments: NS CE MJ DS. Analyzed the data: NS CE MJ DS. Contributed reagents/materials/analysis tools: NS CE MJ DS. Contributed to the writing of the manuscript: NS CE MJ DS HNL.

References

1. Modak S, Cheung NK (2007) Disialoganglioside directed immunotherapy of neuroblastoma. Cancer Invest 25: 67–77.
2. Yang RK, Sondel PM (2010) Anti-GD_2 Strategy in the Treatment of Neuroblastoma. Drugs Future 35: 665.
3. Shuptrine CW, Surana R, Weiner LM (2012) Monoclonal antibodies for the treatment of cancer. Semin Cancer Biol 22: 3–13.
4. Saito M, Yu RK, Cheung NK (1985) Ganglioside GD_2 specificity of monoclonal antibodies to human neuroblastoma cell. Biochem Biophys Res Commun 127: 1–7.
5. Cheresh DA, Rosenberg J, Mujoo K, Hirschowitz L, Reisfeld RA (1986) Biosynthesis and expression of the disialoganglioside GD_2, a relevant target antigen on small cell lung carcinoma for monoclonal antibody-mediated cytolysis. Cancer Res 46: 5112–5118.
6. Simon T, Hero B, Faldum A, Handgretinger R, Schrappe M, et al. (2004) Consolidation treatment with chimeric anti-GD_2-antibody ch14.18 in children older than 1 year with metastatic neuroblastoma. J Clin Oncol 22: 3549–3557.
7. Simon T, Hero B, Faldum A, Handgretinger R, Schrappe M, et al. (2011) Long term outcome of high-risk neuroblastoma patients after immunotherapy with antibody ch14.18 or oral metronomic chemotherapy. BMC Cancer 11: 21.
8. Yu AL, Gilman AL, Ozkaynak MF, London WB, Kreissman SG, et al. (2010) Anti-GD_2 antibody with GM-CSF, interleukin-2, and isotretinoin for neuroblastoma. N Engl J Med 363: 1324–1334.
9. Zeng Y, Fest S, Kunert R, Katinger H, Pistoia V, et al. (2005) Anti-neuroblastoma effect of ch14.18 antibody produced in CHO cells is mediated by NK-cells in mice. Mol Immunol 42: 1311–1319.
10. Ladenstein R, Weixler S, Baykan B, Bleeke M, Kunert R, et al. (2013) Ch14.18 antibody produced in CHO cells in relapsed or refractory Stage 4 neuroblastoma patients: a SIOPEN Phase 1 study. MAbs 5: 801–809.
11. Siebert N, Seidel D, Eger C, Brackrock D, Reker D, et al. (2013) Validated detection of anti-GD_2 antibody ch14.18/CHO in serum of neuroblastoma patients using anti-idiotype antibody ganglidiomab. J Immunol Methods 398–399: 51–59.
12. Siebert N, Eger C, Seidel D, Juttner M, Lode HN (2014) Validated detection of human anti-chimeric immune responses in serum of neuroblastoma patients treated with ch14.18/CHO. J Immunol Methods 407: 108–115.
13. Seeger RC, Rayner SA, Banerjee A, Chung H, Laug WE, et al. (1977) Morphology, growth, chromosomal pattern and fibrinolytic activity of two new human neuroblastoma cell lines. Cancer Res 37: 1364–1371.
14. Bumol TF, Reisfeld RA (1982) Unique glycoprotein-proteoglycan complex defined by monoclonal antibody on human melanoma cells. Proc Natl Acad Sci U S A 79: 1245–1249.
15. Keshelava N, Seeger RC, Groshen S, Reynolds CP (1998) Drug resistance patterns of human neuroblastoma cell lines derived from patients at different phases of therapy. Cancer Res 58: 5396–5405.
16. Biedler JL, Helson L, Spengler BA (1973) Morphology and growth, tumorigenicity, and cytogenetics of human neuroblastoma cells in continuous culture. Cancer Res 33: 2643–2652.
17. Lode HN, Schmidt M, Seidel D, Huebener N, Brackrock D, et al. (2013) Vaccination with anti-idiotype antibody ganglidiomab mediates a GD_2-specific anti-neuroblastoma immune response. Cancer Immunol Immunother 62: 999–1010.
18. DeSilva B, Smith W, Weiner R, Kelley M, Smolec J, et al. (2003) Recommendations for the bioanalytical method validation of ligand-binding assays to support pharmacokinetic assessments of macromolecules. Pharm 20: 1885–1900.
19. Homolya L, Hollo Z, Germann UA, Pastan I, Gottesman MM, et al. (1993) Fluorescent cellular indicators are extruded by the multidrug resistance protein. J Biol Chem 268: 21493–21496.
20. Gelderman KA, Tomlinson S, Ross GD, Gorter A (2004) Complement function in mAb-mediated cancer immunotherapy. Trends Immunol 25: 15164.
21. Sorkin LS, Otto M, Baldwin WM III, Vail E, Gillies SD, et al. (2010) Anti-GD_2 with an FC point mutation reduces complement fixation and decreases antibody-induced allodynia. Pain 149: 135–42.
22. Li S, Schmitz KR, Jeffrey PD, Wiltzius JJ, Kussie P, et al. (2005) Structural basis for inhibition of the epidermal growth factor receptor by cetuximab. Cancer Cell 7: 301–311.
23. Clynes RA, Towers TL, Presta LG, Ravetch JV (2000) Inhibitory Fc receptors modulate in vivo cytotoxicity against tumor targets. Nat Med 6: 443–446.
24. Di GN, Cittera E, Nota R, Vecchi A, Grieco V, et al. (2003) Complement activation determines the therapeutic activity of rituximab in vivo. J Immunol 171: 1581–1587.
25. Ahmed M, Cheung NK (2014) Engineering anti-GD_2 monoclonal antibodies for cancer immunotherapy. FEBS Lett 588: 288–297.
26. Lichtenfels R, Biddison WE, Schulz H, Vogt AB, Martin R (1994) CARE-LASS (calcein-release-assay), an improved fluorescence-based test system to measure cytotoxic T lymphocyte activity. J Immunol Methods 172: 227–239.
27. Lewis SM, Stoddart CT (1971) Effects of anticoagulants and containers (glass and plastic) on the blood count. Lab Pract 10: 787–792.
28. Smolec J, DeSilva B, Smith W, Weiner R, Kelly M, et al. (2005) Bioanalytical method validation for macromolecules in support of pharmacokinetic studies. Pharm Res 9: 1425–1431.
29. Tonini GP, Nakagawara A, Berthold F (2012) Towards a turning point of neuroblastoma therapy. Cancer Lett 326: 128–134.

10

Spermicidal and Contraceptive Potential of Desgalactotigonin: A Prospective Alternative of Nonoxynol-9

Debanjana Chakraborty[1], Arindam Maity[1¤], Tarun Jha[2], Nirup Bikash Mondal[1*]

1 Department of Chemistry, Indian Institute of Chemical Biology, Council of Scientific and Industrial Research, Jadavpur, Kolkata, West Bengal, India, 2 Department of Pharmaceutical Technology, Division of Medicinal and Pharmaceutical Chemistry, Jadavpur University, Kolkata, West Bengal, India

Abstract

Crude decoction of *Chenopodium album* seed showed spermicidal effect at MIC 2 mg/ml in earlier studies. Systematic isolation, characterization and evaluation revealed that the major metabolite Desgalactotigonin (DGT) is the most effective principle in both *in vitro* and *in vivo* studies. The *in vitro* studies comprises (a) rat and human sperm motility and immobilizing activity by Sander-Cramer assay; (b) sperm membrane integrity was observed by HOS test and electron microscopy; (c) microbial potential was examined in *Lactobacillus* broth culture, and (d) the hemolytic index was determined by using rat RBCs. The *in vivo* contraceptive efficacy was evaluated by intra uterine application of DGT in rat. Lipid peroxidation and induction of apoptosis by DGT on human spermatozoa were also studied. The minimum effective concentration (MEC) of DGT that induced instantaneous immobilization *in vitro* was 24.18 μM for rat and 58.03 μM for human spermatozoa. Microbial study indicated DGT to be friendly to *Lactobacillus acidophilus*. Implantation was prevented in DGT treated uterine horn while no hindrance occurred in the untreated contra lateral side. At the level of EC_{50}, DGT induced apoptosis in human spermatozoa as determined by increased labeling with Annexin-V and decreased polarization of sperm mitochondria. Desgalactotigonin emerged 80 and 2×10^4 times more potent than the decoction and Nonoxynol-9 respectively. It possesses mechanism based detrimental action on both human and rat spermatozoa and spares lactobacilli and HeLa cells at MEC which proves its potential as a superior ingredient for the formulation of a contraceptive safer/compatible to vaginal microflora.

Editor: Wei Yan, University of Nevada School of Medicine, United States of America

Funding: Indian Council for Medical Research (ICMR), Delhi project No 59/3/2007/BMS/TRM. The funders had no role in study design, data collection and analysis, decision to publish, or preparation of the manuscript.

Competing Interests: The authors have declared that no competing interests exist.

* Email: nirup@iicb.res.in

¤ Current address: Dr. B. C. Roy College of Pharmacy & AHS, Durgapur, West Bengal, India

Introduction

The world population, which was 2.5 billion in 1950, has crossed the 7 billion mark [1] in 2012 and is projected to touch 9.4 billion by 2050 [2]. Anticipating that 86% of the global population will live in less developed countries by the year 2050 [3], the present-day scenario of world population looks alarming. The demographers and social scientists have recommended drastic family planning programs and emphasized that contraception is the only means to combat this devastating problem; they therefore felt, among others, an urgent need for developing options that allow women to prevent or delay their pregnancies [4]. Although a number of contraceptive methods have been developed, the acceptability of these methods has quite often been limited by their associated untoward side effects, failure rate or irreversibility [5]. Spermicides are biologically obvious ways of interrupting fertility and have the advantage that they do not require highly skilled personnel for their prescription and use. Thus research has focused on the development of safe, highly effective and inexpensive spermicidal agents as one of the several alternative methods for family planning [6].

The currently available spermicidal contraceptive formulations, mostly based on the mixture of oligomers nonoxynol-9 or N-9, [7,8] are effective but their repeated use is associated with vaginal/cervical irritation or even ulceration [9] and disturbance of the normal vaginal microflora; this facilitates microbial infection and renders the subject susceptible to sexually transmitted diseases (STDs) [10]. Several European nations have banned or restricted the use of N-9 related compounds on the basis of health risks and potential environmental toxicity [11,12]. The limitations of N-9 to protect sexually transmitted diseases [13] have encouraged researchers to develop better alternatives that would have dual function of contraception and STD protection for women.

Our group has made concerted efforts to develop novel spermicidal cum microbicidal molecules from synthetic [14,15] and natural [16,17] sources. Previous studies on *Chenopodium album* revealed that the aqueous decoction of the seeds has *in vitro* sperm immobilizing activity [18,19,20]. As the healthcare industry moves towards using either pure compounds or mixtures whose individual components meet safety standards, we undertook the program of separating the active constituent(s) of the decoction *of C. album* seeds. We have thereby succeeded in isolating the active components. In this article we wish to report both the spermicidal and microbial potential of the isolated molecule(s) which appears to possess the dual function of contraception and STD protection for women.

Materials and Methods

Plant material

Matured fruits of *Chenopodium album* (Linn) were collected from the medicinal plant garden of R. K. Mission, Narendrapur, Kolkata, during April 2012. As the plant is not an endangered or protected species rather a small herb that grows all over the garden as a common agricultural weed thus no specific permissions were required for its collection. This plant material was authenticated by Dr. Debjani Basu, Asst. Director, Botanical Survey of India, Howrah (West Bengal, India). A voucher specimen (No. 786) was deposited in the Steroid and Terpenoid Chemistry Department, Indian Institute of Chemical Biology. The black seeds were segregated from the pericarp of the fruits and then ground in an industrial blender.

Preparation of extract

Powdered seeds (3 Kg) were subjected to successive percolation with (i) petroleum ether (60–80°C), (ii) chloroform, (iii) methanol, and (iv) methanol: water (1:1). The solvents were distilled off under reduced pressure (temperature <50°C) using a rotary evaporator (Eyela, Tokyo, Japan). Removal of inorganic salts from the methanol extract was effected by partitioning between n-butanol and water. The n-butanol part was concentrated by reduced pressure distillation to yield 35 g of greenish brown mass.

Purification of extract

The greenish brown mass obtained from the n-butanolic portion was passed through silica gel column (60–120 mesh size) and eluted with solvents in an increasing order of polarity starting with chloroform and ending with methanol. The fractions obtained by column chromatography from different ratios of chloroform: methanol was subjected to screening for spermicidal activity. The active fractions were further purified through repeated column chromatography in conjunction with thin layer chromatography. This ultimately yielded four products, the major one with eluent $CHCl_3$: MeOH (75:25) and the minor three were with (70:30), (65:35) and (50:50) respectively. The major product which was crystallized from MeOH and characterized as Desgalactotigonin (yield 0.004%, on dry weight basis of the plant material) via spectroscopic analysis, viz. mass, ^{13}C NMR, and ^{1}H NMR spectroscopy followed by comparison with data reported in the literature [21]. It is worthy of mention that this compound is being isolated for the first time from *Chenopodium album*. The minor products were also characterized by spectral analysis as glucuronopyranosyl analogues of oleanolic acid viz. (i) 3-*O*-β-D-Glucuronopyranosyl oleanolic acid, (yield 0.0001%) [22] (ii) 3-*O*-[β-D-Glucuronopyranosyl]-28-*O*-β-D-g-lucuronopyranosyl oleanolic acid (yield 0.0006%) and (iii) 3-*O*-[3′-*O*-(2″-*O*-Glycolyl)-glyoxylyl β-D-glucuronopyranosyl] oleanolic acid (yield 0.0005%) [23]. These glucuronopyranosyl analogues of oleanolic acid were also present in trace amounts in methanol: water (1:1) fraction. However, these were not taken into account as they showed less activity in comparison to desgalactotigonin. (See Data S1).

Desgalactotigonin (Fig.1) is an amorphous solid, mp (235-237°C); Q-TOF Mass (m/z) 1057 $[M+Na]^+$; ^{1}H NMR (Pyridine-d_5, 600 MHz) δ 0.51 (1H, m), 0.64 (3H, s), 0.70 (3H, d, J = 4.8 Hz), 0.82 (4H, s), 0.89 (1H, m), 1.05 (3H, m), 1.15 (5H, d, J = 7.2 Hz), 1.38 (4H, m), 1.61 (8H, m), 1.79 (2H, m), 1.99 (2H, m), 3.61 (2H, m), 3.92 (5H, m), 4.08 (6H, m), 4.19 (1H, m), 4.24 (3H, m), 4.43 (3H, m), 4.58 (3H, m), 4.89 (1H, d, J = 7.2 Hz), 5.20 (1H, d, J = 8.4 Hz), 5.25 (1H, d, J = 7.8 Hz), 5.43 (1H, s), 5.59 (1H, d, J = 7.2 Hz); ^{13}C NMR [Pyridine-d_5, 150 MHz] δ 12.5 (CH_3), 15.3 (CH_3), 16.8 (CH_3), 17.7 (CH_3), 21.5 (CH_2), 29.1 (CH_2), 29.5 (CH_2), 30.1(CH_2), 30.8 (CH), 32.0 (CH_2), 32.4 (CH_2), 32.6 (CH_2), 35.0 (CH_2), 35.5 (CH), 36.0 (C), 37.4 (CH_2), 40.4 (CH_2), 41.0 (C), 42.2 (CH), 44.9 (CH), 54.6 (CH), 56.7 (CH), 60.5 (CH_2), 62.7 (CH_2), 63.2 (CH), 63.2 (CH_2), 67.1 (CH_2), 67.6 (CH_2), 70.7 (CH), 70.9 (CH), 71.2 (CH), 73.4 (CH), 75.3 (CH), 75.6 (CH), 75.8 (CH), 76.5 (CH), 77.6 (CH), 77.9 (CH), 78.0 (CH), 78.9 (CH), 79.0 (CH), 80.2 (CH), 81.4 (CH), 81.6 (CH), 86.9 (CH), 102.6 (CH), 105.1 (CH), 105.2 (CH), 105.4 (CH), 109.5 (C).

Chemicals

Chemicals and solvents were of analytical grade and mostly procured from Merck India Ltd. LIVE/DEAD sperm viability kit was from Life Technologies (Invitrogen, India Pvt Ltd) and the other chemicals were from Sigma (St Louise, MO, USA). JC-1 and FITC-Annexin-V/PI assay kits were purchased from Life Technologies (Molecular Probes, USA) and Calbiochem (USA) respectively. Thiobarbituric acid (TBA) and trichloroacetic acid (TCA) were purchased from Merck Specialities Pvt Ltd (Mumbai, India).

Animals

Adult Sprague-Dawley rats (230–270 g) were collected from the animal house of the Indian Institute of Chemical Biology. The animals were maintained under standard husbandry conditions (12:12, dark/light cycle) and fed with standard pellet diet; water was supplied ad libitum. All experiments were performed in accordance with the guidelines recommended and approved by the Indian Institute of Chemical Biology's Animal Care and Use Committee of Laboratory Animals (Animal Ethics Committee) registered with the Ministry of Social Justice &Empowerment for breeding, maintenance and experimentation of animals (IICB Reg. No. is 147/1999/CPCSEA, renewed in 2002 and 2005).

Isolation of rat caudal sperm

Males of proven fertility were used for sperm collection following sexual abstinence. The animals were necropsied following anesthesia with ketamine (100 mg/kg body weight). The caudal portion of the epididymis was dissociated and minced in 2.5 ml of BWW medium (94 mM NaCl, 4.7 mM KCl, 1.7 mM $CaCl_2$, 1.2 mM KH_2PO_4, 1.2 mM $MgSO_4 \cdot 7H_2O$, 25 mM $NaHCO_3$, 0.5 mM sodium pyruvate, 19 mM sodium lactate, 5 mM glucose, 0.4% BSA, 0.1% antibiotic (penicillin/streptomycin) solution, pH 7.2) [24]. The collected spermatozoa exudates were then suspended in the same medium. The spermatozoa were incubated for 30 min under oil cover in a CO_2 chamber. Sperm count was done using a Makler's chamber. Highly motile sperm suspensions with a sperm count of 20–25×10^6/ml were used for further work.

Human spermatozoa

Fresh human semen samples, obtained by masturbation into a sterile vial from healthy, young fertile donors, were liquefied for 45 min at 37°C and used for in vitro spermicidal assays. Samples having >65×10^6/ml sperm count with >70% motility and normal sperm morphology were used in the study. The study protocol was approved by the Institutional Ethics Committee of Institute of Reproductive Medicine, Kolkata, governed by Indian Council of Medical Research, New Delhi (Ref. No.IRM/HEC/

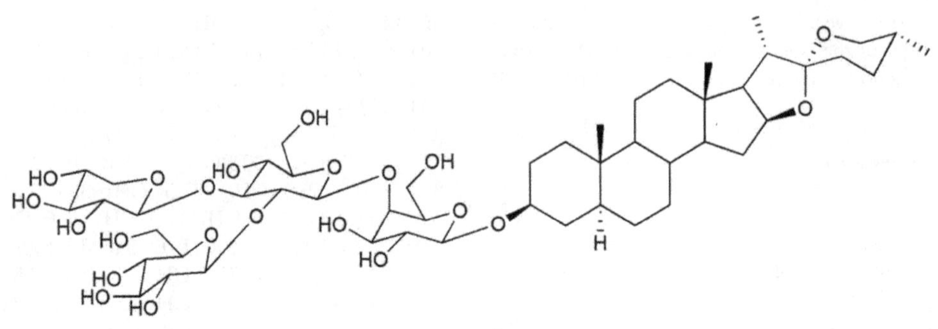

Figure 1. Structure of Isolated Compound. Structure of desgalactotigonin (DGT).

BNC/25-01-2013). Written informed consent was obtained from all the participants prior to enrolling in the study. The highly motile spermatozoa with forward motility were washed with BWW medium and separated from immotile or sluggishly motile spermatozoa by 'swim up' technique and semen characteristic, pH, motility, morphology were determined on the World Health Organization guidelines [25] and finally resuspended in pre-equilibrated BWW medium to obtain working spermatozoa suspension having concentration of $30–35\times10^6$ cells/ml.

Assessment of spermicidal activity

The spermicidal activity of desgalactotigonin (DGT) was assayed according to the modified Sander–Cramer method [26,27]. Varying concentrations of DGT solution (0, 5, 10, 15, 20, 25, 30 μM in case of rat and 0, 15, 30, 45, 60, 65 μM for human) were prepared in physiological saline and 100 μl of each was mixed with a 20 μl aliquot of sperm suspension (25×10^6/ml). The specimens were examined under a phase contrast microscope (×100) after 20 s of treatment and counted for motile spermatozoa. The sperm that lost complete motility within 20 s were subsequently tested for motility revival. About 250 μl of Baker's buffer (glucose 3%, $Na_2HPO_4{\cdot}2H_2O$ 0.31%, NaCl 0.2%, KH_2PO_4 0.01%) was used to show total immobilization of the spermatozoa by incubating at 37°C for 60 min and observing for regeneration of any kind of motility. The minimum concentration of DGT that caused 100% immobilization of spermatozoa within 20 s with no revival of motility after subsequent 60 min of incubation in Baker's buffer at 37°C was considered to be the minimum effective concentration (MEC).

Hypo-osmotic swelling test

Control and DGT-treated (at MEC, i.e. 24.18 μM for rat and 58.03 μM for human) spermatozoa suspensions were exposed to HOS solution (75 mM fructose, 20 mM sodium citrate) for at least 30 min at 37°C. After thorough mixing, a drop of mixture was placed on a glass slide and covered with a cover slip to detect changes in sperm membrane integrity [28,29,30,31]. The number of spermatozoa showing characteristic tail curling or swelling was counted under a phase contrast microscope (×400).

Sperm viability test by fluorescent staining

Sperm viability was assessed by using a sperm viability kit according to the manufacturer's instructions, where live spermatozoa fluoresced green (SYBR-14 dye) and dead spermatozoa fluoresced red [propidium iodide (PI)]. DGT treated (for rat at MEC 24.18 μM and human at MEC 58.03 μM) and untreated sperm samples were subjected to sperm viability assessment [32]. Sperm count was taken from 200 spermatozoa under a phase contrast microscope (×200).

Assessment of irritation potential through hemolytic studies

The irritation potential of the compound was estimated using an RBC hemolytic assay. The RBC from rat blood was isolated by repeated washing (three times) with isotonic phosphate buffered saline (PBS; pH 7.4). These were mixed with varying concentrations of DGT, 0.1% of Triton X-100 and PBS, and used as treated, positive control and negative control, respectively. The test samples were prepared in PBS and incubated at 37°C for 30 min with occasional mild shaking to achieve complete hemolysis. The reaction was quenched in ice, the samples were centrifuged at 1500 rpm for 2 min, and the supernatants were used for spectrophotometer reading at 576 nm. The percentage hemolysis was then calculated by the following formula [33]: $\%H = 100\%\ (Abs - Abs_{control})/(Abs_{100} - Abs_{control})$, where, Abs is the absorbance of the sample, $Abs_{control}$ is the absorbance of the control sample (negative control) and Abs_{100} is the absorbance of the sample where 100% hemolysis occurred. Hemolytic index (50% hemolysis) was determined by comparing control and positive control.

Evaluation of effect on *Lactobacillus acidophilus* NCIM 2285

Inoculum preparation. Bacterial colonies were grown in MRS broth at 37°C for 36 h, adjusted to 0.5 McFarland standard, [34] and diluted with 0.9% sterile saline to a final count of 1.5×10^6 CFU/ml.

The compound (DGT) was first dissolved in 0.4% DMSO, diluted with MRS broth media to give a final concentration of 1000 μg/ml, and then serially diluted two fold to obtain different concentration ranges [35]. An aliquot (0.1 ml) of standardized suspension of bacteria (1.5×10^6 CFU/ml) was added to each well (96 microplate) containing the test compound at a final concentration of 0–1000 μg/ml, and incubated at 37°C for 36 h [36]. Beside each of test sample, one negative control well was taken which contained liquid broth culture without any test sample. N-9 (Sigma-Aldrich) was used as positive control. The absorbance of the solution was measured at 540 nm.

Contraceptive efficacy

The contraceptive efficacy of the compound was assayed in rats via intrauterine administration of DGT and subsequent evaluation of mating outcomes. Sexually mature cyclic adult Sprague-Dawley rats (n = 10) were subjected to light ether anesthesia on the day of proestrous phase of their cycle, then one very small mid-ventral abdominal incision was made through which the uterine horns were gently pulled out carefully. In one horn, 50 µl of DGT solution (3000 µg/ml of sterile physiological saline) was introduced through a tuberculin syringe fitted with a 24-G needle that penetrated through the cervical end (treated horn). The contralateral uterine horn received 50 µl of sterile physiological saline (control horn). The incision was closed by suture and Mitchel's clip. The animals were maintained in individual cages and divided into two groups with five animals per group. In the evening, they were exposed to males of proven fertility in 1:1 ratio. In the next morning the presence of sperm in vaginal lavage confirmed mating. Mated rats of one group were sacrificed on Day 10 of gestation. The uterine horns were examined and the number of implantation sites/fetus was counted. Animals of the other groups were allowed to deliver pups. After parturation, pups were examined visually for any abnormalities.

Ultrastructural study

Transmission electron microscopy. Control and DGT treated human sperm suspensions were fixed in 2.5% glutaraldehyde in 0.1% cacodylate buffer for 3 days following the procedure of Niksirat et al. [37]. After three successive washings in buffer, overnight post-fixation was done using 4% osmium tetroxide solution. Three further washings in buffer were done and samples were dehydrated through graded series of acetone. Finally the samples were embedded in spur resins and polymerized for 48 h. Ultra thin sections were cut, stained with uranyl acetate and lead citrate, and observed under transmission electron microscope (JEOL, Tokyo, Japan) operating at 80 kV. Fifty (50) spermatozoa were scanned from treated and untreated groups for the intactness of sperm head membranes; photograph of one representative sperm from each group has been presented.

Scanning electron microscopy. For scanning electron microscopic (SEM) observation, human spermatozoa were fixed with 2.5 % glutaraldehyde in 0.1% cacodylate buffer. Next, samples were rinsed three times in filtered f/2 medium and immobilized by spreading onto a poly-L-lysine coated glass slide. Samples were then post fixed by 2% osmium tetroxide and dehydrated in graded series of acetone, with 15 min incubation at each step. After drying by the critical point method (CPD2, Pelco TM), glass slides were mounted on an aluminum stub using carbon conductive tape and a silver paste. Specimens were gold coated (SEM Coating Unit E 5100, Polaron) and observed in a field emission scanning electron microscope (JEOL JSM 7401-F).

Determination of lipid peroxidation on human sperm

Lipid peroxidation was measured to determine the extent of oxidative damage induced by DGT on the human sperm membrane as indicated by malondialdehyde (MDA) adduct formation. DGT was serially diluted with BWW medium to make solutions of final concentrations ranging between 29.01 µM and 106.38 µM and treated with the sperm suspension at 5:1 ratio. The sperm suspension (1 ml of $25–30\times10^6$ cells/ml solution), treated with or without different concentration of DGT, was mixed with 2 ml of TBA-TCA reagent (15% w/v TCA, 0.375% w/v TBA, and 0.25 M HCl). The mixture was boiled in water bath for 30 min. After cooling, the suspension was centrifuged at 1500 g for 15 min. The supernatant was separated and the absorbance was measured at 535 nm. The result was expressed as simple concentration of MDA (nmol/10^8 sperm) as determined by specific absorbance coefficient (1.56×10^5/mol per cm^3) [38,39]. MDA produced (µmol/ml) = [OD $\times10^6\times$ total volume (3 ml)]/[$1.56\times10^5\times$ test volume (1 ml)].

Cytotoxicity study against the human cervical cell line (HeLa) by MTT assay

Colorimetric assay can be done using the 3-(4,5-dimethylthiazol-2-yl)-2,5-diphenyltetrazolium bromide (MTT) assay. It was used for evaluation of cytotoxicity of spermicidal compound against the HeLa cell line. In each well of a 96 well culture plate 2×10^5 cells were seeded in triplicate. The cells were incubated for 24 h in a 5% CO_2 incubator at 37°C and then exposed to various concentrations of DGT. At the end of the treatment the drug containing medium was removed and 20 µl of 5 mg/ml MTT dissolved in the same medium was added to each well. The plate was further incubated for an additional 5 h. After removing the supernatant at the end of incubation, the resultant intracellular formazan crystals were solubilised with DMSO and the absorbance of the solution was measured at 595 nm using an ELISA reader. Absorbance (O.D) of the medium containing the different concentrations of the compound and MTT reagents was subtracted from the respective experimental sets and then viability was calculated.

Apoptotic changes in plasma membrane of human spermatozoa

Dual fluorescent labelling with fluorescein isothiocyanate (FITC)-Annexin V and propidium iodide (Calbiochem, USA) was used to study the expression of phosphatidylserine on sperm cell surfaces (apoptotic cells) and the membrane permeabilization of the cells (necrotic cells) respectively. Aliquots of highly motile human sperm (10^7) in triplicate were incubated in BWW-0.4% bovine serum albumin (BSA) containing 94 mM NaCl, 4.7 mM KCl, 1.7 mM $CaCl_2$, 1.2 mM KH_2PO_4, 1.2 mM $MgSO_4\cdot7H_2O$, 25 mM $NaHCO_3$, 0.5 mM sodium pyruvate, 19 mM sodium lactate, 5 mM glucose, 0.1% antibiotic (penicillin/streptomycin) solution, pH 7.2 at 37°C for 3 h with EC_{50} of DGT. Control tubes contained only BWW medium with 0.4% BSA. After incubation, sperms were washed in 1% BSA in Tyrode's buffer and labeled with fluorescent probes. An apoptosis detection kit (Calbiochem, USA) was used to detect apoptosis in sperm cells by following manufacturer's instruction. The percentages of cells positive for Annexin-V and PI were determined in a flow cytometer (Model BD LSRFortessa, BD Biosciences, USA). Four populations of cells (unstained, FITC stained, FITC + PI stained, and PI stained) were identified [40] and designated as viable, apoptotic, necrotic and dead respectively.

Apoptotic changes in mitochondria on human sperm cell

The loss of mitochondrial trans-membrane potential ($\Delta\Psi m$, an early marker for cell apoptosis) was quantified by flow cytometry using the lipophilic cationic dye 5,5′,6,6′-tetrachloro-1,1′,3,3′-tetraethylbenzimidazolylcarbocyanine iodide (JC-1). Concurrently, highly motile human spermatozoa (10^7 in triplicate) were incubated in BWW-0.4% BSA at 37°C for 3 h with EC_{50} of DGT. Positive control tubes contained 50 µM CCCP and control tubes contained BWW-0.4% BSA. After incubations, 10 µg/ml JC-1 (Molecular probes) was added to sperm from a stock solution of 1 mg/ml in DMSO. Spermatozoa were incubated for another 10 min, washed and re-suspended in Tyrode's salt solution. The cells were finally analysed in a flow cytometer (Model BD LSR Fortessa, BD Biosciences, USA) using an argon laser (488 nm) for excitation, and emissions at 530 nm (green) and 575 nm (red/orange) were quantified using the threshold signal for intact cells.

Results

Spermicidal activity

There was a dose-dependent increase in sperm immobilization with an increase in concentration of DGT. (Fig. 2 A and B) depict the effect of varying concentrations of DGT on both human and rat sperm motility. The MEC that induced 100% immobilization of the spermatozoa in 20 s was 24.18 μM for rat and 58.03 μM for human. At MEC of DGT, no revival of motility was observed after subsequent 60 min of incubation in Baker's buffer at 37°C.

Sperm membrane integrity

More than 90% of the control spermatozoa (both rat and human) were HOS responsive, whereas DGT-treated spermatozoa at MEC (both rat and human) was non-HOS responsive as depicted via tail curling (Fig. 3 A, B and E for rat and Fig. 3 C, D and F for human). Loss of HOS responsiveness indicated compromised sperm membrane integrity post DGT treatment, anticipating overall loss of sperm-membrane physiology.

Sperm viability test by fluorescent staining

The fluorescent green (Sybr-14) and red (PI) dyes differently stain live and dead sperm, respectively. At MEC in case of rat (24.18 μM), treated sperm were all dead, which fluoresced red, and control sperm fluoresced green (Fig. 4A–B). In the control set (without DGT) of human spermatozoa, 92% fluoresced green and were viable, while cells treated at MEC (58.03 μM), which fluoresced red (Fig. 4C–D), were all dead.

Irritation potential as measured by hemolytic activity

The hemolytic activity of DGT for rat as depicted in (Fig. 5A) was determined by quantifying the hemoglobin released from the RBC following exposure to varying concentrations of DGT. At 47 μg/mL of DGT, 50% hemolysis occurred. That is one and half fold higher than MEC. RBC treated with 0.1% Triton X-100 served as positive control.

Effect on *Lactobacillus acidophilus in vitro*

For this experiment, the control contains only lactobacillus strain with broth medium, DGT and nonoxynol-9 represents standard. This hour vs optical density graph (Fig. 5B) established that as compared with control, DGT up to 40 fold concentrations (for rat) and 19 fold concentrations (for human) of its MEC did not inhibit the growth of *Lactobacillus acidophilus* during the period of 36 h culture.

Contraceptive efficacy in rats

All the females mated successfully and no deviation of mating efficiency was observed. Not a single implantation site was observed in the DGT-treated horns on Day 10 of gestation. On the contrary, the number (mean±SEM) of implantation sites in the saline treated control horn showed the presence of 5±0.52 beads like embryonic swellings. On the parturation 4 normal pups were delivered by the other groups of rats. This observation (Fig. 6) suggests that even in the uterine milieu, DGT could effectively block sperm potential to reach and/or fertilize oocyte, while fertilization and implantation were unhindered in the control horn. The results suggest that DGT decreased fertility to zero.

Ultrastructural study

Transmission electron microscope. Ultrastructural microphotograph showed considerable membrane damage in 100% of the DGT exposed human sperm. As compared with the intact plasma membrane surroundings the head of 80% of the control spermatozoa (Fig. 7A), all treated spermatozoa exhibited dissolution of the acrosomal cap, and expansion as well as separation of the plasma membrane from the nucleus (Fig. 7B).

Scanning electron microscope. Electron microscopic photographs of human spermatozoa are presented in Fig. 7C–D. As compared with intact plasma membrane and acrosomal vesicles of 92% of the untreated spermatozoa, all (100%) DGT treated spermatozoa exhibited disintegrated plasma membrane with damaged acrosomal cap of various degrees ranging from perforations and vesiculation to complete disintegration.

Effect of lipid peroxidation on human spermatozoa

The spectrophotometric readings demonstrated a dose dependent increase in the concentration of malondialdehyde (MDA; μmol/10^8 sperm) in concert with an increase in DGT concentration

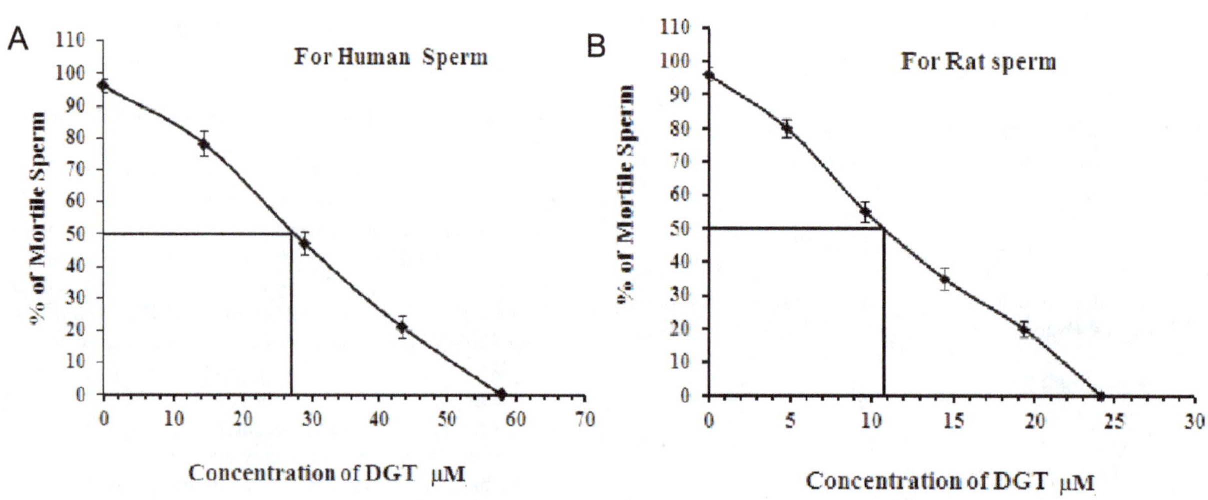

Figure 2. MEC Dose of the compound. Dose-dependent sperm immobilizing activity of DGT. The percentage of motile (A) human spermatozoa and (B) rat spermatozoa were determined after 20s following exposure to the test compounds at different concentrations. All data were adjusted to a normal control motility of 95%. Each point of DGT represents the mean ± SEM. values of five independent experiments.

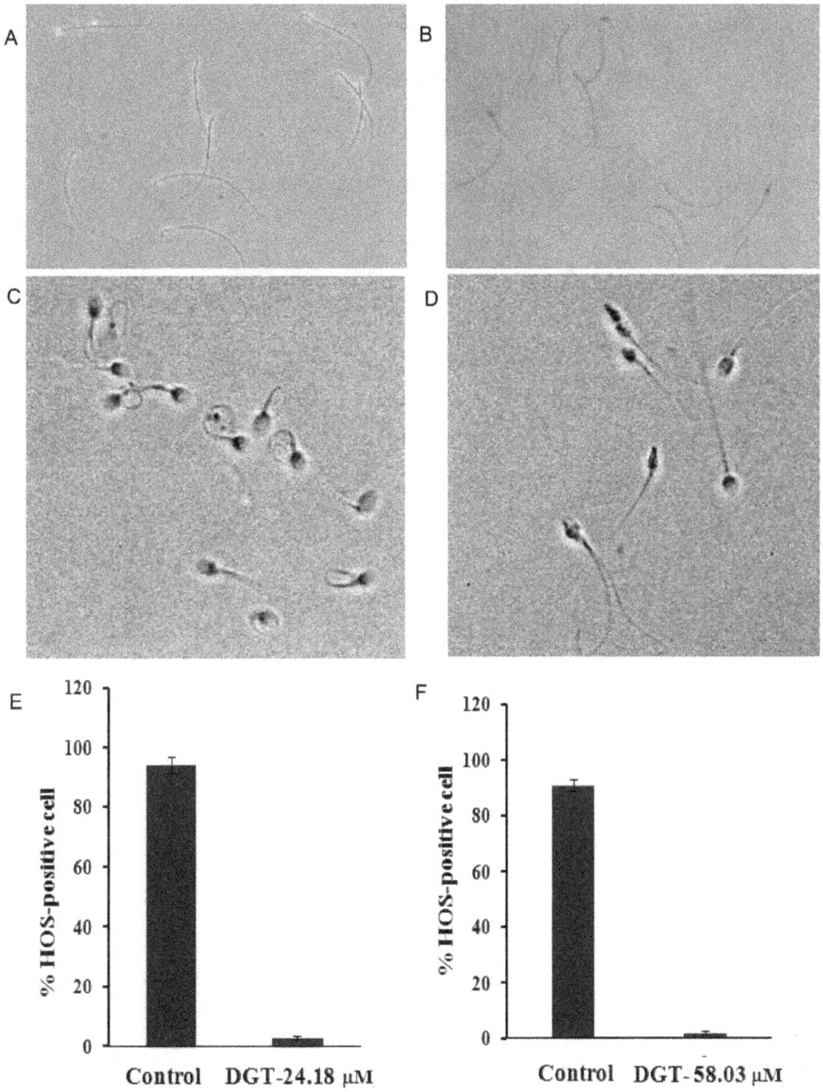

Figure 3. The HOS responsiveness of the sperm, as indicated by tail coiling. HOS responsiveness of rat sperm as tail coiling: (A) Untreated control. (B) DGT-treated rat sperm (24.18 μM) examined under a phase contrast microscope (40×). Response of control (C) and DGT-treated (D) human sperm (58.03 μM) population following exposure to hypo-osmotic solution and evaluation under a phase contrast microscope. Over 90% of control-untreated sperm exhibited HOS response typically characterized by tail coiling, where as sperm exposed to DGT at MEC examined no response under a phase contrast microscope (40×). (E): For rat sperm, (F): For human sperm. Each bar represents the mean ± SEM of five observations ($P<0.05$).

(Fig. 8). As analyzed by ANOVA, the MDA production by spermatozoa treated with DGT at MEC (0.697±0.0150 μmol/10^8 sperm) was significantly higher ($p<0.01$) than that of control spermatozoa (0.563±0.0140 μmol/10^8 sperm).

MTT assay for cytotoxicity

DGT did not show any detectable cytotoxicity towards the human cervical cell line (HeLa) at MEC. The IC_{50} values for cytotoxicity of DGT and N-9 towards HeLa cells were 135.54 and 0.675 μg/ml respectively. The selectivity index of the compounds was calculated as a ratio of cytotoxicity IC_{50} to spermicidal EC_{50}. DGT exhibited a selectivity index of 4.55, much higher than that of N-9. So, this cytotoxicity assay revealed a massive 529.06 level of safety for DGT compared with N-9 (Table 1).

Induction of apoptosis by spermicides on human spermatozoa

The selective spermicidal action of DGT (after 3 h incubation at different concentrations) is shown in Fig. 9 (Dot plot). By labeling with FITC-Annexin V (for detection of phosphatidyl serine on cell surface) and PI (for cell membrane integrity), cells were identified in four quadrants by flow cytometry: live (viable, LL), apoptotic (FITC stained, LR), necrotic (FITC+PI stained, UR), and dead (PI stained, UL). The data from the dual fluorescent labelling with Annexin V- FITC and PI showed that the control sample contained 92.9% viable, 7.0% apoptotic, 0.0% necrotic and 0.1% dead sperm (Fig. 9A). After treatment with DGT at EC_{50} (29.01 μM), the number of apoptotic cells rose significantly to 25.8%, with reduction in the populations of viable (74.2%) sperm cells (Fig. 9B). The figure increased to 29.7% after treatment with 58.03 μM DGT (Fig. 9C). The apoptotic, necrotic and dead cell

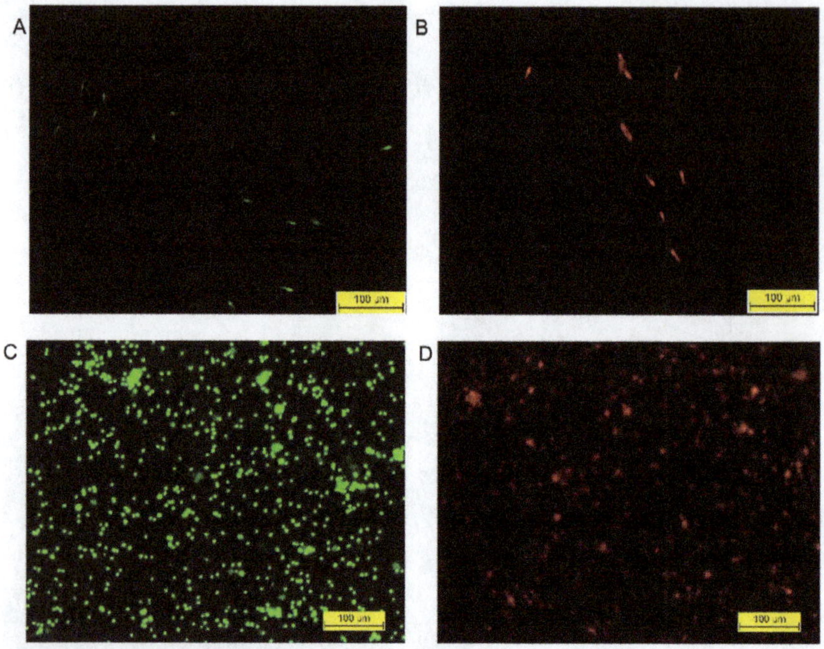

Figure 4. The sperm viability, as assessed by a fluorescent staining method. Rat Sperm viability assessment by SYBR-14/PI staining. (A) Control rat sperm appear green due to uptake of SYBR14 only; (B) DGT-treated rat sperm appear red due to uptake of PI when observed under a fluorescence microscope. Overlaid fluorescence images of (C) control and (D) DGT-treated human spermatozoa, dual stained with SYBR-14 and propidium iodide to distinguish green-fluorescing live from red-fluorescing dead spermatozoa.

populations increased to 20.4%, 2.3%, and 5.2% respectively after treatment with 106.38 μM DGT (Fig. 9D).

Apoptotic changes in mitochondria on human spermatozoa

There was a significant decrease in mitochondrial transmembrane potential ($\Delta\Psi$m) of sperm cells treated with the spermicide as indicated by an increase in the number of sperms exhibiting green fluorescence for JC-1. The decline was greater (79.9%) in case of DGT at 106.38 μM (Fig. 10D), but was 78.8% at 58.03 μM (Fig. 10C), 59.9% at 29.01 μM (Fig. 10B), and 74.5% for CCCP (Fig. 10E).

Discussion

All the above experiments focus on the assessment of desgalactotigonin, which was isolated from seed extract of *Chenopodium album*, for its sperm immobilizing activity. Spermicidal activity, contraceptive efficacy and other related parameters of DGT as spermicidal agent were verified in a series of in vitro and in vivo experiments. Results revealed that the compound has

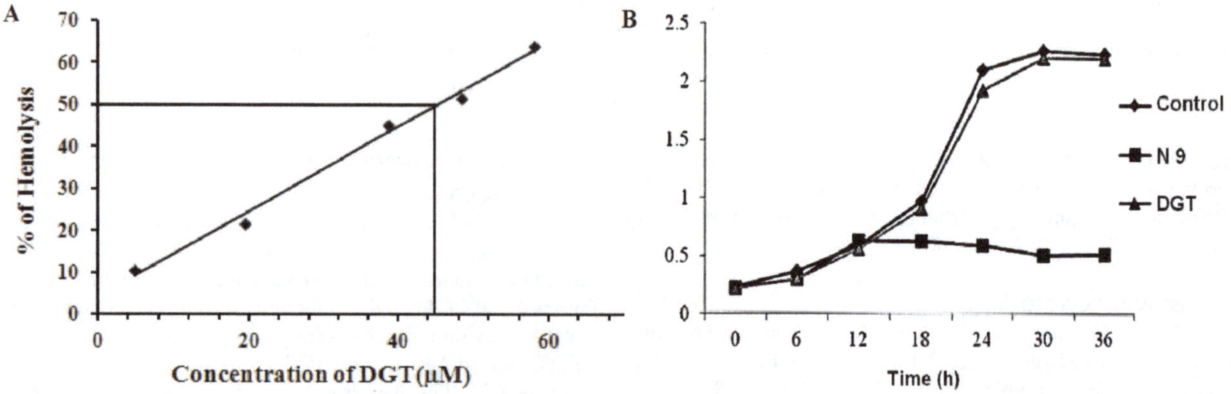

Figure 5. Irritation potential as measured by hemolytic activity and effect on *Lactobacillus acidophilus in vitro.* (A) Dose-dependent effect of DGT in rat RBCs. Isolated RBCs were incubated with varying drug dilutions, Triton X-100 and PBS. The extent of hemolysis was determined spectrophotometrically. (B) Effect of desgalactotigonin (DGT) and nonoxynol-9 on *Lactobacillus acidophilus*. [Optical density as the measure of turbidity denoting growth of bacterial colonies during 36 h of culture in the absence (control) and presence of DGT. There was a gradual increase in the growth of colonies that reached a plateau after 24 h of culture. Irrespective of the dose of DGT (19×MEC), the growth of bacterial colony was comparable with that of the control. N-9, however, exerted constant inhibition of bacterial growth throughout the entire culture period.]

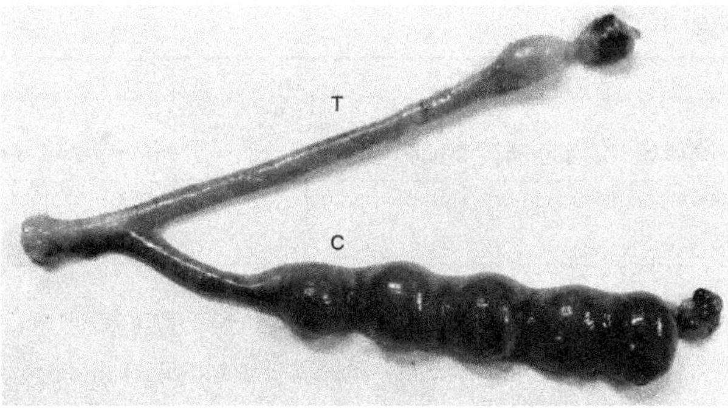

Figure 6. The contraceptive efficacy of DGT in Sprague-Dawley rats. Photograph of a uterus showing the presence or absence of implantation sites in the control [C] and DGT-treated [T] uterine horn of a Sprague–Dawley rat.

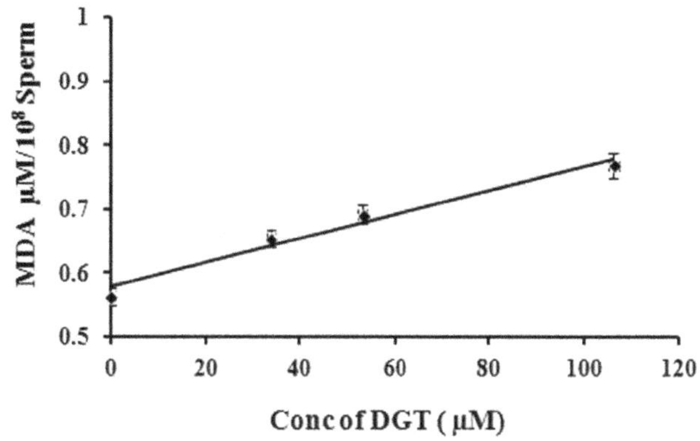

Figure 8. Effect of lipid peroxidation on human sperm. Generation of malondialdehyde (MDA) as a function of lipid peroxidation by human sperm treated with or without DGT at varying concentrations. Values on Y-axis represent mean ± SEM. values of five determinations ($P<0.05$). The graph shows dose-dependent increase in MDA generation following exposure of motile spermatozoa to DGT.

sperm immobilizing property. At a concentration of 24.18 μM in case of rat and 58.03 μM in case of human, DGT caused 100% immobilization of sperm within 20 s with no revival of motility after subsequent 60 min of incubation in Baker's buffer at 37°C. So, the values of 24.18 μM for rat and 58.03 μM for human were considered as minimum effective concentrations (MEC) and used for further studies. DGT thus requires low concentration for the preparation of local vaginal contraceptive.

Plasma membrane integrity is directly dependent on membrane permeability, which is indispensable for effective sperm motility during transport and fertilization. HOS test is an indicator of the structural and functional integrity of sperm membrane [30,31]. Plasma membrane is semi-permeable in living state; in hypo-osmotic condition, intact cell membrane facilitates free entrance of solvent in to the cell to attain osmotic equilibrium causing the cell to swell. Since the plasma membrane around the sperm tail fiber is more loosely bound as compared to the rest of the sperm, sperm cell is particularly susceptible to hypo-osmotic fluctuation and responds by curling. This characteristic feature was exhibited in > 90% of the sperm in control set, while the DGT exposed sperm showed no such morphological distortion. This experiment illustrated that the functional integrity of sperm membrane was totally lost on exposure to DGT. This conclusion was additionally validated by using fluorescent staining method. Sperm viability was assessed by using a membrane permanent nucleic acid dye

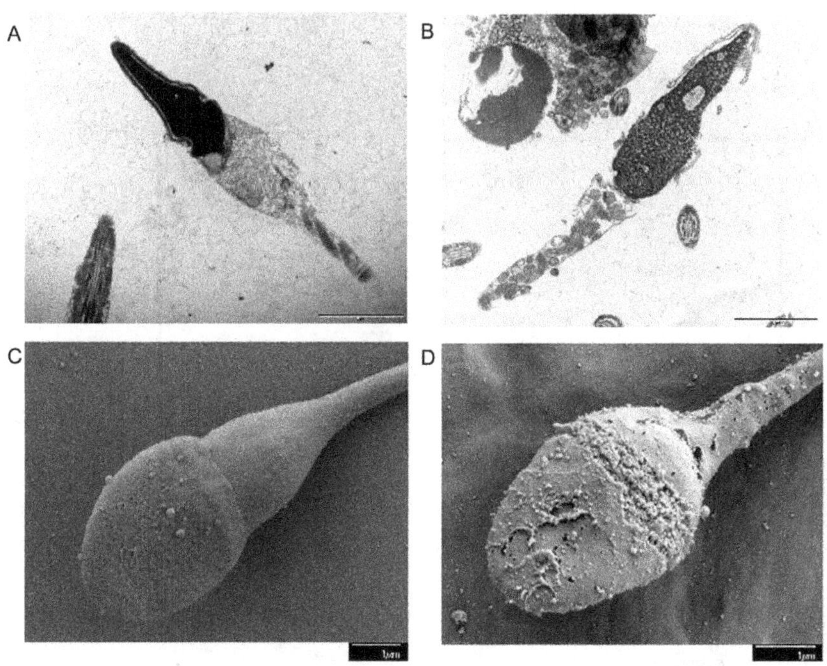

Figure 7. The microscopic ultrastructural changes in the sperm. Transmission electron micrographs of human sperm samples incubated in the absence or presence of DGT (at MEC). (A) Control spermatozoa show proper acrosomal cap with intact plasma membrane, while (B) DGT-treated spermatozoa exhibit dissolution of the acrosomal cap. High resolution scanning electron micrographs (×15000 and ×19000) of human sperm treated without and with DGT at MEC. (C) Control sperm shows intact acrosomal cap and plasma membrane around the head and neck regions, while (D) DGT-treated sperm demonstrates dissolution of the acrosomal cap.

Table 1. Spermicidal potential, cytotoxicity and selectivity index of DGT, N-9 [51].

Treatment	Spermicidal EC_{100} (μg/ml)	Spermicidal EC_{50} (μg/ml)	Cytotoxicity IC_{50} (μg/ml)	Selectivity Index (IC_{50}/EC_{50})	Safety versus N-9
DGT	60	29.8	135.54	4.55	529.06
N-9	486.82	78.34	0.675	0.0086	1

SYBR-14 (green, for live sperm) and PI (red, for dead sperm) [41]. In dual fluorescent staining method control spermatozoa appeared green while treated spermatozoa turned red. DGT treated sperm were almost 100% dead. All these observations reveal that DGT compromised sperm membrane integrity suggesting that there was an ultimate loss of functionality. Both TEM and SEM findings of human spermatozoa also illustrated that DGT treatment affected sperm membrane integrity with dissolution of outer acrosomal cap.

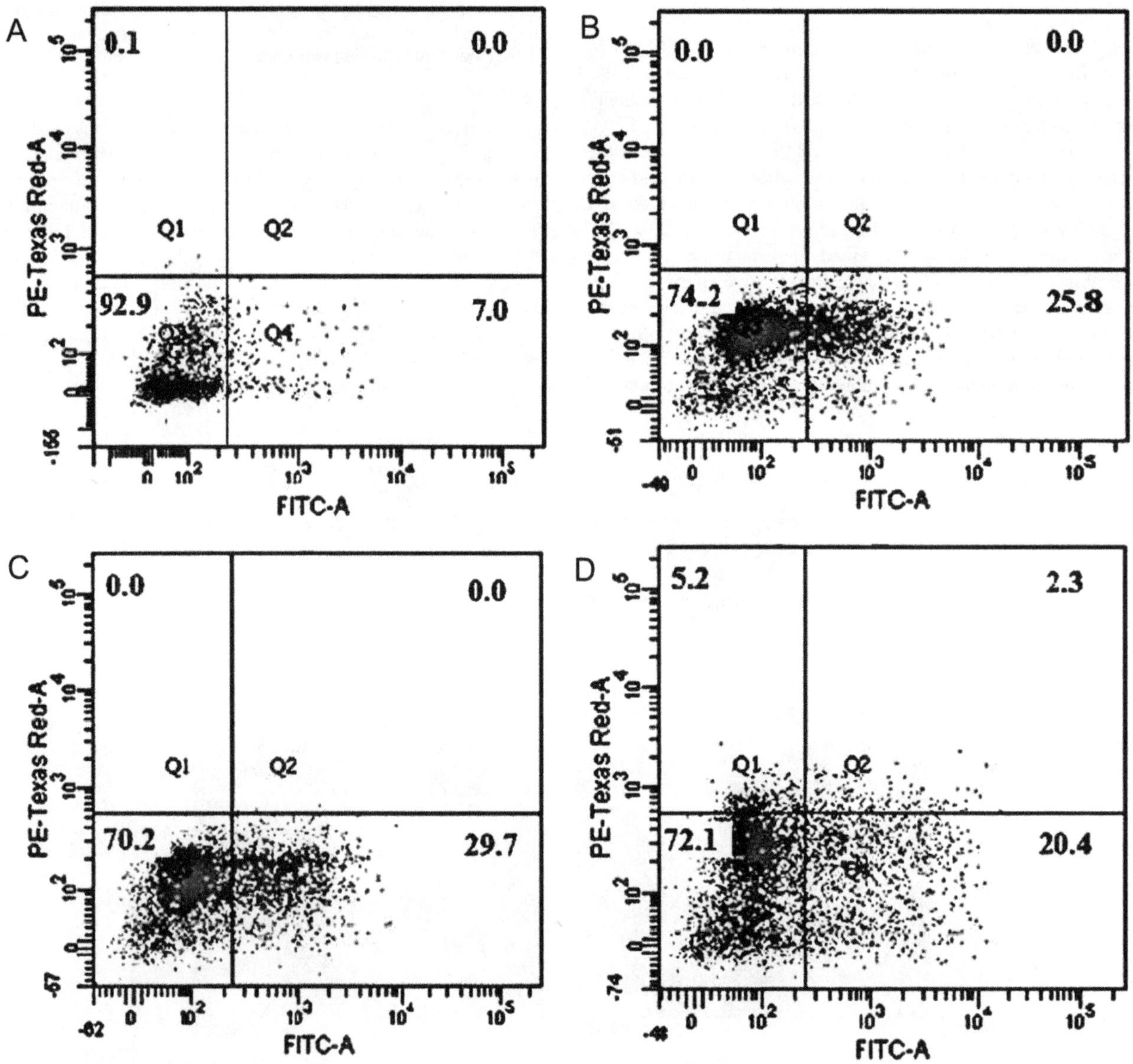

Figure 9. Apoptotic changes in plasma membrane. Representative images of apoptosis/necrosis induction by DGT in sperm cells, measured by Annexin-V/PI labelling and flow cytometry. Concentrations used were 29.01 μM, 58.03 μM and 106.38 μM of DGT against sperm for 3 h. [A. control, medium only, B. 29.01 μM DGT, C. 58.03 μM DGT, D. 106.38 μM DGT]. Cell population in four quadrants identified as: [lower left, live; lower right, apoptotic; upper right, necrotic; upper left, dead].

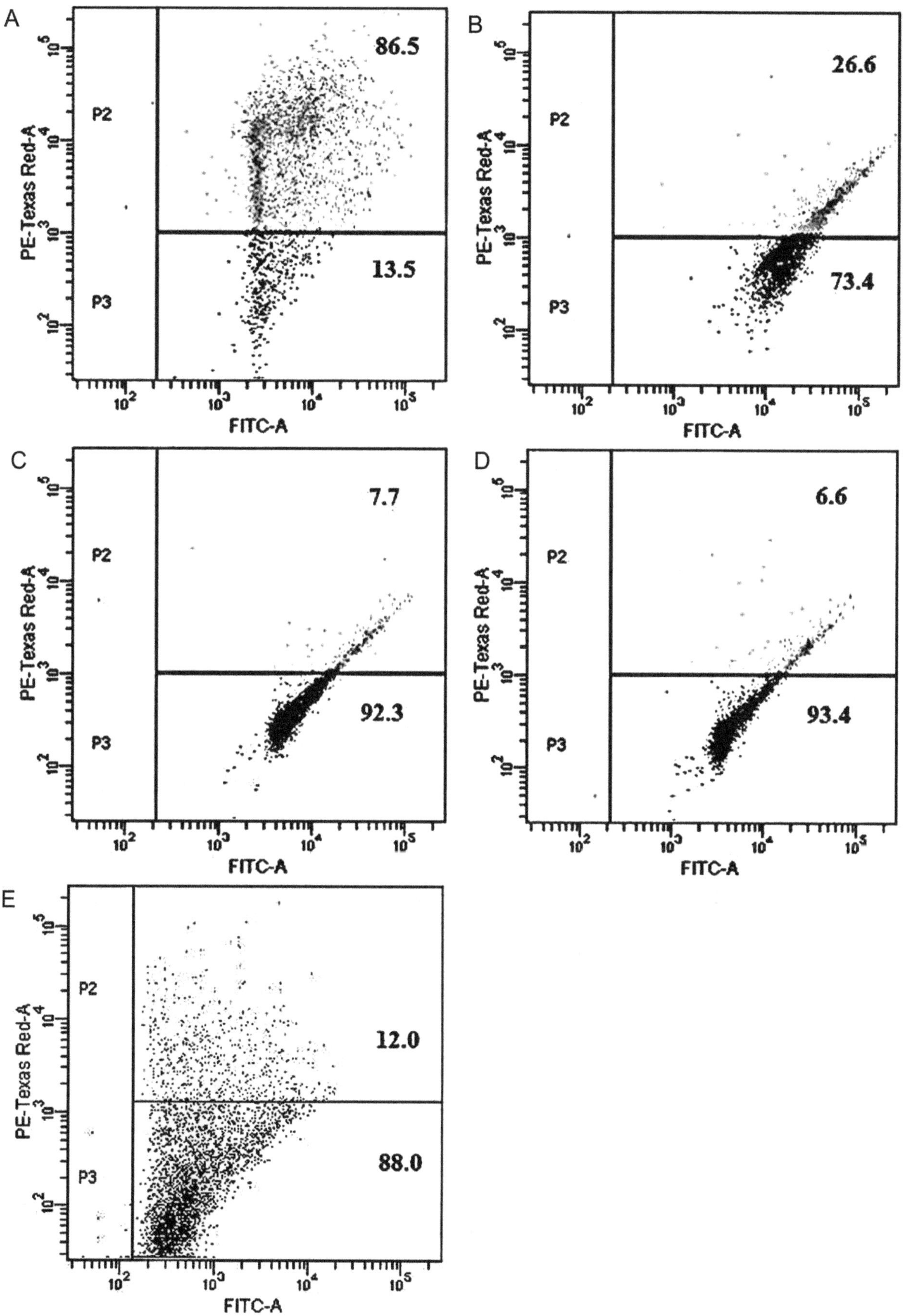
A
B
C
D
E
P2
P3
86.5
13.5
26.6
73.4
7.7
92.3
6.6
93.4
12.0
88.0
PE-Texas Red-A
FITC-A

Figure 10. Apoptotic changes in mitochondria. Representative illustration of the depolarization of mitochondrial transmembrane potential of sperm cells by DGT, measured by lipophilic cationic dye JC-1 staining. Concentrations used were 29.01 μM, 58.03 μM, and 106.38 μM against sperm for 3 h. [A. control, medium only, B. 29.01 μM DGT, C. 58.03 μM DGT, D. 106.38 μM DGT, E. CCCP]. Cell population in quadrants identified as: [upper right, polarized; lower right, depolarized].

The above conclusion was supported biochemically by the observation of increased lipid peroxidation. Mammalian sperm cells present highly specific lipid composition comprising a high proportion of polyunsaturated fatty acids, plasmalogens and sphingomyelins. Malondialdehyde is a product of LPO that appears to be produced in relatively constant proportion to the breakdown of polyunsaturated fatty acids [38,39]. Saponins have previously been reported to induce permeability change [42]. DGT being a saponin exerts similar mode of action. From this mechanism we deduced that DGT treated human spermatozoa totally lost their membrane integrity.

To evaluate the contraceptive efficacy of DGT we undertook in vivo investigation by using rat model. We wanted to utilize the advantage of bi-cornuate uterus with separate cervical opening of two uterine horns in rat. While one horn can serve as control, the other is the experimental one; both are exposed to identical systemic milieu. However, the rat model is not suitable for evaluating the efficacy of DGT as vaginal contraceptive because in this model mating involves disposition of sperm in the cervix, not in vagina [43]. Since sperm passes by the vagina to reach uterus, we introduced DGT directly into the uterine horn. The intrauterine applications of DGT in rats were significantly encouraging as fertility was reduced to zero on comparison with control.

Hemolytic index is a rapid screening assay of first order for the assessment of acute irritation potential of topically applicable microbicides or spermicides [44]. From this index, the subsequent doses which would be used for toxicity studies can be determined. At 45.5 μM of DGT, which is one and a half fold higher than MEC, 50% hemolysis occurred. However, further studies are required to explore the cytotoxicity of DGT.

The normal vaginal flora of healthy women is dominated by lactobacilli. Lactobacillus produces a number of compounds including lactic acid, hydrogen peroxide, lactacin and acidolin that maintain a low acidic pH (3.5–5.0) [45] and thereby protect against the pathogens that cause STIs including HIV [46,47]. Currently used spermicides are mainly N-9 based. The vaginal spermicide nonoxynol-9 does not protect against sexually transmitted diseases and HIV in clinical situation but may in fact increase their incidence due to its non specific, surfactant actions [48]. But, in microbial studies, the effect of DGT on *Lactobacillus* culture was different. From the result it appears that a 20 fold higher concentration of its MEC has no significant inhibitory activity on the growth of *Lactobacillus acidophilus* during 36 h of culture period.

MTT assay was used to evaluate the cytotoxicity in human cervical (HeLa) cell lines. DGT has not only potent sperm immobilizing property but has precise, targeted action that kills 100% spermatozoa in 20 s without affecting human cervical cell line viability for up to 24 h in vitro culture. The IC_{50} concentration of DGT for cytotoxicity towards HeLa cells was much lower than that for N-9. This indicates that, in comparison with N-9, this spermicide specifically and selectively targets sperm cells, which provides a safety index of orders of magnitude in its favour. This is the most notable characteristic of this molecule.

Flow cytometry has been extensively employed for the analysis of acrosomal integrity, mitochondrial function, and motility of spermatozoa to determine the fertilizing potential of human sperm sample. It is an automated approach that can measure the amount of one or more fluorescent stains associated with cells in an unbiased manner, offering properties of precision, sensitivity, accuracy, rapidity, and multiparametric analysis on a statistically relevant number of cells. The finer aspects of spermicidal action on sperm cell were therefore studied at EC_{50} concentration by flow cytometry. The compound DGT induced apoptosis in sperm cells, which was characterized by an increase in FITC-Annexin V labelling of human spermatozoa. DGT treatment induces apoptosis without causing any necrosis (green and red fluorescence) of human sperm cells. This further indicates the mechanism based action of DGT on human spermatozoa that is different from general dissolution of cell membrane.

The mitochondrial transmembrane potential maintains the integrity of mitochondrial polarization for normal energy generation and dissipation, [49] and a significant drop in this potential indicates initiation of apoptotic process [50]. The depolarization of sperm mitochondria and induction of apoptosis by DGT once again reflects the difference in mechanisms of action.

Although this compound belongs to the saponin family, it has no detergent like property and the vaginal ecosystem remains unhampered. The uniqueness of this compound is that it has four sugar moieties and high molecular weight (1034), one and half times that of the synthetic molecule N-9 (MW 617), which indicates a lesser chance of absorption through vaginal epithelia. It has good solubility and MEC of this compound is comparatively low. It is possible that this rendered the compound more effective and bioavailable. Moreover, N-9 hampers the vaginal ecosystem by inhibiting the growth of lactobacilli, leading to an increased risk of developing sexually transmitted diseases and HIV. But DGT at twenty fold higher concentration than its MEC has no harmful effect on vaginal flora. In todays world most women prefer an antimicrobial spermicide. This compound can suitably replace N-9 in vaginal preparations to make them more acceptable for repeated use. The results of this study lead us to propose that this naturally occurring compound selectively kills sperm without hampering lactobacilli and HeLa cells at MEC, indicating its potential as a superior ingredient for a future contraceptive formulation. However, further studies related to pathogen killing, local toxicity and teratogenic properties are to be carried out to prove it as a prophylactic contraceptive agent.

Statistical analysis

All biochemical observations were based on 5 independent experiments. Data were expressed as mean ± SEM or percentage. The results were analyzed by 1-way analysis of variance (ANOVA), and chi-square test, as applicable, using the Graph Pad Prism 3.0 software (Graph Pad software, Inc, San Diego, California). $P<0.05$ was considered significant.

Acknowledgments

The authors express their gratitude to the Director, IICB for laboratory facilities, and the Indian Council for Medical Research (ICMR) for providing the funding and fellowships to DC. NBM is indebted to CSIR for the award of Emeritus Scientist scheme. We express our gratitude to Dr. Sukdeb Banerjee and Dr. B. Achari (Ex. Emeritus Scientist, CSIR) for their valuable suggestions and also gratefully acknowledge the help received from Dr. Anirban Ash in acquiring the pictures on TEM and SEM. We are thankful to Dr. B. N. Chakravarty, Director, Institute of Reproductive Science, for his generous help by providing human semen samples for our study. Special thanks are due to Petra Masařová, Martina Tesařová, Jiří Vaněček (all from the Institute of Parasitology, České Budějovice) for their kind help in electron microscopy.

Author Contributions

Conceived and designed the experiments: DC AM. Performed the experiments: DC AM. Analyzed the data: DC AM. Contributed reagents/materials/analysis tools: NBM TJ. Wrote the paper: NBM TJ DC AM.

References

1. World Population Data-sheet/worldmap.aspx (2013) Available from http://www.prb.org/Publications/Datasheets/2013/2013-world-population-data-sheet/world-map.aspx; and also http://www.infoplease.com/world/statistics/world-population-seven-billion.html.
2. United Nations Population Fund. State of the world population (2011) New York: UNFPA; 2011. Available from http://www.unfpa.org/swp/.
3. Doncel GF (2006) Exploiting common targets in human fertilization and HIVinfection: development of novel contraceptive microbicides, Hum. Reprod 12 (2): 103–117.
4. ICPD '94: Summary of the programme of action. International Conference on Population and Development, United Nations. (1995) Available from:http:/www.un.org/ecosocdev/geninfo/populatin/icpd.htm.
5. Singh KK, Parmar S, Tatke PA (2012) Contraceptive efficacy and safety of HerbOshield™ vaginal gel in rats. Contraception 85: 122–127.
6. Shah HC, Tatke P, Singh KK (2008) Spermicidal agents: A review. Drug Discov Ther 2(4): 200–210.
7. Jain RK, Jain A, Maikhuri JP, Sharma VL, Dwivedi AK, et al. (2008) *In vitro* testing of rationally designed spermicides for selectively targeting human sperm in vagina to ensure safe contraception. Human Reprod 24: 590–601.
8. Shah V, Doncel GF, Seyoum T, Eaton KM, Zalenskaya I, et al. (2005) Sophorolipids, Microbial Glycolipids with Anti-Human Immuno-deficiency Virus and Sperm-Immobilizing Activities. Antimicrob Agents Chemother 49: 4093–4100.
9. Martin HL, Richardson BA, Nyange PM, Lavreys L, Hillier SL, et al. (1999) Vaginal lactobacilli, microbial flora And risk of human immunodeficiency virus type 1 and sexually transmitted disease acquisition. J Infect Dis 180: 1863–1868.
10. D'Cruz OJ, Shih MJ, Yiv SH, Chen CL, Uckun FM, et al. (1999) Synthesis, characterization and preclinical formulation of a dual-action phenyl phosphate derivative of bromo-methoxyzidovudine (compound WHI-07) with potent anti-HIV and spermicidal activities. Mol Hum Reprod 5: 421–432.
11. Renner R (1997) European bans on surfactant trigger transatlantic debate. Environ Sci Technol 31: A316–A320.
12. Thiele B, Gunther K, Schwuger MJ (1997) Alkylphenolethoxylates trace analysis and environmental behavior. Chem Rev 97: 3247–3272.
13. Roddy RE, Zeking L, Ryan KA, Tamoufe U, Weir SS, et al. (1998) A controlled trial of nonoxynol 9 film to reduce male-to-female transmission of sexually transmitted diseases. N Engl J Med 339: 504–510.
14. Paira P, Hazra A, Kumar S, Paira R, Sahu KB, et al. (2009) Efficient synthesis of 3,3-diheteroaromatic oxindole analogues and their in vitro evaluation for spermicidal potential. Bioorg Med Chem Lett 19: 4786–4789.
15. Bhowal SK, Lala S, Hazra A, Paira P, Banerjee S, et al. (2008) Synthesis and assessment of fertility regulating potential of 2-(2″-chloroacetamidobenzyl)-3-(3′-indolyl) quinoline in adult rats as a male contraceptive agent. Contraception 77: 214–222.
16. Bharitkar YP, Banerjee M, Kumar S, Paira R, Meda R, et al. (2013) Search for a potent microbicidal spermicide from the isolates of *Shorearobusta* resin. Contraception 88: 133–140.
17. Kumar S, Naskar S, Hazra A, Sarkar S, Mondal NB, et al. (2009) Evaluation of spermicidal potential of labdanediterpenes from *Andrographispaniculata*. Int J Biol Chem Sci 3: 628-636.
18. Kumar S, Biswas S, Mandal D, Roy HN, Chakraborty S, et al. (2007) *Chenopodium album* seed extract:a potent sperm-immobilizing agent both in vitro and in vivo. Contraception 75: 71–78.
19. Kumar S, Chatterjee R, Dolai S, Adak S, Kabir SN, et al. (2008) *Chenopodium album* seed extract induced sperm cell death: exploration of a plausible pathway, Contraception 77: 456–462.
20. Kumar S, Biswas S, Banerjee S, Mondal NB (2011) Evaluation of safety margins of *Chenopodium album* seed decoction: 14-day subacute toxicity and microbicidal activity studies. Reprod Biol Endocrin 9: 102–110.
21. Yan W, Ohtani K, Kasai R, Yamasaki K (1996) Steroidal saponins from fruits of *Triblusterrestris*. Phytochemistry 42: 1417–1422.
22. Das N, Chandran P, Chakraborty S (2011) Potent spermicidal effect of oleanolic acid 3-beta-D-glucuronide, an active principle isolated from the plant Sesbania sesban Merrill. Contraception 83: 167–175.
23. Lavaud C, Voutquenne L, Bal P, Pouny I (2000) Saponins from *Chenopodium album*. Fitoterapia 71(3): 338–340.
24. Briggers JD, Whitten WK, Whittengham DG (1977) The culture of mouse-embryo in vitro. In: Daniel JD, editor. Methods in mammalion embryology. San Francisco: WH Freeman and Co. 41–54.
25. World Health Organization [WHO] (1999) Laboratory Manual for the Examination of Human Semen and Cervical Mucus Interaction, edn 4. New York: Cambridge University Press.
26. Sander FV, Cramer SD (1941) A practical method for testing the spermicidal action of chemical contraceptives. Hum Fertil 6: 134–137.
27. Green TR, Fellman JH, Wofl DP (2001) Human spermicidal activity of inorganic and organic oxidants. Fertil Steril 76: 157–162.
28. Paul D, Bera S, Jana D, Maiti R, Ghosh D, et al. (2006) *In vitro* determination of the contraceptive spermicidal activity of a composite extract of Achyranthe-saspera and Stephaniahernandifolia on human semen. Contraception 73: 284–288.
29. Maikhuri JP, Dwivedi AK, Dhar JD, Setty BS, Gupta G, et al. (2003) Mechanism of action of some acrylophenones, quinolines and dithiocarbamate as potent, non-detergent spermicidal agents. Contraception 67: 403–408.
30. Lee CH (1996) Review: In vitro spermicidal tests. Contraception 54: 131–147.
31. Cuneo MF, Ruiz RD, Tissera A, Estofan D, Molina RI, et al. (2006) Improving the predictive value of the hypoosmotic swelling test in humans. FertilSteril 85: 1840–1842.
32. Flajshans M, Cosson J, Rodina M, Linhart O (2004) The application of image cytometry to viability assessment in dual fluorescence-stained fish spermatozoa. International Journal of Cell Biology 28: 955–959.
33. Fowler PT, Doncel GF, Bummer PM, Digenis GA (2003) Coprecipitation of nonoxynol-9 with polyvinylpyrrolidone to decrease vaginal irritation potential while maintaining spermicidal potency. AAPS Pharm Sci Tech 4: 1–8.
34. McFarland J (1907) The nephelometer: an instrument for estimating the number of bacteria in suspensions used for calculating the opsonic index and for vaccines. J Am Med Assoc 49: 1176–1178.
35. Chattopadhyay D, Sinha B, Vaid LK (1998b) Antibacterial activity of *Syzygium*species: A report. Fitoterapia 69: 365–367.
36. Kuete V, Ango YP, Fotso WG, Kapche DWFG, Dzoyem PJ, et al. (2011) Antimicrobial activities of the methanol extract and compound from *Artocarpuscommunis* (Moraceae). BMC Complementary and Alternative Medicine 11: 42.
37. Niksirat H, Kouba A, Pšenička M, Kuklina I, Kozak P, et al. (2013) Ultrastructure of spermatozoa from three genera of crayfish Orconectes, Procambarus and Astacus (Decapoda: Astacoidea): New findings and comparisons. ZoologischerAnzeiger – A Journal of Comparative Zoology 252(2): 226–233.
38. Buege JA, Aust SD (1978) Microsomal lipid peroxidation. Eds S Fleischer & L Packer. London: Academic Press, In Methods in Enzymology 52: 302–310.
39. Suleiman SA, Ali ME, Zaki MS, Malik EMEA, Nast MA, et al. (1996) Lipid peroxidation and human sperm motility: protective role of vitamin E. Journal of Andrology17: 530–537.
40. Anzar M, He L, Buhr MM, Kroetsch TG, Pauls KP, et al. (2002) Sperm apoptosis in fresh and cryopreserved bull semen detected by flow cytometry and its relationship with fertility. BiolReprod 66: 354–360.
41. Garner DL, Johnson LA (1995) Viability assessment of mammalian sperm using SYBR-14 and propidium iodide. Biology of Reproduction 53: 276–284.
42. Saha P, Majumdar S, Pal D, Pal BC, Kabir SN, et al. (2010) Evaluation of spermicidal activity of Mi-saponin A. Reprod Sci 17: 454–464.
43. Castle PE, Hoen TE, Whaley KJ, Cone RA (1998) Contraceptive testing of vaginal agents in rabbits. Contraception58: 51–60.
44. Pape W, Pfannenbecker U, Hoppe U (1987) Validation of the red blood cell test system as in vitro assay for the rapid screening of irritation potential of surfactants. Mol Toxicol 88: 525.
45. Hawes SE, Hillier SL, Benedetti J, Stevens CE, Koutsky LA, et al. (1996) Hydrogen peroxide producing lactobacilli and acquisition of vaginal infections. Journal of Infectious Diseases 174: 1058–1063.
46. Kempf C, Jentsch P, Barre-Sinoussi FB, Poirier B, Morgenthaler JJ, et al. (1991) Inactivation of human immunodeficiency virus (HIV) by low pH and pepsin. Journal of Acquired Immune Deficiency Syndromes 4: 828–830.
47. Klebanoff SJ, Coombs RW (1991) Viricidal effect of Lactobacillus acidophilus on human immunodeficiency virus type-1: possible role in heterosexual transmission. Journal of Experimental Medicine 174: 289–292.

48. WHO/CONRAD (2002) Technical Consultation on nonoxynol-9 World Health Organization, Geneva, 9-10 Oct, 2001,Summary Report, Reprod Health Matters 10(20): 175–181.
49. Bains R, Moe MC, Larsen GA, Berg-Johnsen J, Vinje ML, et al. (2006) Volatile anaesthetics depolarize neural mitochondria by inhibition of the electron transport chain. Acta Anaesthesiol Scand 50: 572–579.
50. Chaoui D, Faussat AM, Majdak P, Tang R, Perrot JY, et al. (2006) JC-1, a sensitive probe for a simultaneous detection of P-glycoprotein activity and apoptosis in leukemic cells. Cytometry B Clin Cytom70:189–196.
51. Jain RK, Jain A, Maikhuri JP, Sharma VL, Dwivedi AK, et al. (2009) In vitro testing of rationally designed spermicides for selectively targeting human sperm in vagina to ensure safe contraception. Human Reproduction 24:590–601.

11

Identification of Unprecedented Anticancer Properties of High Molecular Weight Biomacromolecular Complex Containing Bovine Lactoferrin (HMW-bLf)

Fawzi Ebrahim[1☯¶¤], Jayanth Suryanarayanan Shankaranarayanan[1☯¶], Jagat R. Kanwar[1], Sneha Gurudevan[1], Uma Maheswari Krishnan[2], Rupinder K. Kanwar[1]*

1 Nanomedicine-Laboratory of Immunology and Molecular Biomedical Research, School of Medicine, Faculty of Health, Deakin University, Geelong, Victoria, Australia, **2** Centre for Nanotechnology & Advanced Biomaterials (CeNTAB), School of Chemical & Biotechnology, SASTRA University, Thanjavur, India

Abstract

With the successful clinical trials, multifunctional glycoprotein bovine lactoferrin is gaining attention as a safe nutraceutical and biologic drug targeting cancer, chronic-inflammatory, viral and microbial diseases. Interestingly, recent findings that human lactoferrin oligomerizes under simulated physiological conditions signify the possible role of oligomerization in the multifunctional activities of lactoferrin molecule during infections and in disease targeting signaling pathways. Here we report the purification and physicochemical characterization of high molecular weight biomacromolecular complex containing bovine lactoferrin (≥250 kDa), from bovine colostrum, a naturally enriched source of lactoferrin. It showed structural similarities to native monomeric iron free (Apo) lactoferrin (~78–80 kDa), retained anti-bovine lactoferrin antibody specific binding and displayed potential receptor binding properties when tested for cellular internalization. It further displayed higher thermal stability and better resistance to gut enzyme digestion than native bLf monomer. High molecular weight bovine lactoferrin was functionally bioactive and inhibited significantly the cell proliferation ($p<0.01$) of human breast and colon carcinoma derived cells. It induced significantly higher cancer cell death (apoptosis) and cytotoxicity in a dose-dependent manner in cancer cells than the normal intestinal cells. Upon cellular internalization, it led to the up-regulation of caspase-3 expression and degradation of actin. In order to identify the cutting edge future potential of this bio-macromolecule in medicine over the monomer, its in-depth structural and functional properties need to be investigated further.

Editor: Andrea Motta, National Research Council of Italy, Italy

Funding: The work was funded by Australia-India Strategic Research Fund (AISRF, BF 030016). The financial support for Postgraduate Fellowships from Deakin University and Ministry of Higher Education of Libya and BTRC is gratefully acknowledged. The funders had no role in study design, data collection and analysis, decision to publish, or preparation of the manuscript.

Competing Interests: The authors have declared that no competing interests exist.

* Email: rupinder.kanwar@deakin.edu.au

☯ These authors contributed equally to this work.

¶ FE and JSS are shared first authors on this work.

¤ Current address: Biotechnology Research Center (BTRC), Tripoli, Libya

Introduction

Clinical and mechanistic research over the past few decades has indicated significant relationships between nutrition and health. The clinical studies with bovine milk derived cancer preventive multifunctional protein lactoferrin (bLf) are currently a promising field of research. Lactoferrin (Lf) is an iron binding ~78–80 kDa glycoprotein of the transferrin family found to be widely distributed in mammalian milk and most other exocrine secretions such as tears, nasal and bronchial mucous, saliva etc. [1]. Lf comprises of ~700 amino acids with two symmetrical lobes forming a single polypeptide chain. Each lobe is further subdivided into two domains that harbor the iron binding sites [2]. In its natural form, native monomeric-bLf (NM-bLf) is approximately 15-20% saturated with Fe^{3+} ions [3]. bLf's role in mammalian iron homeostasis, organ morphogenesis, and bridging innate and adaptive immune functions has resulted in its potential applications in the medical field, along with its wide use as a current nutraceutical and a safe food supplement [1,4,5]. More recently, based on the success of animal feeding studies and human clinical trials, bLf has gained significant attention for its prospective use as a safer anti-cancer chemopreventive and therapeutic agent [5,6,7].

Because of the worldwide interest in bLf's health and medical applications, investigators for several decades have searched for the most convenient way to produce bLf. Today, native ~78–80 kDa bLf is mostly produced at a commercial scale from skim milk or whey and bovine colostrum (BC) [4]. When compared to milk, BC is a naturally rich source of bLf, known to contain 1.5–5.0 g L^{-1} of bLf. BC is a thick yellow fluid produced during the first few days after calf's birth. It is known to contain immune, and growth factors to support the growth of the young calf, and also to prevent gastrointestinal infections until the calf develops its own active immune defense [8].

Attempts have also been made to explore the multifunctional nature of Lf. Considering Lf's apparently higher concentrations found in mammalian secretions during the acute phase of infection, inflammation, and its interactions with a range of cells and biomacromolecules (proteins, DNA, oligosaccharides, mono-nucleotides), a possible role of oligomerization of Lf has been suggested [9]. Earlier, it has been demonstrated that tetramer is the dominating form of human Lf (hLf) found under physiological conditions [10]. Being an acute phase protein with conformational flexibility, Lf can self-assemble into larger structures. However, molecular level explanation for this process is scarce, and investigations are still underway to unravel this property of Lf. Recently, by employing different techniques such as gel filtration, soft laser ablation, small-angle X-ray scattering (SAXS), and light scattering (LS), hLf has been reported to oligomerize into several high molecular weight (HMW) aggregates (70 kDa–800 kDa). The level of oligomerization was reported to depend on the concentrations of Lf, KCl, NaCl and also on the duration of the protein storage in solution [11]. Interestingly, the addition of oligonucleotides, oligosaccharides, or mononucleotides to hLf in the presence or absence of KCl accelerated the oligomerization rate leading to the formation of associates containing ten or more protein molecules. The presence of ions, ATP, NAD, nucleotides, DNA or polysaccharides can further effect the self-association of Lf molecule under physiological conditions [11]. These findings suggest the importance of oligomerization for the multifunctional activities of Lf during host–pathogen interactions, and also in targeting cellular and molecular components of disease signaling pathways.

Chromatographic analysis of bovine milk reveals that the bLf is also found to elute as high molecular weight (HMW) mass complexes corresponding to its monomers, dimers and trimers [12]. Moreover, thermal treatments have been reported to induce bLf aggregation into high molecular weight polymers, and this self-association depends on iron saturation. The thermal stability of bLf markedly increases with iron saturation leading to decrease in the formation of larger aggregates [13]. The oligomerization of bLf therefore can have, varied implications for its biological functions and iron binding abilities. Whether HMW-bLf aggregates/oligomers retain their functional activities like monomer is presently unknown. Due to extensive health promoting activities of monomeric bLf, it becomes essential to unravel the biological functions of HMW-bLf/oligomers of bLf. In this study, we first investigated if it was possible to purify HMW-bLf/oligomers of bLf from BC which is known to contain a high concentration of bLf. We then tested if the HMW-bLf/oligomeric bLf was structurally and immunochemically similar to a native monomeric bLf (NM-bLf). As a proof of concept, by using robust *in vitro* cell bioassays with human breast (MDA-MB-231) and colon cancer (SW480) cell lines from ATCC, we further determined if HMW-bLf/oligomeric bLf potentially targeted cancer cell proliferation and cell death. Another ATCC cell line FHs 74 Int, derived from normal human fetal intestine has been reported to show mature epithelial-like characteristics [14]. It was also employed to investigate the effects of HMW-bLf on normal cells.

Materials and Methods

i) Purification of HMW-bLf from bovine colostrum whey

The colostrum sample was obtained from an Australian farm, which was milked normally during postpartum/postnatal period (first 2–4 days after calf's birth). The sample was obtained with the permission from the farm to collect and use it for the study. To obtain the whey proteins, the high viscous colostrum sample was diluted with sterile PBS (pH 7.4). Diluted colostrum sample was skimmed by centrifugation at 3000×g at 4°C for 30 min. The fat (yellow layer) was discarded, and the supernatant was collected and processed immediately or kept frozen at −20°C.

Casein removal by acid precipitation. The skimmed diluted bovine colostrum sample as obtained above was acidified by 1 M HCl until it reached pH 4.6 to achieve isoelectric precipitation of casein. The precipitated casein was removed by centrifugation (3500×g for 30 min at 4°C); the supernatant was collected, and the pH was adjusted to pH 7.4.

Cation-exchange chromatography. HMW-bLf was further purified using cation exchange chromatography on SP-Sepharose following the modified procedure of Van Berkel *et al.* [15]. Briefly, the column was packed with SP-Sepharose food grade big beads (Amersham biosciences, 17-0657-03). Before first use, the stationary phase was washed with 5 column volumes of water followed by 5 column volumes of 1 M NaCl. It was left in 1 M NaCl for 12 h and then in 5 column volumes of water. The skimmed colostrum after casein removal was diluted in the ratio of 1:1 with the dilution buffer (0.04 M NaH_2PO_4, 0.8 M NaCl, 0.04% (v/v) Tween 20, pH 7.4), and filtered through 0.45 µm and 0.22 µm filters. The diluted colostrum sample was then loaded in the column and allowed to pass through the column at a flow rate of 0.3 mL min^{-1}. Following this, the SP-Sepharose was repeatedly washed with washing buffer (0.02 M NaH_2PO_4, 0.4 M NaCl, 0.02% (v/v) Tween 20, pH 7.4) to remove the unbound whey proteins. Bovine Lf was then eluted with the elution buffer (0.02 M NaH_2PO_4, 1 M NaCl, pH 7.4). The column was run at a flow rate of 3 mL min^{-1}. The eluted fractions were dialyzed extensively with a 100 kDa cut off dialysis membrane (Spectrum Labs) against sterile Milli-Q water for 24 h. The purity check and the characterization of eluted fractions were further carried out as described in the following section.

ii) Characterization of HMW-bLf

SDS-PAGE and Western blotting. The purity and molecular weight of purified fractions were analyzed by SDS-PAGE. Following electrophoresis, Western blotting was carried out to confirm the purity and identity of HMW-bLf. The protein was transferred on to a PVDF membrane and probed for bLf with goat anti- bLf antibody (Bethyl Laboratories) diluted in the ratio of 1:1000 for 1 h at 37°C and secondary anti-goat HRP (Sigma-Aldrich) for 1 h at 37°C with appropriate washing with TBS-T (137 mM NaCl, 20 mM Tris, 0.1% Tween 20, pH 7.6). The membrane was developed using ECL chemiluminescence reagent (GE) in ChemiDoc XRS gel doc (Bio-Rad). Protein samples were freeze-dried for further characterization studies.

Dissociation of HMW-bLf into monomers and dimers. In order to identify the homogeneity of HMW-bLf, analysis of the components of HMW-bLf was further carried out by dissociating the complex into its dimeric and monomeric forms in the presence of 1 M NaCl as described earlier for hLf [11]. The study reported that hLf oligomers dissociate fast and almost completely to monomers in the presence of high concentrations (≥1.0 M) of Na^+ or K^+. Briefly, 3 mg mL^{-1} of HMW-bLf was dissolved in 50 mM Tris HCl (pH 7.5) containing 1 M NaCl and incubated for 1 day at 37°C. SDS-PAGE was carried out to analyze the dissociation of HMW-bLf complex into its components [11]. Western blotting was carried out to analyze the obtained protein bands by goat anti- bLf (Bethyl Laboratories) diluted in the ratio of 1:1000 to confirm the presence of lactoferrin.

Detection of Lipopolysaccharide (LPS) content. The presence of any LPS activity was measured using E-Toxate assay kit (Sigma-Aldrich). Briefly, 10 mg of purified and freeze-dried

HMW-bLf protein was dissolved in endotoxin-free water to prepare a test stock solution of 10 mg mL^{-1}, from which serial dilutions of the protein were made to obtain 1, 0.5, 0.1 and 0.01 mg mL^{-1} solutions. Endotoxin standards were prepared from the stock solution (400 EU mL^{-1}) to obtain standards of different endotoxin concentrations of 40, 4, 0.4 and 0.04 EU mL^{-1} solutions. Endotoxin free water supplied with the kit was used as a negative control. E-Toxate reagent working solution containing Limulus Amebocyte Lysate (LAL) was prepared according to the manufacturer's instructions. To 0.1 mL of the test/standards/controls, 0.1 mL of E-Toxate reagent working solution was added in 10×75 mm sterile fresh glass tube. The tubes were covered with parafilm and were incubated at 37°C for 1 h without disturbance. After 1 h the tubes were taken out and observed for gelation by tilting them to 120°. The formation of a solid gel was considered a positive result. Semi-solid and watery gels were considered as negative for endotoxin activity. The final endotoxin concentration in the test samples was calculated as; Endotoxin (EU mL-1) = (1/Highest dilution at which the sample was positive)*(Lowest dilution at which endotoxin standard found negative), and it is represented as endotoxin units per mg of the protein.

Determination of iron content in HMW-bLf. The iron saturation level in purified HMW-bLf was determined as described earlier by Kanwar *et al.* (2008) [16]. Briefly, to 1 mL of each sample, 50 µL of ascorbic acid was added and allowed to stand for 10 min. Iron standards representing a range of iron concentrations and blank (Milli-Q water) were used to plot a calibration curve. Samples were then centrifuged at 10000 rpm for 20 min. 500 µL supernatant collected from each sample was added into new tubes containing 100 µL of alkaline acetate solution followed by addition of 75 µL of tripyridyl solution. Two hundred microliters of each solution were then transferred into an optically clear 96 well plate, and the absorbance was read at 550 nm. Commercially obtained native LPS free monomeric bLf (NM-bLf) was used to prepare iron saturated (Fe-bLf) and iron free (Apo-bLf) according to the previously described method developed in our laboratory by Kanwar *et al.* (2008) [5,16]. These forms were used as controls for all the assays.

Differential scanning calorimetry (DSC). 5 mg of bLf was measured accurately by sensitive balance and sealed into an aluminum pan. DSC (TA instrument DSC Q200) scans were programmed in the temperature range of 35–110°C and at heating rate of 10°C min^{-1}. Native monomeric bovine lactoferrin (NM-bLf) ~78 kDa was used as a control, along with its iron depleted (Apo-bLf) and iron saturated (Fe-bLf) forms to determine the thermal stability of these proteins.

Fourier Transform Infrared Spectroscopy (FTIR) analysis. Samples were mixed with 200 mg of KBr (Sigma-Aldrich) powder and pelleted into a KBr disc using a hydraulic press. FTIR spectroscopy (Bio-Rad with OPUS 5.5 software) analysis was performed between 4000 and 450 cm^{-1} at a resolution of 4 cm^{-1} averaging 10 scans.

Gut enzyme intestinal digestion assay. Omnizyme cocktail represents most of the gut enzymes responsible for digestion of proteins, carbohydrates and fats [14]. Omnizyme (Rainrock Nutritionals) enzyme solution was added to the purified HMW-bLf (1:50) to investigate its stability against gut enzymes. The supernatants collected at different time intervals of (4 h, 6 h and 8 h) were heated at 42°C for 7 min to arrest the enzyme activity and all samples were analyzed by SDS-PAGE.

iii) Cell bioassays

MDA-MB-231, SW480 and FHs 74 Int cells were obtained from American Type Culture Collection (ATCC, supplied by Cryosite). MDA-MB-231 has been derived from *Homo sapiens* (female) breast carcinoma while SW480 cell line was derived from *Homo sapiens* (male) colorectal adenocarcinoma. Both MDA-MB-231 and SW480 cell lines were epithelial and had adherent growth properties. Both the cell lines were routinely cultured in L-15 media containing 10% FBS at 37°C without CO_2. FHs 74 Int is a cell line from normal human fetal intestinal tissue, and it was grown in DMEM with 10% FBS at 37°C under 5% CO_2.

Cell cytotoxicity (LDH release) assay. Cytotoxicity caused by treatments with HMW-bLf and other control forms of bLf was measured by release of lactate dehydrogenase (LDH) following cellular injury or cytotoxic insult. The cytotoxicity detection kit (Roche Applied Science) was used according to manufacturer's instructions. The assay is based on calculating the LDH leakage into the culture medium after 24 h following exposure of cells to different treatments. LDH is constitutively present in all cells and is released into supernatant due to cell membrane damage. MDA-MB-231 SW480 and FHs 74 Int cells were treated with media containing different treatment concentrations (800, 1600, 2400, 3200 µg mL^{-1}) of HMW-bLf for 24 h. Each treatment was carried out three times, in triplicates. The absorbance values were measured by using a SH-1000 lab absorbance microplate reader (Corona Electric) at 492 nm with reference wavelength at 620 nm. All values were the product of background subtraction with media alone reacting to the LDH reagent. Addition of Apo-bLf, Fe-bLf and HMW-bLf to the media did not alter the background reading. The % cytotoxicity was calculated by the formula; Cytotoxicity % = [(Exp. value-Low control)/(High control-Low control)] ×100.

Negative control (Low control) used was the cell culture supernatant of untreated cells and positive control (High control) representing the maximum value of LDH release was the cell culture supernatant of the cells treated with 1% (v/v) Triton X-100 (Sigma-Aldrich, Sydney, Australia). All obtained values for treatments are represented relative to untreated control value set to zero.

Cell proliferation assay. The inhibition of cell proliferation caused by bLf treatments was analyzed by determining the DNA content of the cell using CyQuant assay kit (Invitrogen) as per manufacturer's instructions. Briefly, viable MDA-MB-231 and SW480 cells were plated, initially at a concentration of 2×10^5 cells/mL in 96 well microplates and incubated overnight. Cells were then treated with fresh media containing different treatment concentrations (800, 1600, 2400, 3200 µg mL^{-1}) of HMW-bLf for 24 h and the media was aspirated out. The CyQuant reagent was then added to the cell pellet, and the corresponding fluorescence from the DNA was measured using a fluorescence reader at an excitation wavelength of 490 nm and emission of 530 nm. Treatments with different doses of HMW-bLf were carried out in triplicates, and the assay was repeated three times. Media with 20% FBS was used as a positive control. Background measurements for the plate alone with CyQuant reagent were subtracted from the test values.

Measurement of cell death by Flow cytometry. MDA-MB-231, SW480 and FHs 74 Int cells were treated with different concentrations of HMW-bLf for 24 h, and then trypsinized. Cell pellets were washed with sterile PBS and resuspended in 500 µL sterile PBS containing 0.1 mg mL^{-1} Propidium Iodide (PI) solution. PI is a fluorochrome that intercalates into double-stranded nucleic acids. After 15 min of incubation in dark at room temperature, the cells were analyzed for cell death (viability counts) using Flow cytometry (BD FACSCanto II). Untreated unstained cells were used to set up the instrument for acquisition, and the gating was adjusted to have <1% PI positive cells. The test samples were acquired after this under the same settings, and the percentage of cells in the PI positive gate was considered as the percentage dead cells.

Cellular internalization of HMW-bLf. Cellular uptake of HMW-bLf was studied by immunofluorescence and visualized by confocal microscopy. SW480, MDA-MB-231 and FHs 74 Int cells were seeded in an 8-chamber multi-well slide (BD falcon) at a density of 1×10^5 cells/well and were then treated with 800 $\mu g\ mL^{-1}$ of HMW-bLf for different time intervals in assay media (basal cell media with 1% FBS). Cells (to be treated as well as the untreated) were pre-conditioned to the assay media for 24 h before the actual assay by culturing in the assay media and remained healthy. Following treatment, the medium was removed, and the cells were washed thoroughly using PBS (pH 7.4) to remove unbound and non-internalized HMW-bLf from the cell layer, followed by fixation with 4% paraformaldehyde. After fixation, the cells were permeabilized with 0.1% TritonX-100 for 5 min on ice. Blocking was carried out with 2% sterile rabbit serum in PBS and cells were then incubated with primary antibody, goat anti-bovine lactoferrin (Bethyl Laboratories) at a dilution of 1:200 in PBS at 37°C for 1 h. The primary antibody was then removed and after washing, cells were incubated with anti-goat IgG-FITC conjugate (Sigma-Aldrich) and counterstained for actin with Phalloidin-AlexaFluor 568 (Invitrogen) and nucleus with DAPI in fluorshield (Sigma-Aldrich). The slides were imaged using TCS SP5 Leica broadband confocal microscope and processed using LAS-AF software. Media containing 1% FBS was used to avoid any protein-protein interactions during treatments. Because we used the lower FBS concentration in the assay media than the normal growth media, the cell viability was checked with trypan blue exclusion assay, before performing cellular uptake studies. No difference was noted between the cells ability to exclude the trypan blue dye when cells were grown in media containing 10% FBS or of that in 1% FBS for 24 h (Figure S1 in File S1). The 800 $\mu g\ mL^{-1}$ of HMW-bLf concentration was used for its comparatively lower cytotoxic effects on cancer cells. As a result following incubation with these treatments, lesser cell detachment (of dying/dead cells) was observed from the slide, and the cell monolayer survived the staining and imaging procedure.

Caspase-3 assays. Activation of cellular apoptosis was determined by caspase-3 activation assay using the method described by Fujie *et al.* [17]. Cells were treated with different concentrations of HMW-bLf and Fe-bLf (3200 $\mu g\ mL^{-1}$) for 24 h. Cells were lysed, centrifuged, and supernatant containing 100 $\mu g\ mL^{-1}$ protein lysates were taken for analysis from each treatment. 50 µL of mixture reagent (Dithiothreitol (DTT) in radio-immunoprecipitation assay RIPA buffer solution) was added. Finally, 6 µL of substrate acetyl-Asp-Glu-Val- Asp p-nitroanilide (Sigma-Aldrich) dissolved in dimethyl sulfoxide (DMSO) at 10 $mg\ mL^{-1}$ was added to all samples. The plate was then incubated for 180 min at room temperature in dark. Level of caspase-3 expression was quantified by using SH-1000 lab absorbance microplate reader (Corona Electric) at 405 nm.

The activation of cleaved caspase-3 was also confirmed using Western blot for cleaved caspase-3. Cells were treated with different concentrations of HMW-bLf, Apo-bLf and Fe-bLf (3200 $\mu g\ mL^{-1}$) for 24 h. Cells were lysed using RIPA (Radio Immuno-Precipitation Assay) buffer, and 75 µg of total protein was loaded for the SDS-PAGE. The proteins were then transferred to a PVDF membrane using Trans-Blot Turbo (Bio-Rad) semidry transfer instrument. The membrane was blocked using 3% skim milk for one hour after which they were probed using cleaved caspase-3(Asp175) primary antibody (Cell Signaling Technology) in the dilution of 1:500 at 37°C for 1 h. The primary antibody was then removed, and the membranes were washed thrice with TBS-T to remove unbound primary antibodies. It was then incubated with 1:40000 anti-rabbit HRP secondary antibody (Sigma) for 1 h at 37°C. After incubation, the secondary antibody was removed and membrane was washed three times with TBS-T. The membrane was developed using ECL chemiluminescence reagent (Amersham) and viewed under Chemi-doc XRS gel documentation system (Bio-Rad).

Statistical analysis. Data was expressed as mean values (±SD) and Student's t-test was performed for evaluating statistical significance. A value of ($p<0.05$) denotes statistical significance, whereas ($p \leq 0.01$) denotes results that are highly significant. All treatments were tested in triplicate, and each assay was repeated 3 times.

Results and Discussion

HMW biomacromolecular complex containing bLf was purified from skimmed defatted, casein free colostrum whey using cation exchange chromatography with SP Sepharose food grade big beads. Casein from skimmed bovine colostrum was completely precipitated at lower pH and was removed. The whey obtained was therefore casein and fat free. Lactoferrin has an Iso-electric point of pH 8.7 which is the highest among all the milk proteins. Hence bLf remains positively charged even at the near neutral pH of 7.4. It binds very strongly to the cation exchange resin whereas other whey proteins are not strongly bound, and they get washed off during the washing step, leaving only the bLf molecules attached to the resin. This bound bLf was then isolated using a strong cationic 1 M salt solution [18]. The eluted protein fractions were then subjected to extensive dialysis. The purity of the eluted fractions was checked by SDS-PAGE that showed a single HMW band ≥250 kDa (Figure 1A). The HMW protein band on SDS-PAGE was later identified as bLf by Western blotting using anti-bLf antibody (Figure 1B). Native bLf as a monomer has a molecular mass of ~77–80 kDa, depending upon the glycosylation of mature protein, the ≥250 kDa HMW-bLf therefore indicates a trimer or a probably partially degraded tetramer due to its possible interaction with Sepharose resin during purification. This phenomenon has been reported earlier that incubation of hLf with oligosaccharides led to the formation of unstable oligomers as studied by gel filtration chromatography using polysaccharide resins such as Sephadex, Sepharose 4B, etc. [11]. These authors suggested that Sepharose, containing alternating residues of β-D-galactopyranose and 3, 6 anhydrido-α-1-galactopyranose linked by 1-4 bonds, could dissociate hLf oligomers. As explained above, Lf has high affinity for such resins, thereby efficiently interacts with them. Lf bound to these gel filtration/cation exchange chromatographic resins can be eluted at high salt concentrations (KCl or NaCl), since the high ionic strength causes dissociation of oligomers, and Lf then can be mostly eluted as a monomer.

Interestingly, previous Sephadex G-200 chromatographic purification reports reveal that when the concentration of bLf was high in mammary secretions due to infections such as during mastitis, bLf was initially obtained as 77 kDa monomer, and as the infection progressed, it was separated at approximately the size of a trimer (~240 kDa). These observations were therefore concurrent with the increasing bLf concentrations during infections [19]. Another study similarly reported that the bLf, in non-lactating mammary secretions during involution, was mainly present as HMW complexes rather than as monomers, and majority of total bLf existed in ~250 kDa molecular mass fractions [12]. Structural

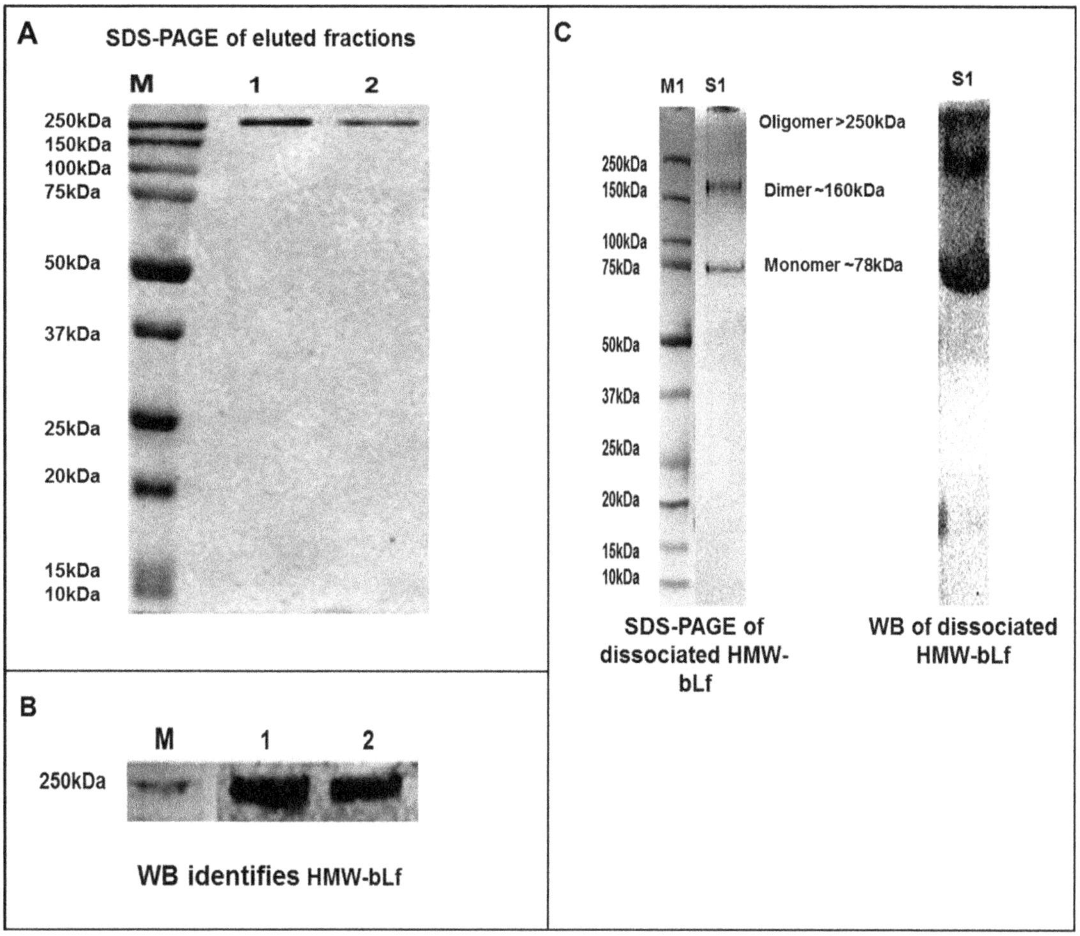

Figure 1. Purification and analysis of components. A) SDS-PAGE analysis of purified HMW-bLf indicating the presence of pure ≥250 kDa protein in elutes (lanes 1 and 2). B) The purified protein was confirmed to be bLf through Western blotting using anti-bLf specific antibody. C) Dissociation of HMW-bLf in 1 M NaCl into the dimeric (~160 kDa) and monomeric (~78 kDa) forms (lane S1). These were confirmed to be bLf bands by Western blot for the same dissociated sample (S1). The absence of any other lower bands and the detection of all the constituent bands by anti-bLf specific antibody indicate that HMW-bLf is an oligomer formed by the interactions of monomeric bLf molecules.

studies employing the method of sedimentation equilibrium in the ultracentrifuge, on purified preparations of bLf obtained from commercial preparations, revealed that the purified protein exhibited heterogeneity with respect to its molecular weight in dilute aqueous salt solutions. The top of the cell had 76 kDa bLf material while >200 kDa material was sedimented at the cell bottom. These findings implied that bLf associated in the native state in a concentration dependent manner, and aggregates as high as trimers were obtained [20]. The nature of these intermolecular interactions in bLf oligomers remained unknown, and mostly investigators in the late last century, did not take bLf oligomeric forms into consideration. There are reports that bLf dimers have also been mistaken for IgG, because of its molecular weight that is twice of the bLf monomer [21,22].

More recently, emerging experimental evidence indicate Lf as an extremely conformationally dynamic protein that is prone to self-association. The macromolecule has a dumbbell shape, well described by a bi-axial ellipsoid with half-axis of 47 Å and 26 Å [11,13,21]. While the levels of self-association were shown to depend on the number of conditions such as Lf concentration, presence of salts, ligands, storage in solutions, iron saturation and temperature, a molecular level explanation remains yet to be understood for this phenomenon. Without salt or at physiological salt concentrations, bLf as well as hLf reportedly self-associate in aqueous solutions as dimers, trimers, and also as tetramers with tetramer being the dominant form [11,21]. In these studies, gel filtration analysis also revealed small peaks of the decamer. For tetramer formation, which is the predominant molecular form of Lf in human serum, tears, and breast milk, calcium dependent oligomerization of hLf has been reported, [23]. Therefore the purification of ≥250 kDa bLf oligomer in our study is in agreement with the aforementioned findings of other investigators. Colostrum is known to contain higher concentrations of bLf and calcium ions than milk [8,24,25] these could have also contributed to the self -association of bLf into HMW oligomeric complex along with the unidentified molecular trigger(s) of self-association.

HMW- bLf molecule was also found to be dissociated into the dimeric (~160 kDa) and monomeric (~78 kDa) forms of bLf when kept for 24 h in the presence of 1 M NaCl. This observation is inconsistent with earlier findings on hLf [11]. As determined by gradient SDS-PAGE (reducing gel) analysis followed by Western blotting with anti-bLf antibody (Figure 1C), all the three bands were identified as bLf protein. More interestingly, a progressive increase in the intensity of monomeric ~78 kDa band with a simultaneous decrease in the remaining HMW-bLf band was observed. This is clearly evident in Western blot (Figure 1C). We

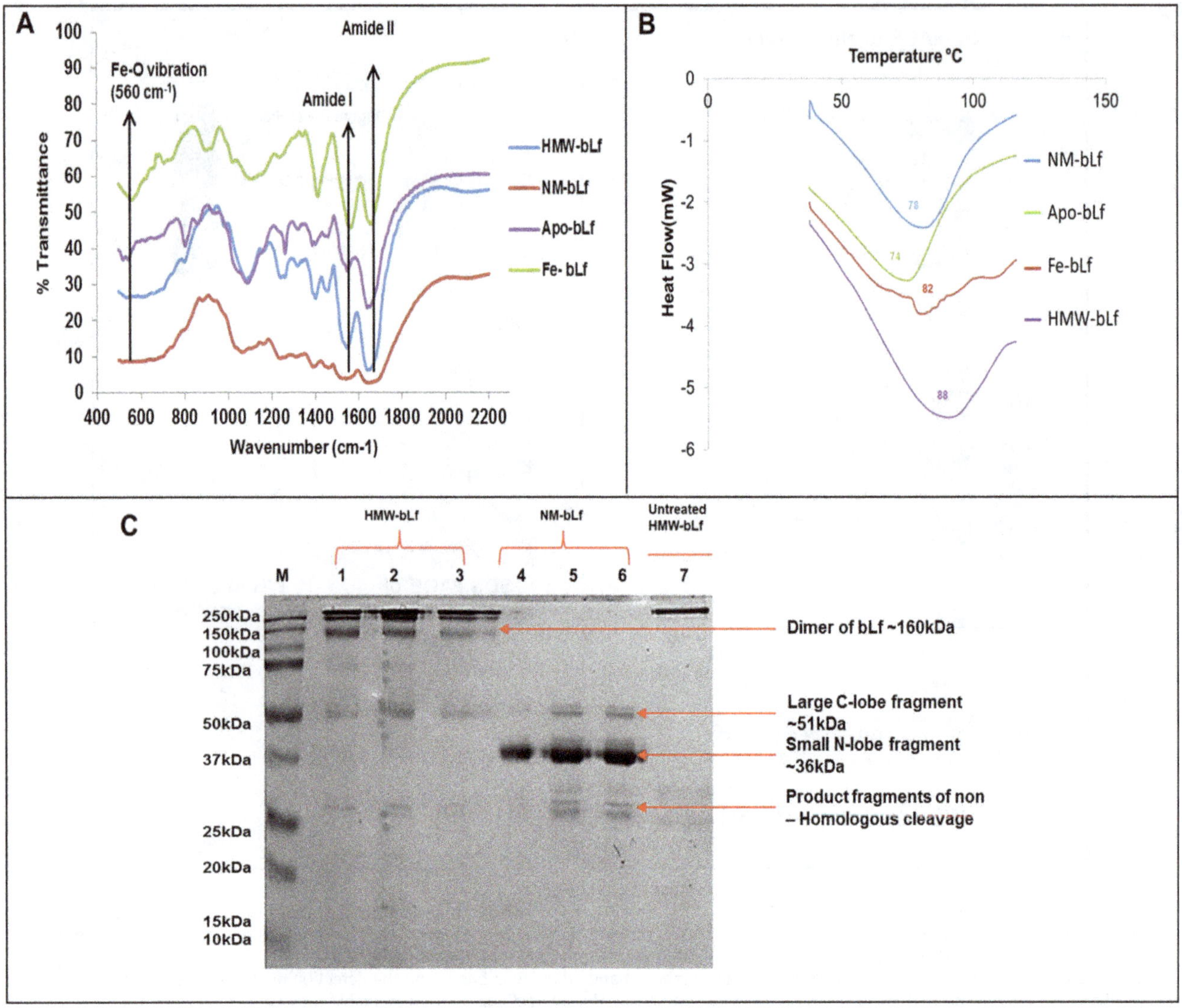

Figure 2. Physico-chemical characterization of HMW-bLf. A) Fourier transform infra-red (FTIR) spectra of HMW-bLf indicating characteristic peaks and compared with other forms of bLf. B) Differential scanning calorimetry thermograms of the different bLf forms C) SDS-PAGE showing the comparative resistance of HMW-bLf to Omnizyme (human digestive enzyme cocktail) treatment. It also gives an indication that HMW-bLf is an oligomer made of bLf monomers; because upon digestion HMW-bLf besides dimers and trimers does not release any other fragments lower than ~78 kDa apart from the ones produced from the digestion of commercially pure NM-bLf.

have also noted that since the purified HMW-bLf sample (Figure 1B) was stored for about a year after purification and lyophilization, a much larger bLf aggregate (polymer) in the stacking gel was identified that showed lower mobility protein material with a comparative decrease in its band density, than the ≥250 kDa oligomeric complex band observed just after the purification (Figure 1A). These observations are also consistent with the earlier oligomerization studies on hLf which report that in the presence of 1 M NaCl, the hLf oligomers dissociate slowly into monomers whereas, during storage of dialyzed and lyophilized protein solutions at neutral pH, the monomeric or oligomeric forms slowly aggregate[11,26]. We also performed Western blotting for bovine IgG to identify dimeric −160 kDa band, and the larger HMW-bLf aggregate band but no immunoreactivity was observed indicating there was no contamination from IgG. Further, no other bands that could correspond to molecular weights of any other milk protein (lysozyme − 14.6 kDa, α-lactalbumin -14.12 kDa, β-lactoglobulin – 22.40 kDa, αs_1-casein – 33.30 kDa, β-casein – 37.50 kDa) in the dissociated sample of HMW-bLf were observed on SDS-PAGE reducing gel (Figure 1 C), indicating their absence in the sample.

The absence of any LPS contamination and endotoxin activity in the purified protein was confirmed using E-Toxate assay kit which indicated the presence less than 0.04 EU/mg (Endotoxin Units/mg) of endotoxin activity in the purified HMW-bLf samples. This was much lower than the FDA accepted standards [27]. Our observations thus indicate that purified HMW-bLf could be made up of bLf molecules forming a multimeric complex due to non- covalent, ionic interactions. These interactions were broken in the presence of strong ionic solution (1 M NaCl) and results in the appearance of more intense low molecular weight monomeric as well as dimeric forms. In the existing literature, despite the emerging data on Lf oligomerization/self-association, little is known about the nature of the chemical linkages/binding interactions that result in the formation of Lf-Lf complexes. Ionic, thiol/disulfide and hydrophobic interactions may all be involved in these intermolecular interactions. Earlier findings on thermal aggregation of bLf molecules proposed that the bLf aggregation proceeded via a combination of non-covalent interactions and intermolecular thiol/disulphide reactions that did not require free thiol residues. Specifically, the thermal aggregation of iron saturated bLf was mainly driven by non-covalent interactions, with intermolecular thiol/disulphide reactions also observed above 80°C [13]. Using force field based molecular modeling of the protein–protein interaction free energy, it was demonstrated that at neutral pH, Lf forms highly stereo-specific dimers. This self-association is driven by a high charge complementarity across the proteins' contact surface [21].

Because of its iron binding properties, Lf is known to exist in two forms: holo-Lf (binds two Fe^{3+} ions, iron saturated), Apo-Lf (iron depleted) [2]. Native Lf is only partially saturated. Therefore, we measured the iron content of HMW-bLf and found that it contained only 0.47% iron and thus, was more like Apo-bLf (1.1%), when compared with other forms of bLf such as NM-bLf (22% iron), and iron saturated bLf (Fe-bLf) >94% iron (Figure S2 in File S1). Figure 2A shows a comparison between the FTIR spectra of HMW-bLf, NM-bLf, Apo-bLf and Fe-bLf. The characteristic amide carbonyl stretching appeared between 1630 and 1650 cm^{-1}, the C-N stretch was observed between 1500 and 1550 cm^{-1} while the O-C-N bend was discernible between 675 and 721 cm^{-1} in the four forms. The Fe-O vibration band appeared at 560 cm^{-1} in the FTIR spectrum of Fe-bLf while it was not pronounced in the other three spectra suggesting high iron content in Fe-bLf (Figure S3 in File S1). This also confirms our iron content estimation results. bLf is classified as a glycoprotein, the bands from 900–1200 cm^{-1} due to C–O, C–C, C–O–H, C–O–C vibrations of the carbohydrate moiety were therefore observed in all the four forms of bLf [28].

Exploring the thermal stability of bLf has been also important because of its bioactivity. In order to develop a practical method for pasteurization of bLf, the heat stability has been studied previously. Several factors can affect the heat stability of bLf such as pH, salts, and other whey proteins [29]. We tested the thermal stability of HMW-bLf, Fe-bLf, Apo-bLf and NM-bLf in lyophilized powder form by DSC. The thermogram of ≥250 kDa HMW -bLf (Figure 2B) showed denaturation peak at 88°C, which was the highest when compared with those of Fe-bLf, Apo-bLf and NM-bLf, and their denaturation peaks were observed at 82°C, 74°C and 78°C, respectively. These findings suggest that the higher thermal stability of HMW-bLf may be due to its structural integrity as an oligomer. Among other bLf forms, the Fe-bLf was comparatively more resistant to heat when compared to the Apo-bLf and the NM-bLf. Similar findings have also been reported, suggesting that an increase in protein stability depends upon the degree of iron saturation [13,30,31]. Increased thermal stability of Fe-bLf (holo-bLf) has been attributed to the more compact conformation, adopted by the molecule by binding a ferric ion in the inter-domain cleft of each lobe [2]. Slightly higher thermal stability of the NM-bLf than the Apo-bLf could thus be attributed to partial iron saturation status of the native protein.

From our results, and the aforementioned discussion, it can be inferred that the interactions between the bLf molecules may largely be ionic to form the HMW-bLf oligomer. Oligomerization/protein aggregation is a concentration dependent process. At high concentration of Lf and of calcium in the bovine colostrum, the equilibrium shifts towards the formation of oligomers, however, under dilution or at high Na^{+}/K^{+} concentration the ionic bonds are broken and they tend to shift towards existence as monomers. We propose that HMW-bLf, which is similar to Apo-bLf and lacks mostly the iron content, and likely contain lot of free aspartate and tyrosine residues. This confers a very open, flexible configuration to HMW-bLf molecule similar to Apo-bLf [32]. Due to this, the ability of the molecule to undergo intermolecular interactions was highly increased when maintained at a high concentration and in the absence of any salt content, especially iron [13]. These complex interactions in HMW-bLf appeared to be very strong [11] and led to the formation of even larger aggregates upon prolonged storage (Figure 1C). We have also noticed that NM-bLf (22% iron saturated), when stored at high concentration, displays trimers and dimers formation visualized on denaturing SDS-PAGE condition (data not shown). In a study that investigated the effect of iron saturation on thermal aggregation of bLf in Apo state, it was shown that Apo-bLf associated into large polymers by non-covalent interactions without the participation of disulphide cross-links. The more unfolded structure of heat sensitive Apo-bLf may have increased the exposure of non-covalent sites normally buried in the core of both lobes of the protein, thereby favoring intermolecular interactions and the formation of larger aggregates [13]. The in-depth molecular and biophysical characterization of the HMW-bLf needs to be investigated further with more powerful proteomics tools such as Mass spectroscopy and Circular Dichroism, in order to identify the chemical as well structural changes/linkages in the oligomer. To determine spontaneous association of bLf in physiologically simulated solution SAXS and LS can be employed to analyze the oligomeric states of HMW-bLf.

The consumption of test drinks containing Apo-bLf and iron saturated bLf in human volunteers has shown that Apo-bLf is more susceptible to *in vivo* gut digestion, than the corresponding iron-saturated form [33]. Similarly, we have reported earlier the resistant nature of Fe-bLf towards Omnizyme (a digestive enzyme cocktail) [5]. In the current study, HMW-bLf was found to be more resistant to Omnizyme digestion *in vitro*, even after 4, 6, and 8 h incubation periods. Figure 2C shows that HMW-bLf in lanes 2, 3 and 4 showed excellent stability to digestion, with digested forms appearing as 150–160 kDa dimers at various intervals of time (4, 6 and 8 h) while faint bands at ~78, 50 and 25 kDa. In the case of NM-bLf, in lanes 5, 6 and 7 the 78 kDa bands have completely disappeared and digested to its peptides that appeared at 51, 37and ~25 kDa. HMW-bLf's comparatively much stronger resistance to gut enzyme digestion despite having far lower iron content than NM-bLf (0.47% versus 22%).This can be explained in terms of the robustness of its structure being a larger biomacromolecule/oligomer. This property will therefore prove beneficial for its potential use as a nutraceutical. In that case, if given orally there will be an increase in the *in vivo* bioavailability of HMW-bLf to the required sites of the action in the body, e.g., tumor/infected and inflammatory tissues as compared to NM-bLf, which is comparatively more prone to digestion. This assay also gives an insight into the components of HMW-bLf and indicates that HMW-bLf appears not to be made up of any other component than that of NM-bLf. The fragments that are generated by the Omnizyme digestion show that NM-bLf (Lanes 4, 5 and 6) can be degraded into a large C- terminal lobe with a part of the N-terminal region and the connector seen as a 51 kDa band. The C-terminal lobe on further digestion produced the band at 36 kDa. This is not a homologous digestion, and it does not produce two equal sized fragments hence resulting in a few smaller fragments seen at 25 kDa [34]. The observation that below ~78 kDa, the HMW-bLf also produces the same set of bands as that of NM-bLf (Figure 2C, Lanes 1–3 and 4–6 respectively) thus is in agreement with our dissociation findings of HMW-bLf (Figure 1C) that it was comprised of bLf monomers.

We have shown earlier that 100% iron-saturated bLf form (Fe-bLf) when given orally to mice prior to chemotherapy caused its augmentation [16]. Significant eradication of large tumors in combination with anticancer drugs was observed. However, 20% iron-saturated (NM-bLf) or Apo-bLf remained ineffective in eradicating these tumors, owing to their high degradation in the gut as compared to Fe-bLf. In order to increase the more bioavailability of Fe-bLf to the tumour sites, more recently, we have developed a novel nanodrug delivery system (alginate-enclosed chitosan–calcium phosphate-loaded Fe-bLf nanocarriers) for oral delivery. By employing human colon xenograft model, we reported that nanoformulated Fe-bLf when fed orally led to the complete inhibition of tumorigenesis in prevention mode. A complete tumor rejection through regression, in the treatment mode was also observed [5]. These nanocarriers thus led to the increased bioavailability of Fe-bLf to the tumor sites, and were found to be safe and nontoxic. Similarly, another study has shown that the anti-tumor effects of NM-bLf on melanoma cells can be enhanced with liposomalization. A lipid delivery system (liposomes) was used to prevent the NM-bLf from proteolysis or neutralization by serum proteins [35]. Considering the findings that tetramer is reported to be the dominating form of hLf observed under physiological conditions [10,23], and bLf self-associates as dimers, trimers and tetramers in mammary secretions during infection and involution [12,19], it may imply that the physiological existence of Lf oligomers, can therefore be a protection strategy acquired by multifunctional Lf against proteolysis or neutralization by serum proteins.

Earlier it has been shown that NM-bLf decreased the viability of breast cancer cell lines HS578T and T47D by inducing a 2-fold increase in apoptosis, and decreased the proliferation rates as well in both the cell lines [36]. A similar effect of bLf was seen on colon carcinoma [37] and *in vivo* on tumors of melanoma, EL-4 T-cell thymic lymphoma and Lewis lung cancer cells [16]. To test the anticancer activities of HMW-bLf, we employed MDA-MB-231 (human breast carcinoma) and SW480 (human colorectal adenocarcinoma) cell lines. Figure 3 (A and B) shows the cytotoxic effects of HMW-bLf. It was assessed by measuring the leaked LDH enzyme (as a cell viability biomarker), from dying or dead cells (early/late apoptotic and necrotic) due to their damaged cell membranes. HMW-bLf was found to be effective in a concentration dependent manner in inducing cell cytotoxicity in both MDA-MB- 231 and SW480 cells. The cytotoxicity values of HMW-bLf and Fe-bLf at the highest concentration used (3200 μg mL^{-1}), were highly significant (*p<0.01*) with 90% and 76% cytotoxicity observed respectively. Similarly, when compared with the other control forms of bLf, 3200 μg mL^{-1} of HMW-bLf also showed significantly highest cytotoxicity in SW-480 cells. Though, among all the concentrations of HWW-bLf tested on SW480 cells, it showed lowest cytotoxicity values at a concentration of 800 μg mL^{-1} but the effect was still statistically significant (p<0.05) when compared to the untreated cells' (value set at zero). The cytotoxicity of HMW-bLf towards non-cancerous human cells (of normal intestinal origin) was also tested by treating FHs 74 Int cells with its different concentrations. A significant increase in the LDH release activity corresponding to 15% cytotoxicity was observed only at the highest concentration (3200 μg mL^{-1}) of HMW-bLf, as shown in Figure 3 C. More importantly, in HMW-bLf treated colon cancer cells (SW480), the corresponding cytotoxicity values at all the concentrations tested were significantly higher (P<0.01) than those obtained with FHs 74 Int cells. Moreover, at HMW-bLf treatments(800 μg mL^{-1}, 1600 μg mL^{-1} and 2400 μg mL^{-1}), LDH release activity from FHs74 Int cells was significantly lower than that of untreated cells. The presence of Lf in mammalian milks and bovine colostrum has an important role for the normal gut cell growth, maturation and repair in young ones. It could thus possibly be a therapeutic action of the HMW-bLf in repairing membrane damage, occurred normally to these normal intestinal cells under *in vitro* culture. A maximum of LDH release corresponding to 33% cytotoxicity (p<0.01) was seen with NM-bLf 3200 μg mL^{-1} treatment to FHs74Int cells. There was no significant difference observed among the cytotoxic activities of Apo-bLf (20±6.5%), NM-bLf (33±15%) and HMW-bLf (15±4.2%) at 3200 μg mL^{-1}. However, when compared at 1600 μg mL^{-1}, NM-bLf caused significantly higher cytotoxic effect on FHs74 Int cells than HMW-bLf at the same concentration. It is important to note here that among all the treatments, NM-bLf induced highest 33% cytotoxicity to the normal intestinal cells. The non-toxicity of bLf to normal cells/ tissues during long-term feeding has been clearly shown through number of *in vivo* animal studies, and oral feeding trials in human volunteers and colon cancer patients [4,5,6,16]. It has been approved by the Food and Drug Administration (FDA) of United States in 2001, and later by European Food Safety Authority as a dietary supplement in food products [38,39]. Moreover, FHs 74 Int is a fetal derived intestinal cell line, known to grow as normal enterocytes. Considering Lf's intense affinity for iron [1,32], it can be explained that FHs 74 Int cells' requirement of iron, for their cell viability, appears to be targeted by both Apo-bLf (iron free) and NM-bLf (partially saturated with iron) thus showing significantly higher cytotoxicity values than Fe-bLf. On the other hand, HMW-bLf although showed very low iron content but having a more robust complex molecular structure, might not bind iron as fiercely as Apo-bLf and NM-bLf do. Therefore, it showed comparatively less cytotoxicity than Apo-bLf and NM-bLf. These observations need follow-up investigations to determine the complete safety profile of HMW-bLf towards the normal cells.

Since recent reports suggest that LDH release measurements can underestimate the cytotoxicity caused by compounds causing cell cycle arrest [40], the cytotoxic effects of HMW-bLF were also studied by Flow cytometry using PI staining. Figures 3 (D and E) and Figure S4 in File S1, show the cell death induced by HMW-bLf in cancer cells and FHs74 Int cells, respectively. PI test values appeared higher (Figure 3 D and E) than the LDH release assay (Figure 3 A and B). However, the results of the two assays were in general agreement and showed that HMW-bLf targeted cell death in a dose-dependent and cell specific manner. Even within cancer cells from different tissues, it was significantly more cytotoxic towards MDA-MB-231 cells than SW480 cells.

To determine the growth inhibitory properties of HMW-bLf, we further assessed the proliferation of MDA-MB-231 and SW480 cells after treatments for 24 h using the CyQuant assay. Figure 4 (A and B) shows that HMW-bLf decreases the rate of cell proliferation in a dose-dependent manner. At the highest dose, it significantly (*p<0.01*) inhibited the proliferation of both MDA-MB- 231 and SW480 cells (up to 90%), a better rate than any other control forms of bLf. Furthermore, observation into the effects of HMW-bLf on cell morphology revealed that cells after treatments for 24 h, exhibited poor growth showed altered morphology with high levels of cellular fragmentation and apoptotic bodies. Both cell lines used in this study showed detachment from culture dish bottom and floating dead cells were mostly observed, when highest concentration of HMW-bLf was employed (Figure 4 C and D).

NM- bLf is known to be internalized into live cells through cell surface (membrane) receptor mediated endocytosis mechanism

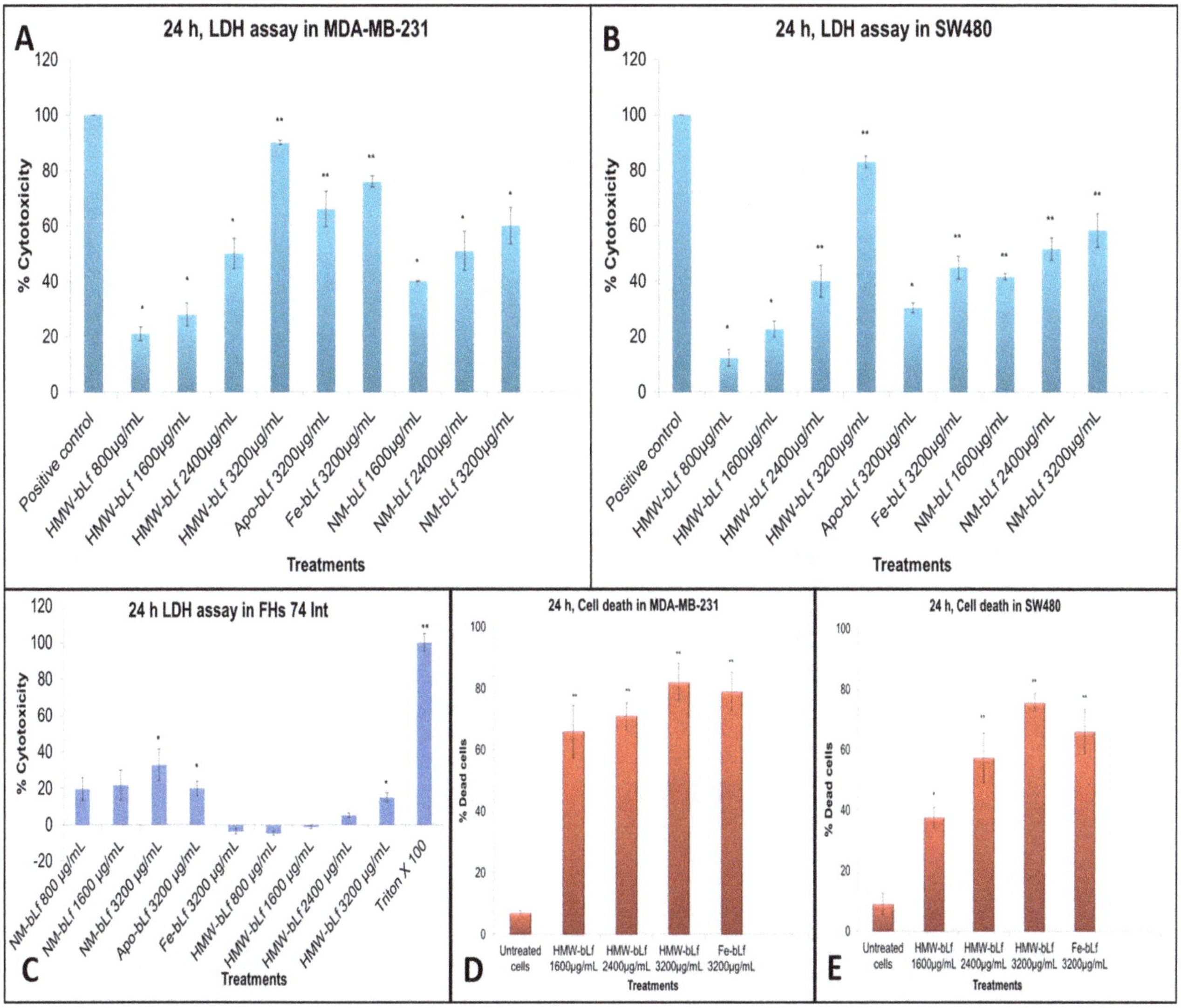

Figure 3. Cytotoxic effects of HMW-bLf. A B and C represent the cellular cytotoxicity measured by LDH release assay induced by HMW-bLf in a concentration dependent manner, in MDA-MB-231 (human breast carcinoma) SW480 (human colorectal adenocarcinoma) and FHs 74 Int (normal intestinal cells) cells. D and E show the cell death (mortality count) as measured by Flow cytometry using propidium iodide staining (* $p<0.05$ and ** $p<0.01$). Other forms of bLf were used for comparison.

[1,41]. The published data report that transferrin receptor (TfR), lactoferrin receptors and low density lipoprotein receptor-related protein receptors (LRPs) play a crucial role in facilitating the internalization of bLf inside cells[42,43]. Using both colon and breast cancer cells it was observedthat bLf internalized into the membrane, cytoplasm and nucleus in a time dependent fashion (unpublished studies from our laboratory). Therefore immunofluorescence was carried out in order to determine whether the oligomerization state of HMW-bLf affects its cellular internalization and receptor binding properties using MDA-MB-231 SW480 and FHs74 Int cells (Figure 5 and Figure S5 in File S1). Since the cytotoxicity of HMW-bLf was observed in a concentration dependent manner, only lowest concentration (800 µg mL^{-1}) was used. Therefore following incubation, lesser cellular detachment (of dying/dead cells) was observed from the slide making the immunostaining and imaging possible. The confocal microscopy images indicate that beginning at 30 min after incubation, there was a rapid internalization of HMW-bLf by the three cell types. The presence of green fluorescence signal of bLf specific antibody immunostaining was mainly seen on the cell surface and cell membrane. Since internalization is a time dependent process, it was more evident at earlier time points of incubation (30 min and 4 h). HMW-bLf was also found to be localized along the perinuclear region in 4 h. In the images obtained after 6 h and 8 h of incubation periods, HMW-bLf was seen to be internalized into the nuclei of cancer cells. This indicates that bLf in its oligomeric state retains its ability to interact with receptors and is taken up by the cells in time dependent fashion, although further investigations are needed to determine the receptor-ligand interactions completely. Taken together, the results of cellular internalization, LDH release and CyQuant assays reveal that cellular uptake of HMW-bLf even at 800 µg mL^{-1} proved effective; where internalized HMW-bLf displayed its functional bioactivity in terms of inducing significant cytotoxicity (LDH release) and anti-cell proliferative activity in cancer cells. Interestingly, the degradation of actin network within the cells

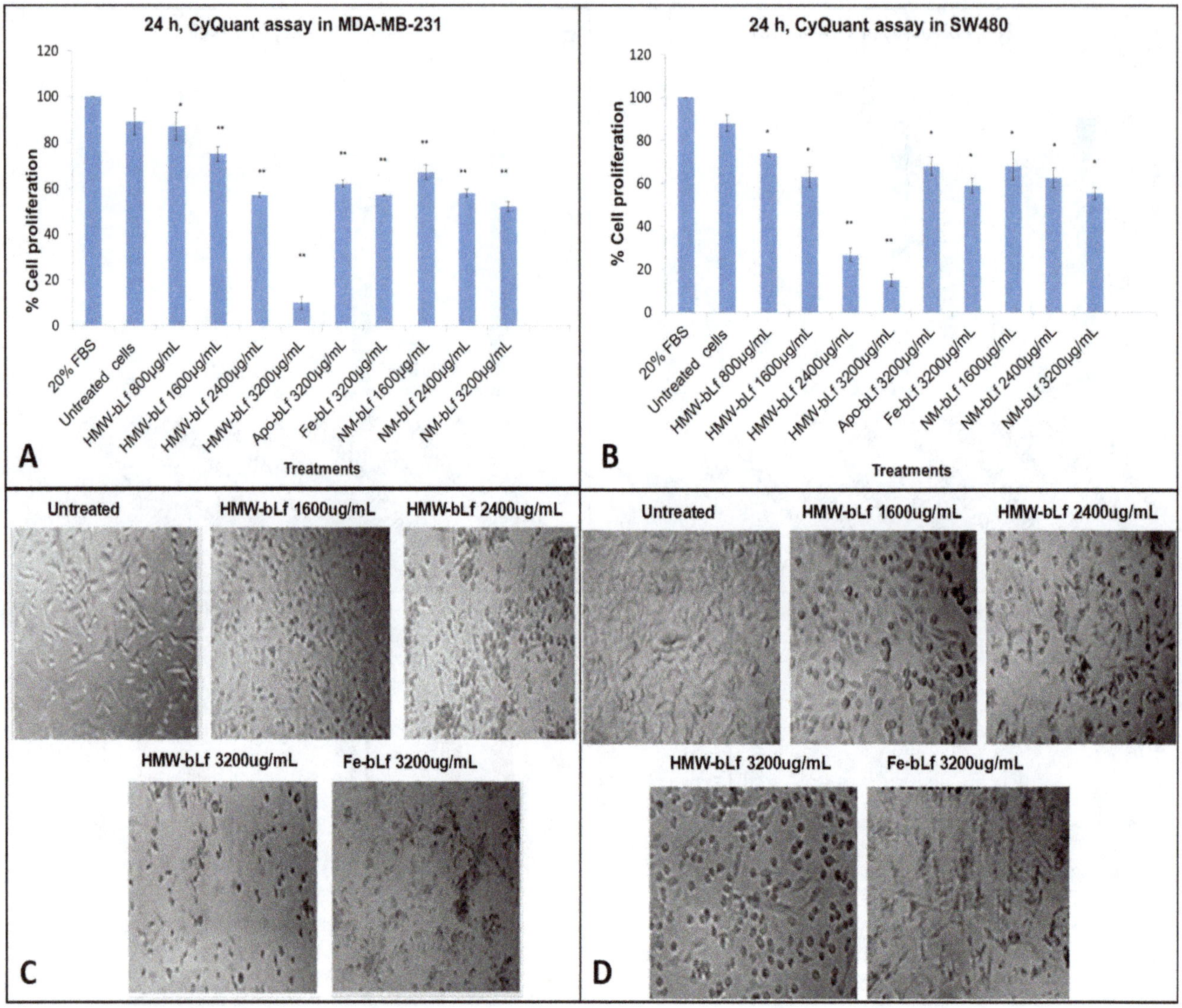

Figure 4. Cell growth inhibition. HMW-bLf decreases the cellular proliferation of MDA-MB-231 and SW480 (A and B respectively) cells in a concentration dependent manner. The cell fate was also monitored by analyzing the cell morphology (C – MDA-MB-231 and D – SW480) which clearly indicates cell death. (* $p<0.05$ and ** $p<0.01$)

was observed by the reduced fluorescence intensity of phalloidin - AlexaFluor 568 stain (red fluorescence). This shows that the cellular uptake of HMW-bLf triggers the process of apoptosis resulting in the loss of actin framework which acts as a substrate for caspase-3 and its downstream products [44]. Figure 5B shows the high magnification image of HMW-bLf internalization in SW480 cells after 4 h with the arrows pointing out at the cells that have internalized HMW-bLf and thereby showing the degradation of actin. An arrow head points to the cell with intact actin structure that has not taken up HMW-bLf. Figure 5C is a high magnification image of HMW-bLf internalization at 6 h showing the beginning of nuclear material degradation which is the final stage in the apoptotic pathway.

This was further confirmed by studying the release of caspase-3, considered as the final executioner enzyme in the apoptotic pathway [45]. Treatment with HMW-bLf induced a statistically significant increase in the levels of caspase-3 secretion in both MDA-MB-231 and SW480 cells, thereby confirming the induction of cell death by apoptosis, (Figure 6 A and B). In both SW480 and MDA-MB-231 cells, HMW-bLf treatment significantly ($p<0.01$) up-regulated caspase-3 levels, and in SW480 cells the effect was also significant when compared with control Fe-bLf at 3200 µg mL^{-1}. The rapid internalization of HMW-bLf into the cytoplasm and nuclei of cancer cells seems to lead to the initiation of gene transcription within the cell to trigger apoptotic signals thereby, resulting in cell death via apoptosis. We and other researchers have also shown that internalization of NM-bLf into the cell and nucleus can regulate gene transcription of its receptors, cytokines such as transforming growth factor-β and survivin [1,46,47]. bLf has been shown to activate both extrinsic and intrinsic apoptotic pathways through activation of different caspases [1,7]. To confirm the results obtained using the caspase-3 activity assay, Western blot was performed for cleaved caspase-3, which is the active form of the apoptosis activator enzyme. Both SW480 and MDA-MB-231 cells show upregulation of the cleaved caspase-3 expression upon treatment with HMW-bLf. Especially, high expression of cleaved caspase-3 is seen in the 3200 µg mL^{-1} treatments of both Fe-bLf and HMW-bLf in MDA-MB-231 and

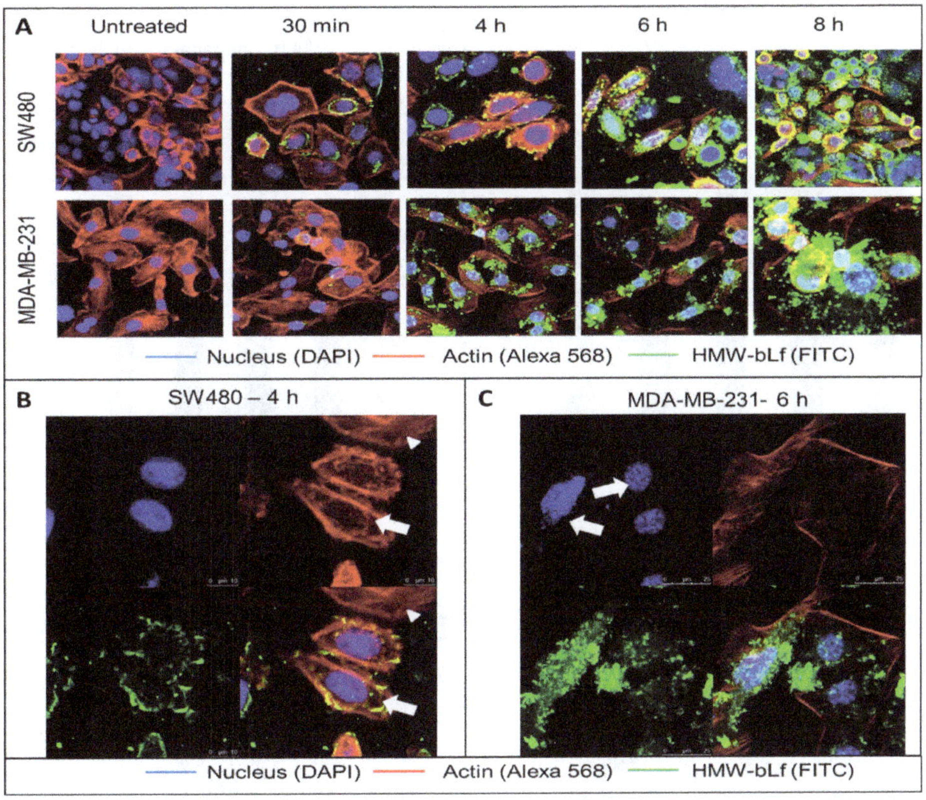

Figure 5. Cellular uptake of HMW-bLf. A – Representative confocal microscopic images show HMW-bLf internalization in MDA-MB-231 and SW480 in a time dependent manner. The degradation of actin an indicator of apoptosis was observed after 6 h of treatment with HMW-bLf. The reduction in the intensity of the Alexa 568 signal indicates the degradation of the actin cytoskeleton. B and C are high magnification images HMW-bLf internalization in SW480 (B) and MDA-MB231(C) with separate panels showing nucleus, actin and HMW-bLf alone. Arrows in 4B points out to the cells that have taken up HMW-bLf showing perturbed actin structure, and arrowhead points out to the cell with intact actin structure and is without HMW-bLf uptake in 4 h (SW480). Arrows in 4C point out to the beginning of nuclear degradation at 6 h (MDA-MB-231).

with 1600 μg mL^{-1} in SW480 (Figure 6C and D). This indicates the ability HMW-bLf to induce apoptosis by activating caspase-3.

Conclusions

In summary, our current *in vitro* study using breast and colon cancer cells showed for the first time the anticancer efficacy of ≥250 kDa HMW-biomacromolecular complex containing bLf. HMW-bLf was purified to homogeneity from Australian bovine colostrum. We have identified its unprecedented and interesting properties. HMW-bLf besides having molecular and structural similarities to Apo-bLf in terms of iron content also retains its antibody, and receptor binding properties. It possesses unique features such as higher thermal stability and better resistance against gut enzyme digestion than other forms of bLf monomer. Furthermore, HMW-bLf displayed stronger anti-cancer properties in terms of cytotoxicity and anti-cell proliferation activity. The possible actin degradation due to increased caspase-3 activity thereby, leading to apoptosis further signifies the need to explore the exact level of interesting interactions exhibited by HMW-bLf in modulating cancer cell death. The purified sample tested for its anticancer activities was obtained through final step of dialysis with 100 kDa MW cut off membrane, and thus devoid of any contamination with bLf monomer and other low molecular weight whey proteins such as lysozyme (14.6 kDa), α-lactalbumin - 14.12(kDa), β-lactoglobulin – (22.40 kDa), αs_1-casein – (33.30 kDa), β-casein – (37.50 kDa). The discovery of functionally bioactive HMW-bLf in this study has opened up greater scope for future research, considering the inherent multifunctional nature of bLf with its potential in improving human health. Through preclinical and clinical studies, we and others have shown that NM-bLf and Fe-bLf can not only inhibit tumor development but also reduce growth and metastasis of solid tumors [5,6,16]. Because of its widely reported multifunctional properties, and approval by FDA (US) and European Food Safety Authority as a dietary supplement in food products [38,39] NM-bLf is gaining recent attention as an important therapeutic and nutraceutical against cancer, chronic inflammatory, viral and microbial diseases. In this regard, further studies are therefore, needed to decipher the structural and functional nature of HMW-bLf with more powerful techniques for its in-depth molecular organization and biophysical characterization. This will lead to the identification of similarities and differences in the activities displayed by these two forms of bLf, and help in understanding the true potential bLf as a multifunctional bio-macromolecule, in meeting the aims of modern medicine.

Supporting Information

File S1 Figures S1–S4. Figure S1. Representative microscopy images showing trypan blue exclusion assay when the cells were grown in their respective growth media with 1% FBS for 24 h, indicating the >98% viability. This indicates that serum deprivation on incubation with bLf treatments for cellular uptake

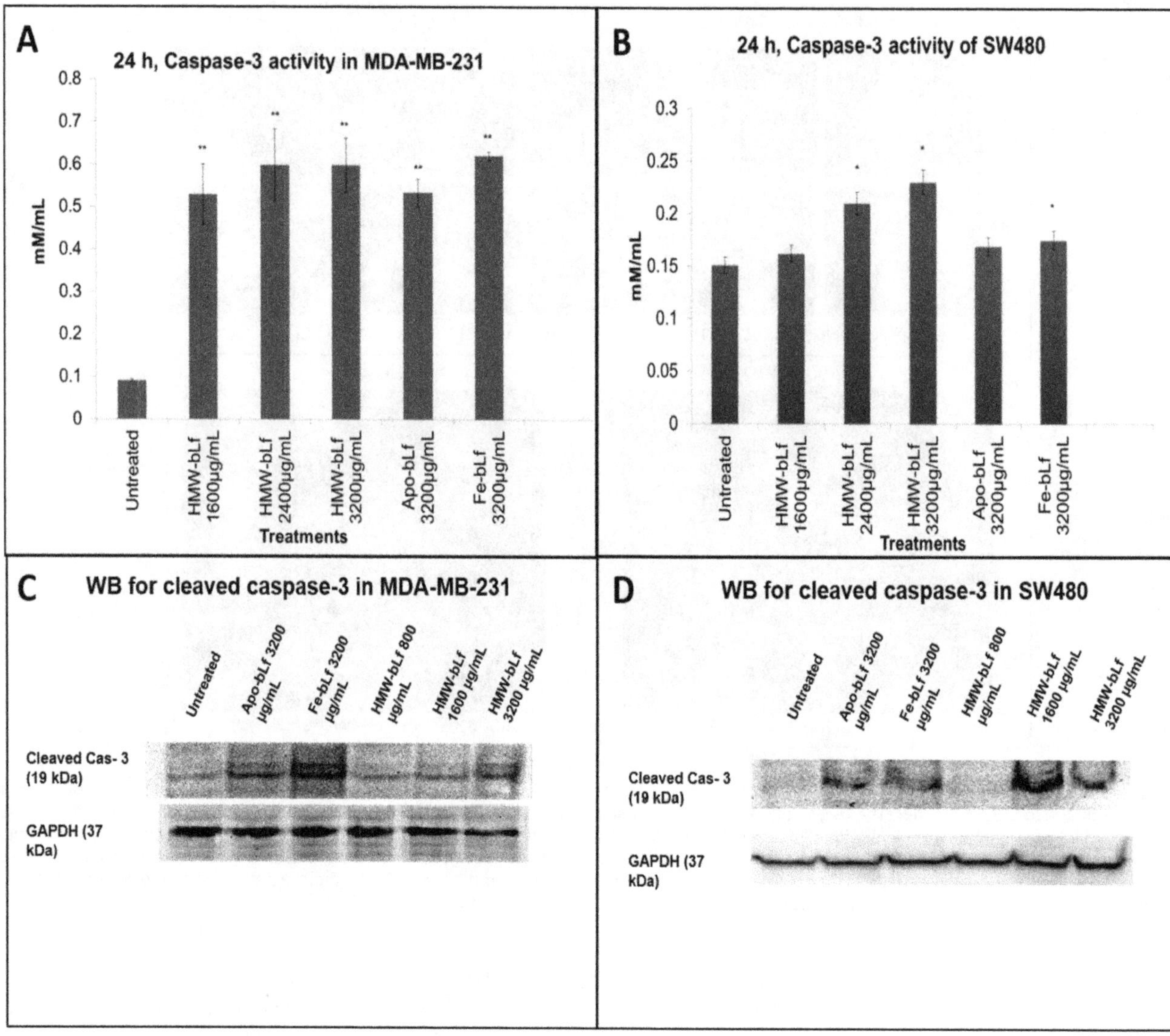

Figure 6. Caspase-3 activation. A and B represent the increased caspase-3 activity measurements upon treatment with HMW-bLf in MDA-MB-231 and SW480 cells, respectively. (* P<0.05 and ** P<0.01). Panels C and D are the respective Western blots showing an increase in cleaved caspase-3 expression upon treatments in MDA-MB-231 and SW480 cells.

in 1% FBS containing assay media does not compromise the ability of the cells to exclude the dye and they remained healthy with intact membranes for cellular uptake of bLf. Magnifications 40X. Figure S2. Representative graph of the percentage iron content in the different forms of bLf. Figure S3. High resolution graph of FTIR spectra. The Fe-O vibration band appears at 560 cm-1 in the FTIR spectrum of Fe-bLf, and it is not pronounced in the other three spectra suggesting the high iron content in Fe-bLf and confirming iron content estimation. Figure S4. Cell death (mortality count) in FHs 74 Int as measured by Flow cytometry using propidium iodide staining (* p<0.05). Fe-bLf was used as a control. Figure S5: Confocal microscopy images showing FHs 74 Int cells (of normal intestinal origin) also take up HMW-bLf in a time dependent fashion. The internalized HMW-bLf was detected by indirect immunofluorescence using goat anti-bovine lactoferrin (Bethyl Laboratories) antibody at a dilution of 1:200 in PBS at 37°C for 1 h. The primary antibody was then removed and after washing, cells were incubated with anti-goat IgG-FITC conjugate (Sigma-Aldrich) and counterstained for nucleus with DAPI (blue) in fluorshield (Sigma-Aldrich). Scale bar = 25 µm.

Acknowledgments

The authors would like to thank Professor Peter Hodgson Director, Institute for Frontier Materials, Deakin University for his support during the work. The authors are grateful to Australian farmer families for providing bovine colostrum.

Author Contributions

Conceived and designed the experiments: RKK. Performed the experiments: FE JSS SG. Analyzed the data: RKK JRK JSS SG UMK FE. Contributed reagents/materials/analysis tools: RKK JRK. Wrote the paper: FE JSS RKK. Acquired funding for the research: RKK JRK.

References

1. Kanwar RK, Kanwar JR (2013) Immunomodulatory lactoferrin in the regulation of apoptosis modulatory proteins in cancer. Protein Pept Lett 20: 450–458.
2. Baker EN, Baker HM (2005) Molecular structure, binding properties and dynamics of lactoferrin. Cell Mol Life Sci 62: 2531–2539.
3. Gutteridge JM, Paterson SK, Segal AW, Halliwell B (1981) Inhibition of lipid peroxidation by the iron-binding protein lactoferrin. Biochem J 199: 259.
4. Tomita M, Wakabayashi H, Shin K, Yamauchi K, Yaeshima T, et al. (2009) Twenty-five years of research on bovine lactoferrin applications. Biochimie 91: 52–57.
5. Kanwar JR, Mahidhara G, Kanwar RK (2012) Novel alginate-enclosed chitosan-calcium phosphate-loaded iron-saturated bovine lactoferrin nanocarriers for oral delivery in colon cancer therapy. Nanomedicine 7: 1521–1550.
6. Tsuda H, Kozu T, Iinuma G, Ohashi Y, Saito Y, et al. (2010) Cancer prevention by bovine lactoferrin: from animal studies to human trial. Biometals 23: 399–409.
7. Gibbons JA, Kanwar RK, Kanwar JR (2011) Lactoferrin and cancer in different cancer models. Front biosci (Scholar edition) 3: 1080.
8. Stelwagen K, Carpenter E, Haigh B, Hodgkinson A, Wheeler T (2009) Immune components of bovine colostrum and milk. J Anim Sci 87: 3–9.
9. Kanyshkova T, Buneva V, Nevinsky G (2001) Lactoferrin and its biological functions. Biochemistry (Moscow) 66: 1–7.
10. Mantel C, Miyazawa K, Broxmeyer HE (1994) Physical characteristics and polymerization during iron saturation of lactoferrin, a myelopoietic regulatory molecule with suppressor activity. Lactoferrin: Springer. pp. 121–132.
11. Nevinskii AG, Soboleva SE, Tuzikov FV, Buneva VN, Nevinsky GA (2009) DNA, oligosaccharides, and mononucleotides stimulate oligomerization of human lactoferrin. J Mol Recognit 22: 330–342.
12. Wang H, Hurley WL (1998) Identification of lactoferrin complexes in bovine mammary secretions during mammary gland involution. J Dairy Sci 81: 1896–1903.
13. Brisson G, Britten M, Pouliot Y (2007) Heat-induced aggregation of bovine lactoferrin at neutral pH: Effect of iron saturation. Int Dairy J 17: 617–624.
14. Kanwar JR, Kanwar RK (2009) Gut health immunomodulatory and anti-inflammatory functions of gut enzyme digested high protein micro-nutrient dietary supplement-Enprocal. BMC immunol 10: 7.
15. Van Berkel P, Geerts M, Van Veen H, Kooiman P, Pieper F, et al. (1995) Glycosylated and unglycosylated human lactoferrins both bind iron and show identical affinities towards human lysozyme and bacterial lipopolysaccharide, but differ in their susceptibilities towards tryptic proteolysis. Biochem J 312: 107–114.
16. Kanwar JR, Palmano KP, Sun X, Kanwar RK, Gupta R, et al. (2008) 'Iron-saturated'lactoferrin is a potent natural adjuvant for augmenting cancer chemotherapy. Immunol cell biol 86: 277–288.
17. Fujie Y, Yamamoto H, Ngan CY, Takagi A, Hayashi T, et al. (2005) Oxaliplatin, a potent inhibitor of survivin, enhances paclitaxel-induced apoptosis and mitotic catastrophe in colon cancer cells. JPN J Clin Oncol 35: 453–463.
18. Sato K, Shiba M, Shigematsu A, Teduka N, Tomizawa A (2004) Method for producing lactoferrin. Google Patents.
19. Harmon RJ, Schanbacher FL, Ferguson LC, Smith KL (1976) Changes in lactoferrin, immunoglobulin G, bovine serum albumin, and alpha-lactalbumin during acute experimental and natural coliform mastitis in cows. Infect Immun 13: 533–542.
20. Castellino FJ, Fish WW, Mann KG (1970) Structural studies on bovine lactoferrin. J Biol Chem 245: 4269–4275.
21. Persson BA, Lund M, Forsman J, Chatterton DE, Akesson T (2010) Molecular evidence of stereo-specific lactoferrin dimers in solution. Biophys Chem 151: 187–189.
22. F.L. Schanbacher KLS, Ferguson LC (1971) The similarity of bovine lactoferrin dimer to IgG2. Fed Proc, 30: p. 532.
23. Bennett RM, Bagby GC, Davis J (1981) Calcium-dependent polymerization of lactoferrin. Biochem biophys res comm 101: 88–95.
24. Klimeš J, Jagoš P, Bouda J, Gajdůšek S (1986) Basic qualitative parameters of cow colostrum and their dependence on season and post partum time. Acta Veterinaria Brno 55: 23–39.
25. Sanchez L, Aranda P, Perez MD, Calvo M (1988) Concentration of lactoferrin and transferrin throughout lactation in cow's colostrum and milk. Biol Chem Hoppe Seyler 369: 1005–1008.
26. Soboleva S, Tuzikov F, Tuzikova N, Buneva V, Nevinsky G (2009) DNA and oligosaccharides stimulate oligomerization of human milk lactoferrin. Mol Biol 43: 142–149.
27. DEPT. OF HEALTH E, AND WELFARE PUBLIC HEALTH SERVICE FOOD AND DRUG ADMINISTRATION *ORA/ORO/DEIO/IB* (1985) Inspection Technical Guides, Bacterial Endotoxins/Pyrogens.
28. Xavier PL, Chaudhari K, Verma PK, Pal SK, Pradeep T (2010) Luminescent quantum clusters of gold in transferrin family protein, lactoferrin exhibiting FRET. Nanoscale 2: 2769–2776.
29. Kussendrager K (1994) Effects of heat treatment on structure and iron-binding capacity of bovine lactoferrin. FIL-IDF. Secretariat general.
30. Conesa C, Sánchez L, Pérez M-D, Calvo M (2007) A calorimetric study of thermal denaturation of recombinant human lactoferrin from rice. J Agr Food Chem 55: 4848–4853.
31. Rüegg M, Moor U, Blanc B (1977) A calorimetric study of the thermal denaturation of whey proteins in simulated milk ultrafiltrate. J Dairy Res 44: 509–520.
32. Baker HM, Baker EN (2004) Lactoferrin and iron: structural and dynamic aspects of binding and release. Biometals 17: 209–216.
33. Troost FJ, Steijns J, Saris WH, Brummer RJ (2001) Gastric digestion of bovine lactoferrin in vivo in adults. J Nutr 131: 2101–2104.
34. Sitaram MP, McAbee DD (1997) Isolated rat hepatocytes differentially bind and internalize bovine lactoferrin N- and C-lobes. Biochem J 323 (Pt 3): 815–822.
35. Roseanu A, Florian PE, Moisei M, Sima LE, Evans RW, et al. (2010) Liposomalization of lactoferrin enhanced its anti-tumoral effects on melanoma cells. Biometals 23: 485–492.
36. Duarte D, Nicolau A, Teixeira J, Rodrigues L (2011) The effect of bovine milk lactoferrin on human breast cancer cell lines. J Dairy Sci 94: 66–76.
37. Iigo M, Kuhara T, Ushida Y, Sekine K, Moore MA, et al. (1999) Inhibitory effects of bovine lactoferrin on colon carcinoma 26 lung metastasis in mice. Clin Exp Metastasis 17: 35–40.
38. Rulis AM (2001) Agency Response Letter GRAS Notice No. GRN 000077.
39. EFSA Panel on Dietetic Products NaAN (2012) Scientific Opinion on bovine lactoferrin. EFSA Journal 10(7):2811 [14 pp.].
40. Smith SM, Wunder MB, Norris DA, Shellman YG (2011) A Simple Protocol for Using a LDH-Based Cytotoxicity Assay to Assess the Effects of Death and Growth Inhibition at the Same Time. PLoS ONE 6: e26908.
41. Lonnerdal B, Jiang R, Du X (2011) Bovine lactoferrin can be taken up by the human intestinal lactoferrin receptor and exert bioactivities. J Pediatr Gastroenterol Nutr 53: 606–614.
42. Samarasinghe RM, Kanwar RK, Kanwar JR (2014) The effect of oral administration of iron saturated-bovine lactoferrin encapsulated chitosan-nanocarriers on osteoarthritis. Biomaterials 35: 7522–7534.
43. Kanwar JR, Mahidhara G, Roy K, Sasidharan S, Krishnakumar S, et al. (2014) Fe-bLf nanoformulation targets survivin to kill colon cancer stem cells and maintains absorption of iron, calcium and zinc. Nanomedicine: 1–21.
44. Kothakota S, Azuma T, Reinhard C, Klippel A, Tang J, et al. (1997) Caspase-3-generated fragment of gelsolin: effector of morphological change in apoptosis. Science 278: 294–298.
45. Wolf BB, Schuler M, Echeverri F, Green DR (1999) Caspase-3 is the primary activator of apoptotic DNA fragmentation via DNA fragmentation factor-45/inhibitor of caspase-activated DNase inactivation. J Biol Chem 274: 30651–30656.
46. Fleet JC (1995) A New Role for Lactoferrin: DNA Binding and Transcription Activation. Nutrition Reviews 53: 226–227.
47. Jiang R, Lonnerdal B (2011) Apo-lactoferrin regulates transcription of the TGF beta 1 gene and may thus stimulate intestinal differentiation. The FASEB Journal 25: 340.346.

12

Silver Wire Amplifies the Signaling Mechanism for IL-1beta Production More Than Silver Submicroparticles in Human Monocytic THP-1 Cells

Hye Jin Jung[1,⁹], Pyo June Pak[1,⁹], Sung Hyo Park[1], Jae Eun Ju[1], Joong-Su Kim[2], Hoi-Seon Lee[3]*, Namhyun Chung[1]*

1 Department of Biosystems and Biotechnology, College of Life Sciences and Biotechnology, Korea University, Seoul, Korea, 2 Bioindustry Process Center, Jeonbuk Branch Institute, Korea Research Institute of Bioscience and Biotechnology, Jeoneup, Korea, 3 College of Agriculture and Life Science, Chonbuk National University, Jeonju, Korea

Abstract

Silver materials have been widely used in diverse fields. However, their toxicity and their mechanism, especially in different forms, have not been studied sufficiently. Thus, cytotoxicity, apoptosis, and interleukin-1beta (IL-1β) production were investigated using macrophage-like THP-1 cells in the presence of Ag microparticles (AgMPs, 2.7 μm), Ag submicroparticles (AgSMPs, 150 nm), and Ag wires (AgWs, 274 nm×5.3 μm). The levels of cytotoxicity, apoptosis, and IL-1β production by AgWs were higher than those by the other two AgSMPs and AgMPs. This trend was also observed with each step of the signaling mechanism for IL-1β production, which is a single pathway affiliated with ROS generation or lysosomal rupture or both, cathepsin B, caspase-1 (NALP3 inflammasome), and finally IL-1β production in THP-1 cells. All these results suggest that, for development of safe and effective silver materials, the shape or form of silver materials should be considered, especially for macrophage cell lines because epithelial cell lines are not overly sensitive to silver materials.

Editor: Wei-Chun Chin, University of California, Merced, United States of America

Funding: Funding provided by the National Research Foundation of Korea; NRF-2011-0017012, www.nrf.re.kr. The funders had no role in study design, data collection and analysis, decision to publish, or preparation of the manuscript.

Competing Interests: The authors have declared that no competing interests exist.

* Email: nchung@korea.ac.kr (NC); hoiseon@jbnu.ac.kr (H-SL)

⁹ These authors contributed equally to this work.

Introduction

Advances in nanotechnology have promoted the use of merchandise containing silver materials with which the public can easily come into contact [1]. Indeed, silver materials are broadly made use of for industrial and biomedical applications since they possess remarkable antimicrobial activity [2,3]. Therefore, the general public can easily be exposed to silver materials from diverse fields. Recently, some studies have demonstrated that silver materials introduced into the systemic blood supply can induce blood-brain barrier dysfunction and astrocyte swelling, in addition to causing neuronal degeneration [4]. Several studies have reported that silver materials significantly decrease mitochondrial function and induce cell necrosis or apoptosis of several cell types [3]. Furthermore, an *in vivo* study by Larese *et al.* has shown that silver materials can penetrate into the upper layers of the epidermis in excised human skin in static diffusion cells [5]. Another *in vivo* study reported that silver materials induce inflammatory responses and tissue damage in the lungs of mice.

Inflammation is a major biological response to harmful stimuli such as pathogens and irritants that occur during infections or after tissue damage [6]. IL-1β is related to some of cytokines, which cause a variety of biological effects associated with infection, inflammation, and autoimmune processes [7]. IL-1β is also an important proinflammatory mediator that is concerned with the generation of systemic and local responses to infection and injury [8]. There is evidence that IL-1β can induce apoptosis and cell proliferation in chondrocytes [9], that is, the inactive precursor pro-IL-1β in the cytosol is converted to mature IL-1β by caspase-1. Caspase-1 itself is synthesized as an inactive pro-caspase-1 (45 kDa zymogen) that undergoes autocatalytic processing in the presence of the stimuli. The activity of caspase-1 is tightly controlled by cytosolic multiprotein complexes called NALP3 inflammasomes (also called cryopyrin or NLRP3).

NALP3 inflammasomes are composed of Nod-like receptor protein NALP3, cardinal, adaptor ASC (apoptosis-associated speck-like protein containing a C-terminal caspase recruitment domain), and caspase-1. NALP3 inflammasomes potently modulate innate immune function by regulating the maturation and secretion of IL-1β [10,11]. NALP3 inflammasome is assembled and activated in the presence of the pathogen-associated molecular patterns (PAMPs) and damage-associated molecular patterns (DAMPs). Though the mechanisms of NALP3 inflammasome activation remain unclear, two separate groups have recently reported on the mediator of NALP3 inflammasome activation. First, lysosomal destabilization and subsequent release of cathepsin B into the cytoplasm induced activation of NALP3 inflammasomes [12]. Second, phagocytosis of crystalline silica by macrophages led to reactive oxygen species (ROS) production, which induces activation of NALP3 inflammasomes [13].

Nowadays, AgWs, and not nanoparticles, are utilized by drug delivery systems [14,15]. AgWs is more preferred for drug delivery system than other silver materials. Above all, AgWs have been suggested for use in nanoscale field-effect transistors, scanning probe microscopy tips, and sensing array elements [14]. In addition, AgWs have been applied in these fields, but even though AgWs are widely applied to living tissues, there is a serious lack of information on the signaling mechanism for the possible toxic effects of AgWs [16,17]. Therefore, the present study aimed to elucidate the signaling mechanism for the cytotoxic effect of silver materials including AgWs, AgSMPs, and AgMPs. We found that the differential degrees of cytotoxicity as observed by apoptosis and IL-1β expression in human monocytic THP-1 cells are correlated to the observed signaling intensity. Our results might provide basic information that helps to design safe and effective forms of silver materials.

Materials and Methods

Cell culture

THP-1 cells (human acute monocytic leukemia cell line; TIB-202, ATCC, USA) were plated at a density of 3.0×10^5 cells/mL with RPMI 1640 (WelGENE, Korea) supplemented with 10% heat-inactivated fetal bovine serum (FBS; JBI, Korea), 0.05 mM 2-mercaptoethanol, 100 U/mL penicillin, and 100 μg/mL streptomycin in 6-well culture plates. The culture was maintained in a 37°C, 5% CO_2 atmosphere.

Characterization of silver materials

The morphologies of silver materials were observed by field-emission scanning electron microscopy (FE-SEM; JEOL 7500, US), equipped with energy-dispersive X-ray spectroscopy (EDS). Each silver material was affixed to the mounts by carbon tape. We investigated the zeta potential of silver materials using the Nanoparticle size & zeta potential analyzer (90plus, Brookhaven Instruments, Germany). To measure the zeta potential, which are a surface electrical characteristic for probing the interaction between particles, all silver materials were freshly prepared in water, FBS, and serum-free RPMI 1640 to a concentration of 100 μg/mL [18].

Treatment of silver materials

Silver materials used in this experiment were AgMPs (2.7 μm; Sigma-Aldrich, USA), AgSMPs (150 nm; Nano Technology Inc., Korea), and AgWs (274 nm×5.3 μm; NanoAmor, USA). THP-1 cells were seeded at a density of 1.0×10^6 cells per well in a 6-well plate. The cells were differentiated into macrophage-like cells by adding 0.5 μM of phorbol 12-myristate 13-acetate (PMA; Sigma-Aldrich, USA) for 24 h prior to use. PMA-primed THP-1 cells were treated with AgWs, AgSMPs, or AgMPs. All silver materials were in serum-free RPMI 1640 to a concentration of 2 mg/mL prior to each experiment. The stock suspension was sonicated for 3 min to disperse silver materials, and then dilutions were made to achieve final test concentrations. The cells were treated with various concentrations (25, 50, 100, and 200 μg/mL) of silver materials according to the time schedule [19].

Morphology of silver materials-treated cells

Cells treated with silver materials were photographed by light optical microscopy. After exposure to 100 μg/mL of silver materials for 24 h, THP-1 cells were gently washed with phosphate-buffered saline and then pictured under light optical microscopy (CK70, Olympus, Japan).

WST-1 cytotoxicity assay

THP-1 cells (5.0×10^4 cells/well) were differentiated by PMA for 24 h in a 96-well cell culture plate and were then washed with a cell culture medium. After differentiation into macrophage, cells were treated with silver materials for 24 h. The cytotoxicity assay was measured by the PreMix WST-1 Cell Proliferation Assay System (Takara Bio Inc., Japan) according to the manufacturer's protocol. Briefly, 10 μL of WST-1 reagent was added per well, and the cells were additionally incubated for 1 h. The absorbance of WST-1-added samples was measured by an EL800 microplate reader (Bio-Tek Instruments, USA) at 490 nm.

Lactate dehydrogenase (LDH) release assay

PMA-primed THP-1 cells were treated with silver materials and evaluated for cytotoxicity using an LDH Cytotoxicity Detection Kit (Takara Bio Inc., Japan) according to the manufacturer's protocol. Supernatant of silver materials-treated cells was separated by centrifugation and analyzed for LDH release. Samples were measured using a microplate reader at a wavelength of 490 nm.

Analysis of sub-G1 DNA content and cell size

DNA fragmentation was analyzed by flow cytometer at an excitation wavelength (Ex) of 488 nm and emission wavelength (Em) of 610 nm. Briefly, after 24 h of exposure to silver materials, the PMA-primed THP-1 cells were collected. Then, the cell pellet was washed in PBS, fixed in ice-cold ethanol (70%), and stored at −20°C for 2 h or longer. Before flow cytometry analysis, ethanol was removed by centrifugation and the cells were washed twice with PBS. The cell pellet was resuspended in a minimal amount of PBS and stained with propidium iodide (PI, 50 μg/mL; Sigma-Aldrich) staining solution containing RNase (0.1 mg/mL; Sigma-Aldrich) and Triton X-100 (0.1%, v/v; Sigma-Aldrich). The PI-stained cells were incubated at 37°C in the dark for 30 min. The sub-G1 DNA content was obtained using the flow cytometer by measuring the amount of PI-labeled DNA in fixed cells. Data was analyzed using the ModiFit LT software program (Verity Software House, USA).

Flow cytometer analysis for apoptosis

PMA-primed THP-1 cells were treated with various concentrations of silver materials for 6 h. After treatment, cells were detached and harvested by centrifugation. Cells were then resuspended in an Annexin V binding buffer, a component of the Apoptosis Detection kit (BD Biosciences, USA). Cells were then mixed with 5 μL of Annexin V-FITC and 5 μL of PI solution. The cell suspension was incubated in the dark for 15 min at room temperature. The fluorescence intensity of Annexin V-FITC and PI was analyzed at an Ex/Em of 488/530 nm and 488/617 nm, respectively.

Enzyme-linked immunosorbent assay (ELISA)

PMA-primed THP-1 cells were treated with various concentrations of silver materials for 24 h. IL-1β production levels in the culture medium were measured using an ELISA kit (R&D Systems, USA) according to the manufacturer's protocol. Plates were read at 450 nm, using an EL800 microplate reader. CA-074-methyl ester (CA-074-Me), diphenyleneiodonium chloride (DPI), and butylated hydroxyanisole (BHA) were purchased from Sigma-Aldrich. For analysis of inhibitor effects, PMA-primed THP-1 cells

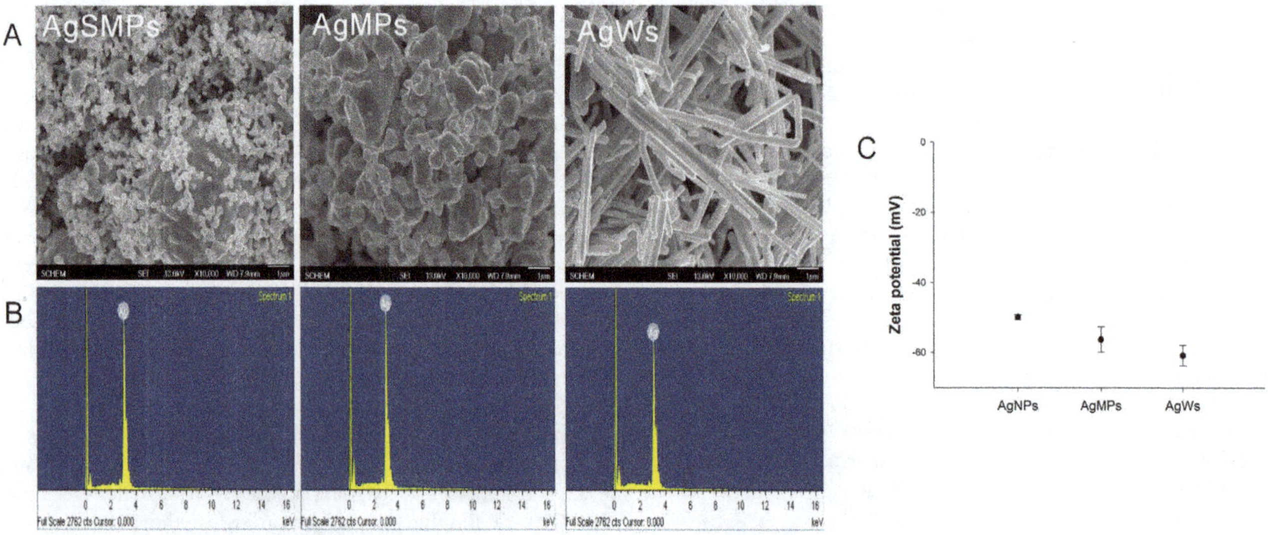

Figure 1. Characterization of silver materials. (A) FE-SEM top-view images of silver materials (10,000×). (B) EDS. (C) Zeta potential of silver materials in serum-free RPMI 1640.

were washed with RPMI 1640 and pre-incubated with CA-074-Me, DPI, and BHA for 30 min. Then, the cells were treated with each silver material for 24 h.

Reverse transcription polymerase chain reaction (RT-PCR)

PMA-primed THP-1 cells (1×10^7) were treated with 100 μg/mL of silver materials for 24 h and then, all RNA was extracted from the cells using an RNeasy Mini Kit (Qiagen, Germany) in accordance with the manufacturer's protocol. Extracted RNA was reverse transcribed using the Reverse Transcription System (Promega, USA). Synthesized cDNA was amplified by PCR using *Taq* polymerase (GeneAll, Korea). The sequence of specific primers for NALP3 (cytoplasmic receptor) and GAPDH was as follows: NALP3 forward: 5′-TGCCTTTGACGAGCACATAG-3′; NALP3 reverse: 5′-GCAGCAAACTGG AAGGAAG-3′; caspase-1 forward: 5′-GAAGGCATTTGTGGGAAGAA-3′; caspase-1 reverse: 5′-CATCTGGCTGCTCAAATGAA-3′; and GAPDH forward: 5′-GAGTCAACGGATTTGGTCGT-3′; GAPDH reverse: 5′-TTGATTTTGGAGGGATCTCG-3′. After 5 min at 95°C, 28 cycles at 95°C for 1 min, 53°C for 1 min (caspase-1; 51°C), and 72°C for 2 min were performed, ending with a final extension step at 72°C for 5 min. Quantification of PCR products was performed by electrophoresis. Data was analyzed using the Image Quant software program (GE Healthcare, USA).

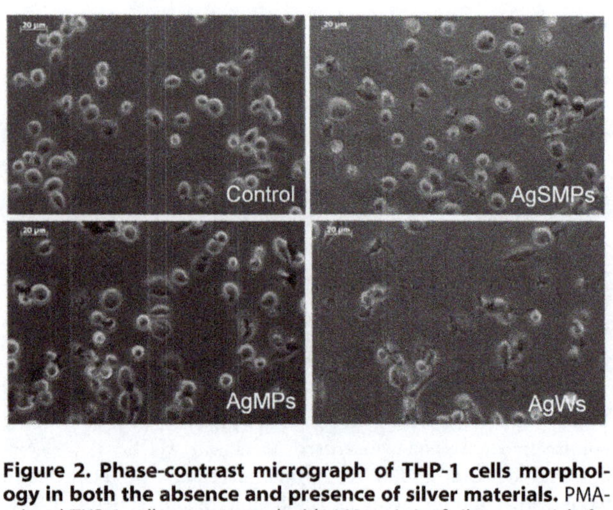

Figure 2. Phase-contrast micrograph of THP-1 cells morphology in both the absence and presence of silver materials. PMA-primed THP-1 cells were treated with 100 μg/mL of silver materials for 24 h. The cells were photographed using a phase-contrast microscope to estimate overall morphology (400×).

Measurement of caspase-1 enzymatic activity

Caspase-1 enzymatic activity was determined by a caspase-1 colorimetric assay kit (R&D Systems, US) according to the manufacturer's protocol. In brief, the PMA-primed THP-1 cells (1×10^7) were treated with 200 μg/mL of silver materials for 24 h, and then the cells were lysed in 250 μL of cold lysis buffer. The cell lysates were incubated on ice for 10 min and centrifuged at 10,000×g for 1 min, and then the supernatants were collected. A volume of 50 μL of cell lysate was added to 50 μL of caspase-1 reaction buffer with 40 mM dithiothreitol (DTT). Each sample was combined with 5 μL of 4 mM caspase-1 colorimetric substrate (WEHE-pNA), followed by a 2-h incubation at 37°C. The enzymatic activity of caspase-1 was measured by an EL800 microplate reader at 405 nm [20].

Acridine orange staining

Change in lysosomal permeability was measured by acridine orange (Sigma-Aldrich) staining using flow cytometry [21]. Briefly, PMA-primed THP-1 cells were preloaded with 0.5 μg/mL acridine orange in RPMI 1640 for 30 min at 37°C and then washed three times with RPMI 1640 and treated with silver materials for 24 h. After exposure, cells were detached and harvested. The fluorescence intensity was analyzed using a FACSCalibur flow cytometer at an Ex/Em of 488/620 nm. Fluorescent photomicrographs of lysosomes in THP-1 cells upon exposure to silver materials were examined using a fluorescence microscope (Axio Observer D1, Carl-Zeiss, Germany). The cells were washed 3 times with phosphate buffer saline after incubation with silver materials and were stained with 20 μg/mL acridine orange for 15 min.

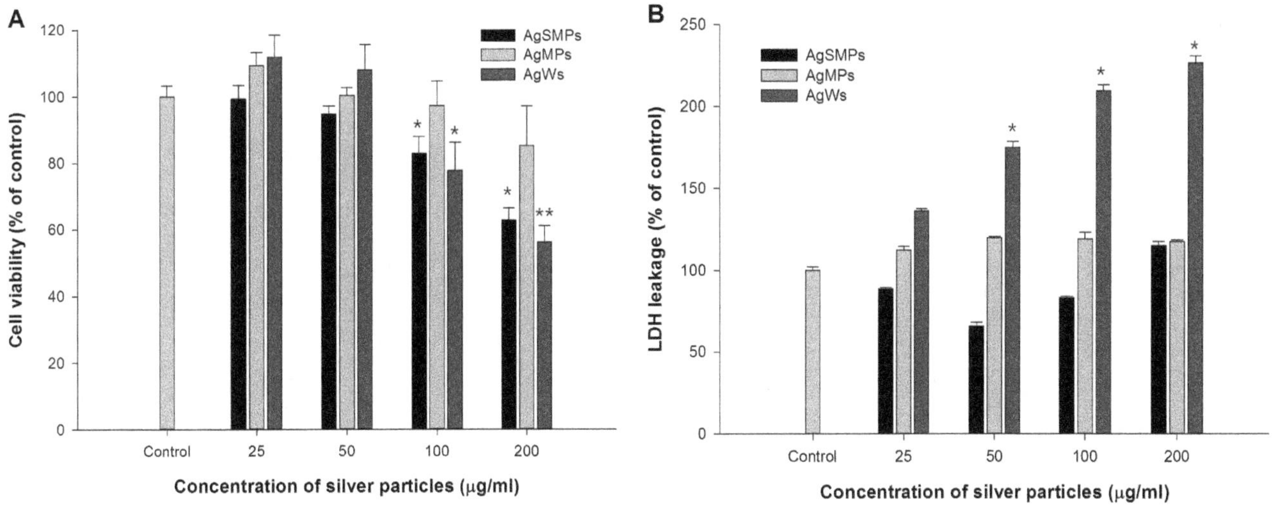

Figure 3. Cytotoxicity induced by different forms of silver materials. (A) Cell viability was measured by WST-1 assay. PMA-primed THP-1 cells were treated with different forms of silver materials for 24 h and the extents of viability for the treated groups (25, 50, 100, and 200 μg/mL) were expressed as a percentage of the control group. Data are represented as the mean ±SD (n = 5). (B) LDH leakage assay due to membrane damage was measured using an LDH Cytotoxicity Detection Kit. PMA-primed THP-1 cells were treated with different forms of silver materials for 24 h and the extents of LDH leakage for the treated groups were expressed as a percentage of the control group. Data are represented as the mean ±SD (n = 5). *$p<0.05$, **$p<0.01$.

Measurement of cellular ROS production

Intracellular formation of ROS was measured as described previously using oxidation-sensitive dye 2′,7′-dichlorofluorescin diacetate (DCFH-DA) as the substrate [22]. THP-1 cells growing in black 96-well microplates were loaded with 100 μM DCFH-DA in phosphate-buffered saline and incubated for 30 min in the dark. Cells were then treated with different concentrations of each silver material and incubated for 24 h after washing the cells with phosphate-buffered saline three times. The formation of 2′,7′-dichlorofluorescin (DCF) due to oxidation of DCFH in the presence of various ROS was read every 30 min at an Ex of 485 nm and an Em of 535 nm using a multilabel plate reader (Victor3, Perkin Elmer, USA). Fluorescent photomicrographs of ROS in THP-1 cells upon exposure to silver materials were obtained using a fluorescence microscope. The cells were washed 3 times with PBS after incubation with silver materials and were stained with 40 μg/mL DCFH-DA for 30 min.

Statistical analyses

Data were expressed as mean ±SD. The data were analyzed using Student's t-test where statistical significance was calculated for silver treated samples against untreated (control). Statistical significance was determined in level of *$p<0.05$ or **$p<0.01$.

Results

Particle characterizations

The shapes of silver materials were examined using FE-SEM images (Fig. 1A). The images showed that AgMPs are larger than AgSMPs and that AgWs have an expected aspect ratio of about 19. Purity of the particles was confirmed by ion analysis of silver materials using EDS. The major constituent of silver materials was silver (Fig. 1B) and the atomic percentages of the particles were 100% (data not shown). We investigated the zeta potential to confirm the stability of silver materials in water, FBS, serum-free RPMI 1640. If particles have high zeta potentials of the same polarity, this can prevent agglomeration among particles because of the repulsive force between each particle. Values for zeta potential were similar in three solvents. Therefore, stability of silver materials was estimated in serum-free RPMI 1640 that was used for this present experiment. The values of silver materials were less than −40 mV (AgWs: −60.82±2.89 mV; AgSMPs: −49.91±0.76 mV; AgMPs: −56.26±3.60 mV) (Fig. 1C). Therefore, the particles were stable in the serum-free RPMI 1640.

Induction of cytotoxicity by silver materials

To assess the cytotoxicity of silver materials on THP-1 cells, overall morphologies of PMA-primed THP-1 cells in both the absence and presence of different forms of silver materials were observed using a phase-contrast microscope (Fig. 2). Unlike control, the cells cultured with AgWs were more elongated or had more of a crushed morphology than those cultured with the other silver materials.

Cell proliferation in the presence of silver materials was measured by WST-1 assay (Fig. 3A). As the concentration of silver materials increased (25–200 μg/mL) for 24 h, the viability of PMA-primed THP-1 cells decreased gradually. The degree of cytotoxicity in higher concentrations (100 and 200 μg/mL) decreased more with AgWs and AgSMPs than with AgMPs. Next, extracellular LDH levels were measured to evaluate the cell membrane damage elicited by silver materials (Fig. 3B). As the concentration of silver materials increased, the LDH level of PMA-primed THP-1 cells became much higher with AgWs than with the others. This result suggests that AgWs induced more membrane damage or LDH leakage than the others.

Induction of apoptosis by silver materials

Cell death induced by silver materials could occur either by an abrupt process called necrosis or by a tightly regulated process called apoptosis [23]. Characteristics of cell death by silver materials can be detailed by studying DNA damage, cell shrinkage, and apoptosis. DNA damage was detected by measuring sub-G1 DNA in cell cycle analysis. The results revealed that the extents of sub-G1 DNA were increased in a dose-

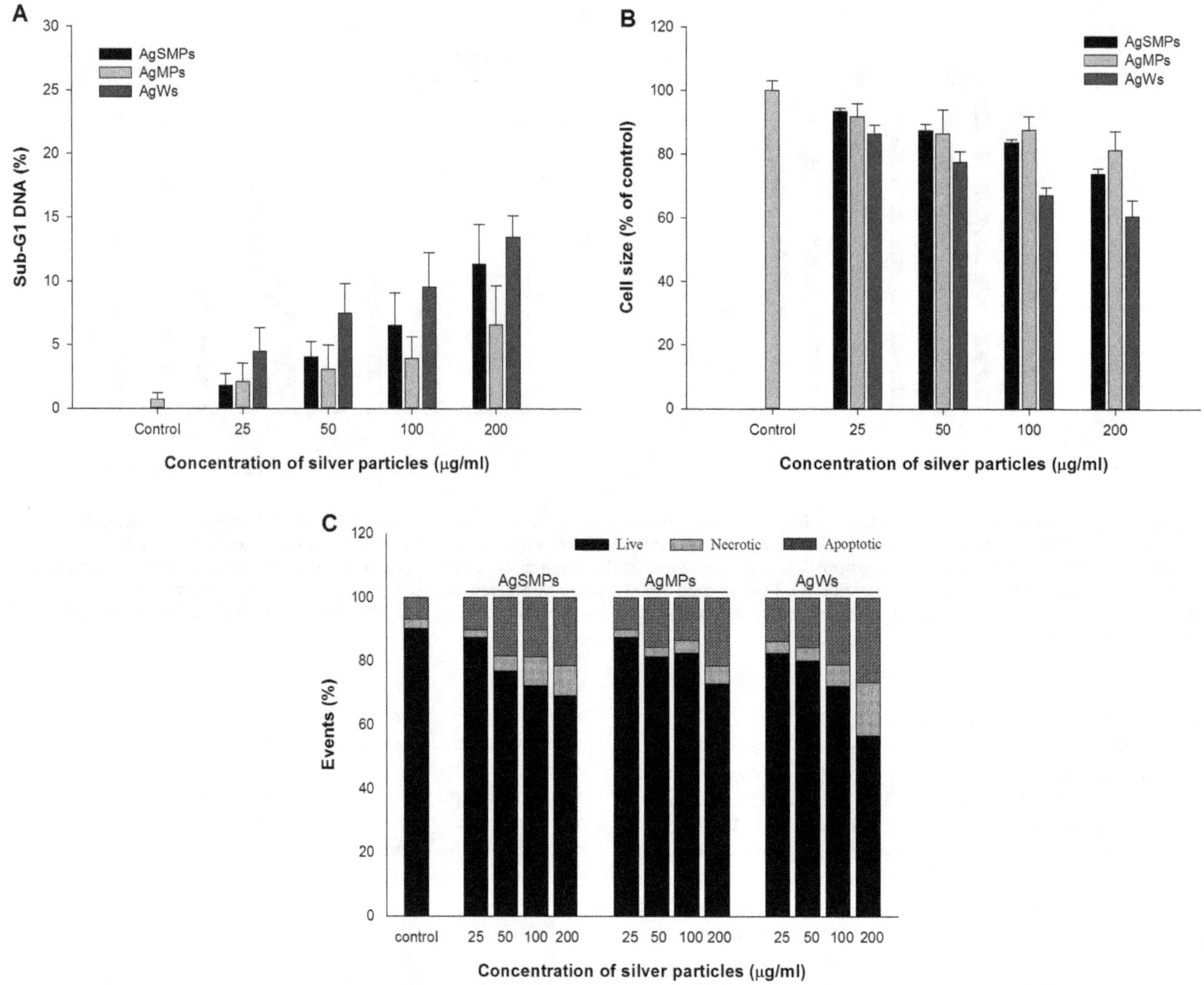

Figure 4. Various evidences of cell death induced by different forms of silver materials. (A) The Sub-G1 DNA analysis for PMA-primed THP-1 cells after treatment with silver materials for 24 h. The extent of the sub-G1 peak was determined by flow cytometry using PI staining. Data are represented as the mean ±SD (n = 3). (B) The decrease in the extent of relative cell size as measured using forward scattering of flow cytometry. PMA-primed THP-1 cells were treated with different forms of silver materials for 24 h. Data are represented as the mean ±SD (n = 3). (C) Annexin-V staining of PMA-primed THP-1 cells to detect the mode of cell death in the presence of different forms of silver materials for 6 h. AnnexinV/PI analysis was performed to assess the percentage of viable, apoptotic, and necrotic cells.

dependent manner (Fig. 4A). The extents of sub-G1 DNA with different forms of silver materials were in the overall order of AgWs>AgSMPs>AgMPs. A significant decrease in the extent of forward scatter (indication of cell shrinkage) in flow cytometry was monitored after treatment with different types of silver materials. A dose course study showed that the treatment caused a rapid decrease in cell size, the degree of which was in the overall order of AgWs>AgSMPs≈AgMPs (Fig. 4B). Cells with irreversible damage undergo apoptosis. Apoptosis has been regarded as a major mechanism for cell death upon exposure to silver materials [24]. To unveil the extent and mode of cell death, annexin-V/PI staining and FACS analysis were performed (Fig. 4C). The results showed that the extent of apoptotic and necrotic cells increased in a dose-dependent manner with all types of silver materials. However, the rates of cells undergoing apoptosis were obviously higher than the rates of cells undergoing necrosis.

Induction of IL-1β maturation and caspase-1 activation by NALP3 inflammasome in the presence of silver materials

Proinflammatory response including release of mature IL-1β was induced by inhalation of AgSMPs [25]. Additionally, IL-1β production depended dramatically on the characteristics of silver materials [26]. Based on these two pieces of information, the association between the characteristics of silver materials and inflammatory response was hypothesized. THP-1 cells were incubated using different silver materials and the level of IL-1β production was analyzed with ELISA. PMA-primed THP-1 cells responded dose-dependently to the addition of silver materials, with AgWs inducing much higher IL-1β production than the other two particles at all concentrations tested (Fig. 5A).

The protease caspase-1, which regulates the cleavage and maturation of the precursor form of IL-1β, is made up of NALP3 inflammasome complex [8,27]. After assembly of NALP3 inflam-

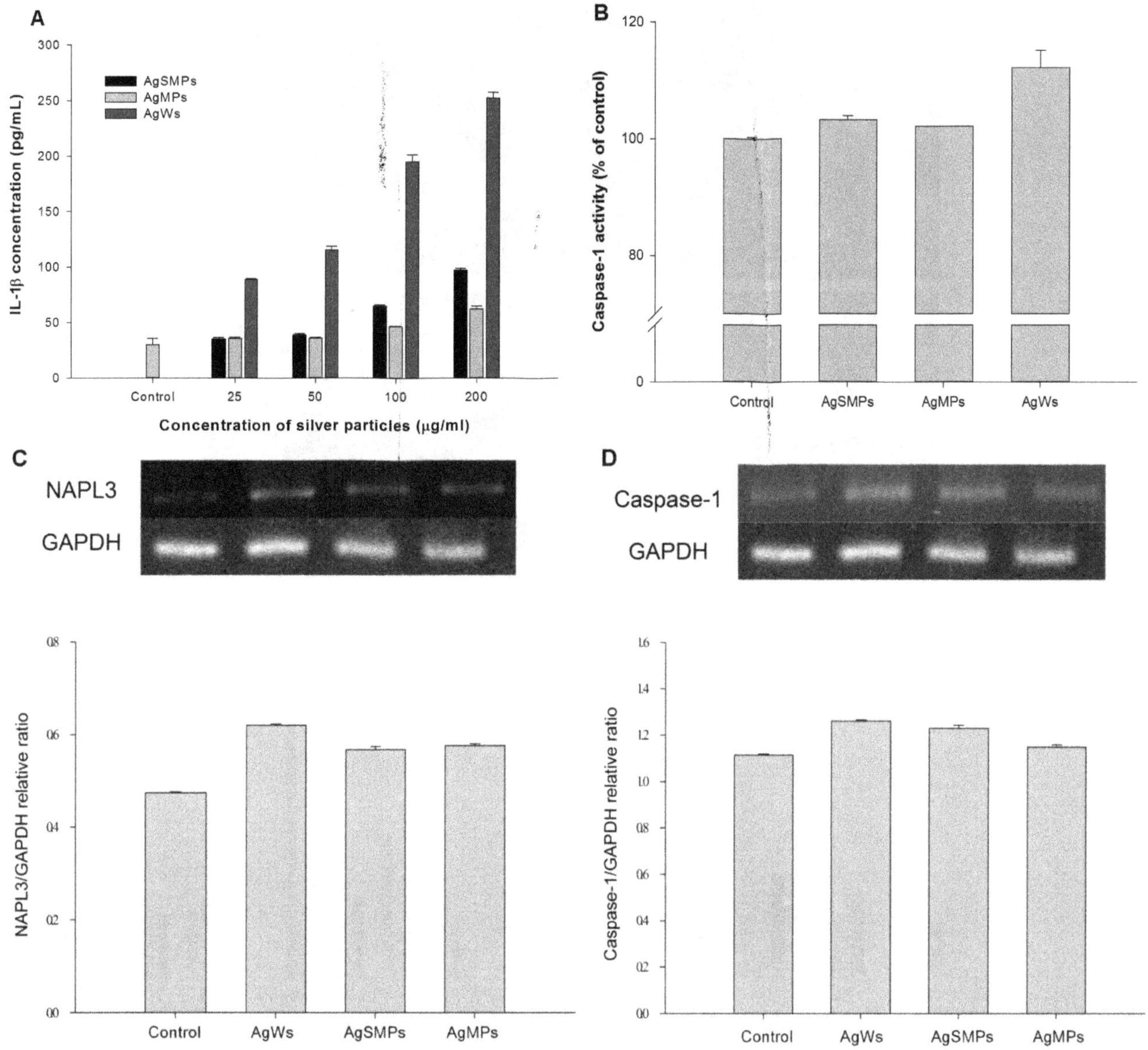

Figure 5. Extent of IL-1β production and active caspase-1 by PMA-primed THP-1 cells in the presence of silver materials. (A) Differences in the levels of IL-1β production induced by different forms of silver materials. The cells were treated with different silver materials for 24 h. Data are represented as the mean ±SD (n = 3). (B) Difference in the levels of caspase-1 activity. The cells were treated with 200 μg/mL of silver materials for 24 h. Data are represented as the mean ±SD (n = 3). (C) Differences in the levels of caspase-1 mRNA expression levels. The cells were treated with 100 μg/mL of silver materials for 24 h. (D) Differences in the levels of caspase-1 mRNA expression. The cells were treated with 100 μg/mL of silver materials for 24 h.

masome, caspase-1 regulates IL-1β maturation. On the other hand, NALP3 inflammasome is required for the activation of procaspase-1 in response to several types of danger signals. We hypothesized that the extent of IL-1β induction is affected by the differential activity of caspase-1 in the presence of silver materials. Caspase-1 enzyme activity was measured in the cell lysate. As a result, although the difference in the extent was small, caspase-1 activity was higher with AgWs than with the others (Fig. 5B). We also examined the mRNA gene expression extent of caspase-1 and NALP3 by PMA-primed THP-1 cells in the presence of silver materials. We found that caspase-1 gene expression was higher with AgWs than with the others (Fig. 5C). Furthermore, NALP3 mRNA gene expression was higher with AgWs than with the others (Fig. 5D). These findings indicate that the level of NALP3 gene expression has relevance to the level of caspase-1 enzyme activation and gene expression. These results collectively indicate that AgWs activates the NALP3 inflammasome complex more than the others, thus leading to the stronger activation of caspase-1.

Activation of NALP3 inflammasome via lysosomal destabilization and cathepsin B activation in the presence of silver materials

The activator of NALP3 inflammasome, for example crystalline or particulate materials, causes phagocytosis and then leads to lysosomal damage, resulting in cytosolic release of lysosomal contents [8]. Cathepsin B, a lysosomal protease, triggers the

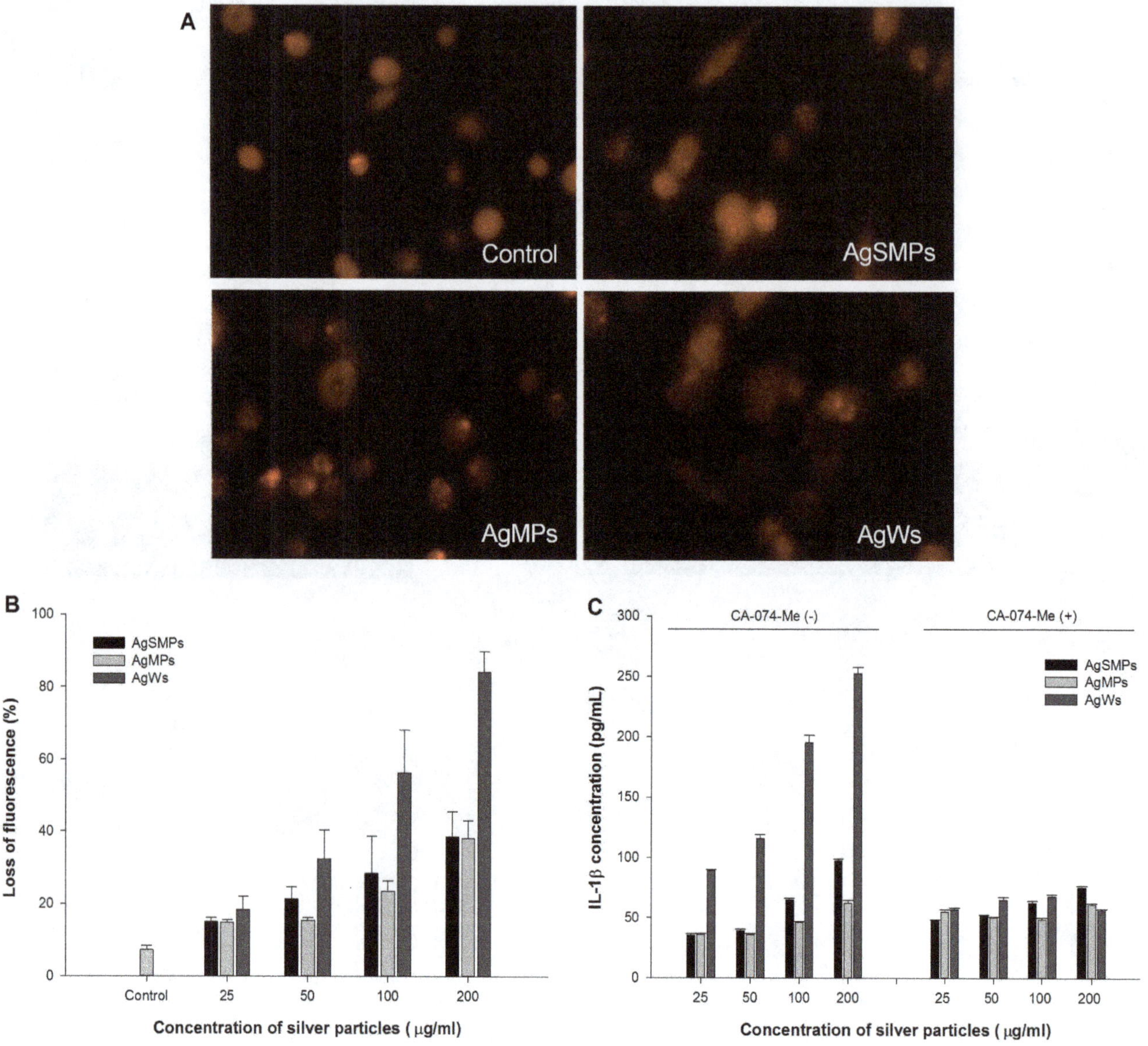

Figure 6. Involvement of lysosomal destabilization and cathepsin B activity with IL-1β production in the presence of silver materials. (A) PMA-primed THP-1 cells were treated with each of the silver materials (100 μg/mL) for 24 h. At the end of exposure, the cells were loaded with acridine orange (20 μg/mL) for 15 min at 37°C and photographed using a fluorescence microscope (400×). (B) Lysosomal destabilization as measured by loss of fluorescence with increasing concentration of silver materials. The cells were preloaded with acridine orange (0.5 μg/mL) for 30 min, treated with silver materials, and analyzed using FACS to determine the loss of acridine orange from lysosome. Data are represented as the mean ±SD (n = 3). (C) Involvement of cathepsin B in silver materials-induced IL-1β production. The cells were treated with different forms of silver materials for 24 h in both the absence and presence of cathepsin B inhibitor (CA-074-Me; 10 μM). IL-1β levels were measured using ELISA. Data are represented as the mean ±SD (n = 3).

NALP3 inflammasome directly. To evaluate the lysosomal destabilization by silver materials, cell staining was conducted with acridine orange and pictured using a fluorescence microscope (Fig. 6A). Acridine orange reacts with the acidic content of organelles after the silver materials incurs membrane damage and then the fluorescence intensity decreases. As can be observed in Fig. 6A, the fluorescent intensity with AgWs was lower or weaker than that with the others. The fluorescent intensity of PMA-primed THP-1 cells treated with silver materials showed a very similar trend (Fig. 6B). These results demonstrate that different forms of silver materials induced the destabilization of lysosomal membranes dose-dependently and that AgWs caused more lysosomal membrane damage than the others.

Next, we hypothesized that cathepsin B was involved in the process of activation of NALP3 inflammasome and caspase-1. PMA-primed THP-1 cells were treated with silver materials in both the absence and presence of a cathepsin-B-specific inhibitor (CA-074-Me). The presence of CA-074-Me significantly suppressed the extent of IL-1β production in all concentrations tested, regardless of the type of silver materials (Fig. 6C). However, in the absence of CA-074-Me, the extent of IL-1β production increased in a dose-dependent manner and was in the order of AgWs>AgSMPs>AgMPs. This result suggests that more cathepsin B was

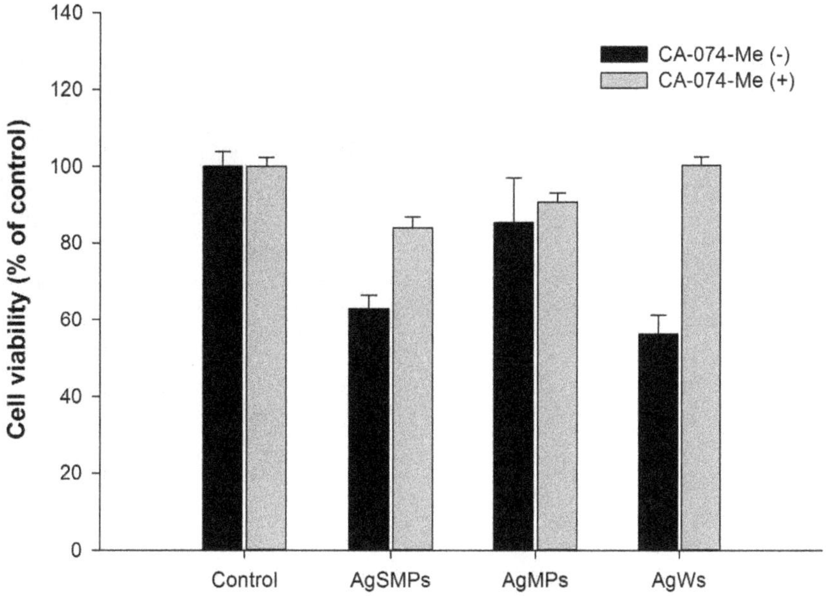

Figure 7. Involvement of cathepsin B in cytotoxicity induced by silver materials. Cell viability was measured by WST-1 assay. PMA-primed THP-1 cells were treated with 200 μg/mL of each of the silver materials for 24 h in both the absence and presence of cathepsin B inhibitor (CA-074-Me; 10 μM). Data are represented as the mean ±SD (n = 5). *p<0.05.

released into the cytoplasm with AgWs than with the others, resulting in the higher activation of NALP3 inflammasome and IL-1β production with AgWs than with the others.

Additionally, PMA-primed THP-1 cells were treated with silver materials both with and without CA-074-Me. Then, WST-1 assay was performed to observe cell viability (Fig. 7). The results demonstrate that CA-074-Me significantly suppressed the cytotoxicity by silver materials, especially in the presence of AgWs. These data suggest that cathepsin B released from damaged lysosome by the action of AgSMPs or AgWs was a cause of the observed phenomenon.

Correlation between ROS generation and NALP3 inflammasome activation

Like cathepsin B, ROS are widely linked to signaling pathways and are known to induce activation of NALP3 inflammasome. To test the hypothesis that the generation of ROS correlates with toxicity and inflammatory response by different types of silver materials, the relationship between the level of ROS generation and the IL-1β production was investigated in the both the absence and presence of ROS inhibitors. First, the levels of ROS with PMA-primed THP-1 cells were measured in the presence of different forms of silver materials (Fig. 8A). The results showed that, in the presence of silver materials, more ROS was produced than with control and that the extent of ROS production was in the order of AgWs>AgSMPs>AgMPs. Photographs taken using a fluorescence microscope (Fig. 8B) supported the previous data in Fig. 8A.

ROS inhibitor BHA (a broad ROS scavenger) or DPI (a specific inhibitor of NADPH oxidase) was employed to suppress ROS production by PMA-primed THP-1 cells in the presence of silver materials. Then, when IL-1β production was measured, IL-1β production was suppressed significantly more in the presence of ROS inhibitors than in the absence of ROS inhibitors (Figs. 8C and D). The extent of IL-1β production was in the order of AgWs>AgSMPs>AgMPs. Considering the report that found that NADPH oxidase generated inflammasome-activating ROS [10], these results imply that ROS as well as cathepsin B are linked to the signaling pathway of IL-1β production through NALP3 inflammasome in the presence of silver materials, especially AgWs or AgSMPs.

Discussion

Engineered silver materials, such as AgSMPs and AgWs, are being developed and used in a variety of applications [28], and thus, people can easily be exposed to these silver materials. However, what is still required is a) a detailed description of the molecular mechanism induced by silver materials and b) a risk assessment for using them. This present study aimed to identify the mechanisms of inflammatory responses to silver materials, including AgWs. Many previous studies reported about the risks of wire-structured metal. AgWs induced cytotoxicity at concentrations ≥190 μg/mL in Hela cells and HEp-2 cells and resulted in the up-regulation in macrophages of inflammatory cytokines such as IL-1α and IFN-γ and the down-regulation of IL-6 [29,30]. Also PVP-coated Ag wire causes cytotoxicity but that PVP-coated spherical Ag has no cytotoxicity in A549 cell lines [31].

Based on these previous studies, we employed AgSMPs of 150 nm in the present study. As expected and known in other studies, if the particle size become smaller than 150 nm, we believe that the cytotoxicity of sphere-shaped particle increases up to certain point since many studies indicated that nanoparticle with too small size (for example, <10 nm) is not toxic any more [32]. So, we hypothesized that AgWs might induce more cytotoxicity and inflammatory responses than AgSMPs and AgMPs.

In the present study, silver materials were diluted and sonicated before addition to the culture medium RPMI 1640 containing 10% FBS. It is known that silver materials can be stabilized in the presence of FBS [33]. Thus, complexation between silver materials and FBS may help silver materials to be stabilized and dispersed so that silver materials can enter inside the macrophage cells. In analogy, silver materials in the environment are not supposed to be

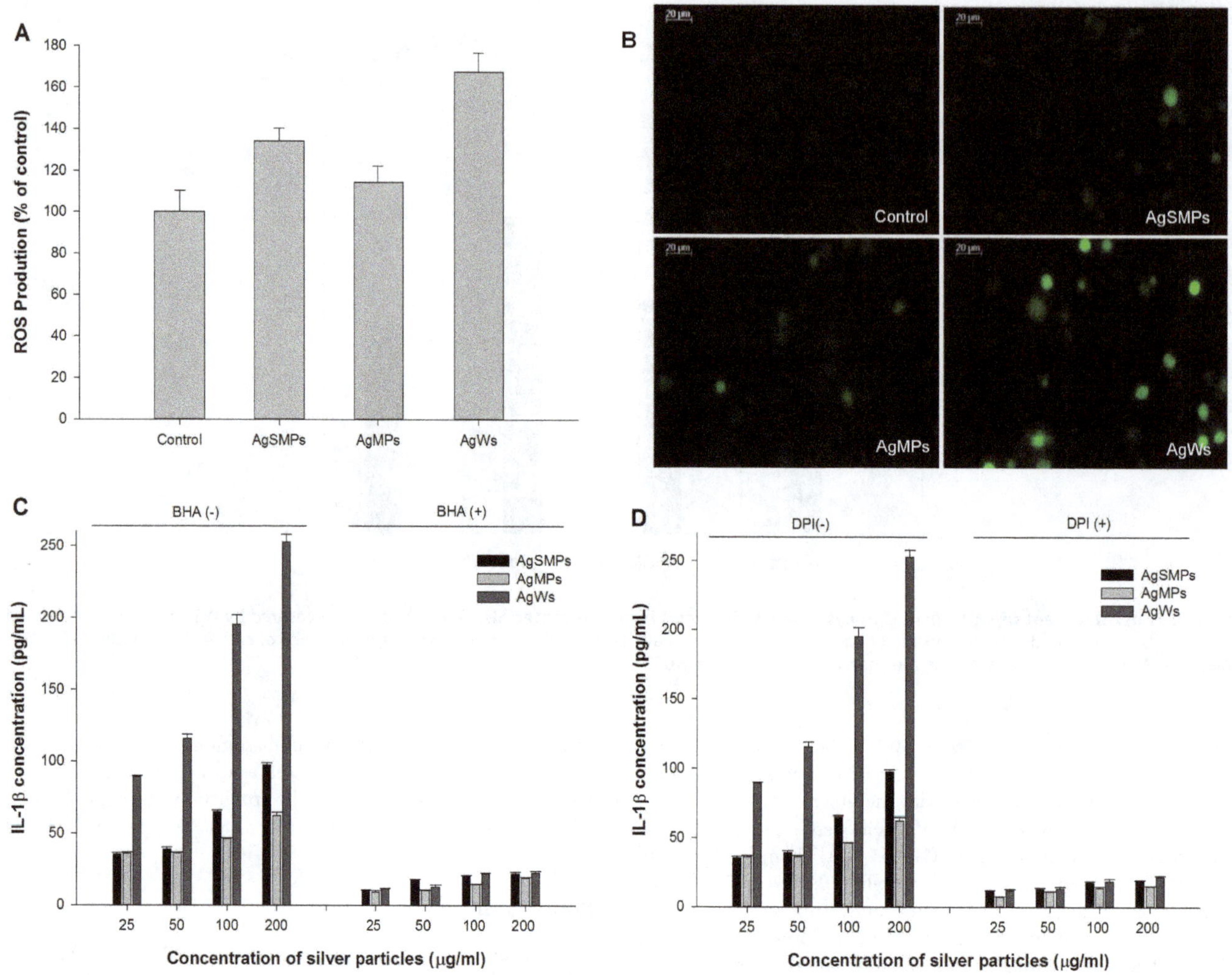

Figure 8. The association between silver materials-induced ROS generation and IL-1β production. (A) PMA-primed THP-1 cells were treated with each of the silver materials (100 μg/mL) for 24 h. At the end of exposure, the cells were loaded with DCFH-DA (100 μM) for 30 min and the fluorescence intensity was measured using a fluorometer. Data are represented as the mean ±SD (n = 5). (B) The cells were treated with each of the silver materials (100 μg/mL) for 24 h. At the end of exposure, the cells were loaded with DCFH-DA (40 μM) for 30 min at 37°C and photographed using a fluorescence microscope (400×). (C) The cells were treated with different forms of silver materials for 24 h in both the absence and presence of BHA (150 μM). IL-1β levels were measured using ELISA. Data are represented as the mean ±SD (n = 3). (D) The cells were treated with different forms of silver materials for 24 h in both the absence and presence of DPI (200 μM). IL-1β levels were measured using ELISA. Data are represented as the mean ±SD (n = 3).

coated. However, when the silver materials come into contact with human cells, they are exposed to human serum to be coated. On the other hand, silver materials containing no surface modifiers or stabilizers could enter the macrophage cells by pinocytosis [3]. In a cytotoxicity test of selected silver materials, the cytotoxicity measured by WST-1 and LDH release assay noticeably decreased and increased, respectively, in a dose-dependent manner. In particular, the cells treated with AgWs exhibited the highest degree of cytotoxicity and membrane damage (Fig. 3). As shown in Fig. 4A, all types of silver materials elicited DNA fragmentation as evidenced by occurrence of a sub-G1 peak, and again AgWs induced a higher degree of sub-G1 DNA content than the others. Cell shrinkage, a hallmark of apoptotic cell death, showed almost the same trend after exposure to silver materials (Fig. 4B). As apoptosis has been suggested as a major mechanism for cell death by silver materials [34], we attempted to determine the mode of cell death (Fig. 4C). The data indicated that although apoptosis is the major mode of cell death, necrosis might be the second mode of cell death in the presence of silver materials, especially in the presence of a high concentration of AgWs.

IL-1β production via caspase-1 is presently considered to play a crucial role in initial inflammation [9,35]. Both IL-1β production and caspase-1 activation were the highest with AgWs among the tested silver materials (Figs. 5A, B, and C). Caspase-1, a component NALP3 inflammasome, induces release of active IL-1β only after NALP3 inflammasomes are activated by environmental irritants [36]. As expected, NALP3 mRNA expression levels were highest with AgWs among the silver materials tested (Fig. 5D). The mechanism for NALP3 inflammasome-mediated IL-1β secretion by silver materials is not yet known, making the creation of safe silver materials difficult. A few studies reported that cathepsin B leakage after lysosomal rupture and cytoplasmic ROS play a critical role in the activation of NALP3 inflammasome [10,12]. Thus, we demonstrated here that silver material-induced

IL-1β production was mediated by cathepsin B release and ROS production (Figs. 6, 7, and 8). AgWs caused more serious damage to lysosomal membrane than the others (Figs. 6A and 6B). The specific inhibitor of cathepsin B, CA-074-Me, suppressed IL-1β production by THP-1 cells more evidently in the presence of AgWs than in the presence of the others (Fig. 6C), indicating that active cathepsin B is one of the most important activators of the inflammasome upon stimulation by silver materials.

The NALP3 activators, including ATP, asbestos, and silica, trigger the generation of ROS. Treatment with various ROS scavengers blocks NALP3 activation [11]. In the present study, AgWs generated more intracellular ROS than the others (Figs. 8A and B). Figs. 8C and D proved that silver material-induced IL-1β production is related to this increase in intracellular ROS. This result indicated that not only cathepsin B released from lysosome but also ROS generated by silver materials play crucial roles and possibly interact with each other in silver materials-induced IL-1β production. We believe that the silver materials are phagocyto-sized. Then, while producing ROS, the reactive silver material surface may interact with phagolysosomal membranes, leading to lysosomal rupture. However, as evidenced with the higher LDH values, AgWs might cause more membrane damage and rupture and more ROS production than AgSMPs (150 nm; nominal surface area $=7.065\times10^{-2}$ μm^2) and AgMPs (2.7 μm; nominal surface area $=2.289\times10^{-2}$ μm^2) since AgWs (274 nm×5.3 μm; nominal surface area $=4.677$ μm^2) have more surface area than the others. As further study, we plan to elucidate on how cytotoxicity and signaling intensity are affected by the aspect ratio between the diameter and length of AgWs.

Conclusions

In summary, we suggest that silver materials induce different levels of IL-1β production and cytotoxicity depending on their form. Furthermore, AgWs induced more apoptosis and IL-1β production than AgSMPs and AgMPs because AgWs cause more membrane damage than the others. We also speculated that silver material-induced IL-1β production is affected by a single pathway affiliated with ROS and lysosomal rupture, cathepsin B, caspase-1 (NALP3 inflammasome), and IL-1β production in THP-1 cells. For our healthy lives, the development of safe and effective metal materials should be advanced. However, it is necessary to obtain more information about the association between the shape of metal materials and their biological effects. These results may provide essential basic information for the development of safe forms of silver materials.

Author Contributions

Conceived and designed the experiments: HJJ PJP HSL NHC. Performed the experiments: HJJ PJP JEJ JSK SHP. Analyzed the data: JSK SHP HSL NHC. Contributed reagents/materials/analysis tools: SHP. Wrote the paper: HJJ PJP HSL NHC.

References

1. Samberg ME, Oldenburg SJ, Monteiro-Riviere NA (2010) Evaluation of silver nanoparticle toxicity in skin in vivo and keratinocytes in vitro. Environ Health Persp 118: 407–413.
2. Miura N, Shinohara Y (2009) Cytotoxic effect and apoptosis induction by silver nanoparticles in HeLa cells. Biochem Bioph Res Co 390: 733–737.
3. Yen HJ, Hsu SH, Tsai CL (2009) Cytotoxicity and immunological response of gold and silver nanoparticles of different sizes. Small 5: 1553–1561.
4. Sharma HS, Ali SF, Hussain SM, Schlager JJ, Sharma A (2009) Influence of engineered nanoparticles from metals on the blood-brain barrier permeability, Cerebral Blood Flow, Brain Edema and Neurotoxicity. An experimental study in the rat and mice using biochemical and morphological approaches. J Nanosci Nanotechno 9: 5055–5072.
5. Larese FF, D'Agostin F, Crosera M, Adami G, Renzi N, et al. (2009) Human skin penetration of silver nanoparticles through intact and damaged skin. Toxicology 255: 33–37.
6. Stutz A, Golenbock DT, Latz E (2009) Inflammasomes: too big to miss. J Clin Invest 119: 3502–3511.
7. Netea MG, Simon A, van de Veerdonk F, Kullberg BJ, Van der Meer JWM, et al. (2010) IL-1 beta processing in host defense: beyond the inflammasomes. Plos Pathog 6.
8. Schroder K, Tschopp J (2010) The Inflammasomes. Cell 140: 821–832.
9. Zhang HY, GharaeeKermani M, Phan SH (1997) Regulation of lung fibroblast alpha-smooth muscle actin expression, contractile phenotype, and apoptosis by IL-1 beta. J Immunol 158: 1392–1399.
10. Dostert C, Petrilli V, Van Bruggen R, Steele C, Mossman BT, et al. (2008) Innate immune activation through Nalp3 inflammasome sensing of asbestos and silica. Science 320: 674–677.
11. Tschopp J, Schroder K (2010) NLRP3 inflammasome activation: the convergence of multiple signalling pathways on ROS production? Nat Rev Immunol 10: 210–215.
12. Hornung V, Bauernfeind F, Halle A, Samstad EO, Kono H, et al. (2008) Silica crystals and aluminum salts activate the NALP3 inflammasome through phagosomal destabilization. Nat Immunol 9: 847–856.
13. Cassel SL, Eisenbarth SC, Iyer SS, Sadler JJ, Colegio OR, et al. (2008) The Nalp3 inflammasome is essential for the development of silicosis. P Natl Acad Sci USA 105: 9035–9040.
14. Portney NG, Ozkan M (2006) Nano-oncology: drug delivery, imaging, and sensing. Anal Bioanal Chem 384: 620–630.
15. Uskokovic V, Lee K, Lee PP, Fischer KE, Desai TA (2012) Shape effect in the design of nanowire-coated microparticles as transepithelial drug delivery devices. ACS nano 6: 7832–7841.
16. Trickler WJ, Lantz SM, Murdock RC, Schrand AM, Robinson BL, et al. (2010) Silver nanoparticle induced blood-brain barrier inflammation and increased Permeability in primary rat brain microvessel endothelial cells. Toxicol Sci 118: 160–170.
17. Timko BP, Cohen-Karni T, Qing Q, Tian BZ, Lieber CM (2010) Design and implementation of functional nanoelectronic interfaces with biomolecules, cells, and tissue using nanowire device arrays. Ieee T Nanotechnol 9: 269–280.
18. Zhang Y, Yang M, Portney NG, Cui DX, Budak G, et al. (2008) Zeta potential: a surface electrical characteristic to probe the interaction of nanoparticles with normal and cancer human breast epithelial cells. Biomed Microdevices 10: 321–328.
19. Ghasempour S, Shokrgozar M, Ghasempour R, Alipour M (2014) The acute toxicity of urea coated ferrous oxide nanoparticles on L929 cell line, evaluation of biochemical and pathological parameters in rat kidney and liver. Physiol Pharmacol. 17: 423–436.
20. Niyonsaba F, Ushio H, Nagaoka I, Okumura K, Ogawa H (2005) The human beta-defensins (-1,-2,-3,-4) and cathelicidin LL-37 induce IL-18 secretion through p38 and ERK MAPK activation in primary human keratinocytes. J Immunol 175: 1776–1784.
21. Boya P, Andreau K, Poncet D, Zamzami N, Perfettini JL, et al. (2003) Lysosomal membrane permeabilization induces cell death in a mitochondrion-dependent fashion. J Exp Med 197: 1323–1334.
22. Okimoto Y, Watanabe A, Niki E, Yamashita T, Noguchi N (2000) A novel fluorescent probe diphenyl-1-pyrenylphosphine to follow lipid peroxidation in cell membranes. Febs Lett 474: 137–140.
23. Hussain S, Thomassen LCJ, Ferecatu I, Borot MC, Andreau K, et al. (2010) Carbon black and titanium dioxide nanoparticles elicit distinct apoptotic pathways in bronchial epithelial cells. Part Fibre Toxicol 7.
24. Hsin YH, Chena CF, Huang S, Shih TS, Lai PS, et al. (2008) The apoptotic effect of nanosilver is mediated by a ROS- and JNK-dependent mechanism involving the mitochondrial pathway in NIH3T3 cells. Toxicol Lett 179: 130–139.
25. Park EJ, Choi K, Park K (2011) Induction of Inflammatory Responses and Gene Expression by Intratracheal Instillation of Silver Nanoparticles in Mice. Arch Pharm Res 34: 299–307.
26. Morishige T, Yoshioka Y, Inakura H, Tanabe A, Yao XL, et al. (2010) The effect of surface modification of amorphous silica particles on NLRP3 inflammasome mediated IL-1 beta production, ROS production and endosomal rupture. Biomaterials 31: 6833–6842.
27. Halle A, Hornung V, Petzold GC, Stewart CR, Monks BG, et al. (2008) The NALP3 inflammasome is involved in the innate immune response to amyloid-beta. Nat Immunol 9: 857–865.
28. Scanlan LD, Reed RB, Loguinov AV, Antczak P, Tagmount A, et al. (2013) Silver Nanowire Exposure Results in Internalization and Toxicity to Daphnia magna. Acs Nano 7: 10681–10694.
29. Adili A, Crowe S, Beaux MF, Cantrell T, Shapiro PJ, et al. (2008) Differential cytotoxicity exhibited by silica nanowires and nanoparticles. Nanotoxicology 2: 1–8.

30. Ainslie KM, Bachelder EM, Sharma G, Grimes CA, Pishko MV (2007) Macrophage cell adhesion and inflammation cytokines on magnetostrictive nanowires. Nanotoxicology 1: 279–290.
31. Stoehr LC, Gonzalez E, Stampfl A, Casals E, Duschl A, et al. (2011) Shape matters: effects of silver nanospheres and wires on human alveolar epithelial cells. Part Fibre Toxicol 8.
32. Carlson C, Hussain SM, Schrand AM, Braydich-Stolle LK, Hess KL, et al. (2008) Unique cellular interaction of silver nanoparticles: size-dependent generation of reactive oxygen species. J Phys Chem B. 112: 13608–13619.
33. Lok CN, Ho CM, Chen R, He QY, Yu WY, et al. (2007) Silver nanoparticles: partial oxidation and antibacterial activities. J Biol Inorg Chem 12: 527–534.
34. Rauch J, Kolch W, Laurent S, Mahmoudi M (2013) Big Signals from Small Particles: Regulation of Cell Signaling Pathways by Nanoparticles. Chem Rev 113: 3391–3406.
35. Morishige T, Yoshioka Y, Tanabe A, Yao XL, Tsunoda S, et al. (2010) Titanium dioxide induces different levels of IL-1 beta production dependent on its particle characteristics through caspase-1 activation mediated by reactive oxygen species and cathepsin B. Biochem Bioph Res Co 392: 160–165.
36. Misawa T, Takahama M, Kozaki T, Lee H, Zou J, et al. (2013) Microtubule-driven spatial arrangement of mitochondria promotes activation of the NLRP3 inflammasome. Nat Immunol 14: 454–460.

13

Autophagy and Apoptosis in Hepatocellular Carcinoma Induced by EF25-$(GSH)_2$: A Novel Curcumin Analog

Tao Zhou[1], Lili Ye[1], Yu Bai[1], Aiming Sun[2,3], Bryan Cox[2], Dahai Liu[1,5], Yong Li[1,5], Dennis Liotta[2,3], James P. Snyder[2,3], Haian Fu[4], Bei Huang[1,5]*

1 School of life Sciences, Anhui University, Hefei, China, **2** Department of Chemistry, Emory University, Atlanta, Georgia, United States of America, **3** Emory Institute for Drug Development (EIDD), Emory University, Atlanta, Georgia, United States of America, **4** Department of Pharmacology and Emory Chemical Biology Discovery Center, Emory University, Atlanta, Georgia, United States of America, **5** Center for Stem Cell and Translational Medicine, Anhui University, Hefei, China

Abstract

Curcumin, a spice component as well as a traditional Asian medicine, has been reported to inhibit proliferation of a variety of cancer cells but is limited in application due to its low potency and bioavailability. Here, we have assessed the therapeutic effects of a novel and water soluble curcumin analog, 3,5-bis(2-hydroxybenzylidene)tetrahydro-4*H*-pyran-4-one glutathione conjugate [EF25-$(GSH)_2$], on hepatoma cells. Using the MTT and colony formation assays, we determined that EF25-$(GSH)_2$ drastically inhibits the proliferation of hepatoma cell line HepG2 with minimal cytotoxicity for the immortalized human hepatic cell line HL-7702. Significantly, EF25-$(GSH)_2$ suppressed growth of HepG2 xenografts in mice with no observed toxicity to the animals. Mechanistic investigation revealed that EF25-$(GSH)_2$ induces autophagy by means of a biphasic mechanism. Low concentrations ($<$5 μmol/L) induced autophagy with reversible and moderate cytoplasmic vacuolization, while high concentrations ($>$10 μmol/L) triggered an arrested autophagy process with irreversible and extensive cytoplasmic vacuolization. Prolonged treatment with EF25-$(GSH)_2$ induced cell death through both an apoptosis-dependent and a non-apoptotic mechanism. Chloroquine, a late stage inhibitor of autophagy which promoted cytoplasmic vacuolization, led to significantly enhanced apoptosis and cytotoxicity when combined with EF25-$(GSH)_2$. Taken together, these data imply a fail-safe mechanism regulated by autophagy in the action of EF25-$(GSH)_2$, suggesting the therapeutic potential of the novel curcumin analog against hepatocellular carcinoma (HCC), while offering a novel and effective combination strategy with chloroquine for the treatment of patients with HCC.

Editor: Yu-Jia Chang, Taipei Medicine University, Taiwan

Funding: Support was provided by the Natural Science Foundation of the Education Department in Anhui Province, China (KJ2012A030, to Bei Huang) and NCI 5 P50 CA128613 SPORE in Head and Neck Cancer (to Haian Fu and J. P. Snyder). The funders had no role in study design, data collection and analysis, decision to publish, or preparation of the manuscript.

Competing Interests: The authors have declared that no competing interests exist.

* Email: beihuang@163.com

Introduction

Hepatocellular carcinoma (HCC) is the fifth most common cancer and the third leading cause of cancer death worldwide [1]. Certain regions in Asia and Africa are disproportionally affected, while China alone accounted for half of the new liver cancer cases occurring worldwide during 2008 [2]. Chemotherapy plays a crucial role in the treatment of HCC especially at advanced stages when curative therapies like resection and liver transplantation are inapplicable [3,4]. However, since most widely used chemotherapeutic drugs show severe side effects, development of novel and safe agents is mandatory.

Curcumin, a natural compound isolated from the commonly used spice turmeric, has been shown to inhibit cell proliferation in various types of cancer cells *in vitro* and *in vivo* [5]. Numerous curcumin derivatives and analogues have been developed in recent years in order to enhance anti-tumor efficacy and overcome limitations such as poor aqueous solubility, relative low bioavailability and intense yellow staining [6,7]. The compounds 3,5-bis(2-flurobenzylidene)piperidin-4-one (EF24) and 3,5-bis(pyridin-2-ylmethylene)piperidin-4-one (EF31), synthetic structural analogues of curcumin [8], exhibit improved anticancer activity and a safety profile similar to curcumin [8–11]. Synthetic manipulation of these agents generates EF24-$(GSH)_2$ and EF31-$(GSH)_2$, double glutathione conjugates with no less anticancer capability compared to EF24 and EF31. However the conjugates exhibit superior stability in solution, water solubility and lack of color [8]. The structurally related compound 3,5-bis(2-hydroxybenzylidene)tetrahydro-4*H*-pyran-4-one (EF25) and its double glutathione conjugate EF25-$(GSH)_2$, are under investigation and reported here for the first time.

Although much of the research into the anti-cancer mechanisms of curcumin has focused on its ability to induce apoptosis, curcumin has also been found to induce other types of cell death including autophagic cell death, mitosis catastrophe and paraptosis [5,12–14]. By testing different cell lines, it has been found that the mode of cell death induced by curcumin varies among different cell lines, and the mechanisms of different cellular responses remains a mystery [14].

Here we show that *in vitro* EF25-$(GSH)_2$ exhibits preferential toxicity to malignant liver cancer cells compared with immortalized human hepatic cells. In parallel, *in vivo* EF25-$(GSH)_2$ significantly suppresses the growth of hepatocellular carcinoma

(HepG2) xenografts and is relatively nontoxic to mice. Further investigation into the mechanism of action reveals that EF25-$(GSH)_2$ induces a mixed mode of cell death in hepatoma cells in which autophagy, cell cycle arrest, cytoplasmic vacuolization, caspase-dependent and caspase-independent apoptosis all take place.

Materials and Methods

1. Ethics Statement

All procedures involving mice were approved by Anhui Medical University Animal Care Committee, which follows the protocol outlined in The Guide for the Care and Use of Laboratory Animals published by the USA National Institute of Health (NIH publication No. 85-23, revised 1996). The details of animal welfare and steps taken to ameliorate suffering were in accordance with the recommendations in The Guide for the Care and Use of Laboratory Animals, and all efforts were made to minimize suffering.

2. Reagents

Cisplatin was purchased from the National Institutes for Food and Drug Control (China). Curcumin and other reagents were purchased from Sigma-Aldrich. Antibodies against microtubule-associated protein 1 light chain 3B (LC3B), caspase-3, caspase-8 and actin were obtained from Cell Signaling Technology. mCherry-GFP-LC3B plasmid was kindly provided by Dr. Mian Wu (University of Science and Technology of China). Lentivirus-based shRNA constructs targeting the human Atg5 gene (pLKO.1-shAtg5-D8 and pLKO.1-shAtg5-D9, targeting different sequences), human Beclin-1 gene (pLKO.1-shBeclin-1-C2 and pLKO.1-shBeclin-1-C3, targeting different sequences) were kindly provided by Dr. Qinghua Shi (University of Science and Technology of China), and negative control targeting LacZ (pLKO.1-shLacZ) was obtained from the National RNAi Core Facility (Taiwan). Three helper plasmids (pLP1, pLP2 and pLP/VSVG) of lentiviral systems were kindly provided by Dr. Yong Li (Anhui University).

3. Synthesis of EF25 and EF25-$(GSH)_2$

EF25 was prepared as previously reported where it was originally named "compound 11" [15], while EF25-$(GSH)_2$ was obtained by a procedure identical to that for EF24-$(GSH)_2$ [8]. It should be noted that EF25 combined with glutathione much more slowly by comparison with EF24. EF25 (64.0 mg, 0.2 mmol, 1.0 eq.) in CH_3CN (0.2 ml) was added dropwise to a solution of GSH (123.0 mg, 0.4 mmol, 2.0 eq.) in water at room temperature. The reaction mixture was refluxed for 2 hr until the disappearance of both the yellow color and EF25 by LC/MS. Evaporation of the solvent delivered the product as a white powder in quantitative yield. HR-ESI-MS (*m/z*): $[M+H]^+$ calcd for $C_{39}H_{51}O_{16}N_6S_2$ 923.28053, found, 923.28121 (= 00068 amu) (Fig. S1).

The ^1H NMR spectrum of EF25-$(GSH)_2$ in DMSO-*d6* and D_2O (buffer pH7) are complex due to the presence of diastereoisomers resulting from GSH conjugation at the two C = C bonds of EF25. The ^1H NMR spectrum of the unconjugated EF25 in DMSO-*d6* exhibits a sharp singlet at 7.89 ppm assigned to the olefinic(C =)C–H proton and sharp aromatic signals at 6.8–7.3 ppm. The intensity of the olefinic signal decreases for the conjugated EF25-$(GSH)_x$, and the sharp aromatic signals observed for unconjugated EF25 are broadened for EF25-$(GSH)_x$. These observations indicate a mixture of the mono- and bis-conjugates EF25-(GSH) and EF25-$(GSH)_2$, respectively, and possibly rapid exchange between them (Fig. S2). The comparison of the ^1H NMR spectra of EF25 in DMSO-*d6* and EF25-$(GSH)_2$ in D_2O (pH7) illustrates the absence of observable quantities of unconjugated EF25 (Fig. S3). Thus, in these solvents, the equilibrium lies primarily on the side of the conjugates, although in biological tissues it is shifted to the unconjugated form as the hydrophobic EF25 interacts with its target proteins.

4. Cell culture

The three human hepatocellular carcinoma cell lines (HepG2, SMMC-7721 and BEL-7402) and one immortalized human hepatic cell line (HL-7702) were kindly supplied by Dr. Hui Zhong (Academy of Military Medical Sciences) [16–19]. The other three human tumor cell lines (HCT116 human colon cancer cell line, A549 human lung carcinoma cell line and Hela human cervical carcinoma cell line) and HEK293FT cell line were kindly supplied by Dr. Qinghua Shi (University of Science and Technology of China) [20,21]. The HepG2, HCT116, A549, Hela, BEL-7402 and HEK293FT cells were grown in DMEM (Gibco). The SMMC-7721 cells and HL-7702 cells were grown in RPMI 1640 (Gibco). Both media were supplemented with 10% fetal bovine serum (FBS; Gibco), 100 units/mL penicillin and 100 µg/mL streptomycin at 37°C in a humidified incubator containing 5% CO_2.

5. Cell viability assay

Cells (8×10^3 per well) were seeded onto 96-well plates in supplemented DMEM and incubated overnight. Then the cells were treated in triplicate for the indicated time with increasing doses of EF25-$(GSH)_2$ in 10% FBS containing DMEM or RPMI 1640 without antibiotic. Treated cells were then incubated in the presence of 0.5 mg/mL 3-(4,5-Dimethylthiazol-2-yl)-2,5-diphenyltetrazoliumbromide (MTT) for 4 h. The formazan crystals were dissolved in DMSO and monitored at an absorbance of 490 nm. Absorbance values were normalized to those obtained for the untreated cells to determine percentage survival. All experiments were repeated at least three times. IC_{50} values (50% inhibition concentration) were then calculated using the Statistical Package for the Social Sciences (SPSS, Inc.).

6. Colony formation assay

Twenty-four-well plates were seeded with 500 viable cells in complete medium and incubated overnight. The cells were then treated in triplicate with EF25-$(GSH)_2$ in 10% FBS containing DMEM without antibiotic for 24 h. The compound-containing medium was then removed, and the cells were washed with PBS twice and incubated in complete medium for another two weeks. Medium was replaced once at the end of the first week. The cell colonies formed were fixed in 10% formalin for 10 min and visualized by staining with Giemsa [22].

7. DNA content analysis

5×10^6 HepG2 cells were seeded into six-well plates and incubated overnight. The cells were treated with EF25-$(GSH)_2$ and then collected by trypsinization and fixed in precooled 70% ethanol overnight. Cells were then stained with 50 µg/mL propidium iodide (PI) in the presence of 100 µg/mL RNase A. DNA content was analyzed by FACSCalibur (Becton Dickinson), and data were analyzed by the Flowjo software. The percentage of cells in sub-G_1-G_0 was used to represent the apoptosis rate.

8. HepG2 cell tumor xenograft in mice

Five-week-old male athymic mice were obtained from Beijing Vital River Laboratory Animal Co., Ltd. Animals were given ad

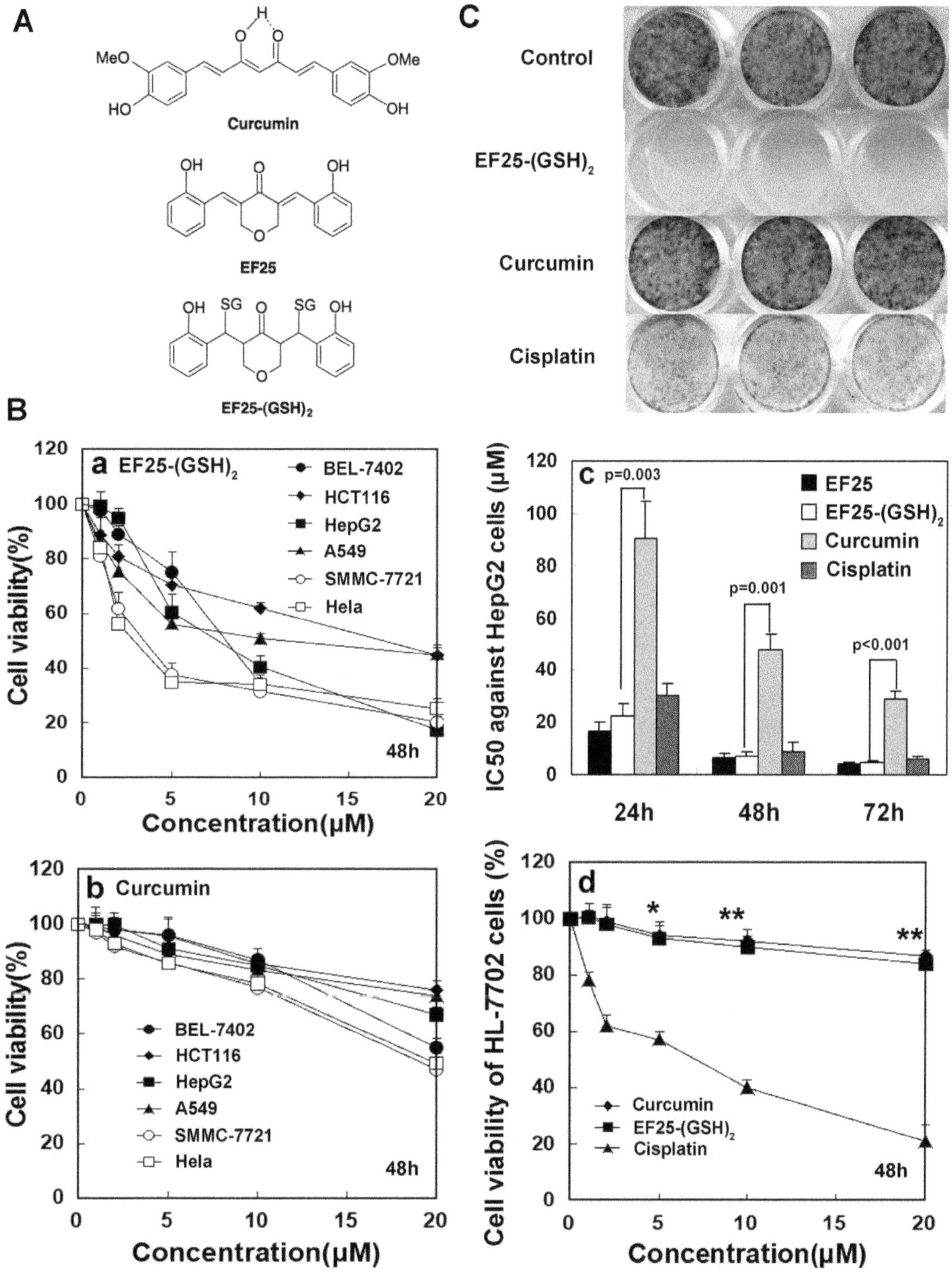

Figure 1. EF25-(GSH)2 inhibited proliferation of tumor cells *in vitro*. (A) The structures of curcumin, EF25 and EF25-$(GSH)_2$. (B) *a and b*, EF25-$(GSH)_2$ showed similar toxicity towards six human tumor cells (BEL-7402, HCT116, HepG2, A549, SMMC-7721 and Hela) (*a*) and the toxicity of curcumin was much lower than that of EF25-$(GSH)_2$ (*b*). *c*, cells were incubated with increasing doses of indicated compounds for 24-, 48-, and 72-h periods and analyzed by MTT assay. The IC_{50} of each agent at each time period was calculated and compared using SPSS. The IC_{50} of EF25-$(GSH)_2$ is much lower than that of curcumin and essentially equivalent to that of cisplatin. *d*, the cytotoxicity of EF25-$(GSH)_2$ to HL-7702 cells was much lower than that of cisplatin and similar to curcumin after 48-hour incubation as determined by MTT assay (*, $p<0.01$, **, $p<0.001$). (C) Cells were incubated with 0.5 μmol/L of the indicated compound for 24 h and subsequently allowed to grow into colonies (2 weeks). EF25-$(GSH)_2$ totally inhibited colony formation leading to clean plates, while curcumin and cisplatin did not. Results are representative of three independent experiments.

libitum access to water and standard mouse chow. 5×10^6 HepG2 cells were injected subcutaneous into the left flank and allowed to form a xenograft. Treatment was initiated when the tumor reached a group mean of 100 mm^3. EF25-$(GSH)_2$ was dissolved in PBS and administrated i.p. daily at a dose of 1.5 mg/kg body weight for 30 days [23,24]. The control group was given the same

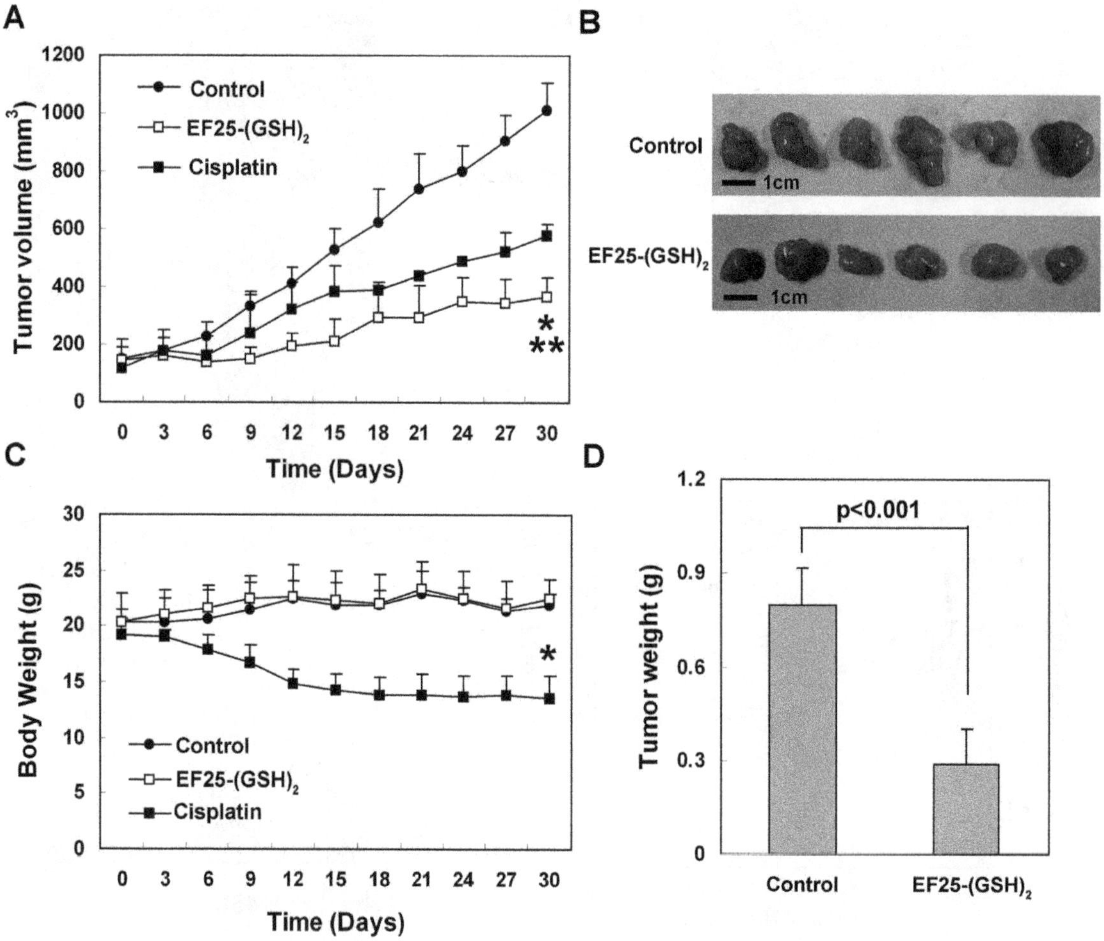

Figure 2. EF25-(GSH)$_2$ suppressed HepG2 xenograft growth *in vivo*. (A) HepG2 cells were injected into the left flank of nude mice and tumors were allowed to grow to a size of about 100 mm^3. Subsequently, EF25-(GSH)$_2$ (dissolved in PBS, 1.5 mg/kg body weight) was injected daily i.p. for 30 d (n = 6). The cisplatin group (dissolved in PBS, 0.5 mg/kg body weight) was injected every other day i.p. (n = 4), and the control group was injected with the same volume of PBS daily i.p. (n = 6). Tumor growth was significantly suppressed in the EF25-(GSH)$_2$-treated group compared to either control (**, $p<0.001$) or cisplatin-treated group (*, $p<0.01$). (B) At the end of the treatment, tumor volume in the EF25-(GSH)$_2$-treated group was much smaller than that of the control group. (C) The EF25-(GSH)$_2$-treated group maintained normal weight gain while the cisplatin-treated group suffered a remarkable weight loss throughout the treatment (*, $p<0.001$). (D) At the end of the treatment, EF25-(GSH)$_2$ treatment resulted in significantly lower tumor weight when compared with control group.

volume of PBS only. Tumor volume was calculated using the formula $V = a^2 \times b/2$, where a and b represent the shorter and longer diameters of the tumor, respectively. At the end of the treatment, the mice were sacrificed under etherization, and the tumors were weighed.

9. Transmission electron microscopy

Treated cells were collected by trypsinization, washed twice with PBS, and then fixed with ice-cold 3% glutaraldehyde in 0.1 mol/L cacodylate buffer at 4°C overnight. Cells were then postfixed in osmium tetroxide and embedded in Polybed resin. Ultrathin sections were double stained with uranyl acetate and lead citrate and examined with a JEM-2100 electron microscope.

10. 4, 6-diamidino-2-phenylindole (DAPI) staining

At the end of the EF25-(GSH)$_2$ treatment, DAPI was added to the medium at a final concentration of 1 µg/mL. After staining with DAPI for 15 min, cell morphology was examined by laser confocal microscopy. Uniformly stained nuclei with clear margins were regarded as normal, while condensed or fragmented nuclei with strengthened fluorescence were considered apoptotic.

11. Transient transfection

HepG2 cells were seeded in six-well plates and incubated overnight. mCherry-GFP -LC3 was transfected using Lipofectamine 2000 according to the manufacturer's instructions. The transfection mixture was replaced with 10% FBS containing DMEM without antibiotic 6 hours after transfection and incubated for another 24 hours. Cells were then treated with EF25-(GSH)$_2$ for the indicated time. Green (GFP) and red (mCherry) fluorescence was observed under a laser confocal microscope.

12. Knockdown of Atg5 and Beclin-1 expression by lentivirus-delivered shRNA

For lentivirus preparation, HEK293FT cells were transfected with pLKO.1-shRNA and three helper plasmids (pLP1, pLP2 and pLP/VSVG) with Fugene 6 Reagent (Roche). To generate human Atg5-knockdown or Beclin-1-knockdown cells, HepG2 cells were

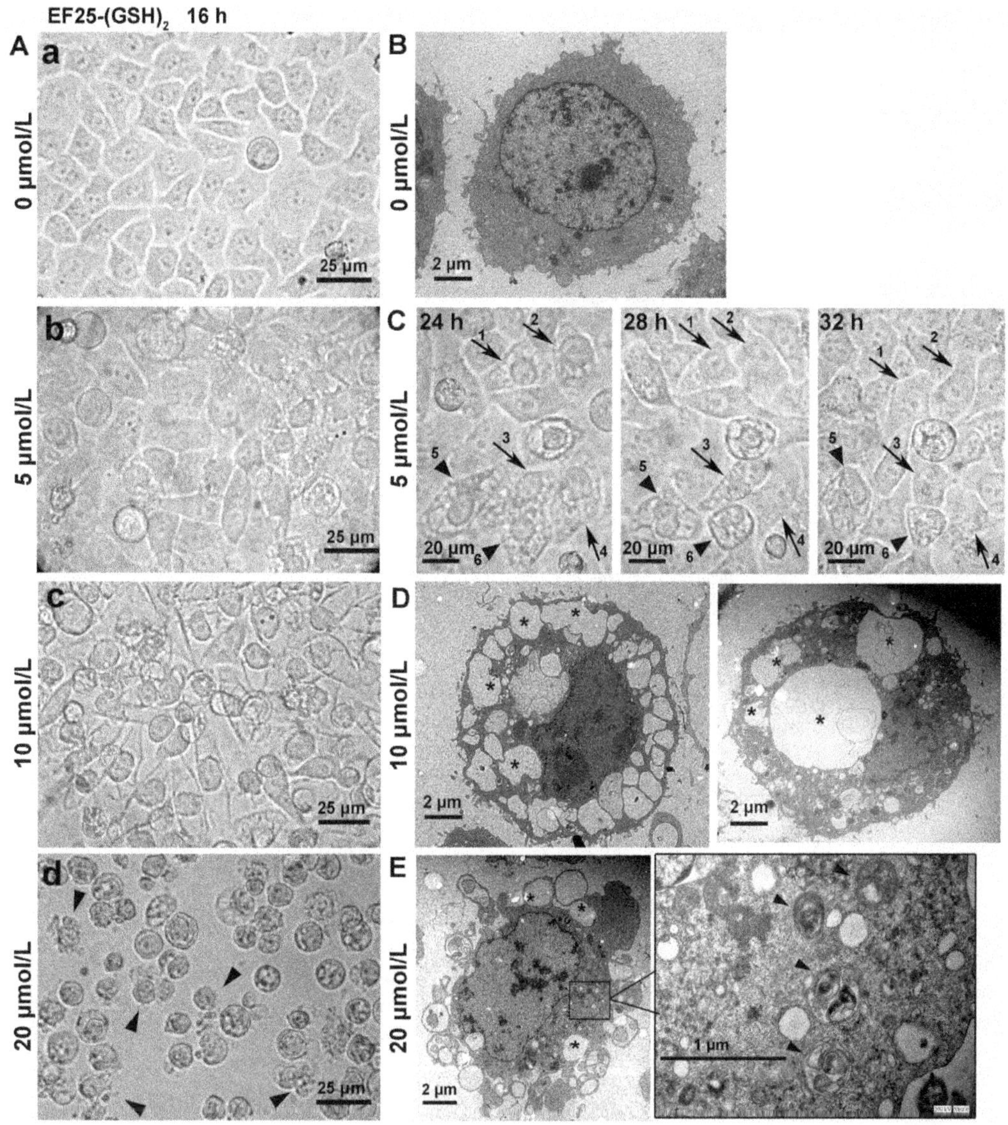

Figure 3. The morphological appearance of EF25-(GSH)$_2$-treated HepG2 cells. (A) HepG2 cells treated with increasing concentrations of EF25-(GSH)$_2$ for 16 h were observed under a light microscope and representative images were visualized. EF25-(GSH)$_2$-treated cells underwent vacuolization, the extent of which varied when treated with different concentrations of EF25-(GSH)$_2$. At 20 μmol/L, apoptotic-like cell membrane blebbing was observed (arrowheads). (B) A representative transmission electron microscopy (TEM) image of untreated HepG2 cells. (C) In 5 μmol/L EF25-(GSH)$_2$-treated cells, most vacuolated cells regained normal morphology at 32 h post-treatment (arrows, 1-4) while some did not (arrow heads, 5 and 6). (D) Representative TEM images of cells treated with 10 μmol/L EF25-(GSH)$_2$ for 16 h. *, large empty vacuoles with varying size. (E) Representative TEM images of cells treated with 20 μmol/L EF25-(GSH)$_2$ for 16 h. *, large empty vacuoles; arrows, autophagic vacuoles.

transduced with lentivirus expressing shAtg5 or shBeclin-1, respectively, and selected with 2 μg/ml puromycin.

13. Western blot assay

Cell lysates were subjected to SDS-PAGE and blotted onto polyvinylidene difluoride (PVDF) membranes. The membranes were then incubated with the each primary antibody and appropriate secondary antibody. The immunoblots were visualized by a chemiluminescence HRP substrate.

14. Statistical analysis

All values are expressed as the mean±SE. Data were analyzed using two-tailed student's t test. P≤0.05 was considered statistically significant. Statistical analysis was performed using SPSS.

Results

1. EF25-(GSH)$_2$ inhibited proliferation of tumor cells

The structures of curcumin analogues, EF25 and EF25-(GSH)$_2$, examined in this study are presented in Figure 1A. We first determined the effect of EF25, EF25-(GSH)$_2$ and curcumin on cell proliferation of HepG2 cells. Cisplatin, a widely used chemotherapeutic drug, was also examined under the same conditions. EF25-(GSH)$_2$, which is far more effective than curcumin, showed similar cytotoxicity to cell lines derived from three types of hepatomas (HepG2, SMMC-7721 and BEL-7402) and three other carcinomas (HCT116, A549 and Hela) (Fig. 1B a, b). EF25 and EF25-(GSH)$_2$ exhibit similar cytotoxicity in a dose- and time-dependent manner, indicating that GSH association does not change the cell-

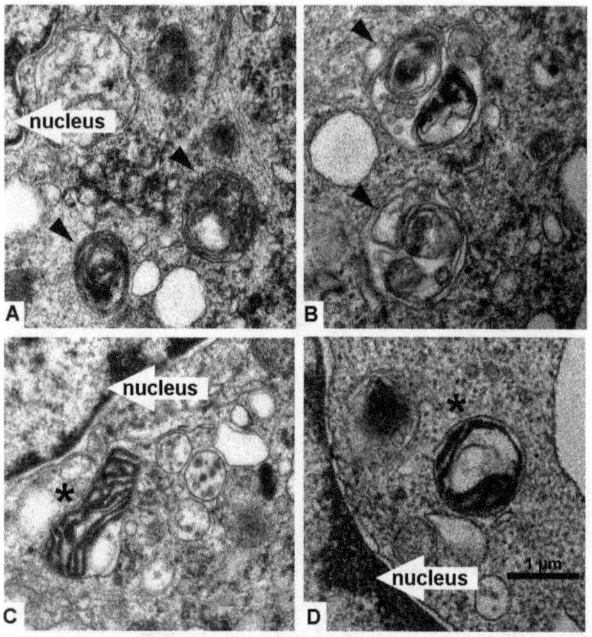

Figure 4. Morphology of autophagosomes in EF25-(GSH)$_2$-treated HepG2 cells. HepG2 cells were treated with 20 μmol/L EF25-(GSH)$_2$ for 16 h and observed under transmission electron microscopy. (A) and (B), multimembranous autophagic vacuoles engulfing cytoplasmic components are indicated with black arrowheads. (C) and (D), autophagic vacuoles containing a mitochondrion are indicated with black asterisk.

kill capacity of the EF25 conjugate. The mechanism of this phenomenon was elucidated in our previous investigation showing that the conjugate is reversible [8]. Thus, the active agent in both cases would appear to be EF25. That the latter showed slightly better activity than EF25-(GSH)$_2$ at 24 h, and that the difference between them diminished as time prolonged to 72 h (Fig. 1B c), is mostly likely due to differential cell penetration regulated in part by the equilibrium shift from conjugate to free EF25. In effect, EF25-(GSH)$_2$ serves as a pro-drug capable of releasing the active agent EF25 by reversal of the well-known Michael reaction in cells [8]. The cytotxicity of EF25-(GSH)$_2$ to HepG2 cells is much greater than that of curcumin as characterized by its much lower IC_{50} value (7.2 μmol/L at 48 h), which is close to that of cisplatin (9.1 μmol/L at 48 h) (Fig. 1B c). In order to examine if EF25-(GSH)$_2$ can preferentially kill malignant cells, cytotoxicities of the conjugate and cisplatin against immortalized human hepatic cell line HL-7702 were examined at 48 h post-treatment by the MTT assay. The results show that the cytotoxicity of EF25-(GSH)$_2$ to HL-7702 cells was much lower than that of cisplatin (Fig. 1B d).

To examine the long-term effect of EF25-(GSH)$_2$ treatment, the colony formation assay was performed. A quantity of 0.5 μmol/L EF25-(GSH)$_2$ totally inhibited colony formation, while 0.5 μmol/L curcumin had nearly no effect. An 0.5 μmol/L cisplatin treatment also caused a significant reduction in colony number, but was much less efficiently by comparison with EF25-(GSH)$_2$ (Fig. 1C).

2. EF25-(GSH)$_2$ suppresses HepG2 xenograft growth

To assess the antitumor potential of EF25-(GSH)$_2$ *in vivo*, HepG2 xenograft-bearing mice were given EF25-(GSH)$_2$ i.p. daily for 30 days (1.5 mg/kg body weight, PBS as vehicle, n = 6). For comparison, cisplatin was dissolved in PBS and given i.p. every other day at a dose of 0.5 mg/kg body weight (n = 4). Compared with vehicle treatment (n = 6), EF25-(GSH)$_2$ treatment significantly suppressed the growth of tumor volume which was much more efficient than cisplatin treatment (Fig. 2A, B). Notably, while the EF25-(GSH)$_2$-treated group maintained normal weight gain, the cisplatin-treated animals suffered a remarkable weight loss throughout the treatment (Fig. 2C). The tumor weights of EF25-(GSH)$_2$-treated mice were also significantly lower than that of the control group (Fig. 2D). There was no apparent change in liver, kidney and spleen weight in the EF25-(GSH)$_2$-treated group, while

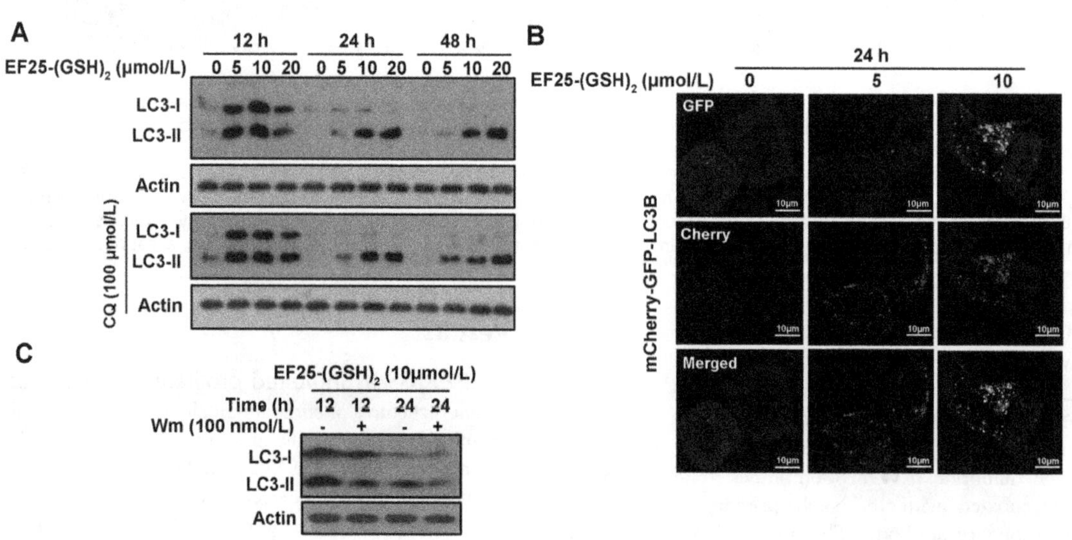

Figure 5. EF25-(GSH)$_2$ induced autophagy in HepG2 cells. (A) Western blot analysis of the LC3B expression in HepG2 cells treated with EF25-(GSH)$_2$ at varying concentrations for 12 to 48 h with or without chloroquine (CQ, 100 μmol/L). (B) The cellular distribution of mCherry-GFP-LC3B in HepG2 cells treated with EF25-(GSH)$_2$ at different concentrations for 24 h was examined under a laser confocal microscope. (C) Lysates from HepG2 cells incubated with 10 μmol/L EF25-(GSH)$_2$ for 12 or 24 h pretreated with or without wortmannin (Wm, 100 nmol/L, pretreated for 2 h) were analyzed by Western blotting for LC3B expression level.

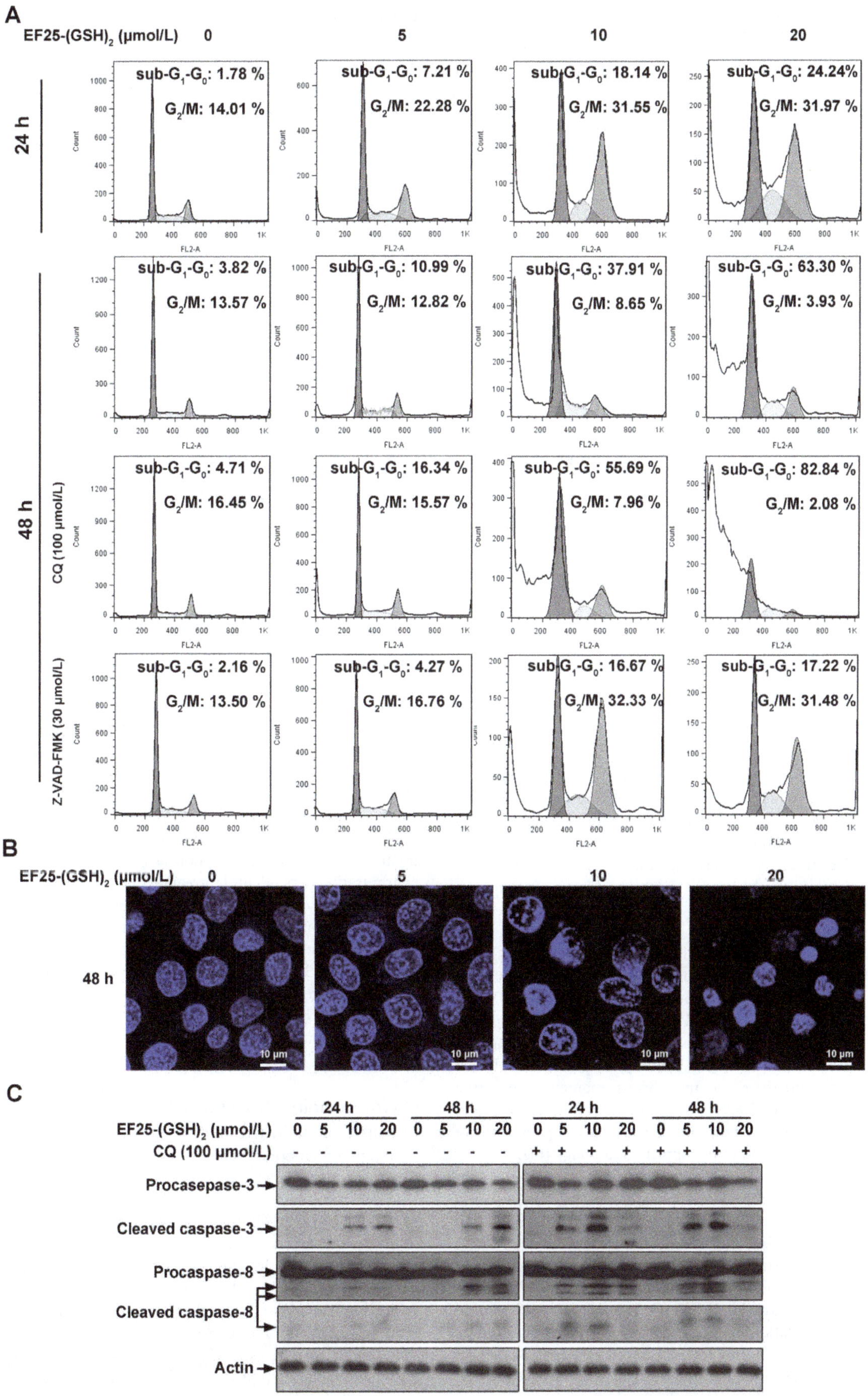
A
EF25-(GSH)$_2$ (µmol/L) 0 5 10 20
24 h
48 h
CQ (100 µmol/L)
Z-VAD-FMK (30 µmol/L)
sub-G$_1$-G$_0$: 1.78 %
G$_2$/M: 14.01 %
sub-G$_1$-G$_0$: 7.21 %
G$_2$/M: 22.28 %
sub-G$_1$-G$_0$: 18.14 %
G$_2$/M: 31.55 %
sub-G$_1$-G$_0$: 24.24%
G$_2$/M: 31.97 %
sub-G$_1$-G$_0$: 3.82 %
G$_2$/M: 13.57 %
sub-G$_1$-G$_0$: 10.99 %
G$_2$/M: 12.82 %
sub-G$_1$-G$_0$: 37.91 %
G$_2$/M: 8.65 %
sub-G$_1$-G$_0$: 63.30 %
G$_2$/M: 3.93 %
sub-G$_1$-G$_0$: 4.71 %
G$_2$/M: 16.45 %
sub-G$_1$-G$_0$: 16.34 %
G$_2$/M: 15.57 %
sub-G$_1$-G$_0$: 55.69 %
G$_2$/M: 7.96 %
sub-G$_1$-G$_0$: 82.84 %
G$_2$/M: 2.08 %
sub-G$_1$-G$_0$: 2.16 %
G$_2$/M: 13.50 %
sub-G$_1$-G$_0$: 4.27 %
G$_2$/M: 16.76 %
sub-G$_1$-G$_0$: 16.67 %
G$_2$/M: 32.33 %
sub-G$_1$-G$_0$: 17.22 %
G$_2$/M: 31.48 %
Count
FL2-A
B
EF25-(GSH)$_2$ (µmol/L) 0 5 10 20
48 h
10 µm
C
24 h 48 h 24 h 48 h
EF25-(GSH)$_2$ (µmol/L) 0 5 10 20 0 5 10 20 0 5 10 20 0 5 10 20
CQ (100 µmol/L) - - - - - - - - + + + + + + + +
Procasepase-3
Cleaved caspase-3
Procaspase-8
Cleaved caspase-8
Actin

Figure 6. The apoptosis in HepG2 cells triggered by EF25-$(GSH)_2$ in the presence or absence of CQ/Z-VAD-FMK. (A) HepG2 cells were treated with various concentrations of EF25-$(GSH)_2$ for 24 h and 48 h with or without chloroquine (CQ, 100 μmol/L)/Z-VAD-FMK (30 μmol/L, pretreated for 2 h) and then analyzed for DNA content (propidium iodide, PI) and cell cycle distribution. Apoptosis was measured as the percentage of cells containing hupodiploid quantities of DNA (sub-G_1-G_0 peak). Percentage of cells within the sub-G_1-G_0 and G_2/M stages is shown for each data point. Graphs are representative of data collected from three independent experiments. (B) HepG2 cells incubated with increasing concentrations of EF25-$(GSH)_2$ for 48 h were stained with 4, 6-diamidino-2-phenylindole (DAPI) and examined by laser confocal microscopy. Untreated HepG2 cells showed uniformly stained nuclei, while EF25-$(GSH)_2$-treated cells exhibited chromatin condensation in a concentration-dependent manner. (C) Lysates from HepG2 cells incubated with increasing concentrations of EF25-$(GSH)_2$ for 24 or 48 h with or without chloroquine (CQ, 100 μmol/L) were analyzed by Western blotting for both full length and cleaved caspase-3 and caspase-8 expression levels.

the weight of these organs dropped dramatically in the cisplatin-treated group (data not shown).

3. The morphological appearance of EF25-$(GSH)_2$-treated HepG2 cells

The morphological changes in EF25-$(GSH)_2$-treated cells were observed under a light microscope to observe apparent vacuolization in the cytoplasm. The number of cells that suffered cytoplasmic vacuolization and its extent varied when treated with different concentrations of EF25-$(GSH)_2$, but all reached a maximum at about 16 hours post-treatment (Fig. 3A). When treated with 5 μmol/L EF25-$(GSH)_2$, the cells experienced moderate vacuolization which regained normal morphology after about 8 hours (Fig. 3C). In contrast, most cells exposed to 10 μmol/L EF25-$(GSH)_2$ showed extensive and irreversible vacuolization in the cytoplasm. At 20 μmol/L, EF25-$(GSH)_2$ not only induced massive cytoplasmic vacuolization but also caused apoptotic membrane blebbing (Fig. 3A).

In the cytoplasm of HepG2 cells treated with 10 or 20 μmol/L EF25-$(GSH)_2$ for 16 hours, large vacuoles of varying size were content-free and single membrane bounded, while the small vacuoles resemble autophagic vacuoles (Fig. 3D, E).

4. EF25-$(GSH)_2$ induced autophagy in HepG2 cells

The ultrastructural details of HepG2 cells treated with 20 μmol/L EF25-$(GSH)_2$ for 16 hours were further examined by transmission electron microscopy. Typical multimembrane autophagic vesicles engulfing cytoplasmic components and organelles were identified in the cytoplasm (Fig. 4).

To further confirm whether EF25-$(GSH)_2$ triggered autophagy in HepG2 cells, we examined the expression of the two forms of microtubule-associated protein 1 light chain 3 (LC3). In the process of autophagy, LC3-I residing in the cytosol is modified to LC3-II, which binds to the autophagosome membrane. Thus, the degree of LC3-I to LC3-II conversion correlates to the extent of autophagosome formation [25]. EF25-$(GSH)_2$ treatment obviously increased the expression level of both LC3-I and LC3-II as early as 12 hours post-treatment, but the bands corresponding to LC3-I were weakened and there was no obvious augmentation in the LC3-II expression when EF25-$(GSH)_2$ treatment was prolonged or the dosage was increased, indicating that the lack of conversion of LC3-I to LC3-II may due to incomplete autophagy (Fig. 5A).

The increase in LC3-II expression can be associated with either an enhanced formation of autophagosome or an impaired autophagic degradation [26]. Chloroquine (CQ) is a lysosomal trophic agent that raises the lysosomal pH and, hence, blocks autophagy at the late stages [27]. Accordingly, CQ was used to test if EF25-$(GSH)_2$ can induce complete autophagic flux [28,29]. In cells treated with 5 μmol/L EF25-$(GSH)_2$, the LC3-II showed progressive accumulation in the presence of CQ at 24 h and 48 h. However, at 10 and 20 μmol/L, EF25-$(GSH)_2$-treated samples with and without CQ were indistinguishable with respect to LC3-II expression (Fig. 5A). This data indicates that autophagy flux was achieved at 5 μmol/L EF25-$(GSH)_2$ but was blocked at 10 and 20 μmol/L.

In addition, we examined the localization of autophagosome-specific protein LC3B in HepG2 cells treated with EF25-$(GSH)_2$ for 24 hours using Cherry-GFP-LC3B plasmid. When autophagy is induced, exogenous LC3 distributes to the membrane of autophagosomes and shows characteristic green (GFP) or red (mCherry) dots. Because GFP is acid-labile, only mCherry red fluorescence can be seen in autophagolysosmes, while the neutral structures display both green and red fluorescence [30]. In untreated cells, mCherry-GFP-LC3B showed a homogeneous distribution, whereas the EF25-$(GSH)_2$-treated cells showed fluorescent dots. At 5 μmol/L, the cells exhibit mostly only red dots, suggestive of autophagic degradation. Meanwhile, at 10 μmol/L, cells expressed double-tagged fusion proteins indicating that autophagic degradation was blocked (Fig. 5B). The data coincide well with the immunoblot analysis of LC3B in the presence of CQ.

5. EF25-$(GSH)_2$ induced G_2/M cell cycle arrest and apoptosis in HepG2 cells

Curcumin and its analogs have consistently been reported to induce apoptosis [31,32]. To determine whether EF25-$(GSH)_2$ acts similarly in HepG2 cells, the DNA content of permeabilized PI-stained cells was examined by flow cytometry at 24 h and 48 h post-treatment. The cell cycle analysis showed obvious G_2/M cell cycle arrest at 24 h, and the percentage of cells in sub-G_1-G_0 was greatly augmented at 48 h in a concentration-dependent manner (Fig. 6A).

DAPI staining of the nuclei also indicated that EF25-$(GSH)_2$-treated cells underwent apoptosis, the extent of which was concentration dependent. Untreated HepG2 cells showed uniformly stained nuclei, while nuclei of EF25-$(GSH)_2$-treated cells were condensed or fragmented with strengthened fluorescence (Fig. 6B).

These findings were further confirmed by analysis of the expression level of cleaved caspase-8 and caspase-3, both of which were augmented at 24 h post-treatment and maintained a high level up to 48 h at concentrations of 10 μmol/L and 20 μmol/L, whereas caspase activation was undetectable at 5 μmol/L (Fig. 6C).

6. Wortmannin advanced EF25-$(GSH)_2$ induced cell death in HepG2 cells in the early period

Autophagy modulation is a double edged sword in cancer treatment, possibly due to various cellular settings [33]. To test whether autophagy contributed to or hampered EF25-$(GSH)_2$ promoted HepG2 cell death, an inhibitor of autophagic sequestration (wortmannin (Wm)) was used to block autophagy at the early stages [26]. In the presence of 100 nmol/L Wm, the expression levels of both LC3B I and II types were largely reduced, indicating that Wm was effective in inhibiting EF25-$(GSH)_2$-induced autophagy formation (Fig. 5C). Wm at 100 nmol/L was only slightly toxic to HepG2 cells but clearly promoted the EF25-$(GSH)_2$-indued death process in the first 24 hours as evidenced by earlier cell shrinkage, rounding up (data not shown) and a 7–12%

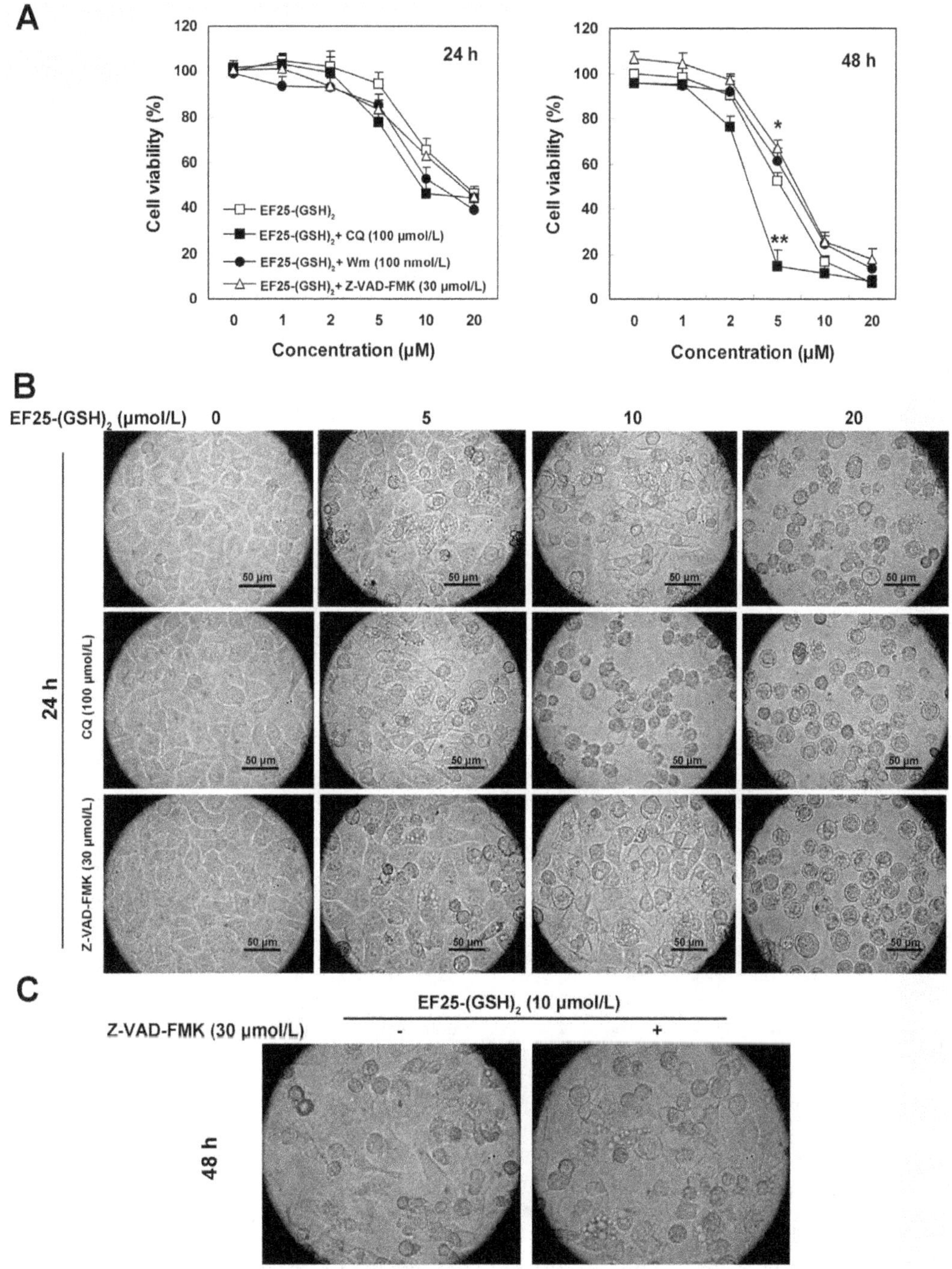

Figure 7. The effect of Wm, CQ and Z-VAD-FMK on the cytotoxicity and morphological changes induced by EF25-(GSH)$_2$ in HepG2 cells. (A) Cell viability was determined by the MTT assay after treatment with increasing concentrations of EF25-(GSH)$_2$ for 24 h or 48 h in the absence or presence of CQ (100 μmol/L)/Wm (100 nmol/L, pretreated for 2 h)/Z-VAD-FMK (30 μmol/L, pretreated for 2 h). *, $p<0.001$, EF25-(GSH)$_2$ plus Z-VAD-FMK vs. EF25-(GSH)$_2$ alone. **, $p<0.001$, EF25-(GSH)$_2$ plus CQ vs. EF25-(GSH)$_2$ alone. (B) Representative light microscopic images of HepG2 cells treated with various concentrations of EF25-(GSH)$_2$ for 24 h in the absence or presence of CQ (100 μmol/L)/Z-VAD-FMK (30 μmol/L, pretreated for 2 h). (C) Representative light microscopic images of HepG2 cells treated with 10 μmol/L EF25-(GSH)$_2$ for 48 h in the absence or presence of Z-VAD-FMK (30 μmol/L, pretreated for 2 h).

fall in cell viability examined by the MTT assay. However, as time progressed, the MTT assay at 48 h showed a slight increase rather than a further decrease of cell viability in Wm-pretreated cells. This indicates that Wm treatment advanced cell death only in the early period but had no obvious effect on the ultimate cytotoxicity of EF25-(GSH)$_2$ (Fig. 7A).

7. Knockdown of Atg5 and Beclin-1 expression did not rescue EF25-(GSH)$_2$-treated HepG2 cells

In order to avoid the non-specific effect of Wm, we knocked down the cellular expression of two autophagy essential genes, Atg5 and Beclin-1, separately, using specific small hairpin RNAs (shRNA) delivered by the lentiviral expression system. The cells

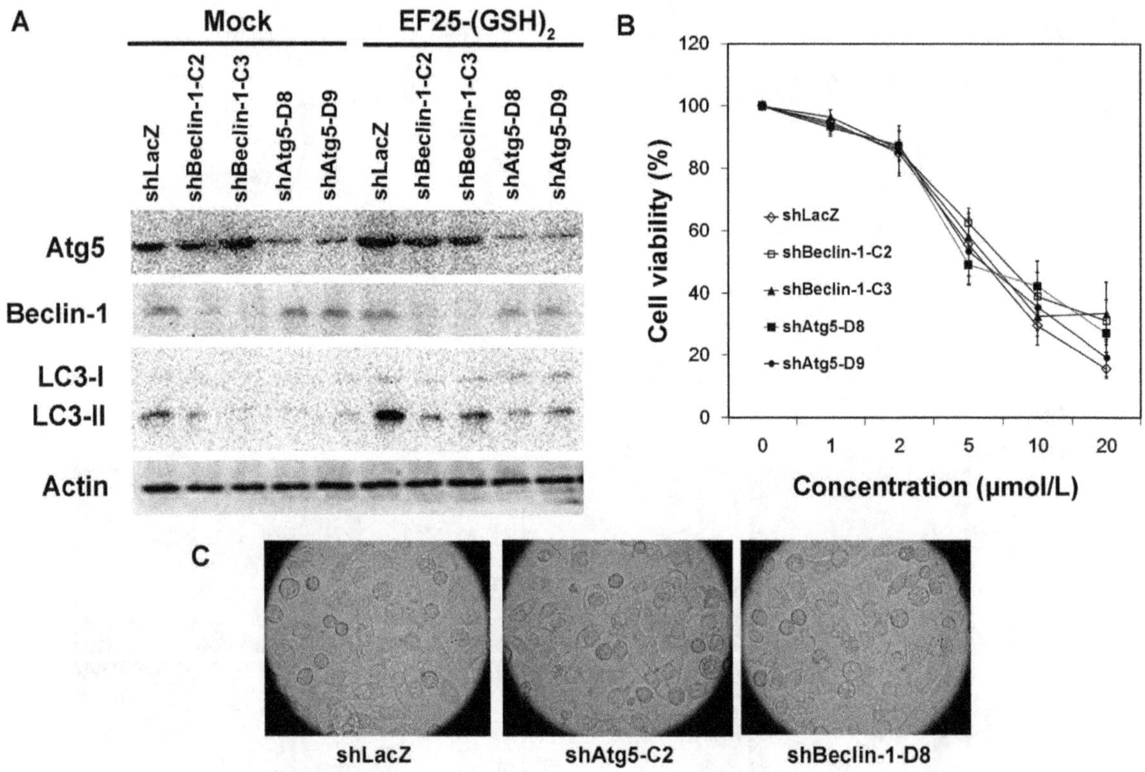

Figure 8. Knockdown of Atg5 and Beclin-1 expression does not rescue EF25-$(GSH)_2$-treated HepG2 cells. (A) HepG2 cells respectively transduced with shLacZ-, shBeclin-1-C2-, shBeclin-1-C3-, shAtg5-D8- and shAtg5-D9-lentivirus were mock-, or treated with 10 μmol/L EF25-$(GSH)_2$ for 24 h. Cells lysates were analyzed by Western blotting with antibodies against Atg5, Beclin-1, LC3 or actin, as indicated. (B) For HepG2 cells respectively transduced with shLacZ-, shBeclin-1-C2-, shBeclin-1-C3-, shAtg5-D8- and shAtg5-D9-lentivirus, cell viability was determined by MTT assay after treatment with increasing concentrations of EF25-$(GSH)_2$ for 48 h. (C) HepG2 cells respectively transduced with shLacZ-, shBeclin-1-C2- and shAtg5-D8-lentivirus were treated with 10 μmol/L EF25-$(GSH)_2$ for 24 h and observed under the light microscope.

were transduced with lentivirus expressing the shRNA targeting LacZ, Atg5 or Beclin 1, and were selected with puromycin. Puromycin-selected cells were then treated with 10 μmol/L EF25-$(GSH)_2$ for 24 h. Atg5- and Beclin-1-knockdown was evident by reduced expression level of Atg5 and Beclin-1, respectively. Furthermore, both Atg5- and Beclin-1-knockdown resulted in the attenuated expression level of LC3II visualized with immunoblotting (Fig. 8A). The MTT assay showed no obvious distinction in cell viability between LacZ-knockdown and Atg5/Beclin-1-knockdown HepG2 cells, which produced similar results with Wm (Fig. 8B). Furthermore, Atg5/Beclin-1-knockdown did not prevent the extensive cytoplasmic vacuolization induced by EF25-$(GSH)_2$, suggesting that this phenomenon is not directly induced by autophagic degradation (Fig. 8C).

8. CQ promoted cytoplasmic vacuolization, apoptosis and cell death induced by EF25-$(GSH)_2$ in HepG2 cells

It has been previously reported that inhibition of autophagy at different stages of the process can lead to distinct results [34,35]. In our study, inhibition of autophagy at an early stage by Wm did not significantly alter either the extent of cytoplasmic vacuolization or the final cell viability at 48 h. However, the late stage inhibitor CQ not only advanced the cell death process but also significantly enhanced cytoplasmic vacuolization, apoptosis and cytotoxicity induced by EF25-$(GSH)_2$. This combination effect of CQ was most dramatic by treatment of EF25-$(GSH)_2$ at 5 μmol/L.

When exposed to 5 μmol/L EF25-$(GSH)_2$ alone, only a small portion of cells was moderately vacuolated, but in the presence of CQ the majority of cells underwent extensive vacuolization to an extent similar to that caused by 10 μmol/L EF25-$(GSH)_2$ (Fig. 7B). This observation indicates that EF25-$(GSH)_2$-induced autophagy exhibits a cytoprotective role at lower concentration.

The MTT assay showed that CQ enhanced the effectiveness of EF25-$(GSH)_2$ within a 24-h period, continued to 48 h and proved especially clear-cut at the concentration of 5 μmol/L where cell viability dramatically dropped from 52.4% to 14.5% after 48 h treatment (Fig. 7A).

We also found that combining CQ with EF25-$(GSH)_2$ greatly augmented the apoptosis rate evidenced by a large increase in the percentage of cells in the sub-G_1-G_0 stage in a concentration-dependent manner (Fig. 6A).

In the presence of CQ, the expression level of activated caspase-3 increased at concentrations of 5 μmol/L and 10 μmol/L, but unexpectedly decreased at 20 μmol/L. Similarly, the expression level of cleaved caspase-8 was clearly increased by CQ treatment except at a concentration of 20 μmol/L EF25-$(GSH)_2$ at 48 h (Fig. 6C).

9. Z-VAD-FMK prolonged vacuolization and G2/M cell cycle arrest partially rescues HepG2 cells from EF25-(GSH)2 toxicity

To determine whether caspase activation plays a crucial role in EF25-$(GSH)_2$-induced cytotoxicity, the pan caspase inhibitor Z-VAD-FMK was employed. In the presence of this compound at 48 h post-treatment, cell cycle analysis showed a clear decrease of cells in the sub-G_1-G_0 stage especially at concentrations of 10 (from 37.9% to 16.7%) and 20 μmol/L (from 63.3% to 17.2%) (Fig. 6A). These data indicate that apoptosis induced by EF25-$(GSH)_2$ is primarily caspase- and concentration-dependent and partially caspase-independent to the extent of about 17%.

However, compared to the 21.2% (10 μmol/L) and 46.1% (20 μmol/L) decrease of apoptotic cells in the presence of Z-VAD-FMK at 48 h, only a 6.3% (10 μmol/L) and 19.3% (20 μmol/L) rise in cell viability was observed when pretreated with Z-VAD-FMK as examined by the MTT assay at 48 h (Fig. 7A), indicating the operation of non-apoptotic cell death. The latter was accompanied by prolonged cytoplasmic vacuolization and G_2/M cell cycle arrest.

The extent of cytoplasmic vacuolization was not significantly enhanced in the presence of Z-VAD-FMK (Fig. 7B), but the period of vacuolization was prolonged beyond the 48 h treatment. Cells exposed to 10 μmol/L EF25-$(GSH)_2$ alone avoided vacuolization and begin to shrink at 48 h. In contrast, cells exposed to co-treatment of 10 μmol/L EF25-$(GSH)_2$ and 30 μmol/L Z-VAD-FMK exhibited extensive vacuolization (Fig. 7C).

Cell cycle analysis showed obvious G_2/M cell cycle arrest in the presence of Z-VAD-FMK at 48 h post-treatment, which is similar to what was observed at 24 h post-treatment with EF25-$(GSH)_2$ alone, indicating that Z-VAD-FMK prolonged the status of G_2/M cell cycle arrest induced by the EF25 conjugate (Fig. 6A).

Discussion

Effective and less toxic alternative chemotherapeutic agents against HCC are needed to address the emerging problem of drug resistance and severe side effects [2]. Widely used drugs like cisplatin exhibit no selectivity for malignant cells, while natural compounds like curcumin, which possess a good safety profile, exert inadequate effectiveness [7].

By contrast, our *in vitro* and *in vivo* data show the novel compound EF25-$(GSH)_2$ to exert preferential toxicity toward HCC cells, offering potential as a promising anti-HCC therapeutic agent. In addition, the double GSH conjugation successfully solves the problems of instability and water insolubility which limits the usage of curcumin and its analogues [8].

Basic and clinical studies have clearly established the importance of apoptosis in therapeutic tumor-cell death, but many notable studies have confirmed that other forms of cell death are crucial for effective cancer therapy, and that apoptosis is not the comprehensive answer especially when dealing with the whole tumor instead of isolated tumor cells [36]. We found that the action of EF25-$(GSH)_2$ is complex in terms of which death pathways are involved. In EF25-$(GSH)_2$ treated HepG2 cells, autophagy and apoptosis were detected and extensive cytoplasmic vacuolization was observed. These events do not occur independently, but are closely connected.

The role of autophagy in cancer therapy is complex and depends on the specific cellular setting and treatment scenario. Under some circumstances, autophagy rescues cells under stress conditions and, in this sense, may suppress apoptosis and/or other

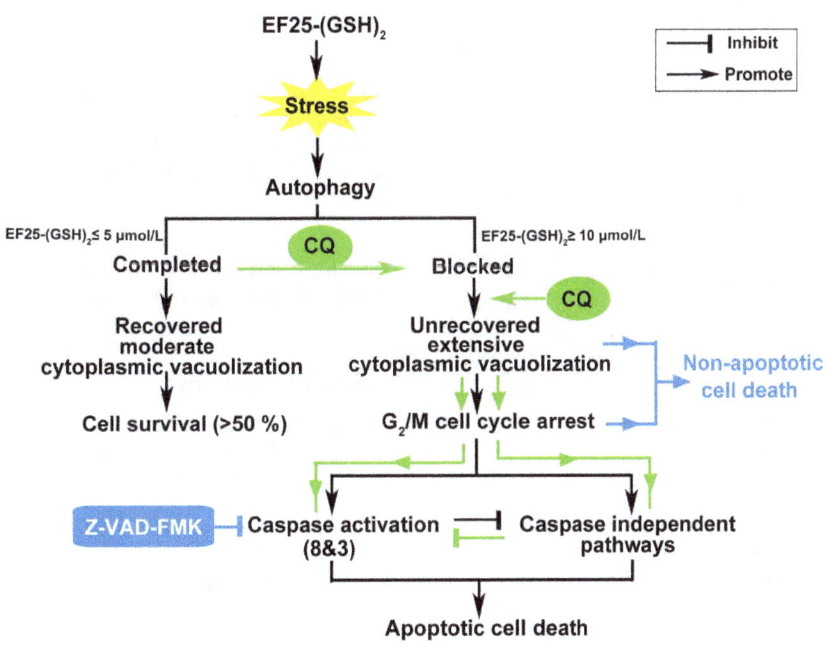

Figure 9. Working model of the mechanisms of EF25-$(GSH)_2$-induced cell death in HepG2 cells. Stress induced by EF25-$(GSH)_2$ promotes autophagy in HepG2 cells. When treated with EF25-$(GSH)_2$ at concentrations of 5 μmol/L or lower, cells experienced full-scale autophagy that displayed moderate cytoplasmic vacuolization, ultimate recovery and partial rescue of cells from the resulting stress. In contrast, the protective autophagy was blocked in cells treated with EF25-$(GSH)_2$ at concentrations of 10 μmol/L or higher which led to massive cytoplasmic vacuolization. The latter cells arrested in the G_2/M phase succumbed to both caspase-dependent and caspase-independent cell death. EF25-$(GSH)_2$ treatment alone led mainly to caspase-dependent apoptotic cell death, but also to a significant proportion of caspase-independent apoptosis. The action of EF25-$(GSH)_2$ could be modulated by CQ (green) and Z-VAD-FMK (blue). Co-treatment of EF25-$(GSH)_2$ with CQ promoted autophagy blockage and cytoplasmic vacuolization, which then enhanced apoptosis for both caspase-dependent and caspase-independent mechanisms. Co-treatment of EF25-$(GSH)_2$ with Z-VAD-FMK inhibited caspase activation and subsequently blocked the caspase-dependent apoptotic death route. Thus, cells were trapped by cytoplasmic vacuolization and G_2/M cell cycle arrest, which eventually led to non-apoptotic cell death.

types of cell death. In other scenarios, irreversible self-destruction caused by massive autophagy leads to cell demise [33]. To investigate the exact role of autophagy in chemotherapy, autophagy inhibitors at different stages have been previously employed. Interestingly, the blockade of autophagy at an early or late stage has been reported by some groups to cause different effects. For example, the late stage inhibition by Bafilomycin A1 was found to enhance apoptosis and cell death, whereas inhibition of autophagy at early stages using 3-MA failed to do so [34,35].

Our autophagy inhibitor data using Wm and CQ also show different effects. Inhibition of autophagy at early stages by Wm advanced the cell death process during early phases of EF25-$(GSH)_2$ treatment, but altered the final toxicity insignificantly. In contrast, CQ greatly enhanced cytoplasmic vacuolization, apoptosis and cell death. These data suggest that autophagy does not directly execute cell death through extensive digestion of cellular cytoplasm, but exhibits a cytoprotective role and functions as a fail-safe response to the stressful condition induced by EF25-$(GSH)_2$. In spite of this, protective autophagic degradation is only operative at low concentrations and is blocked by the action of the compound itself at higher and more cytotoxic concentrations.

However, we found that blocked autophagy contributes to cell death induced by EF25-$(GSH)_2$. In EF25-$(GSH)_2$-treated HepG2 cells, autophagy degradation blockage is accompanied by extensive cytoplasmic vacuolization. The latter phenomenon was found in tumor cells under various chemotherapeutic treatments. Although the cells present with a common morphology, various mechanisms were proposed [14,37–39]. Hence, we conclude that accumulation of autophagosomes instead of autophagic degradation promotes the formation of extensive cytoplasmic vacuolization and subsequent cell death. In some effective cancer therapies, impaired autophagy has been observed [40], which may cause metabolic dysfunction and make cells more susceptible to other types of cell death. Notably, preclinical investigations combining the autophagy late stage inhibitor hydroxychloroquine (HCQ) with various chemotherapies has already entered clinical trials [41].

With EF25-$(GSH)_2$ alone, the number of cells within the G_2/M stage was found to be augmented at a 24 h post-treatment and then largely diminished at 48 h when the number of apoptotic cells greatly soared. Non-apoptotic cell death occurs when the process from G_2/M stage arrest to caspase-dependent apoptosis is blocked by Z-VAD-FMK, implying that cells arrested at G_2/M have already reached a "point of no return" in the lethal process and that caspase activation may not be necessary. Notably, this result suggests that for cells failed to undergo apoptosis, EF25-$(GSH)_2$ induced cell death through non-apoptotic mechanisms, although less effectively without the participation of caspase activation.

As expected, activation of both caspase-3 and caspase-8 was enhanced under co-treatment of CQ and 5 μmol/L or 10 μmol/L EF25-$(GSH)_2$. However, caspase activation was undetectable with co-treatment of CQ and 20 μmol/L EF25-$(GSH)_2$, whereupon the apoptosis rate soared, indicating that the apoptosis in this scenario is mainly caspase-independent. Cell cycle analysis in the presence of the pan-caspase inhibitor Z-VAD-FMK suggests that EF25-$(GSH)_2$ alone causes mainly caspase-dependent apoptosis, but also partially caspase-independent apoptosis.

To sum up, we propose an anti-hepatoma mechanistic model for EF25-$(GSH)_2$ in Figure 9. When treated with EF25-$(GSH)_2$ at a concentration of no more than 5 μmol/L, cells experience successful autophagic degradation. In this case, moderate cytoplasmic vacuolization takes place followed by subsequent recovery, which partially rescues cells from a stressed condition. However, EF25-$(GSH)_2$ at a concentration of 10 μmol/L or higher leads to impaired autophagy during which the autophagic degradation step is blocked and followed by massive cytoplasmic vacuolization. At this point, cells undergo both caspase-dependent and caspase-independent apoptosis. EF25-$(GSH)_2$ treatment alone leads mainly to caspase-dependent apoptosis accompanied by partial caspase-independent apoptosis. Co-treatment with CQ stimulates autophagosome accumulation and cytoplasmic vacuolization, which then promotes both caspase-dependent and caspase-independent apoptosis. Z-VAD-FMK inhibits caspase activation and subsequently blocks the path to apoptotic death. In this case, the status of vacuolization and G_2/M cell cycle arrest is prolonged and eventually leads to non-apoptotic cell death.

In conclusion, our results show that the novel curcumin analog EF25-$(GSH)_2$ has promising potential as a low toxicity chemotherapeutic agent for HCC. Similar to curcumin, the anti-tumor action of EF25-$(GSH)_2$ involved in autophagic, apoptotic and non-apoptotic mechanisms would broaden its application. The combination of EF25-$(GSH)_2$ with chloroquine is suggested to provide a safer and more effective treatment for HCC.

Supporting Information

Figure S1 MS/HR-ESI-MS spectra of EF25-$(GSH)_2$.

Figure S2 Overlay of EF25 (blue) and EF25-$(GSH)_2$ (green) 1H NMR spectra in DMSO-d6. EF25 1H NMR spectrum in DMSO-d6: solvent peak at 2.5 ppm (light yellow); 10.2(s) (OH), 7.9 (=C–H), 6.8–7.3 (aromatic) ppm.

Figure S3 Overlay of EF25 in DMSO-d6 (blue) and EF25-$(GSH)_2$ in D20 (green), buffer pH7, 1H NMR spectra.

Acknowledgments

We thank Dr. Hui Zhong (Academy of Military Medical Sciences, China), Dr. Qinghua Shi (University of Science and Technology of China), Dr. Mian Wu (University of Science and Technology of China) for providing the cell lines and plasmids, Dr. Jun Wang and Mr. Yonglong Zhuang (Anhui University) for technical assistance.

Author Contributions

Conceived and designed the experiments: BH HF. Performed the experiments: TZ LY YB AS BC. Analyzed the data: TZ LY YB AS BC. Contributed reagents/materials/analysis tools: D. Liotta JPS D. Liu YL. Wrote the paper: TZ BH JPS HF.

References

1. Fattovich G, Stroffolini T, Zagni I, Donato F (2004) Hepatocellular carcinoma in cirrhosis: incidence and risk factors. Gastroenterology 127: 35–50.
2. Llovet JM, Bruix J (2008) Novel advancements in the management of hepatocellular carcinoma in 2008. J Hepatol 48: 20–37.
3. Bruix J, Sherman M (2011) Management of hepatocellular carcinoma: an update. Hepatology 53: 1020–1022.
4. Bunchorntavakul C, Hoteit M, Reddy KR (2012) Staging of Hepatocellular Carcinoma. In: N Reau and F. F Poordad, editors. Primary Liver Cancer. New York: Springer Science+Business Media. pp. 161–175.
5. Aoki H, Takada Y, Kondo S, Sawaya R, Aggarwal BB, et al. (2007) Evidence that curcumin suppresses the growth of malignant gliomas in vitro and in vivo through induction of autophagy: role of Akt and extracellular signal-regulated kinase signaling pathways. Mol Pharmacol 72: 29–39.

6. Anand P, Thomas SG, Kunnumakkara AB, Sundaram C, Harikumar KB, et al. (2008) Biological activities of curcumin and its analogues (Congeners) made by man and Mother Nature. Biochem Pharmacol 76: 1590–1611.
7. Steward WP, Gescher AJ (2008) Curcumin in cancer management: recent results of analogue design and clinical studies and desirable future research. Mol Nutr Food Res 52: 1005–1009.
8. Sun A, Lu YJ, Hu H, Shoji M, Liotta DC, et al. (2009) Curcumin analog cytotoxicity against breast cancer cells: exploitation of a redox-dependent mechanism. Bioorg Med Chem Lett 19: 6627–6631.
9. Thomas SL, Zhong D, Zhou W, Malik S, Liotta D, et al. (2008) EF24, a novel curcumin analog, disrupts the microtubule cytoskeleton and inhibits HIF-1. Cell Cycle 7: 2409–2417.
10. Kasinski AL, Du Y, Thomas SL, Zhao J, Sun SY, et al. (2008) Inhibition of IκB Kinase-Nuclear Factor-κB Signaling Pathway by 3,5-Bis(2-flurobenzylidene)piperidin-4-one (EF24), a Novel Monoketone Analog of Curcumin. Mol Pharmacol 74: 654–661.
11. Thomas SL, Zhao J, Li Z, Lou B, Du Y, et al. (2010) Activation of the p38 pathway by a novel monoketone curcumin analog, EF24, suggests a potential combination strategy. Biochem Pharmacol 80: 1309–1316.
12. O'Sullivan-Coyne G, O'Sullivan GC, O'Donovan TR, Piwocka K, McKenna SL (2009) Curcumin induces apoptosis-independent death in oesophageal cancer cells. Br J Cancer 101: 1585–1595.
13. Shinojima N, Yokoyama T, Kondo Y, Kondo S (2007) Roles of the Akt/mTOR/p70S6K and ERK1/2 signaling pathways in curcumin-induced autophagy. Autophagy 3: 635–637.
14. Yoon MJ, Kim EH, Lim JH, Kwon TK, Choi KS (2010) Superoxide anion and proteasomal dysfunction contribute to curcumin-induced paraptosis of malignant breast cancer cells. Free Radic Biol Med 48: 713–726.
15. Adams BK, Ferstl EM, Davis MC, Herold M, Kurtkaya S, et al. (2004) Synthesis and biological evaluation of novel curcumin analogs as anti-cancer and anti-angiogenesis agents. Bioorg Med Chem 12: 3871–3883.
16. Hui IC, Tung EK, Sze KM, Ching YP, Ng IO (2010) Rapamycin and CCI-779 inhibit the mammalian target of rapamycin signalling in hepatocellular carcinoma. Liver international: official journal of the International Association for the Study of the Liver 30: 65–75.
17. Lu B, Ma Y, Wu G, Tong X, Guo H, et al. (2008) Methylation of Tip30 promoter is associated with poor prognosis in human hepatocellular carcinoma. Clinical cancer research 14: 7405–7412.
18. Gao J, Li X, Gu G, Sun B, Cui M, et al. (2011) Efficient synthesis of trisaccharide saponins and their tumor cell killing effects through oncotic necrosis. Bioorg Med Chem Lett 21: 622–627.
19. Tang B, Yu F, Li P, Tong L, Duan X, et al. (2009) A near-infrared neutral pH fluorescent probe for monitoring minor pH changes: imaging in living HepG2 and HL-7702 cells. J Am Chem Soc 131: 3016–3023.
20. Kuck D, Caulfield T, Lyko F, Medina-Franco JL (2010) Nanaomycin A selectively inhibits DNMT3B and reactivates silenced tumor suppressor genes in human cancer cells. Molecular cancer therapeutics 9: 3015–3023.
21. Prause M, Christensen DP, Billestrup N, Mandrup-Poulsen T (2014) JNK1 protects against glucolipotoxicity-mediated beta-cell apoptosis. PloS one 9: e87067.
22. Lin Y, Peng S, Yu H, Teng H, Cui M (2012) RNAi-mediated downregulation of NOB1 suppresses the growth and colony-formation ability of human ovarian cancer cells. Med Oncol 29: 311–317.
23. Yang CH, Yue J, Sims M, Pfeffer LM (2013) The curcumin analog EF24 targets NF-kappaB and miRNA-21, and has potent anticancer activity in vitro and in vivo. PloS one 8: e71130.
24. Yadav VR, Sahoo K, Roberts PR, Awasthi V (2013) Pharmacologic suppression of inflammation by a diphenyldifluoroketone, EF24, in a rat model of fixed-volume hemorrhage improves survival. The Journal of pharmacology and experimental therapeutics 347: 346–356.
25. Kabeya Y, Mizushima N, Ueno T, Yamamoto A, Kirisako T, et al. (2000) LC3, a mammalian homologue of yeast Apg8p, is localized in autophagosome membranes after processing. EMBO J 19: 5720–5728.
26. Klionsky DJ, Abeliovich H, Agostinis P, Agrawal DK, Aliev G, et al. (2008) Guidelines for the use and interpretation of assays for monitoring autophagy in higher eukaryotes. Autophagy 4: 151–175.
27. Choi M-J, Jung KH, Kim D, Lee H, Zheng H-M, et al. (2011) Anti-cancer effects of a novel compound HS-113 on cell growth, apoptosis, and angiogenesis in human hepatocellular carcinoma cells. Cancer letters 306: 190–196.
28. Steele S, Brunton J, Ziehr B, Taft-Benz S, Moorman N, et al. (2013) Francisella tularensis harvests nutrients derived via ATG5-independent autophagy to support intracellular growth. PLoS Pathog 9: e1003562.
29. Shea FF, Rowell JL, Li Y, Chang TH, Alvarez CE (2012) Mammalian alpha arrestins link activated seven transmembrane receptors to Nedd4 family e3 ubiquitin ligases and interact with beta arrestins. PloS one 7: e50557.
30. Pankiv S, Clausen TH, Lamark T, Brech A, Bruun JA, et al. (2007) p62/SQSTM1 binds directly to Atg8/LC3 to facilitate degradation of ubiquitinated protein aggregates by autophagy. J Biol Chem 282: 24131–24145.
31. Adams BK, Cai J, Armstrong J, Herold M, Lu YJ, et al. (2005) EF24, a novel synthetic curcumin analog, induces apoptosis in cancer cells via a redox-dependent mechanism. Anti-Cancer Drugs 16: 263–275.
32. Selvendiran K, Tong L, Vishwanath S, Bratasz A, Trigg NJ, et al. (2007) EF24 induces G2/M arrest and apoptosis in cisplatin-resistant human ovarian cancer cells by increasing PTEN expression. J Biol Chem 282: 28609–28618.
33. Maiuri MC, Zalckvar E, Kimchi A, Kroemer G (2007) Self-eating and self-killing: crosstalk between autophagy and apoptosis. Nat Rev Mol Cell Biol 8: 741–752.
34. Shingu T, Fujiwara K, Bögler O, Akiyama Y, Moritake K, et al. (2009) Inhibition of autophagy at a late stage enhances imatinib-induced cytotoxicity in human malignant glioma cells. Int J Cancer 124: 1060–1071.
35. Kanzawa T, Germano I, Komata T, Ito H, Kondo Y, et al. (2004) Role of autophagy in temozolomide-induced cytotoxicity for malignant glioma cells. Cell Death Differ 11: 448–457.
36. Okada H, Mak TW (2004) Pathways of apoptotic and non-apoptotic death in tumour cells. Nat Rev Cancer 4: 592–603.
37. Chen TS, Wang XP, Sun L, Wang LX, Xing D, et al. (2008) Taxol induces caspase-independent cytoplasmic vacuolization and cell death through endoplasmic reticulum (ER) swelling in ASTC-a-1 cells. Cancer Lett 270: 164–172.
38. Sy LK, Yan SC, Lok CN, Man RY, Che CM (2008) Timosaponin A-III induces autophagy preceding mitochondria-mediated apoptosis in HeLa cancer cells. Cancer Res 68: 10229–10237.
39. Bhanot H, Young AM, Overmeyer JH, Maltese WA (2010) Induction of nonapoptotic cell death by activated Ras requires inverse regulation of Rac1 and Arf6. Mol Cancer Res 8: 1358–1374.
40. Kyoko O, Yoko S, Katsuyuki I, Haruki S, Yoshihiro S (2011) Induction of an incomplete autophagic response by cancer-preventive geranylgeranoic acid (GGA) in a human hepatoma-derived cell line. Biochem J 440: 63–71.
41. Amaravadi RK, Lippincott-Schwartz J, Yin X-M, Weiss WA, Takebe N, et al. (2011) Principles and current strategies for targeting autophagy for cancer treatment. Clin Cancer Res 17: 654–666.

14

A Simple and Rapid Method for Standard Preparation of Gas Phase Extract of Cigarette Smoke

Tsunehito Higashi[1], Yosuke Mai[1], Yoichi Noya[2], Takahiro Horinouchi[1], Koji Terada[1], Akimasa Hoshi[1], Prabha Nepal[1], Takuya Harada[1], Mika Horiguchi[1], Chizuru Hatate[1], Yuji Kuge[2], Soichi Miwa[1]*

1 Department of Cellular Pharmacology, Graduate School of Medicine, Hokkaido University, Sapporo, Hokkaido, Japan, 2 Central Institute of Isotope Science, Hokkaido University, Sapporo, Hokkaido, Japan

Abstract

Cigarette smoke consists of tar and gas phase: the latter is toxicologically important because it can pass through lung alveolar epithelium to enter the circulation. Here we attempt to establish a standard method for preparation of gas phase extract of cigarette smoke (CSE). CSE was prepared by continuously sucking cigarette smoke through a Cambridge filter to remove tar, followed by bubbling it into phosphate-buffered saline (PBS). An increase in dry weight of the filter was defined as tar weight. Characteristically, concentrations of CSEs were represented as virtual tar concentrations, assuming that tar on the filter was dissolved in PBS. CSEs prepared from smaller numbers of cigarettes (original tar concentrations ≤15 mg/ml) showed similar concentration-response curves for cytotoxicity versus virtual tar concentrations, but with CSEs from larger numbers (tar ≥20 mg/ml), the curves were shifted rightward. Accordingly, the cytotoxic activity was detected in PBS of the second reservoir downstream of the first one with larger numbers of cigarettes. CSEs prepared from various cigarette brands showed comparable concentration-response curves for cytotoxicity. Two types of CSEs prepared by continuous and puff smoking protocols were similar regarding concentration-response curves for cytotoxicity, pharmacology of their cytotoxicity, and concentrations of cytotoxic compounds. These data show that concentrations of CSEs expressed by virtual tar concentrations can be a reference value to normalize their cytotoxicity, irrespective of numbers of combusted cigarettes, cigarette brands and smoking protocols, if original tar concentrations are ≤15 mg/ml.

Editor: Thomas H. Thatcher, University of Rochester Medical Center, United States of America

Funding: This work was supported by Grant-in-Aids for Scientific Research (B) 24390059 (SM), Scientific Research (C) 25460326 (KT) and Challenging Exploratory Research 25670123 (SM) from Japan Society for the Promotion of Science (http://www.jsps.go.jp/english/index.html), by a grant from the SRFJ (SM), and by a grant from the Akiyama Life Science Foundation (THi). The funders had no role in study design, data collection and analysis, decision to publish, or preparation of the manuscript.

Competing Interests: The authors have declared that no competing interests exist.

* Email: smiwa@med.hokudai.ac.jp

Introduction

Cigarette smoking is a major risk factor for cardiovascular diseases such as stroke and coronary artery disease [1,2], for chronic pulmonary obstructive diseases [3,4] and for several forms of cancer [5–7]. Cigarette smoke is reported to contain more than 4,000 chemical compounds [8,9]. Among these are reactive oxygen species (ROS) such as peroxynitrate and free radicals of organic compounds [1,10]. Although the free radicals are highly reactive to induce cell injury, their lifetime is too short to reach lung of smokers [10]. Recent studies indicate that cigarette smoke contain stable components which have the potential to stimulate cellular ROS production not only in the lung but also in tissues remote from the lung [11–13].

Cigarette smoke consists of two phases; the tar (particle) phase containing nicotine and the gas phase. In view of human health, the gas phase is important, because it can pass through the lung alveolar epithelium to reach the circulating blood and to induce damage in tissues remote from the lung [14,15]. In fact, the gas phase extract contains stable toxic compounds which exert various cytotoxic effects in a wide range of cells [16–18]. In this context, we have recently shown that the gas phase extract of cigarette smoke induces cell death and plasma membrane damage through ROS generation, which is in turn induced by protein kinase C (PKC)-mediated activation of NADPH oxidase (NOX) [19,20]. In addition, the gas phase extract of cigarette smoke can oxidize LDL in vitro, while it can promote atherosclerotic changes in aortas in vivo [14,21,22]. Recently, using LC/MS and GC/MS in combination with functional assays in cultured cells, we have identified several stable cytotoxic compounds responsible for cytotoxicity in the gas phase extract of cigarette smoke: among these compounds are acrolein (ACR), methyl vinyl ketone (MVK), and 2-cyclopentene-1-one (CPO) [23]. We have also shown that like the gas phase extract, these stable cytotoxic compounds induce cell damage in a PKC- and NOX-dependent manner [20,23].

In spite of its importance for human health, no standard method for preparation of the gas phase extract of the cigarette smoke has been established, although the protocols for standard smoking protocols are established by the International Organization for Standardization (ISO) [24] and Health Canada (HC) [25]. Therefore, researchers have performed experiments using the gas phase extracts prepared by their own methods. The gas phase extracts are generally made by passing cigarette smoke through the

Cambridge filter and subsequently bubbling the smoke in aqueous solution. The methods for preparation of the gas phase extracts differ mainly in terms of smoking protocols (puff smoking vs continuous smoking), bubbling conditions (pore sizes of glass ball filters for generating bubbles and temperatures of the aqueous solution) and the number of combusted cigarettes. The most serious problem is the absence of the definition for concentration of the gas phase extracts of cigarette smoke, which makes it difficult to compare the experimental data on the cigarette smoke extract from different laboratories.

In the present study, we attempt to establish a standard method for preparation of gas phase extracts of cigarette smoke, which is simple and rapid. For this purpose, we use continuous smoking protocol, because it does not require an expensive smoking machine and it is rapid. Using that smoking protocol, we optimize methods for extraction of cytotoxic activities from cigarette smoke into aqueous solution. As a measure of concentrations of the gas phase extracts of cigarette smoke, we introduce the virtual tar concentration (w/v), which is calculated on the assumption that the tar phase trapped on the Cambridge filter is dissolved in the aqueous solution used for extraction of cigarette smoke. We show that the virtual tar concentration can be used as a reference value to normalize the cytotoxic activities of gas phase extracts of cigarette smoke, irrespective of smoking conditions (continuous smoking or puff smoking), cigarette brands and the number of combusted cigarettes, as long as the original tar concentrations in the gas phase extracts are ≤15 mg/ml.

Materials and Methods

Materials

The cigarette used was, unless otherwise specified, the Hi-Lite (JT, Tokyo, Japan) containing 17 mg of tar and 1.4 mg of nicotine per cigarette. In some experiments, other brands such as Peace (JT, 28 mg of tar and 2.3 mg of nicotine), Seven Stars (JT, 14 mg of tar and 1.2 mg of nicotine), Mevius (JT, 10 mg of tar and 0.8 mg of nicotine), Mevius Super Light (JT, 6 mg of tar and 0.5 mg of nicotine), Marlboro (Phillip Morris, 12 mg of tar and 1.0 mg of nicotine), Lucky Strike (British American Tobacco, 11 mg of tar and 1.0 mg of nicotine), Kent 9 mg (British American Tobacco, 9 mg of tar and 0.8 mg of nicotine) were used. The materials and reagents were purchased from the following sources: Cambridge filters from Heinr Borgwaldt GmbH (Hamburg, Germany); CellTiter96 Aqueous One Solution Proliferation Assay Kit and CytoTox-One^{TM} Homogenous Membrane Integrity Assay Kit from Promega Corporation (Madison, WI, USA); acetone, CPO and propionaldehyde from WAKO Pure Chemical Industries (Osaka, Japan); Hoechst 33342, O-(2,3,4,5,6-pentafluorobenzyl) hydroxylamine hydrochloride (PFBOA) and diphenyleneiodonium chloride (DPI) from Sigma Aldrich (St Louis, MO, USA); propidium iodide (PI) from Dojindo Laboratories (Kumamoto, Japan); ACR and MVK from Tokyo Chemical Industry (Tokyo, Japan); bisindolylmaleimide I (BIS I) from Calbiochem (San Diego, CA, USA).

Preparation of the gas phase extract of cigarette smoke

The gas phase extract of cigarette smoke (from now on, we refer to this extract as the cigarette smoke extract [CSE]) was prepared using continuous smoking protocol, unless specified otherwise: this CSE was designated cCSE. The preparation of the cCSE was performed as previously described [19,23] with slight modifications. As shown in Fig. 1, one cigarette per trial was combusted, and the main stream of the cigarette smoke was continuously sucked through a standard glass-fiber Cambridge filter with a constant flow rate of 1.050 l/min by an aspiration pump to remove the tar phase and nicotine. According to the rules of ISO4387, cigarettes with and without filters were combusted up to 3 mm from the tipping paper and 23 mm from the end of cigarette, respectively, while the aspiration rate was set at the average flow rate of the 2-seconds puff duration of the puff smoking defined by ISO3308. The remaining gas phase of cigarette smoke was bubbled into 15 ml of phosphate buffered saline (PBS) in a 100 ml graduated cylinder (the diameter is 28 mm) at 25°C (Fig. 1). To increase the bubbling efficiency, bubbling was performed through a Kinoshita-type glass ball filter with the pore size of 20–30 μm (Kinoshita Industry, Tokyo, Japan). After combustion of cigarettes, the Cambridge filter was dried in air at 25°C for 12 h and an increase in the dry weight of the filter was regarded as the amount of the tar phase. The combustion of cigarette (usually Hi-Lite brand) was repeated, unless otherwise specified, until the dry weight of the tar phase trapped on the Cambridge filter reached 150 mg. The concentration of cCSE was expressed in terms of the virtual tar concentration which was calculated on the assumption that the tar trapped on the Cambridge filter is dissolved in the PBS used for cCSE preparation. The cCSE preparations were aliquoted and stored at −80°C until use.

For preparation of the other type of the gas phase extract of cigarette smoke by puff smoking condition (designated pCSE), smoking was performed using conditions as recommended by ISO (ISO3308). In this case, smoke was generated with a mechanical smoking machine (RM200, Heinr Borgwaldt GmbH) according to ISO3308 rules (2 s puff duration, 35 ml puff volume, bell-shaped puff profile, 60 s puff cycle). The procedures after generation of smoke were the same as those for the cCSE. To avoid the inhalation of cigarette smoke, the devices for CSE preparation were put in the fume hood.

Cell culture

Human embryonic kidney HEK293T cells, human cervical carcinoma HeLa cells, C6 rat glioma cells, A7r5 rat aorta smooth muscle cells, EA.hy926 immortalized human umbilical vein endothelial cells (HUVEC), human lung small cell carcinoma SBC-3 cells, human lung squamous cell carcinoma H1299 cells, and human lung adenocarcinoma A549 cells were maintained in Dulbecco's modified Eagle medium (DMEM) supplemented with 10% (v/v) heat-inactivated fetal bovine serum (FBS), 100 units/ml penicillin G, and 100 μg/ml streptomycin sulfate at 37°C in humidified air with 5% CO_2. U937 human monocytes and RAW264.7 mouse macrophages were maintained in RPMI1640 supplemented with 10% (v/v) FBS, 10 μM 2-mercaptoethanol, 100 units/ml penicillin G, and 100 μg/ml streptomycin sulfate at 37°C in humidified air with 5% CO_2. Chinese hamster ovary (CHO) cells were maintained in F-12 Ham medium supplemented with 10% (v/v) FBS, 100 units/ml penicillin G, and 100 μg/ml streptomycin sulfate at 37°C in humidified air with 5% CO_2.

HEK293T cells, HeLa cells, and CHO cells were purchased from RIKEN CELL BANK (Wako, Japan). C6 cells, A7r5 cells, U937 cells, RAW264.7 cells, and H1299 cells were purchased from American Type Culture Collection (Manassas, VA, USA). SBC-3 cells were purchased from Japanese Collection of Research Bioresources (Ibaraki, Japan). HUVEC were provided from Dr. Cora Jean S. Edgell, University of North Carolina at Chapel Hill [26].

Evaluation of cytotoxicity

We used 3-(4,5-dimethylthiazol-2-yl)-5-(3-carboxymethyl)-2-(4-sulfophenyl)-2H-tetrazolium (MTS) reduction assay for evaluation

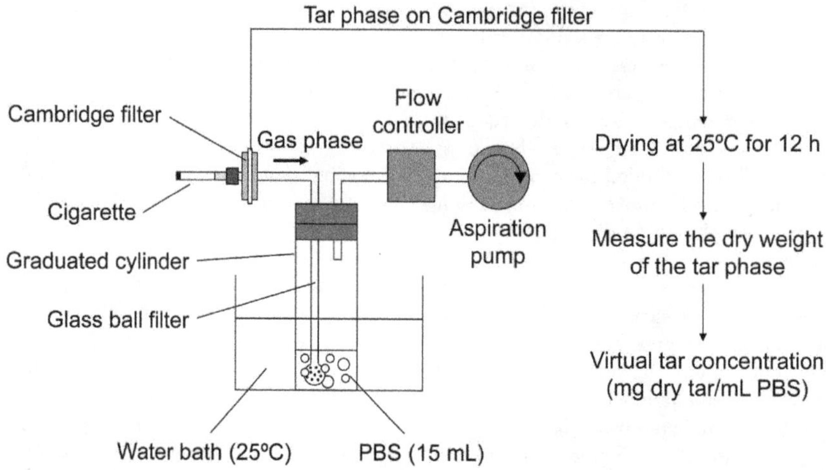

Figure 1. Schematic diagram of an apparatus for preparation of gas phase extracts of cigarette smoke. A standard method for preparation of the gas phase extract of cigarette smoke is as follows. Four cigarettes of Hi-Lite brand, unless otherwise specified, were sequentially combusted and the main-stream smoke was continuously sucked through a Cambridge filter at a constant flow rate of 1.050 l/min by an aspirator, to remove the tar phase. The remaining gas phase was bubbled through a glass ball filter (pore size: 20–30 μm) into phosphate buffered saline (PBS, 15 ml) in a graduated cylinder kept at 25°C. After combustion of cigarette, the filter was dried in air for 12 h at 25°C, and the dry weight of the tar phase trapped on the Cambridge filter was obtained by subtracting the weight of filter before use from that after use. The concentration of the gas phase extract was expressed as the virtual tar concentration (mg tar/ml PBS), assuming that the tar phase trapped on the Cambridge filter is dissolved in the PBS. Four cigarettes of Hi-Lite brand gave the dry tar weight of approximately 150 mg. Notably, cytotoxicity of the gas phase extracts depends not on cigarette brands but on the virtual tar concentration.

of cell viability, PI uptake assay and lactate dehydrogenase (LDH) leakage assay for evaluation of cell membrane damage, and DNA fragmentation assay for evaluation of cell apoptosis.

MTS reduction assay was performed using CellTiter96 Aqueous One Solution Cell Proliferation Assay Kit, as described recently [19,23]. Briefly, the cells were inoculated onto a 96-well plate at a density of 1×10^4 cells per well. After incubation with CSE for 4 h, 20 μl of kit reagent was added to the culture medium (100 μl), and incubated for a further 1 h. The amount of reduced form of MTS was measured by absorbance at 490 nm using a microplate reader (SPECTRA MAX 250, Molecular Devices Corp., Sunnyvale, CA, USA). MTS reduction activity of the CSE-treated cells was represented as a percentage of the absorbance obtained from non-treated cells. MTS reduction activity in culture medium without cells was regarded as zero.

PI uptake assay was performed as recently described [19,20,23]. The cells were incubated with CSE for 4 h in culture medium containing 1 μg/ml PI and 1 μg/ml Hoechst 33342. The fluorescent images of PI and Hoechst 33342 were captured by IX-71 inverted fluorescent microscope (Olympus, Tokyo, Japan) equipped with ×40 objective lens (LUCPlanFL N, NA = 0.60, Olympus).

LDH leakage assay was performed using CytoTox-One™ Homogenous Membrane Integrity Assay Kit according to the manufacture's protocols as recently described [19,20]. The cells were inoculated onto a 96-well plate at a density of 1×10^4 cells per well. After incubation with CSE for 4 h, culture media (100 μl) were transferred to a new 96-well plate (Black Cliniplate; Thermo Fisher Scientific Inc., Rockford, IL, USA) for measurement LDH activity leaked into media. For measurement of total LDH activity, the cells cultured in parallel were disrupted by adding 2 μl of Lysis Buffer to the culture media, and the whole lysates were transferred to the 96-well plate. The enzyme reaction was started by adding 100 μl of CytoTox-ONE™ reagent. After 10-min incubation, at room temperature, the reaction was terminated by adding 50 μl of Stop Solution. The amount of the reaction product (rezorufin) was measured using a microplate spectrofluorometer (Varioscan, Thermo Fisher Scientific Inc.). LDH leakage was represented as a percentage of the total LDH activity. LDH activity in culture media without cells was regarded as zero.

For DNA fragmentation assay, the cells were inoculated onto 6-cm dish at the density of 1×10^6 cells per dish. After 24-h incubation with CSE, the cells were lysed by incubation with lysis buffer (10 mM Tris-HCl [pH 7.4], 5 mM EDTA, 0.5% Triton X-100) for 30 min at 4°C, and centrifuged at 15,000× g for 30 min at 4°C to remove cell debris. The supernatants were transferred to new tubes, and incubated with 40 μg/ml proteinase K for 1 h at 37°C. After purification by phenol/chloroform extraction and ethanol precipitation, the DNA was reconstituted in Tris-EDTA buffer (10 mM Tris-HCl [pH 8.0], 1 mM EDTA) containing 40 μg/ml RNaseA, and incubated for 30 min at 37°C. The purified DNA was subjected to 1.8% agarose gel electrophoresis.

Analysis of CSE by HPLC and GC/MS

Identification of cytotoxic compounds in the CSE was performed using HPLC and GC/MS as described recently [23]. Briefly, the CSE was fractionated by HPLC equipped with a reverse-phase column, each fraction was analyzed for cytotoxic activity using PI uptake assay, and two active fractions inducing PI uptake into cultured C6 glioma cells were analyzed for identification of cytotoxic compounds using GC/MS. Before analysis by GC/MS, the active fractions from HPLC were derivatized with a carbonyl reagent PFBOA to stabilize carbonyl compounds as described [23].

Data analysis

For evaluation of cytotoxic activities of CSEs (cCSE or pCSE) using MTS reduction assay and LDH leakage assay, concentration-response curves were constructed by plotting the activities against virtual tar concentrations of CSEs. MTS reduction activity in the presence of CSEs was represented as a percentage of control value in the absence of CSEs, while LDH activity leaked into culture medium was represented as a percentage of control value in culture medium of cells lysed by 0.2% Triton X-100 in the absence of CSEs. From the concentration-response curves, the values for EC_{50} and maximum inhibition were obtained. The data for experiments performed with or without cultured cells were presented as means ± SE or means ± SD., respectively. The significance of the differences between mean values was evaluated with GraphPad PRISM™ (version 4.0, GraphPad Software Inc., San Diego, CA, USA) by student's unpaired *t*-test or one-way ANOVA, followed by Tukey's multiple comparison test. A *P* value less than 0.05 was considered to indicate statistically significant differences.

Results

Validation of quantification of tar amount

In the present study, we attempted to represent the concentration of the cCSE in terms of the virtual tar concentration which was calculated on the assumption that the tar phase (dry weight [mg]) trapped on the Cambridge filter is dissolved in the PBS (15 ml). Since the tar phase was reported to contain water [27], we first investigated conditions for vaporizing the water in the tar phase on Cambridge filters to estimate the dry weight of the tar phase. To minimize vaporization of volatile chemical components in the tar phase, we tested relatively low temperatures such as 25°C and 55°C for vaporization of water.

For evaluation of vaporizing conditions, smoke from 4 cigarettes of Hi-Lite brand was passed through a Cambridge filter, and the filter was dried at 25°C or 55°C for various lengths of time, and the weight of the filter was measured. The increase in the weight of the filter following smoking was regarded as the weight of the tar phase. As shown in Fig. 2A, the weight of the tar phase on the filter decreased up to 2 h following drying at 25°C, and thereafter, it reached a plateau up to 12 h. Following drying at 55°C, the weight of the tar phase on the filter also decreased in a similar time course, and thereafter, it reached a plateau up to 12 h. Notably, the weight of the tar phase on the filter following drying at 55°C for 12 h is significantly lower than that following drying at 25°C for 12 h, indicating that part of volatile components in the tar phase might have been vaporized. Therefore, in the following experiments, Cambridge filters were dried at 25°C for 12 h.

As shown in Fig. 2B, the weight of the tar phase trapped on the Cambridge filter increased linearly with an increase in the number of combusted cigarettes up to 6 cigarettes (of Hi-Lite brand), which gave approximately 225 mg of tar on the filter. During combustion of cigarettes, the aspiration speed was continuously monitored by a Kofloc flowmeter, and it was found to be constant (1.050 l/min) up to 6 cigarettes. These results indicate that the Cambridge filter functions normally without being saturated with the tar phase at least up to 225 mg. In the following experiments, we usually used 4 cigarettes for preparation of the cCSE. When more than 4 cigarettes were combusted for cCSE preparation, a new Cambridge filter was used every 4 cigarettes to avoid saturation of the filter with tar phase.

Effects of the temperature of PBS and the pore size of the glass ball filter on the cytotoxicity of the gas phase extract of cigarette smoke

Since the water-solubility of chemical compounds is generally affected by temperature, we examined the effect of the temperature of PBS in the graduated cylinder on the cytotoxicity of cCSE preparation. cCSE was prepared by continuous smoking of four cigarettes of Hi-Lite brand which gave 150 mg of tar on the Cambridge filter. The concentrations of the cCSE were expressed in terms of the virtual tar concentration, assuming that the tar trapped on the Cambridge filter was dissolved in cCSE. The tar concentration of the original cCSE was calculated to be 10 mg/ml. The cCSEs prepared with PBS (15 ml) kept at 0°C and 25°C showed similar concentration-response curves for inhibition of MTS reduction activity (Fig. 3A), indicating that the temperature of the PBS has little effect on the recovery of cytotoxic compounds.

The pore size of the glass ball filter used for bubbling smoke might affect the cytotoxicity of cCSE by changing the size of bubbles and hence the efficiency of transfer of cytotoxic compounds from bubbles to PBS. To optimize the pore size of the glass ball filter, we compared the cytotoxicity of cCSEs prepared using glass ball filters with different pore sizes. The cCSEs prepared with glass ball filters of normal pore size (20–30 μm) or large pore size (100–120 μm) showed similar concentration-response curves for inhibition of MTS reduction activity (Fig. 3B), indicating that the pore size of glass ball filters has little effect on the recovery of cytotoxic compounds. Therefore, in the following experiments, we used PBS kept at 25°C and a glass ball filter of normal pore size for preparation of the cCSE.

Effects of the original tar concentrations of cCSEs on their cytotoxic potency

To examine how much cigarette smoke will saturate the PBS (15 ml), we constructed the concentration-response curves for cytotoxicity of cCSEs prepared from varying numbers of cigarettes (Fig. 4A and Table 1). In this experiment, 2–40 cigarettes of Hi-Lite brand were combusted by continuous smoking protocol, and a new Cambridge filter was used every 4 cigarettes, to avoid the saturation of the filter with tar. Again, the concentrations of the cCSE were expressed in terms of the virtual tar concentration, based on the dry weight of tar trapped on the Cambridge filter.

The concentration-response curves for inhibition of MTS reduction activity were similar among cCSEs which were made from 2–6 cigarettes (equivalent to the original tar concentration of 5–15 mg/ml), as demonstrated by comparable values for the EC_{50} and maximal inhibition (Fig. 4A and Table 1). However, the concentration-response curves began to be shifted to the right, when more than 8 cigarettes (equivalent to the original tar concentration ≥20 mg/ml) were used (Fig. 4A and Table 1). The rightward shift of the curves was more marked with an increase in the number of cigarettes, indicating that the cytotoxic activities of cCSEs prepared from larger numbers of cigarettes were lower than expected at a given tar concentration. These results taken together strongly demonstrate that cytotoxic activity in the smoke is efficiently extracted into PBS up to 6 cigarettes of Hi-Lite brand (equivalent to the original tar concentration of ≤15 mg/ml), whereas some part of the cytotoxic activity is leaked with more than 8 cigarettes (equivalent to the original tar concentration of ≥ 20 mg/ml).

To confirm the leakage of the cytotoxic activity, another reservoir containing 15 ml of PBS was incorporated downstream of the first reservoir, and the cytotoxic activity of the PBS in the second reservoir was analyzed using MTS reduction assay. As shown in Fig. 4B, the PBS in the second reservoir showed no cytotoxic activity, when four cigarettes of Hi-Lite brand (equivalent to the original tar concentration of 10 mg/ml) were used for cCSE preparation, but it showed significant cytotoxic activity, when 14 cigarettes (equivalent to the original tar concentration of 35 mg/ml) were used, demonstrating that some part of cytotoxic activity has actually leaked.

These findings taken together show that as long as ≤6 cigarettes of Hi-Lite brand (equivalent to the original tar concentration of ≤ 15 mg/ml) are used for preparation of the original cCSE, nearly

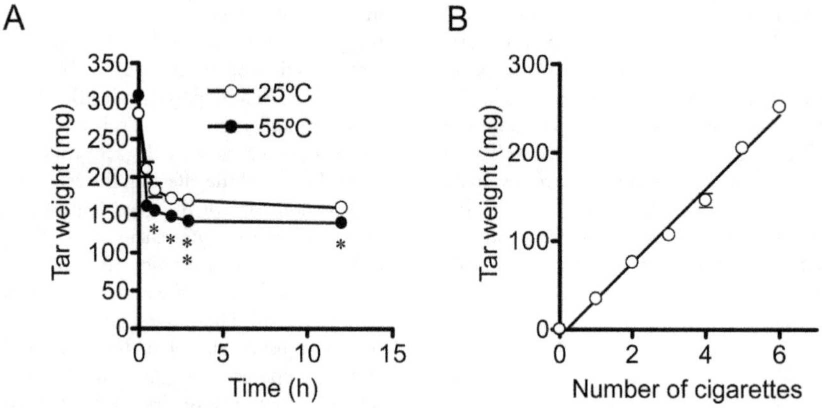

Figure 2. Quantification of the weight of the tar of cigarette smoke trapped on the Cambridge filter. (A) Time-course of a decrease in the weight of the tar phase of cigarette smoke trapped on the Cambridge filter after drying at 25°C (open circle) or 55°C (closed circle). Four cigarettes of Hi-Lite brand were sequentially combusted and the main-stream smoke was sucked through a Cambridge filter at a constant flow rate of 1.050 l/min by an aspiration pump. After combustion of cigarette, the filter was dried for various lengths of time at 25°C (open circle) or 55°C (closed circle), and the weight of the tar phase of cigarette smoke trapped on the Cambridge filter was obtained by subtracting the filter weight before combustion of cigarette from the weight after combustion. (B) The relationship between the number of combusted cigarettes and the dry weight of the tar phase trapped on the Cambridge filter. Various numbers of Hi-Lite brand cigarettes were sequentially combusted as described in A. After combustion, the filter was dried for 12 h at 25°C, and the dry weight of the tar phase on the Cambridge filter was determined as described in A. Values represent means ± SD of three experiments. *, $P<0.05$; **, $P<0.01$ versus 25°C.

100% of the cytotoxic activity is extracted into the PBS, but that with ≥8 cigarettes of Hi-Lite brand (equivalent to the original tar concentration of ≥20 mg/ml), part of cytotoxic activity leaks probably because of saturation of PBS. This means that when cCSEs are prepared at the original tar concentrations of ≤15 mg/ml, the tar concentrations are linearly related with the cytotoxic potency of cCSEs, and hence, that the tar concentrations can be used as a universal measure of cytotoxic potency of cCSE.

To exclude the possibility that the cytotoxicity is caused by a pH change in culture medium (DMEM) following addition of cCSE, we measured the pH values of the medium containing varying concentrations of cCSE. The pH values of DMEM containing cCSE at final tar concentrations of 0, 0.5 and 1.0 mg/ml were 7.48±0.02, 7.45±0.03 and 7.46±0.04, respectively (n = 3 for each group), which were not significantly different from each other. These results suggest that addition of cCSE to culture medium at least up to the virtual tar concentration of 1.0 mg/ml had no effect on the pH of culture medium.

Effects of cigarette brands on the cytotoxicity of cCSE

To clarify whether the potency of cytotoxic activities of cCSE varies depending on cigarette brands, we examined the cytotoxicity of 8 representative cigarette brands (5 brands from JT, Japan, 3 brands from other countries) with different tar contents (Table 2). To prepare the original cCSEs at comparable tar concentrations from various brands of cigarettes, we first determined the dry weight of tar per cigarette which was trapped on the Cambridge filter after combustion of one cigarette by

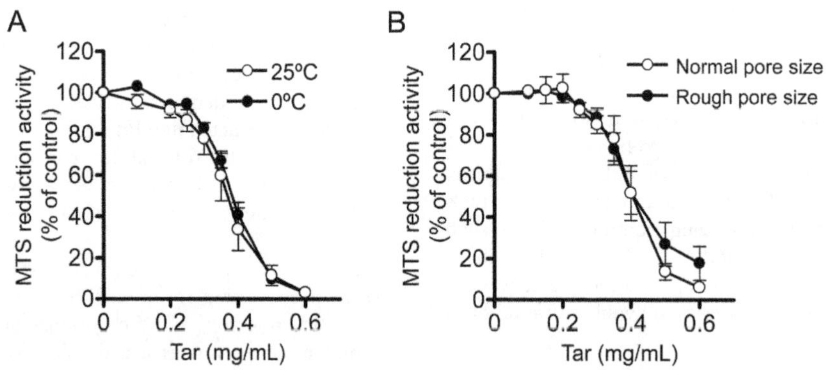

Figure 3. Effects of the bubbling condition on gas phase extracts of cigarette smoke. Effects of the temperature of phosphate-buffered saline (PBS) (A) and pore size of a glass ball filter for bubbling the gas phase of cigarette smoke into PBS (B) on the cytotoxic activities of the gas phase extract were examined. The gas phase extract of cigarette smoke (designated cCSE) was prepared as described in the legend for Fig. 1, by continuous smoking of four cigarettes of Hi-Lite brand which gave the virtual tar concentration of approximately 10 mg/ml PBS. In panel A, the temperature of PBS for extraction of cigarette smoke was kept at either 25°C (open circle) or 0°C (closed circle), and in panel B, the pore size of the glass ball filter was either normal (pore size, 20–30 μm; open circle) or rough (pore size, 100–120 μm; closed circle). For evaluation of the cytotoxicity of cCSE, C6 glioma cells were incubated for 4 h with various concentrations of cCSE and MTS reduction activity was determined as described in Materials and methods. MTS reduction activity in the absence of cCSE was represented as 100%. Values represent means ± SE of three experiments, each in triplicate.

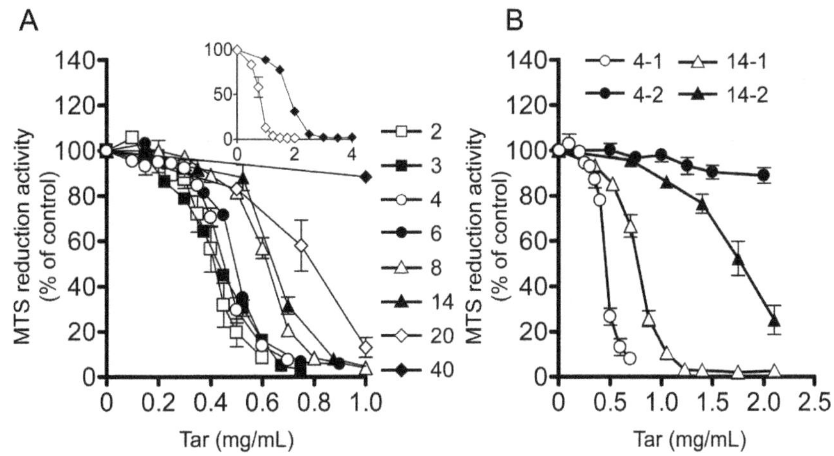

Figure 4. Cytotoxic activities of gas phase extracts of cigarette smoke and the number of cigarette. Concentration-response curves of the gas phase extracts of cigarette smoke prepared from varying numbers of cigarettes (Hi-Lite brand) (A) and of the phosphate buffered saline (PBS) in the second graduated cylinder (B) for inhibition of MTS reduction activity. (A) The gas phase extract of cigarette smoke (designated cCSE) was prepared from varying numbers (2–40) of cigarettes (Hi-Lite brand) based on continuous smoking protocol, while a new Cambridge filter was used every 4 cigarettes. Inset: Concentration-response curves of the cCSE prepared from 20 or 40 cigarettes with a change in scale of concentrations on x axis. (B) In the apparatus for preparation of cCSE, the second graduated cylinder with 15 ml of PBS was incorporated downstream of the first one, and cCSE was prepared from either 4 or 14 cigarettes (Hi-Lite brand). The cytotoxicity of PBS in the original and second graduated cylinders was evaluated using MTS reduction assay. MTS reduction activity in the absence of the gas phase extract was represented as 100%. Values represent means ± SE of three experiments, each in triplicate. 4-1 (14-1) and 4-2 (14-2) represent the cytotoxic activities of the PBS in the first (original) and second graduated cylinders prepared from 4 (14) cigarettes, respectively.

continuous smoking protocol (Table 2). The dry weight of tar per cigarette varied from 18.8 mg to 53.1 mg, which were two to three times larger than the tar content provided by the tobacco company: the difference is mainly due to that the tar content is determined by puff smoking according to the regulation of ISO3308, which discards cigarette smoke during the time interval except puff.

From these cigarettes, we prepared cCSEs, whose original tar concentration was 10 mg/mL (equivalent to the tar concentration of cCSE prepared from four cigarettes of Hi-Lite brand). The concentration-response relationships for inhibition of MTS reduction activity were not significantly different among the cCSEs prepared from different cigarette brands, as demonstrated by comparable values for the EC_{50} and maximal inhibition (Fig. 5 and Table 2). These results demonstrate that the cytotoxic activities of cCSEs depend on the tar concentration but not on either cigarette brands or nominal tar contents of cigarettes. Furthermore, the present results suggest that although cigarettes are highly engineered products containing differing tobacco leave composition and chemical additives [28,29], those factors have little effect on the cytotoxic activities from the toxicological viewpoint.

Comparison of cytotoxic potency of cCSE and pCSE

We compared the cytotoxic potency of two types of CSE, i.e. cCSE and pCSE, which were prepared by continuous or puff smoking protocols, respectively. For both CSEs, the original solutions were prepared at the virtual tar concentration of 10 mg/

Table 1. The EC_{50} and maximal values for inhibition of MTS reduction activity of the cCSEs prepared from varying numbers (2–40) of cigarettes (Hi-Lite brand).

Number of cigarette	EC_{50} (mg/ml)[a]	Maximum inhibition (%)[a]
2	0.411±0.022	91.45±0.70
3	0.431±0.083	96.66±0.54
4	0.451±0.011	92.57±0.66
6	0.494±0.001	94.30±0.46
8	0.618±0.012**	96.95±0.61
14	0.643±0.013**	97.72±0.03
20	0.784±0.059**	97.76±0.53
40	1.797±0.024**	98.17±0.06

[a]The cCSEs at the original tar concentration of 10 mg/ml were subjected to MTS reduction assay in C6 glioma cells. The concentration-response curves for inhibition of MTS reduction activity were constructed, and the EC_{50} values and maximal inhibition were determined. The concentrations of cCSEs were represented by the virtual tar concentrations. MTS reduction activity in the absence of the cCSEs was represented as 100%. Values represent means ± SE of three experiments, each in triplicate. **$P<0.01$ vs the value for 2 cigarettes.

Table 2. Tar content per cigarette of various brands, the dry weight of tar trapped on the Cambridge filter after combustion of one cigarette and the EC_{50} values of cCSEs for inhibition of MTS reduction activity.

Cigarette brand	Nicotine content per cigarette (mg)[a]	Tar content per cigarette (mg)[a]	Dry tar weight per cigarette (mg)[b]	EC_{50} (mg/ml) for MTS reduction activity[c]
Peace	2.3	28	53.1±2.6	0.521±0.025
Hi-Lite	1.4	17	35.5±1.8	0.463±0.014
Seven Stars	1.2	14	35.6±0.4	0.502±0.023
Mevius	0.8	10	25.9±3.1	0.520±0.019
Mevius Super Light	0.5	6	18.8±2.5	0.534±0.006
Marlboro	1.0	12	26.1±1.1	0.496±0.028
Lucky Strike	1.0	11	22.7±2.4	0.495±0.029
Kent 9 mg	0.8	9	26.4±2.4	0.521±0.025

[a]Nicotine and tar content per cigarette is the value reported by its manufacturer and determined by puff smoking based on ISO regulation.
[b]For determination of dry tar weight per cigarette, smoke of one cigarette from either brand was continuously sucked through the Cambridge filter, and the increase in the dry weight of the filter was determined (represented as means ± SD of three experiments).
[c]For determination of the EC_{50} values, cCSEs at the original tar concentration of 10 mg/ml were prepared from cigarettes of various brands by continuous smoking, and subjected to MTS reduction assay in C6 glioma cells for construction of concentration-response curves from which the EC_{50} values (means ± SE of three experiments, each in triplicate) were determined.

ml and their cytotoxic activities were examined using MTS reduction assay and DNA fragmentation assay for cell death, and LDH leakage assay and PI uptake assay for plasma membrane damage. For preparation of 15 mL of cCSE at that tar concentration, four cigarettes of Hi-Lite brand were required, while nine cigarettes were required for preparation of the same amount of pCSE.

cCSE and pCSE showed similar concentration-response relationships for inhibition of MTS reduction activity (Fig. 6A), induction of LDH leakage (Fig. 6B), induction of DNA fragmentation (Fig. 6C) and induction of PI uptake (Figs. 6D and 6E):

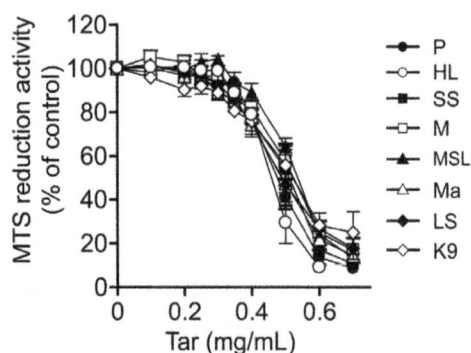

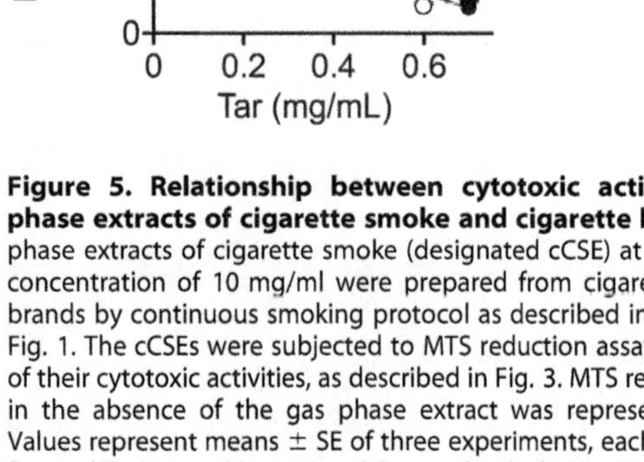

Figure 5. Relationship between cytotoxic activities of gas phase extracts of cigarette smoke and cigarette brand. The gas phase extracts of cigarette smoke (designated cCSE) at the original tar concentration of 10 mg/ml were prepared from cigarettes of various brands by continuous smoking protocol as described in the legend for Fig. 1. The cCSEs were subjected to MTS reduction assay for evaluation of their cytotoxic activities, as described in Fig. 3. MTS reduction activity in the absence of the gas phase extract was represented as 100%. Values represent means ± SE of three experiments, each in triplicate. P, Peace (JT, Japan; 28 mg tar, 2.3 mg nicotine), HL, Hi-Lite (JT, Japan; 17 mg tar, 1.4 mg nicotine), SS, Seven Stars (JT, Japan; 14 mg tar, 1.2 mg nicotine), M, Mevius (JT, Japan; 10 mg tar, 0.8 mg nicotine), MSL, Mevius Super Light (JT, Japan; 6 mg tar, 0.5 mg nicotine), Ma, Marlboro (Phillip Morris, USA; 12 mg tar, 1.0 mg nicotine), LS, Lucky Strike (British American Tobacco, UK; 11 mg tar, 0.9 mg nicotine), K9, Kent 9 mg (British American Tobacco, UK; 9 mg tar, 0.8 mg nicotine).

there was no significant difference between cCSE and pCSE regarding the EC_{50} values for inhibition of MTS reduction activity (0.454±0.004 mg/ml vs 0.469±0.009 mg/ml, respectively) and the EC_{50} values for induction of LDH leakage (0.465±0.035 mg/ml and 0.524±0.025 mg/ml). These results indicate that the cytotoxic potency and property of the gas phase extracts do not depend on smoking protocol.

Comparison of pharmacological properties of cCSE and pCSE

In our recent paper [19,20], we have reported that cCSE induces the plasma membrane damage and cell death in cultured C6 glioma cells, and that total of the plasma membrane damage and part of cell death are induced by ROS which are produced by PKC-dependent activation of NADPH oxidase (NOX), based on the sensitivities to a PKC inhibitor (BIS I) and a NOX inhibitor (DPI). To get insights into the molecular mechanism of action of both types of CSEs, we compared the effects of BIS I and DPI on the cCSE- and pCSE-induced changes in MTS reduction activity (Fig. 7A) and LDH leakage (Fig. 7B).

Following exposure for 4 h to cCSE (final tar concentration, 0.6 mg/ml), MTS reduction activity was decreased to about 10% of the control value without the exposure, and the cCSE-induced decrease in MTS reduction activity was partially recovered (to approximately 70% of the control value) by pretreatment with the maximally effective concentration of BIS I or DPI (Fig. 7A), as reported recently [19,20]. Exposure for 4 h to pCSE (final tar concentration, 0.6 mg/ml) also induced a decrease in MTS reduction activity to the same extent as exposure to cCSE, and the decrease was partially recovered by pretreatment with BIS I or DPI to the extent comparable to that induced by cCSE (Fig. 7A).

LDH leakage was increased to about 100% following exposure for 4 h to cCSE (final tar concentration, 0.6 mg/ml), and the increase was almost totally abrogated by pretreatment with the maximally effective concentration of BIS I or DPI (Fig. 7B), as reported [19,20]. Exposure for 4 h to pCSE (final tar concentration, 0.6 mg/ml) also induced an increase in LDH leakage to the same extent as exposure to cCSE, and the increase induced by pCSE was suppressed by pretreatment with BIS I or DPI to the extent comparable to that induced by cCSE (Fig. 7B). These

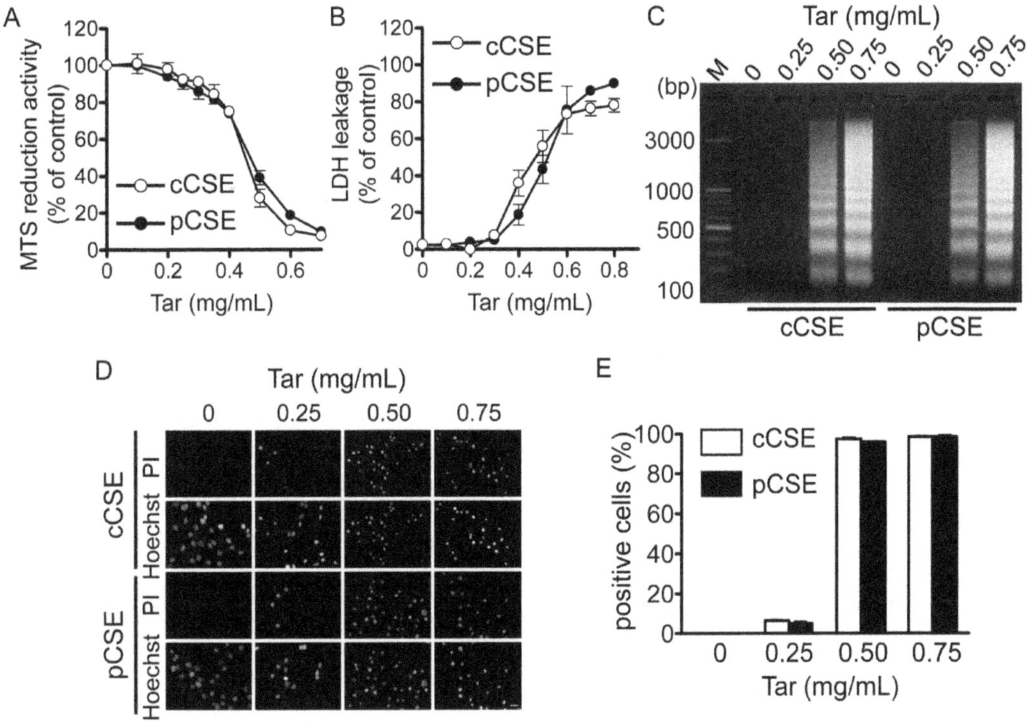

Figure 6. Cytotoxic activities of gas phase extracts of cigarette smoke and smoking methods. The gas phase extracts of cigarette smoke were prepared from Hi-Lite brand cigarettes by either continuous smoking protocol (cCSE) as described in the legend for Fig. 1 or puff smoking (pCSE) as described in Materials and Methods. The original gas phase extracts at the virtual tar concentration of 10 mg/ml PBS were prepared, and they were subjected to MTS reduction assay (A), LDH leakage assay (B), DNA fragmentation assay (C) and PI uptake assay (D, E) in cultured C6 glioma cells for evaluation of their cytotoxic activities. In MTS reduction assay, substrate reduction activity was represented as a percentage of the value in the absence of the gas phase extract; in LDH leakage assay, LDH activity leaked into culture medium was represented as a percentage of total activity in the medium of cells lysed by 0.2% Triton X-100; in PI uptake assay, the number of the cells positive for PI uptake was represented as a percentage of total number of cells identified by Hoechst 33342 for nuclear staining. Values in panels A, B and E represent means ± SE of three experiments, each in triplicate. The results in panels C and D are representative of three separate experiments.

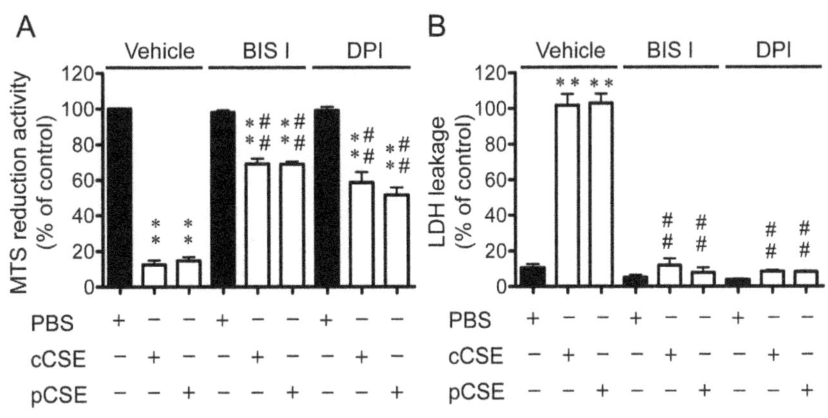

Figure 7. Pharmacological properties of cytotoxic activities of two types of gas phase extracts of cigarette smoke. The gas phase extracts of cigarette smoke at the virtual tar concentration of 10 mg/ml PBS were prepared from Hi-Lite brand cigarettes by either continuous (cCSE) or puff smoking protocol (pCSE), and they were subjected to MTS reduction assay (A) and LDH leakage assay (B). For determination of the effects of inhibitors of protein kinase C or NADPH oxidase, 5 μM BIS I or 1 μM DPI was added to the culture medium of C6 glioma cells, respectively, 30 min before the start of 4-h incubation with cCSE or pCSE. In panel A, MTS reduction activity was represented as a percentage of the control value in the absence of CSEs (PBS) within the vehicle-treated group. In panel B, LDH activity leaked into culture medium was represented as a percentage of total activity in the medium of cells lysed by 0.2% Triton X-100. Values represent means ± SE of three experiments, each in triplicate. **P<0.01 vs PBS-treated cells within either of three groups (Vehicle-, BIS I- and DPI-treated groups); ##P<0.01 vs cCSE- or pCSE-treated cells within the vehicle-treated group.

results taken together indicate that the action mechanisms of two types of CSEs (cCSE and pCSE) for cytotoxicity such as cell death and plasma membrane damage are similar from the pharmacological viewpoint.

Comparison of the concentrations of carbonyl compounds in cCSE and pCSE

In our recent paper [23], we fractionated cCSE into nine fractions with HPLC, found two HPLC fractions to possess cytotoxic activities with functional assays in cultured cells and in those active HPLC fractions, identified ACR, MVK and CPO as stable cytotoxic factors responsible for the cytotoxic activities of cCSE. In addition, in the active HPLC fractions, we identified other carbonyl compounds such as acetone and propionaldehyde which do not possess cytotoxic activities. Therefore, we compared the concentrations of these carbonyl compounds in cCSE with those in pCSE (Table 3). For determination of the concentrations of these carbonyl compounds, both CSEs were first fractionated by reversed-phase HPLC and each fraction was analyzed for cytotoxicity. The fractions showing cytotoxic activities detected by PI uptake assay were subjected to GC/MS after derivatization with a carbonyl reagent PFBOA. As shown in Table 3, there was no significant difference between both types of CSE regarding the concentrations of cytotoxic carbonyls such as ACR and MVK and of noncytotoxic carbonyls such as acetone and propionaldehyde. These results demonstrate that the chemical composition of cCSE and pCSE is equivalent in terms of the concentrations of the major carbonyl compounds.

The sensitivity of various cell lines to cCSE

Finally, we examined the sensitivity to cCSE of various cell lines which are widely used, using MTS reduction assay (Fig. 8). Among these cell lines, CHO cells were the most sensitive to cCSE only in the low tar concentration range (up to 0.2 mg/ml), but they became relatively resistant in the higher tar concentration range. U937 human monocytes, A7r5 rat aorta smooth muscle cells and SBC-3 cells were the second sensitive: the EC_{50} values of cCSE for inhibition of MTS reduction activity were 0.285 ± 0.021 mg/ml, 0.299 ± 0.018 mg/ml and 0.300 ± 0.010 mg/ml (represented by the tar concentration), respectively. C6 rat glioma cells and HEK293T cells were the third in the sensitivity, with the EC_{50} values of 0.423 ± 0.019 mg/ml and 0.446 ± 0.015 mg/ml, respectively. In contrast, HeLa cells, RAW264.7 mouse macrophages, HUVEC, H1299 cells and A549 cells were resistant to CSE up to the tar concentration of 0.6 mg/ml.

Discussion

The gas phase of cigarette smoke is considered to be important from the viewpoint of human health, because it is the gas phase but not the tar phase that can pass through the alveolar epithelium of the lung to enter the circulation, exerting cytotoxic effects in tissues remote from the lung [14,15,30]. However, no standard method for preparation of the gas phase extracts of cigarette smoke has so far been established, and hence, researchers have performed experiments using the gas phase extracts prepared by their own methods. Because of the potential variability in the composition and concentration of those extracts, the comparison of the data from different laboratories has been difficult. In the present study, we have standardized a simple and rapid method for preparation of the gas phase extract of cigarette smoke based on continuous smoking protocol (referred to as cCSE).

The protocol for preparation of cCSE established in the present study is as follows. 1) Cigarette smoke of any brand is continuously sucked through a Cambridge filter with a constant flow rate of 1.050 l/min. 2) The smoke is subsequently bubbled through a glass ball filter of normal pore size into 15 mL of PBS kept at 25°C. 3) The dry weight of the tar phase trapped on the Cambridge filter is determined after drying at 25°C for 12 h, 4) The concentration of cCSE is expressed in terms of the virtual tar concentration which is calculated on the assumption that the tar trapped on the Cambridge filter is dissolved in the PBS used for cCSE preparation, 5) Combustion of cigarette can be repeated as long as the dry weight of tar trapped on the Cambridge filter is $\leq$ 225 mg.

The most important finding is that the concentration of cCSE expressed in terms of the virtual tar concentration can be used as a reference value to normalize the cytotoxic activities of cCSE, irrespective of the number of combusted cigarettes, cigarette brands and smoking protocols (continuous smoking vs puff smoking), as long as the tar concentrations in the original cCSEs are $\leq$15 mg/ml of PBS: over this concentration range, part of the cytotoxic activity in the smoke escapes without being extracted into the PBS, causing a lower cytotoxic potency than expected from the tar concentration.

Amongst cigarette brands, the ratio of tar to other gas phase components might vary. Indeed, the ratio of tar to nicotine varies among brands (Table 2). Given this, a given virtual tar concentration may expose cells to differing levels of specific gas phase components despite standardizing by the virtual tar concentration. However, as shown in Figure 5, the concentration-response curves for the cytotoxic activities of the cCSEs prepared from different cigarette brands are not significantly different from each other, when the concentrations of cCSEs are normalized in terms of the virtual tar concentration. This result strongly indicates that the

Table 3. Comparison of concentrations of carbonyl compounds in cCSE and pCSE.

	cCSE[a]	pCSE[a]
Acetone (μM)	287.9±29.2	326.1±20.3
Acrolein (μM)	36.7±1.3	41.7±2.8
Propionaldehyde (μM)	24.4±3.5	28.7±6.9
Methyl vinyl ketone (μM)	17.5±3.0	13.8±0.5

[a]The cCSE and pCSE at the original tar concentration of 10 mg/ml were prepared from Hi-Lite brand cigarettes by either continuous (cCSE) or puff smoking protocol (pCSE). cCSE and pCSE were fractionated by HPLC and each fraction was analyzed for cytotoxic activities using PI uptake assay. The positive fractions were analyzed by GC/MS after derivatization with a carbonyl reagent PFBOA. Values represent means ± SD of three experiments.

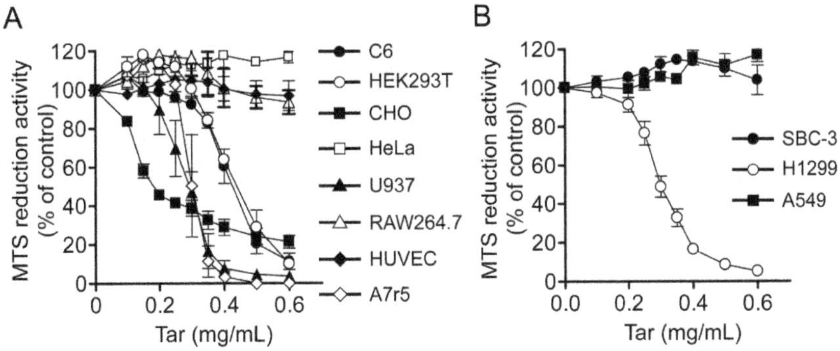

Figure 8. Sensitivities of various cultured cells to the gas phase extracts of cigarette smoke. The gas phase extracts of cigarette smoke (cCSE) at the virtual tar concentration of 10 mg/ml were prepared from Hi-Lite brand cigarettes by continuous smoking protocol, and they were subjected to MTS reduction assay using various cultured cells. MTS reduction activity was represented as a percentage of the control value in the absence of cCSE. Values represent means ± SE of three experiments, each in triplicate. (A) C6, rat glioma cells; HEK293T, human embryonic kidney cells; CHO, Chinese hamster ovary cells; HeLa, human cervical carcinoma cells; U937, human monocytes; RAW264.7, mouse macrophages; HUVEC, immortalized human umbilical vein endothelial cells; A7r5, rat aorta smooth muscle cells. (B) SBC-3, human lung small cell carcinoma; H1299, human lung squamous cell carcinoma; A549, human lung adenocarcinoma.

concentrations of cytotoxic compounds in the CSEs are actually normalized by the virtual tar concentration, and hence that the ratio of cytotoxic compounds to tar is independent of the ratio of nicotine to tar.

Another important finding is that the toxicological properties of cCSE are equivalent to those of pCSE, in terms of potency of cytotoxicity, pharmacology of the cytotoxicity and the concentrations of major cytotoxic compounds such as ACR and MVK. Although there are no experimental data, it has so far been believed that the chemical composition and hence the property of the cytotoxicity of the smoke generated by continuous and puff smoking protocols might be different, mainly based on the consideration that the combustion temperature of cigarette might be different between the two smoking protocols, leading to generation of different spectrum of chemicals [31,32].

The standard method for cCSE preparation established in the present study makes possible the comparison of the experimental data on cCSE from various laboratories, and is expected to accelerate the research on toxicity of smoking and pathophysiology of smoking-related diseases, leading to development of methods for prevention and treatment of smoking-related diseases. However, because cytotoxicity is only one measure of the effects of cigarette smoke, it is noted that other measures such as protease/cytokine expression or mucin production [33,34] might vary among brands despite the virtual tar concentration being controlled.

In the present study, we have proposed a standardized method for preparation of nicotine- and tar-free CSE, i.e. the gas phase extract of cigarette smoke. The other phase (tar phase) containing tar and nicotine is reported to be also important for human health [35–37]. However, a standardized method for preparation of the tar phase extract which is simple and rapid is also absent. Therefore, as a next step, it is important to establish such standardized method and to accelerate the investigation on the cytotoxic effects of nicotine and tar and their molecular mechanisms of action.

In summary, we introduced the virtual tar concentration as a measure of cytotoxic potency of the gas phase extract of cigarette smoke, and established a simple and rapid method for standard preparation of the gas phase extract of cigarette smoke based on continuous smoking protocol. We also demonstrated that from the toxicological viewpoint, the gas phase extract prepared by the present method is equivalent to the extract prepared by a puff smoking machine.

Acknowledgments

We thank Dr. Cora Jean S. Edgell, University of North Carolina at Chapel Hill for providing us with HUVEC.

Author Contributions

Conceived and designed the experiments: T. Higashi SM. Performed the experiments: T. Higashi YM YN AH PN T. Harada MH CH. Analyzed the data: T. Higashi T. Horinouchi KT. Contributed reagents/materials/analysis tools: YK. Contributed to the writing of the manuscript: T. Higashi SM.

References

1. Ambrose JA, Barua RS (2004) The pathophysiology of cigarette smoking and cardiovascular disease: an update. J Am Coll Cardiol 43: 1731–1737.
2. Steenland K, Thun M, Lally C, Heath C, Jr. (1996) Environmental tobacco smoke and coronary heart disease in the American Cancer Society CPS-II cohort. Circulation 94: 622–628.
3. Erhardt L (2009) Cigarette smoking: an undertreated risk factor for cardiovascular disease. Atherosclerosis 205: 23–32.
4. Nussbaumer-Ochsner Y, Rabe KF (2011) Systemic manifestations of COPD. Chest 139: 165–173.
5. D'Agostini F, Balansky R, Steele VE, Ganchev G, Pesce C, et al. (2008) Preneoplastic and neoplastic lesions in the lung, liver and urinary tract of mice exposed to environmental cigarette smoke and UV light since birth. Int J Cancer 123: 2497–2502.
6. Hecht SS, Kassie F, Hatsukami DK (2009) Chemoprevention of lung carcinogenesis in addicted smokers and ex-smokers. Nat Rev Cancer 9: 476–488.
7. Tauler J, Mulshine JL (2009) Lung cancer and inflammation: interaction of chemokines and hnRNPs. Curr Opin Pharmacol 9: 384–388.
8. Burns DM (1991) Cigarettes and cigarette smoking. Clin Chest Med 12: 631–642.
9. Church DF, Pryor WA (1985) Free-radical chemistry of cigarette smoke and its toxicological implications. Environ Health Perspect 64: 111–126.
10. Pryor WA, Stone K (1993) Oxidants in cigarette smoke. Radicals, hydrogen peroxide, peroxynitrate, and peroxynitrite. Ann N Y Acad Sci 686: 12–27; discussion 27–18.
11. Csiszar A, Podlutsky A, Wolin MS, Losonczy G, Pacher P, et al. (2009) Oxidative stress and accelerated vascular aging: implications for cigarette smoking. Front Biosci (Landmark Ed) 14: 3128–3144.

12. Jaimes EA, DeMaster EG, Tian RX, Raij L (2004) Stable compounds of cigarette smoke induce endothelial superoxide anion production via NADPH oxidase activation. Arterioscler Thromb Vasc Biol 24: 1031–1036.
13. Orosz Z, Csiszar A, Labinskyy N, Smith K, Kaminski PM, et al. (2007) Cigarette smoke-induced proinflammatory alterations in the endothelial phenotype: role of NAD(P)H oxidase activation. Am J Physiol Heart Circ Physiol 292: H130–139.
14. Kunitomo M, Yamaguchi Y, Kagota S, Yoshikawa N, Nakamura K, et al. (2009) Biochemical evidence of atherosclerosis progression mediated by increased oxidative stress in apolipoprotein E-deficient spontaneously hyperlipidemic mice exposed to chronic cigarette smoke. J Pharmacol Sci 110: 354–361.
15. Yamaguchi Y, Nasu F, Harada A, Kunitomo M (2007) Oxidants in the gas phase of cigarette smoke pass through the lung alveolar wall and raise systemic oxidative stress. J Pharmacol Sci 103: 275–282.
16. Lambert C, McCue J, Portas M, Ouyang Y, Li J, et al. (2005) Acrolein in cigarette smoke inhibits T-cell responses. J Allergy Clin Immunol 116: 916–922.
17. Su Y, Han W, Giraldo C, De Li Y, Block ER (1998) Effect of cigarette smoke extract on nitric oxide synthase in pulmonary artery endothelial cells. Am J Respir Cell Mol Biol 19: 819–825.
18. Takano S, Matsuoka I, Magami W, Watanabe C, Nakanishi H (1997) Possible existence of platelet aggregation inhibitor(s) in a gas-phase extract of cigarette smoke. Fukushima J Med Sci 43: 1–11.
19. Asano H, Horinouchi T, Mai Y, Sawada O, Fujii S, et al. (2012) Nicotine- and tar-free cigarette smoke induces cell damage through reactive oxygen species newly generated by PKC-dependent activation of NADPH oxidase. J Pharmacol Sci 118: 275–287.
20. Mai Y, Higashi T, Terada K, Hatate C, Nepal P, et al. (2012) Nicotine- and tar-free cigarette smoke extract induces cell injury via intracellular Ca2+-dependent subtype-specific protein kinase C activation. J Pharmacol Sci 120: 310–314.
21. Frei B, Forte TM, Ames BN, Cross CE (1991) Gas phase oxidants of cigarette smoke induce lipid peroxidation and changes in lipoprotein properties in human blood plasma. Protective effects of ascorbic acid. Biochem J 277 (Pt 1): 133–138.
22. Yamaguchi Y, Kagota S, Haginaka J, Kunitomo M (2002) Participation of peroxynitrite in oxidative modification of LDL by aqueous extracts of cigarette smoke. FEBS Lett 512: 218–222.
23. Noya Y, Seki K, Asano H, Mai Y, Horinouchi T, et al. (2013) Identification of stable cytotoxic factors in the gas phase extract of cigarette smoke and pharmacological characterization of their cytotoxicity. Toxicology 314: 1–10.
24. Hammond D, Wiebel F, Kozlowski LT, Borland R, Cummings KM, et al. (2007) Revising the machine smoking regime for cigarette emissions: implications for tobacco control policy. Tob Control 16: 8–14.
25. Stephens WE (2007) Dependence of tar, nicotine and carbon monoxide yields on physical parameters: implications for exposure, emissions control and monitoring. Tob Control 16: 170–176.
26. Edgell CJ, McDonald CC, Graham JB (1983) Permanent cell line expressing human factor VIII-related antigen established by hybridization. Proc Natl Acad Sci U S A 80: 3734–3737.
27. Purkis SW, Cahours X, Rey M, Teillet B, Troude V, et al. (2011) Some consequences of using cigarette machine smoking regimes with different intensities on smoke yields and their variability. Regul Toxicol Pharmacol 59: 293–309.
28. Connolly GN, Wayne GD, Lymperis D, Doherty MC (2000) How cigarette additives are used to mask environmental tobacco smoke. Tob Control 9: 283–291.
29. Rabinoff M, Caskey N, Rissling A, Park C (2007) Pharmacological and chemical effects of cigarette additives. Am J Public Health 97: 1981–1991.
30. Canales L, Chen J, Kelty E, Musah S, Webb C, et al. (2012) Developmental cigarette smoke exposure: liver proteome profile alterations in low birth weight pups. Toxicology 300: 1–11.
31. Kozlowski LT, O'Connor RJ (2002) Cigarette filter ventilation is a defective design because of misleading taste, bigger puffs, and blocked vents. Tob Control 11 Suppl 1: I40–50.
32. Purkis SW, Troude V, Duputie G, Tessier C (2010) Limitations in the characterisation of cigarette products using different machine smoking regimes. Regul Toxicol Pharmacol 58: 501–515.
33. Tamimi A, Serdarevic D, Hanania NA (2012) The effects of cigarette smoke on airway inflammation in asthma and COPD: therapeutic implications. Respir Med 106: 319–328.
34. Yu H, Li Q, Kolosov VP, Perelman JM, Zhou X (2012) Regulation of cigarette smoke-mediated mucin expression by hypoxia-inducible factor-1alpha via epidermal growth factor receptor-mediated signaling pathways. J Appl Toxicol 32: 282–292.
35. Hecht SS (1999) Tobacco smoke carcinogens and lung cancer. J Natl Cancer Inst 91: 1194–1210.
36. Le Houezec J, McNeill A, Britton J (2011) Tobacco, nicotine and harm reduction. Drug Alcohol Rev 30: 119–123.
37. Valavanidis A, Vlachogianni T, Fiotakis K (2009) Tobacco smoke: involvement of reactive oxygen species and stable free radicals in mechanisms of oxidative damage, carcinogenesis and synergistic effects with other respirable particles. Int J Environ Res Public Health 6: 445–462.

15

Codelivery of Chemotherapeutics via Crosslinked Multilamellar Liposomal Vesicles to Overcome Multidrug Resistance in Tumor

Yarong Liu[1]◑, Jinxu Fang[1]◑, Kye-Il Joo[1], Michael K. Wong[2], Pin Wang[1,3,4]*

1 Mork Family Department of Chemical Engineering and Materials Science, University of Southern California, Los Angeles, California, United States of America, 2 Division of Medical Oncology, Norris Comprehensive Cancer Center, Keck School of Medicine, University of Southern California, Los Angeles, California, United States of America, 3 Department of Biomedical Engineering, University of Southern California, Los Angeles, California, United States of America, 4 Department of Pharmacology and Pharmaceutical Sciences, University of Southern California, Los Angeles, California, United States of America

Abstract

Multidrug resistance (MDR) is a significant challenge to effective cancer chemotherapy treatment. However, the development of a drug delivery system that allows for the sustained release of combined drugs with improved vesicle stability could overcome MDR in cancer cells. To achieve this, we have demonstrated codelivery of doxorubicin (Dox) and paclitaxel (PTX) *via* a crosslinked multilamellar vesicle (cMLV). This combinatorial delivery system achieves enhanced drug accumulation and retention, in turn resulting in improved cytotoxicity against tumor cells, including drug-resistant cells. Moreover, this delivery approach significantly overcomes MDR by reducing the expression of P-glycoprotein (P-gp) in cancer cells, thus improving antitumor activity *in vivo*. Thus, by enhancing drug delivery to tumors and lowering the apoptotic threshold of individual drugs, this combinatorial delivery system represents a potentially promising multimodal therapeutic strategy to overcome MDR in cancer therapy.

Editor: Bing Xu, Brandeis University, United States of America

Funding: This work was supported by National Institutes of Health grants (R01AI068978, R01CA170820 and P01CA132681), a translational acceleration grant from the Joint Center for Translational Medicine, the National Cancer Institute (P30CA014089), and a grant from the Ming Hsieh Institute for Research on Engineering Medicine for Cancer. The funders had no role in study design, data collection and analysis, decision to publish, or preparation of the manuscript.

Competing Interests: The authors have declared that no competing interests exist.

* Email: pinwang@usc.edu

◑ These authors contributed equally to this work.

Introduction

The development of multidrug resistance (MDR) against a variety of conventional and novel chemotherapeutic agents has been a major impediment to the success of cancer therapy [1,2]. One of the most important mechanisms involved in MDR is the overexpression of P-glycoprotein (P-gp) in the plasma membrane of various cancer cells. P-gp, an active drug efflux transporter, is capable of effluxing a broad range of anticancer agents, such as taxanes and anthracyclines [3]. For example, the efficacy of doxorubicin (Dox) and paclitaxel (PTX), two of the most widely used agents for the treatment of various cancers, is often compromised by P-gp-mediated MDR [4,5]. Therefore, a strategy to inhibit P-gp expression has been developed to overcome MDR. For instance, a large number of P-gp inhibitors and siRNAs targeting the gene encoding P-gp have been delivered in combination with anticancer agents to downregulate P-gp expression, thereby enabling drugs to reach sufficient concentrations to induce cytotoxicity [6,7]. However, P-gp inhibitors, either functional inhibitors or siRNA, have yielded disappointing clinical trials resulting from their high systemic toxicities and enhanced side effects of chemotherapy in normal cells [8,9].

Combination therapy with multiple chemotherapeutics provides an alternative strategy to suppress MDR. Different drugs may attack cancer cells at varying stages of their growth cycles, thus decreasing the concentration threshold for individual drugs that is otherwise required for cytotoxicity [10]. It has been reported that various drug combinations have successfully induced synergistic antitumor activities and prevented disease recurrence [11,12]. For example, a Dox and PTX cocktail is now considered a standard anthracycline-taxane combination treatment for various tumors by their ability to overcome drug resistance [13,14,15]. However, a major challenge of combination therapy is coordinating the pharmacokinetics and cellular uptake of combined therapeutics. This obstacle has limited the clinical success of combination therapy [16,17].

To overcome this challenge, novel strategies that allow loading of multiple therapeutics into a single drug-delivery vehicle for concurrent delivery at the site of action have been extensively explored [18,19]. Several drug delivery systems have been able to intercalate multiple drugs for site-specific delivery to tumors and, hence, improve antitumor activities, potentially overcoming drug resistance, while, at the same time, reducing the dosage of individual drugs [20,21,22]. Indeed, nanoparticle delivery systems are known to deliver therapeutics efficiently to the tumor sites through the enhanced permeability and retention (EPR) effect, thereby enhancing the concentration of therapeutics in tumors [23,24]. Moreover, these nanoparticles can enter cancer cells through endocytosis in a manner independent of the P-gp pathway, thereby enhancing cellular accumulation of therapeutics [25,26,27]. Thus, a nanoparticle delivery system capable of mediating high efficiency of cellular entry and subsequent triggering of intracellular release of multiple anticancer drugs to overcome MDR is highly desirable.

Liposomes are one of the most popular nanoparticle delivery systems for combinatorial delivery of multiple drugs based on their ability to efficiently load both hydrophilic and hydrophobic drugs [24,28]. We previously developed a robust crosslinked multilamellar liposomal vesicle (cMLV), with enhanced vesicle stability, to efficiently codeliver hydrophilic (Dox) and hydrophobic (PTX) drugs and induce ratio-dependent synergistic antitumor activity, both *in vitro* and *in vivo* [29,30,31]. Moreover, it was shown that cMLV particles are mainly internalized by cells through caveolin-dependent endocytosis and are then trafficked through the endosome-lysosome network for release of drugs [30]. In this study, we have examined the potential of cMLV as a combinatorial delivery system aimed at overcoming P-gp-mediated drug resistance, both *in vitro* and *in vivo*. Indeed, we have demonstrated that the combination of Dox and PTX, when administered at 1:1 weight ratio in cMLV formulations, shows significant enhancement of cytotoxicity and antitumor activities. Combining these drugs through the use of cMLV formulations contributes to these antitumor activities by enhancing systemic delivery efficiency and lowering tumor apoptotic threshold.

Materials and Methods

Mice

Female BALB/c mice (6–10 weeks old) were purchased from Charles River Breeding Laboratories (Wilmington, MA). All mice were held under specific pathogen-reduced conditions in the Animal Facility of the University of Southern California (USA). All experiments were performed in accordance with the guidelines set by the National Institutes of Health and the University of Southern California on the Care and Use of Animals. This study was approved by the Committee on the Ethics of Animal Experiments of the University of Southern California.

Cell culture

B16 tumor cells (B16–F10, ATCC number: CRL-6475) and 4T1 tumor cells (ATCC number: CRL-2539) were maintained in a 5% CO_2 environment with Dulbecco's modified Eagle's medium (Mediatech, Inc., Manassas, VA) supplemented with 10% FBS (Sigma-Aldrich, St. Louis, MO) and 2 mM of L-glutamine (Hyclone Laboratories, Inc., Omaha, NE). B16-R and 4T1-R cells were produced by continuously treating B16 and 4T1 cells with 5 µg/ml PTX for 4 days. The cells were then recovered by replacing medium with fresh medium without drugs for 7 days. The remaining cells formed drug resistance for PTX. JC cells (ATCC number: CRL-2116) were used as a model drug-resistant tumor cell line because it has been shown that JC cells overexpress P-gp and exhibit a drug-resistant phenotype, both *in vitro* and *in vivo* [32].

Synthesis of cMLVs

Liposomes were prepared based on the conventional dehydration-rehydration method. All lipids were obtained from the NOF Corporation (Japan). 1.5 µmol of lipids 1,2-dioleoyl-sn-glycero-3-phosphocholine (DOPC), 1,2-dioleoyl-sn-glycero-3-phospho-(1′-rac-glycerol) (DOPG), and maleimide-headgrouplipid1,2-dioleoyl-sn-glycero-3-phosphoeth-anolamine-N-[4-(p-maleimidophenyl) butyramide (MPB-PE) were combined in chloroform at a molar lipid ratio of DOPC:DOPG:MPB = 4:1:5, and the organic solvent in the lipid mixture was evaporated under argon gas. The lipid mixture was further dried under vacuum overnight to form dried thin lipid films. To prepare cMLV(PTX) and cMLV(Dox+PTX) at a molar ratio of 0.2:1 (drugs:lipids), paclitaxel in organic solvent was mixed with the lipid mixture to form dried thin lipid films. The resultant dried film was hydrated in 10 mM Bis-Tris propane at pH 7.0 with (cMLV(Dox) or cMLV(Dox+PTX)) or without doxorubicin (cMLV(PTX)) at a molar ratio of 0.2:1 (drugs:lipids) with vigorous vortexing every 10 min for 1 h, followed by applying 4 cycles of 15-s sonication (Misonix Microson XL2000, Farmingdale, NY) on ice in 1-min intervals of each cycle. To induce divalent-triggered vesicle fusion, $MgCl_2$ was added at a final concentration of 10 mM. The resulting multilamellar vesicles were further crosslinked by addition of Dithiothreitol (DTT, Sigma-Aldrich) at a final concentration of 1.5 mM for 1 h at 37°C. The resulting vesicles were collected by centrifugation at 14,000 g for 4 min and then washed twice with PBS. For pegylation of cMLVs, the particles were incubated with 1 µmol of 2 kDa PEG-SH (Laysan Bio Inc., Arab, AL) for 1 h at 37°C. The particles were then centrifuged and washed twice with PBS. The final products were stored in PBS at 4°C. The mean diameter of all cMLVs is around 220 nm determined by dynamic light scattering (DLS), and around 160 nm estimated by cryo-electron microscopy. The loading efficiency, and stability of cMLVs were similar to that demonstrated previously [30,31].

In vitro cytotoxicity and data analysis

B16–F10, 4T1, B16–R, 4T1-R, and JC cells were plated at a density of 5×10^3 cells per well in D10 media in 96-well plates and grown for 6 h. The cells were then exposed to a series of concentrations of cMLV (single drug) or cMLV (drug combinations) for 48 h. The cell viability was assessed using the Cell Proliferation Kit II (XTT assay) from Roche Applied Science according to the manufacturer's instructions. Slope m and IC_{50} were obtained from median effect model, and IIP_{Cmax} was calculated via the following equation: $IIP_{Cmax} = \log(1+(Cmax/IC_{50})^m)$. Cmax is the maximum plasma drug concentrations for the commonly recommended dose for each drug.

Cellular uptake of doxorubicin and paclitaxel in cells

4T1 cells were seeded in 24-well plates at a density of 2×10^5 cells per well and grown overnight. The cells were then exposed to empty cMLVs (control), cMLV(Dox), cMLV(PTX), cMLV(Dox+PTX), and Dox+PTX. The final concentrations of Dox and PTX were 1 µg/ml for each group. JC cells were seeded at a density of 10^5 cells per well in D10 media in 96-well plates. The cells were exposed to empty cMLVs, cMLV(Dox), cMLV(PTX), cMLV(Dox+PTX), and Dox+PTX. The final concentrations of Dox and PTX were 5 µg/ml for each group. At 48 h after treatment, the cells were washed twice with PBS and lysed with PBS containing 1% Triton X-100. Doxorubicin and paclitaxel in cell lysates were extracted by 1:1 (v/v) Chloroform/isopropyl alcohol or ethyl acetate, respectively. Paclitaxel concentrations in cell lysates were measured by HPLC C18 column and detected at 227 nm (flow rate 1 ml/min), and doxorubicin was detected by fluorescence with 480/550 nm excitation/emission. The concentrations of Dox and PTX were normalized for protein content as measured with BCA assay (Pierce).

In vivo antitumor activity study

BALB/c female mice (6–10 weeks old) were inoculated subcutaneously with 0.2×10^6 4T1 breast tumor cells. The tumors were allowed to grow for 8 days to a volume of $\sim$50 mm^3 before treatment. After 8 days, the mice were injected intravenously through the tail vein with cMLV(2 mg/kg Dox), cMLV(2 mg/kg PTX), cMLV(2 mg/kg Dox)+cMLV(2 mg/kg PTX), or cMLV(2 mg/kg Dox + 2 mg/kg PTX) every three days (six mice per group). Tumor growth and body weight were monitored for 40 days or to the end of the experiment. The length and width of the tumor masses were measured with a fine caliper every three days after injection. Tumor volume was expressed as 1/2 × (length × $width^2$). Survival end point was set when the tumor volume reached 1000 mm^3. The survival rates are presented as Kaplan-Meier curves. The survival curves of individual groups were compared by a log-rank test.

Immunohistochemistry of tumors and confocal imaging

BALB/c female mice (6–10 weeks old) were inoculated subcutaneously with 0.2 × 10^6 4T1 or JC tumor cells. The tumors were allowed to grow for 20 days to a volume of $\sim$500 mm^3 before treatment. On day 20, the mice were injected intravenously through the tail vein with cMLV (5 mg/kg Dox), cMLV(5 mg/kg PTX), 5 mg/kg Dox + 5 mg/kg PTX, or cMLV(5 mg/kg Dox + 5 mg/kg PTX). Three days after injection, tumors were excised, fixed, frozen, cryo-sectioned, and mounted onto glass slides. Frozen sections were fixed and rinsed with cold PBS. After blocking and permeabilization, the slides were washed by PBS and then incubated with TUNEL reaction mixture (Roche, Indianapolis, Indiana) for 1 h. For P-gp expression, the slides were stained after permeabilization with mouse monoclonal anti-P-gp antibody (Abcam, Cambridge, MA) for 1 h, followed by staining with Alexa488-conjugated goat anti-mouse immunoglobulin G (IgG) antibody (Invitrogen, Carlsbad, CA) and counter-staining with DAPI (Invitrogen, Carlsbad, CA). Fluorescence images were acquired by a Yokogawa spinning-disk confocal scanner system (Solamere Technology Group, Salt Lake City, UT), using a Nikon Eclipse Ti-E microscope. Illumination powers at 405, 491, 561, and 640 nm solid-state laser lines were provided by an AOTF (acousto-optical tunable filter)-controlled laser-merge system with 50 mW for each laser. All images were analyzed using Nikon NIS-Elements software. To quantify TUNEL and P-gp-positive cells, 4 regions of interest (ROI) were randomly chosen per image at ×2 magnification. Within one region, area of TUNEL, or P-gp-positive nuclei, and area of nuclear staining were counted by Nikon NIS-Element software. The data are expressed as % total nuclear area stained by TUNEL or P-gp in the region.

Hematoxylin and Eosin staining of heart sections

Mice bearing 4T1 tumors were i.v. injected with 5 mg/kg Dox + 5 mg/kg PTX or cMLV(5 mg/kg Dox+5 mg/kg PTX). Three days after injection, heart tissues were harvested and fixed in 4% formaldehyde. The tissues were frozen, cut into sections, and mounted onto glass slides. The frozen sections were stained with hematoxylin and eosin. Histopathologic specimens were examined by light microscopy.

Statistics

Differences between two groups were determined with Student's *t* test. The differences among three or more groups were determined with a one-way ANOVA.

Results

In vitro efficacy study by XTT assay

To achieve combination delivery of doxorubicin (Dox) and paclitaxel (PTX), a previously developed crosslinked multilamellar liposomal vesicle (cMLV) was used to incorporate PTX in the lipid membrane and encapsulate Dox in the aqueous core at a 1:1 ratio to form cMLV(Dox+PTX) [30]. We chose this combination ratio because our previous study showed that it could induce synergy combination effect both *in vitro* and *in vivo* [31]. It has been reported that drug combinations can overcome drug resistance that would otherwise limit the potential application of various monotherapeutics [10]. To determine whether codelivery of Dox and PTX could overcome drug resistance, an *in vitro* cytotoxicity assay was performed at a wide range of concentrations of single drug-loaded or dual drug-loaded cMLVs. As shown in Figure 1A and 1B (left panel), both B16 cells and 4T1 cells developed drug resistance to single drug-loaded cMLVs, but this resistance was inhibited by applying the combined formulation, cMLV(Dox+PTX). The maximal cytotoxicity of single drug-loaded cMLV observed in these two tumor cells was between 60%–80%, while cells treated with dual drug-loaded cMLV(Dox+PTX) showed significantly more growth inhibition ($\sim$95%).

To further confirm the efficiency of dual drug-loaded cMLVs in overcoming drug resistance, drug-resistant cell lines B16-R and 4T1-R were generated by continuously treating parental B16 or 4T1 with a high concentration of paclitaxel (5 μg/ml). Various concentrations of single drug-loaded cMLV and dual drug-loaded cMLV(Dox+PTX) were incubated with these two drug-resistant cell lines for 48 h, and the cytotoxicity was measured by a standard XTT assay. As shown in Figure 1D and 1E, both B16-R and 4T1-R cells showed a high tolerance when treated with cMLV(PTX) or cMLV(Dox), indicating that multidrug resistance had been developed in these cells. In contrast, cMLV(Dox+PTX) triggered significantly more cell death (90–100%) compared to that of single drug-loaded cMLVs, confirming that a codelivery system could overcome drug resistance induced by a high concentration of single drug. Furthermore, *in vitro* cytotoxicity studies demonstrated therapeutic efficacy of cMLV(Dox+PTX) in JC cells, a model drug-resistant tumor cell line, corroborating the weaker potency of single drug-loaded cMLVs compared to the dual drug-loaded cMLVs. As shown in Figure 1C (left panel), the maximal cytotoxicity of cMLV(Dox) and cMLV(PTX) was in the range of 60–70%, while peak cMLV(Dox+PTX) cytotoxicity was about 90% in JC cells.

IC_{50}, which indicates drug concentration that causes 50% inhibitory effect on cell proliferation, can provide information on the efficacy of drugs. The IC_{50} values of the individual drugs and combined drugs through cMLVs in B16, 4T1 and JC cells are provided in Figure S1. However, it has also been reported that slope m, a parameter mathematically analogous to the Hill coefficient, may also have a significant effect on cytotoxicity [33,34]. Therefore, a new model has been developed to evaluate drug activity by incorporating three parameters (IC_{50}, drug concentration, and m) from the median effect model into a single-value IIP (potential inhibition) with an intuitive meaning, i.e., the log reduction in inhibitory effect [34]. Accordingly, to increase the trustworthiness of our experiment, IIP was used to evaluate the efficiency of dual drug-loaded cMLVs on cell viability. As shown in Figure 1A to 1C (middle and right panels), Dox and PTX in the dual drug-loaded cMLVs displayed a significantly larger IIP_{Cmax} value in the cell lines studied compared to that of the single drug-loaded cMLVs, indicating that

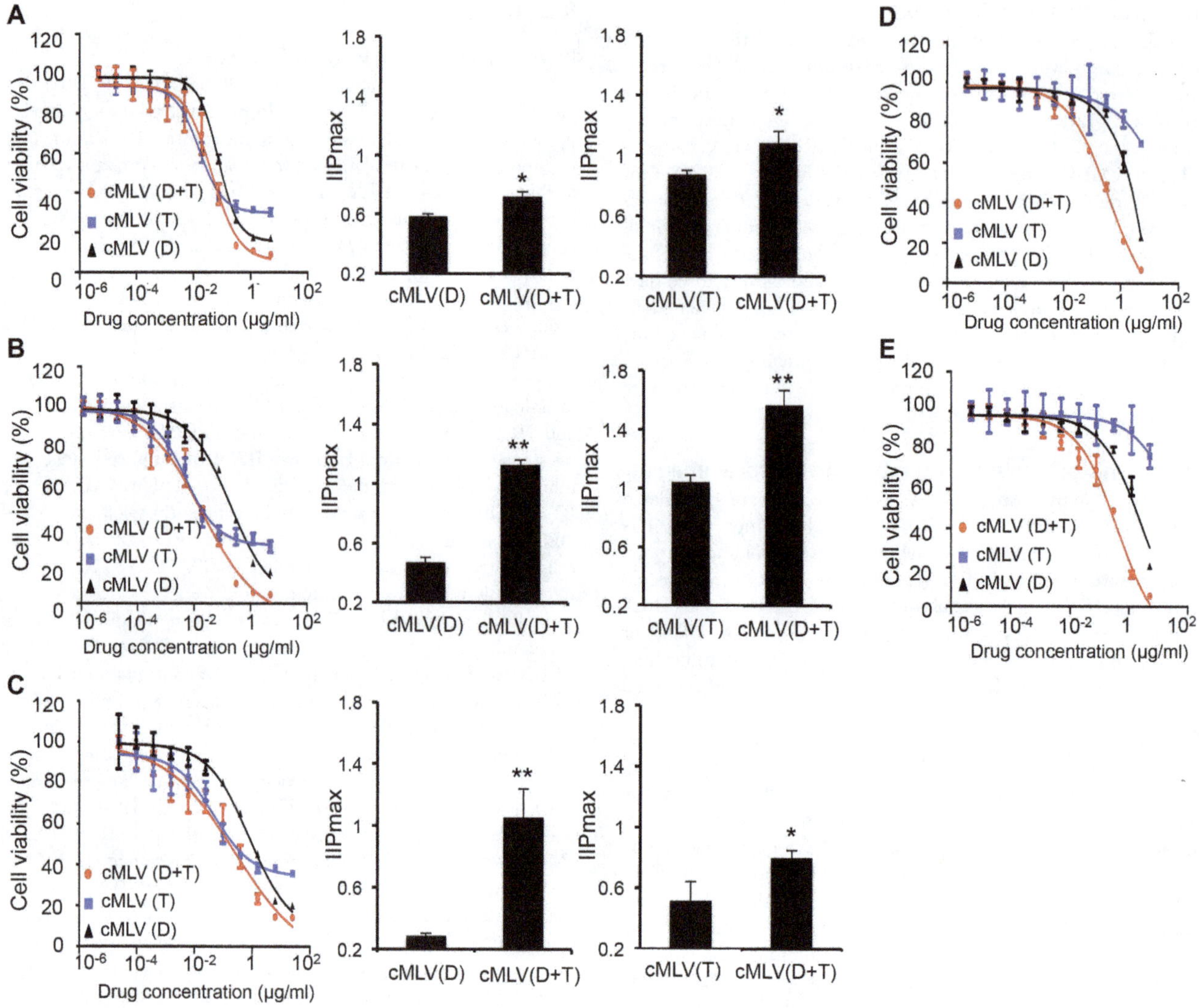

Figure 1. Overcoming drug resistance by codelivery of Dox and PTX via cMLVs (D: Dox; T: PTX). (A, B) *In vitro* cytotoxicity of cMLV(single drug) and cMLV(drug combinations) in B16 melanoma tumor cells (A) and 4T1 breast tumor cells (B). (C, D, E) *In vitro* cytotoxicity of cMLV(single drug) and cMLV(drug combinations) in drug-resistant JC cells (C), B16-R cells (D) and 4T1-R cells (E). IIP_{Cmax} was determined by incorporating three parameters (IC_{50}, *D* and m) in the median effect model into the following equation: $IIP_{Cmax} = \log(1+(Cmax/IC_{50})^m)$. Data are represented as mean ± SD (n = 3). Asterisks indicate statistical significance between two groups (*$P < 0.05$, **$P < 0.01$).

combinatorial cMLVs were more potent in cancer treatment than single drug-loaded cMLVs.

Cellular uptake study of doxorubicin and paclitaxel

To investigate the mechanism of enhanced cytotoxicity observed with cMLV combination therapy, we evaluated the effect of dual drug-loaded cMLVs on rates of drug influx/efflux in cells. The intracellular accumulation of Dox and PTX was examined by HPLC in 4T1 cells following exposure to Dox (1 μg/ml) and PTX (1 μg/ml) in cMLVs, both individually and in combination, and in JC cells with higher dose of Dox and PTX (5 μg/ml). After 3 h incubation, the extracellular medium was discarded, and intracellular drug (Dox or PTX) accumulation was quantitatively determined by drug concentration in the cell lysates, normalized by total cellular protein content of the cells. As seen in Figure 2A and 2B, cMLV(Dox+PTX) significantly increased both Dox and PTX accumulation in 4T1 cells compared to that of single drug-loaded cMLVs ($p < 0.05$), suggesting that combination treatments may overcome drug resistance. In addition, compared to the administration of drug in solution, cMLV combination treatment resulted in higher cellular accumulation of Dox and PTX, an outcome most likely resulting from the internalization of cMLVs by cells through endocytosis [30] and, consequently, effectively bypassing the P-gp efflux pumps. The enhanced cellular accumulation of drugs in dual drug-loaded cMLVs was also observed in drug-resistant JC cells (Figure 2C and 2D) compared to single drug-loaded cMLVs and drug combination in solution. These data suggest that cMLV(Dox+PTX) significantly enhanced the intracellular accumulation of anticancer drugs through mechanisms involving both combination treatment and nanoparticle delivery.

Effect of codelivered nanoparticles on P-gp expression

Having shown that dual drug-loaded cMLVs enhance cellular accumulation of drugs, we next sought to verify that this did, indeed, result from the modulation of membrane pumps, which

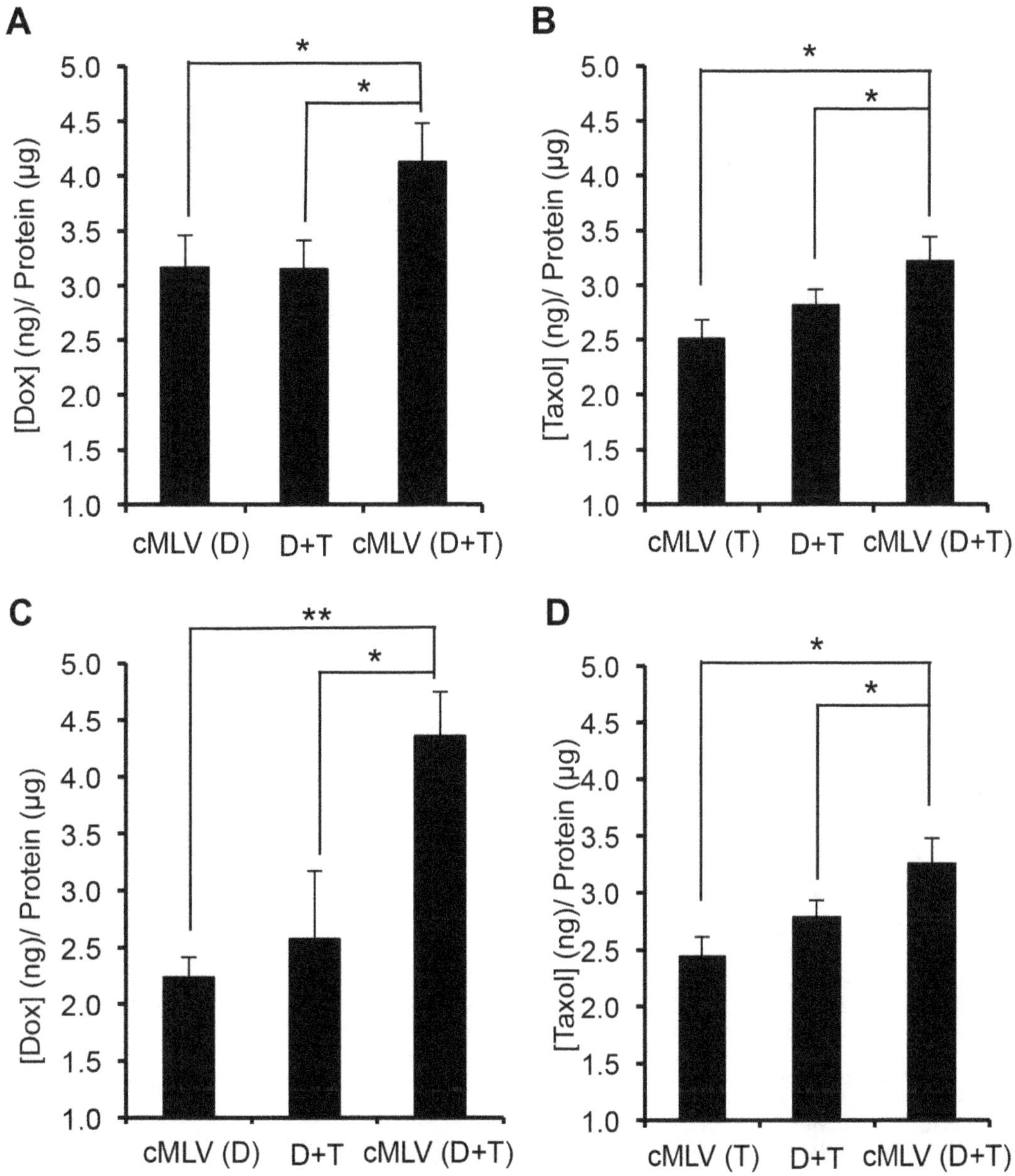

Figure 2. Cellular uptake of Dox and PTX (D: Dox; T: PTX). (A, B) Total cellular uptake of Dox (A) and PTX (B) into 4T1 cells. 4T1 cells were exposed to cMLV(D), cMLV(T), cMLV(D+T), and D+P in solution. The final concentrations of Dox and PTX were 1 μg/ml for each group. (C, D) Total cellular uptake of Dox (C) and PTX (D) in JC cells. JC cells were exposed to cMLV(D), cMLV(T), cMLV(D+T), and D+T. The final concentrations of Dox and PTX were 5 μg/ml for each group. The uptake of Dox and PTX was normalized to protein content measured with the BCA assay. All data are shown as the means of triplicate experiments from three different nanoparticle preparations. Asterisks indicate statistical significance between two groups (*$P < 0.05$, **$P < 0.01$).

are responsible for multidrug resistance. We first measured the expression of P-gp by flow cytometry in 4T1 cells treated with various nanoparticle formulations for 48 h to test if these cMLV formulations were responsible for altering P-gp involvement in multidrug resistance, along with decreased drug accumulation, in cells [3,35]. As shown in Figure 3A, with the single drug-loaded cMLV treatment, the expression of P-gp (in terms of integrated mean fluorescence intensity) increased significantly in 4T1 cells ($p < 0.01$), possibly leading, in turn, to the development of drug resistance in 4T1 cells. However, dual drug-loaded cMLVs significantly inhibited expression of P-gp when compared to that of the single drug-loaded cMLVs and drug combination in solution ($p < 0.01$), suggesting that the combinatorial delivery of Dox and PTX *via* cMLVs could efficiently suppress P-gp expression, thereby overcoming MDR. We next investigated whether cMLV(Dox+PTX) could inhibit multidrug resistance in JC cells, which exhibit drug-resistant phenotype by overexpression of P-gp [32]. As shown in Figure 3B, the expression of P-gp decreased after 48 h of incubation with JC cells ($p < 0.05$) when treated with single drug-loaded cMLV, indicating that the nanoparticle drug delivery system could, at least partially, suppress MDR. However, the codelivery formulation of cMLV(Dox+PTX) significantly inhibited P-gp expression compared to that of single drug-loaded cMLVs and drug combination in solution ($p < 0.01$).

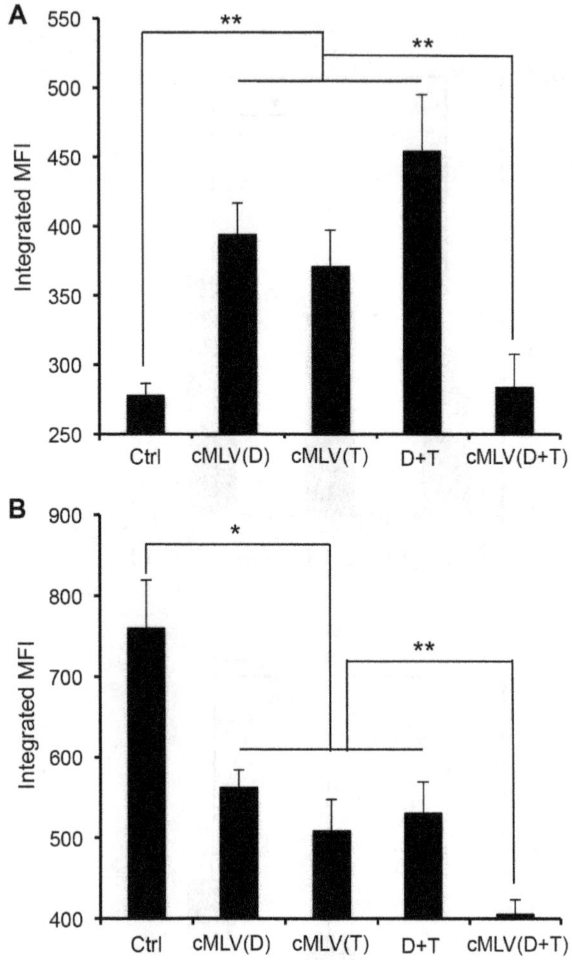

Figure 3. Effect of codelivered nanoparticles on P-gp expression (D: Dox; T: PTX). (A) 4T1 cells were exposed to empty cMLVs (Ctrl), cMLV(D), cMLV(T), cMLV(D+T), and D+T with the same concentration of Dox and PTX (1 μg/ml). (B) JC cells were exposed to empty cMLVs (Ctrl), cMLV(D), cMLV(T), cMLV(D+T), and D+T with the same concentration of Dox and PTX (5 μg/ml). P-gp expression was detected by P-gp-specific antibody *via* flow cytometry. Data are represented as mean ± SD (n = 3). Asterisks indicate statistical significance between two groups (*$P < 0.05$, **$P < 0.01$).

Taken together, these results indicated that the codelivery of Dox and PTX via cMLVs could inhibit the expression of P-gp and increase cellular accumulation of drugs, leading to enhanced drug action in cells, including drug-resistant cells.

Efficacy of dual drug-loaded cMLVs against a murine breast cancer model

It has been demonstrated that codelivery of Dox and PTX via cMLVs is able to overcome drug resistance *in vitro*. However, since the *in vivo* environment is considerably more complicated, it remains unknown if this effect could be translated to an animal cancer model. Therefore, in this experiment, a mouse breast tumor model was used to evaluate the therapeutic efficacy of dual drug-loaded cMLVs compared with that of single-drug liposomal formulations. At day 0, BALB/c mice were inoculated subcutaneously with 4T1 breast tumor cells. On day 8, mice bearing tumors were randomly sorted into six groups, and each group was treated with one of the following: PBS (control), cMLV(2 mg/kg Dox), cMLV(2 mg/kg PTX), cMLV(2 mg/kg Dox)+ cMLV(2 mg/kg PTX), or cMLV(2 mg/kg Dox + 2 mg/kg PTX) every three days. Tumor growth and body weights were monitored until the end of the experiment (Figure 4A).

As shown in Figure 4B, mice in groups receiving cMLV(Dox), cMLV (PTX) or cMLV(Dox)+cMLV(PTX) exhibited tumor inhibition compared to those in the control group ($p < 0.01$). Even more significantly, cMLV(Dox+PTX) treatment induced a greater inhibition than that of cMLV encapsulating a single drug and that of cMLV(Dox)+cMLV(PTX), indicating that codelivery of Dox and PTX through single nanoparticle is essential for overcoming drug resistance ($p < 0.01$). As one indication of systemic toxicity, no weight loss was seen for the cMLV formulation over the duration of the experiment (Figure 4C). The *in vivo* efficacy of dual drug-loaded cMLVs against the 4T1 tumor model was further confirmed by a survival test. As shown in Figure 4D, the groups treated with cMLV(Dox), cMLV(PTX), or cMLV(Dox)+cMLV(PTX) had a prolonged lifespan compared to the control group, while the mice in the group treated with cMLV(Dox+PTX) had a significantly increased lifespan compared to the groups treated with single drug-loaded cMLVs and the group treated with cMLV(Dox) + cMLV(PTX) ($p < 0.01$).

Histology study

To study the antitumor mechanism *in vivo*, a TUNEL assay was carried out to detect tumor cell apoptosis in tumors treated with Dox (5 mg/kg) and/or PTX (5 mg/kg) in various formulations for 3 days. As shown in Figure 5A and Figure 5C, 4T1 tumors treated with cMLV(Dox), cMLV(PTX), and Dox+PTX in solution showed significantly more apoptotic cells compared with controls ($p < 0.01$). The apoptosis index was also significantly higher in the cMLV(Dox+PTX)-treated group as compared with other groups ($p < 0.05$). Thus, the efficacy of cMLV(Dox+PTX) as an antitumor treatment could be explained by data suggesting increased tumor cell apoptosis. To further confirm the induction of cell apoptosis in treated groups, the TUNEL assay was performed in drug-resistant JC tumors treated with various formulations for 3 days. As shown in Figure 5B and 5D, cMLV(Dox), cMLV(PTX), and Dox+PTX induced more apoptotic cells compared to control JC tumors ($p < 0.01$). Dual drug-loaded cMLV-treated JC tumors showed a remarkably higher apoptosis index compared with other groups ($p < 0.01$), again confirming the enhanced antitumor activity of cMLV(Dox+PTX).

To further investigate the innate characteristics of treated tumors, both 4T1 and JC tumor sections from each treatment group were analyzed for the expression of P-gp protein. As shown in Figure 6A, P-gp expression level was moderate in the control group. There appeared to be a significant enhancement of P-gp expression in the cMLV(Dox) and cMLV(PTX) groups, with an even more significant enhancement in Dox+PTX group compared to controls. However, a marked decrease was observed in the cMLV(Dox+PTX)-treated group when compared to the cMLV(Dox), cMLV(PTX), and Dox+PTX groups, as further confirmed by the quantification data in Figure 6C ($p < 0.01$). Interestingly, P-gp was very high in the JC tumor control group, as shown in Figure 6B. However, a significant decrease appeared in the cMLV(Dox), cMLV(PTX), and Dox+ PTX groups, as further confirmed by the quantification data in Figure 6D ($p < 0.05$). An even more significant decrease of P-gp expression was seen in the cMLV(Dox+PTX) group ($p < 0.01$), indicating that dual drug-loaded cMLVs might be able to alter the innate characteristics of the multidrug-resistant tumor cells such as JC cells. Taken together, these data show that drug-loaded nanoparticles can partially bypass the P-gp efflux

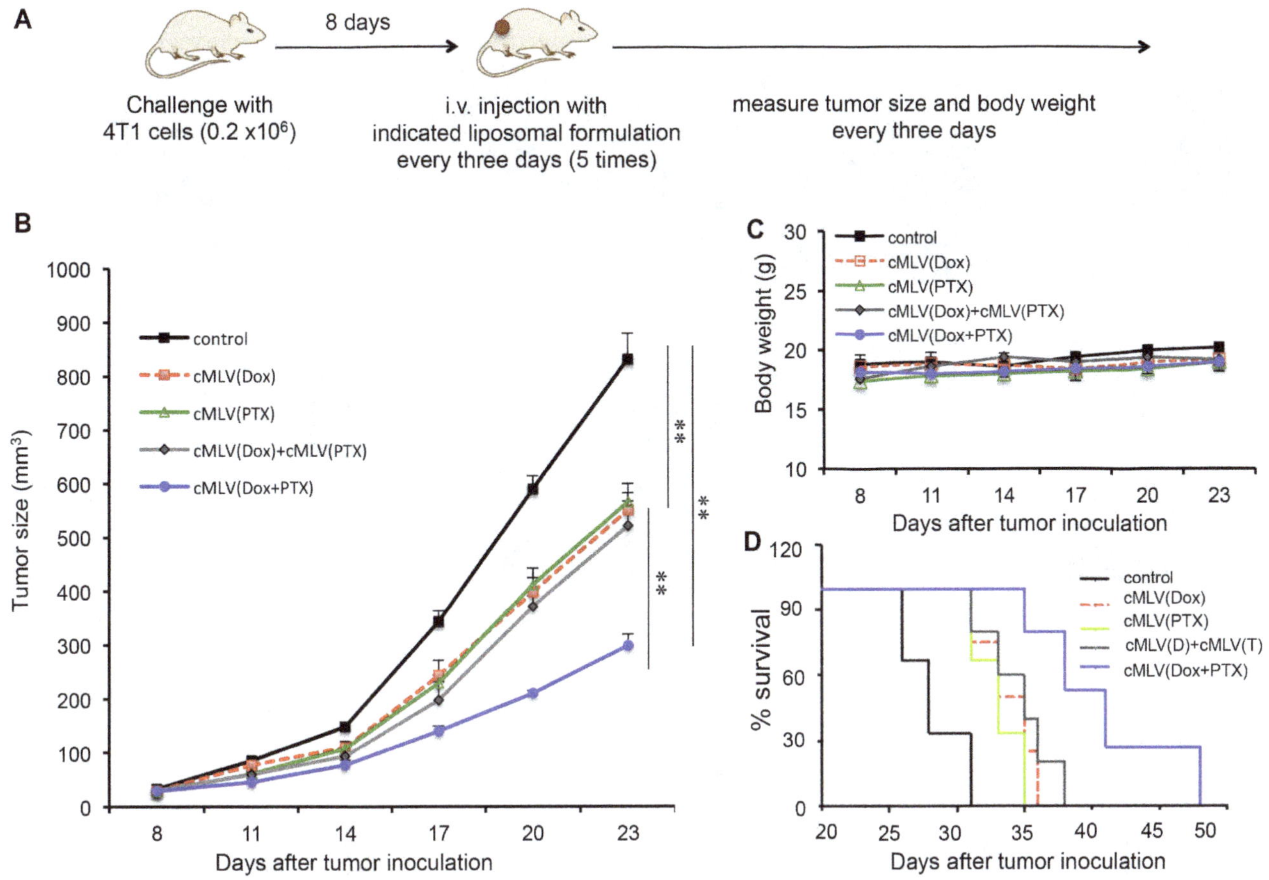

Figure 4. ***In vivo* efficacy of drug combinations *via* cMLVs in a 4T1 tumor model.** (A) Schematic diagram of the experimental protocol for *in vivo* 4T1 tumor study in BALB/c mice. (B) Tumor growth was measured after treatment with PBS (control, black solid line), cMLV (2 mg/kg Dox) (red dashed line), cMLV (2 mg/kg PTX) (green solid line), cMLV(2 mg/kg Dox)+cMLV(2 mg/kg PTX) (grey solid line), or cMLV (2 mg/kg Dox+2 mg/kg PTX) (blue solid line). Error bars represent standard error of the mean, n = 6 for each treatment group (**$p < 0.01$). (C) Average mouse weight loss over the duration of the experiment. (D) Survival curves for 4T1-bearing mice treated with PBS (black solid line), cMLV 2 mg/kg Dox) (red dashed line), cMLV (2 mg/kg PTX) (green solid line), cMLV(2 mg/kg Dox)+cMLV(2 mg/kg PTX) (grey solid line), or cMLV (2 mg/kg Dox+2 mg/kg PTX) (blue solid line). Survival end point was set when the tumor volume reached 1000 mm^3. The survival rates were presented as Kaplan-Meier curves. The survival curves of individual groups were compared by a log-rank test.

pumps to increase cellular uptake of Dox and PTX, sufficiently inducing cytotoxicity in cancer cells.

It has been reported that Dox treatment results in severe irreversible cardiotoxicity, leading to myocyte apoptosis [36]. In addition, cardiac toxicity, an unexpected clinical outcome of combinatorial Dox and PTX treatment, has been reported [37]. Therefore, systemic toxicity of free Dox+PTX and cMLV(Dox+PTX) was evaluated to determine whether codelived cMLVs could decrease this side effect of combination drug treatment. To accomplish this, a single intravenous dose of either Dox+PTX in solution or cMLV(Dox+PTX) was administered to mice bearing 4T1 tumors. Next, hematoxylin and eosin-stained cardiac tissue sections from each treatment group were examined (Figure S2). Treatment with free Dox (5 mg/kg) and PTX (5 mg/kg) in solution did cause cardiac toxicity, as indicated by myofibril loss, disarray, and cytoplasmic vacuolization. However, when cMLV(5 mg/kg Dox+5 mg/kg PTX) was administered under the same experimental conditions *via* cMLVs, no visible loss of myocardial tissue was observed.

Discussion

Chemotherapeutics are crucial to combating a variety of cancers; however, clinical outcomes are always poor, as cancer cells develop a multidrug resistance (MDR) phenotype after several rounds of exposure to the chemotherapeutics. Many efforts have been made to develop a therapeutic strategy to overcome tumor MDR through the use of combined therapeutics to enhance the efficiency of systemic drug delivered to the tumor site and lower the apoptotic threshold. In this study, we have examined augmentation of therapeutic efficacy upon co-administration of Dox and PTX using a crosslinked multilamellar liposomal vesicle (cMLV) in breast cancer cells and drug-resistant JC cells. We demonstrated that combination therapy of Dox and PTX, especially when codelivered in cMLV formulations, was effective in enhancing the cytotoxicity in both wild-type and drug-resistant cells by elevating the cellular accumulation and retention of the drugs. We also showed that the dual therapeutic strategy efficiently suppressed tumor growth by enhancing apoptotic response.

P-glycoprotein (P-gp), a membrane-bound active drug efflux pump, is considered one of the most important mechanisms involved in MDR [3,35]. As a result, growing interest has been

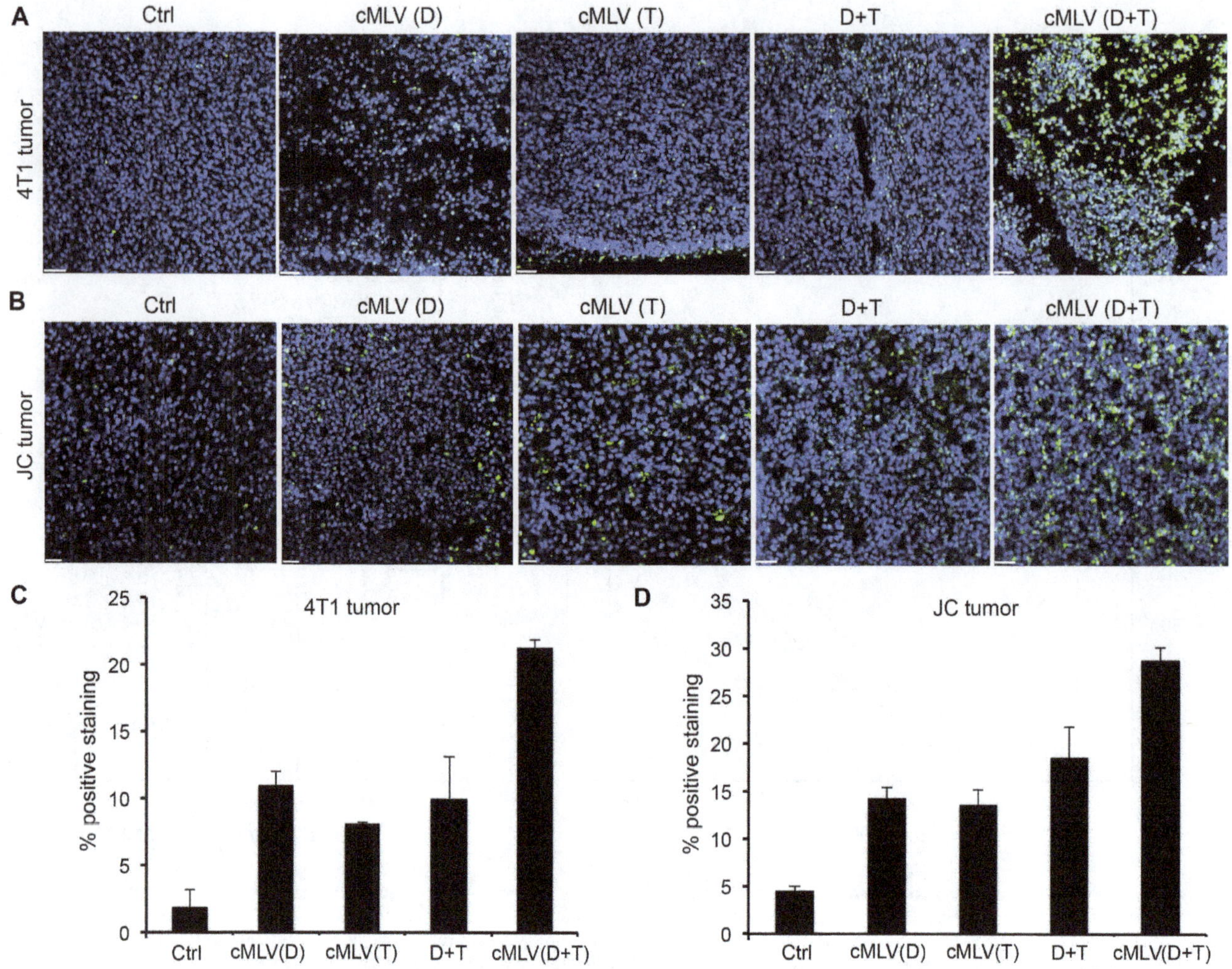

Figure 5. Effect of codelivered cMLVs on tumor apoptosis (D: Dox; T: PTX). (A, B) Mice bearing either 4T1 tumor (A) or multidrug-resistant JC tumor (B) were injected intravenously through the tail vein with cMLV (5 mg/kg Dox), cMLV (5 mg/kg PTX), 5 mg/kg Dox + 5 mg/kg PTX, or cMLV (5 mg/kg Dox+5 mg/kg PTX). Three days after injection, tumors were excised. Apoptotic cells were detected by a TUNEL assay (green), followed by nuclear costaining with DAPI (blue). Scale bar represents 50 μm. (C, D) Quantification of apoptotic cells in 4T1 (C) and JC (D) tumors. To quantify TUNEL-positive cells, 4 regions of interest (ROI) were randomly chosen per image at ×2 magnification. Within one region, area of TUNEL-positive nuclei and area of nuclear staining were counted. The data are expressed as % total nuclear area stained by TUNEL in the region. Data are represented as mean ± SD (n = 3).

shown in the development of nanoparticle drug delivery systems to overcome MDR. With their unique properties, nanoparticles are able to passively target the tumor mass through the enhanced permeability and retention (EPR) effect, enhancing the accumulation of chemotherapeutics at target sites [23,24]. In addition, nanoparticles can enter cells through the endocytosis pathway, which is thought to be independent of the P-gp pathway, thus increasing the cellular uptake and retention of therapeutics in resistant cancer cells [26,27]. Previously, we demonstrated the advantage of cMLVs in cancer therapy over conventional liposomal formulations based on their sustained drug release, enhanced vesicle stability and improved drug release, resulting in improved therapeutic activity with reduced systemic toxicity [30]. Further investigation of this novel liposomal formulation showed that it enable to translate the synergistic combination effect from in vitro to in vivo antitumor efficiency [31]. Moreover, cMLVs are internalized by tumor cells through caveolin-mediated endocytosis [30], suggesting that cMLVs could be an efficient drug carrier to overcome MDR. In this study, our *in vitro* and *in vivo* results demonstrated that the co-administration of Dox and PTX at the synergistic ratio (1:1) *via* cMLVs efficiently suppressed P-gp expression in both wild-type and drug-resistant cancer cells.

In addition to nanodelivery, another potential strategy to overcome MDR has resulted from combining multiple drugs. For example, the combination of Dox and PTX in a cocktail is a standard anthracycline-taxane treatment regimen and was found to be efficacious in treating a variety of tumors by reducing the individual drug concentration that would otherwise be required to achieve cytotoxicity, thus overcoming drug resistance [13,14,15]. However, its clinical outcome was limited by the un-coordinated biodistribution of combined drugs [16,17] and increase in cardiac cytotoxicity [37]. In this study, the pharmacokinetics of Dox and PTX was unified through the encapsulation of both drugs into a single cMLV particle, resulting in dual drug-loaded cMLVs which successfully reduced P-gp expression, increased the cellular accumulation of drugs, and enhanced cytotoxicity in cancer cells, including drug-resistant cells, as compared to single drug-loaded cMLVs. Moreover, combination therapy of Dox and PTX

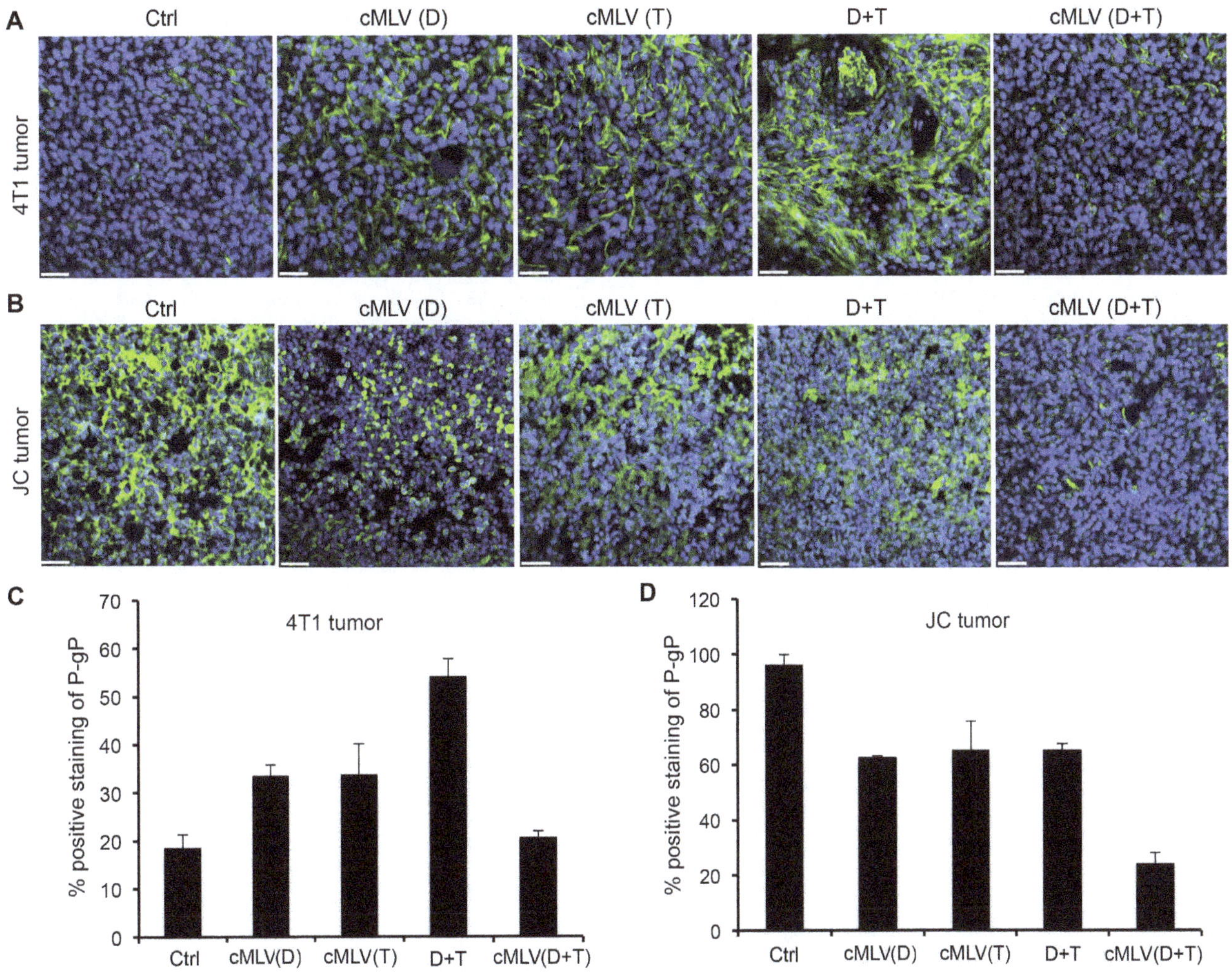

Figure 6. Effect of codelivered cMLVs on P-gp expression in tumors. (A, B) Mice bearing 4T1 tumor (A) and multidrug-resistant tumor JC (B) were injected intravenously through the tail vein with cMLV (5 mg/kg Dox), cMLV (5 mg/kg PTX), 5 mg/kg Dox + 5 mg/kg PTX, or cMLV (5 mg/kg Dox+5 mg/kg PTX). Three days after injection, tumors were excised, and stained by P-gp-specific antibody (green), followed by nuclear costaining with DAPI (blue). Scale bar represents 50 μm. (C, D) Quantification of P-gp-positive cells in 4T1 (C) and JC (D) tumors. To quantify P-gp-positive cells, 4 regions of interest (ROI) were randomly chosen per image at ×2 magnification. Within one region, area of P-gp-positive nuclei and area of nuclear staining were counted. The data are expressed as % total nuclear area that is P-gp-positive in the region. Data are represented as mean ± SD (n = 3).

administered in cMLV formulations showed increased efficacy over cMLV monotherapy in the suppression of tumor growth by promoting apoptotic response *in vivo*.

Conclusion

In summary, we have developed a multimodal therapeutic strategy to overcome tumor MDR by codelivery of Dox and PTX *via* a crosslinked multilamellar liposomal vesicle. We demonstrated that such combinatorial delivery system increased therapeutic efficacy by enhancing delivery efficiency to tumors and lowering the apoptotic threshold of individual drugs, thus overcoming drug resistance. The properties of cMLVs, such as improved stability and sustained release of drugs, enable the nanoparticles to sufficiently accumulate at tumor sites, subsequently entering tumor cells *via* endocytosis to release therapeutics, thus potentially bypassing the P-gp pathway to enhance cellular retention of therapeutics. Moreover, cMLVs enable multidrug delivery to the same action site, thereby lowering the tumor apoptotic threshold of individual therapeutics and potentially inhibiting the MDR. Taken together, this dual drug-loaded cMLV approach shows promise for reducing MDR in cancer therapeutics.

Supporting Information

Figure S1 IC50 values of cMLV(Dox), cMLV(PTX) and cMLV(Dox+PTX) in B16 melanoma, 4T1 breast tumor cells, or drug-resistant JC cancer cells.

Figure S2 Histologic appearance (hematoxylin and eosin staining) of heart tissues by light microscopy isolated on day 3 after a single intravenous injection of PBS (left), 5 mg/kg Dox+5 mg/kg PTX in solution (middle) and cMLV(5 mg/kg Dox+5 mg/kg PTX) (right).

Acknowledgments

We thank the USC NanoBiophysics Core Facility. We also thank Jennifer Rohrs for critical reading of the manuscript.

Author Contributions

Conceived and designed the experiments: YL PW. Performed the experiments: YL JF KJ. Analyzed the data: YL JF KJ. Contributed reagents/materials/analysis tools: MW PW. Contributed to the writing of the manuscript: YL PW.

References

1. Szakács G, Paterson JK, Ludwig JA, Booth-Genthe C, Gottesman MM (2006) Targeting multidrug resistance in cancer. Nat Rev Drug Discov 5: 219–234.
2. Teicher BA (2009) Acute and chronic in vivo therapeutic resistance. Biochem Pharmacol: 1665–1673.
3. Fletcher JI, Haber M, Henderson MJ, Norris MD (2010) ABC transporters in cancer: more than just drug efflux pumps. Nat Rev Cancer 10: 147–156.
4. Schöndorf T, Kurbacher C, Göhring U, Benz C, Becker M, et al. (2002) Induction of MDR1-gene expression by antineoplastic agents in ovarian cancer cell lines. Anticancer Res 22: 2199–2203.
5. Lespine A, Ménez C, Bourguinat C, Prichard RK (2012) P-glycoproteins and other multidrug resistance transporters in the pharmacology of anthelmintics: Prospects for reversing transport-dependent anthelmintic resistance. Int J Parasitol Drugs Drug Resist 2: 230–270.
6. Chen Y, Bathula SR, Li J, Huang L (2010) Multifunctional nanoparticles delivering small interfering RNA and doxorubicin overcome drug resistance in cancer. J Biol Chem 285: 22639–22650.
7. Xu D, McCarty D, Fernandes A, Fisher M, Samulski RJ, et al. (2005) Delivery of MDR1 small interfering RNA by self-complementary recombinant adeno-associated virus vector. Mol Ther 11: 523–530.
8. Hubensack M, Müller C, Höcherl P, Fellner S, Spruss T, et al. (2008) Effect of the ABCB1 modulators elacridar and tariquidar on the distribution of paclitaxel in nude mice. J Cancer Res Clin Oncol 134: 597–607.
9. Liu Y, Rohrs J, Wang P (2014) Development and challenges of nanovectors in gene therapy. Nano LIFE 4: 1441007.
10. Lehar J, Krueger AS, Avery W, Heilbut AM, Johansen LM, et al. (2009) Synergistic drug combinations tend to improve therapeutically relevant selectivity. Nat biotechnol 27: 659–666.
11. Calabrò F, Lorusso V, Rosati G, Manzione L, Frassinet iL, et al. (2009) Gemcitabine and paclitaxel every 2 weeks in patients with previously untreated urothelial carcinoma. Cancer 115: 2652–2659.
12. Mamounas EP, Sledge GW Jr (2001) Combined anthracycline-taxane regimens in the adjuvant setting. Semin Oncol 28: 24–31.
13. Dean-Colomb W, Esteva F (2008) Emerging agents in the treatment of anthracycline- and taxane-refractory metastatic breast cancer. Semin Oncol 35(2 Suppl 2): S31–38.
14. De Laurentiis M, Cancello G, D'Agostino D, Giuliano M, Giordano A, et al. (2008) Taxane-based combinations as adjuvant chemotherapy of early breast cancer: a meta-analysis of randomized trials. J Clin Oncol 26: 44–53.
15. Kataja V, Castiglione M (2008) ESMO Guidelines Working Group Locally recurrent or metastatic breast cancer: ESMO clinical recommendations for diagnosis, treatment and follow-up. Ann Oncol 19(2 suppl): ii11–ii13.
16. Grasselli G, Viganò L, Capri G, Locatelli A, Tarenzi E, et al. (2001) Clinical and pharmacologic study of the epirubicin and paclitaxel combination in women with meta-static breast cancer. J Clin Oncol 19: 2222–2231.
17. Gustafson DL, Andrea L Merz, Long ME (2005) Pharmacokinetics of combined doxorubicin and paclitaxel in mice. Cancer Letters 220: 161–169.
18. Ahmed F, Pakunlu RI, Brannan A, Bates F, Minko T, et al. (2006) Biodegradable polymersomes loaded with both paclitaxel and doxorubicin permeate and shrink tumors, inducing apoptosis in proportion to accumulated drug. J Control Release 116: 150–158.
19. Sengupta S, Eavarone D, Capila I, Zhao G, Watson N, et al. (2005) Temporal targeting of tumour cells and neovasculature with a nanoscale delivery system. Nature 436: 568–572.
20. Wang H, Zhao Y, Wu Y, Hu Y-l, Nan K, et al. (2011) Enhanced anti-tumor efficacy by co-delivery of doxorubicin and paclitaxel with amphiphilic methoxy PEG-PLGA copolymer nanoparticles. Biomaterials 32: 8281–8290.
21. Gao H, Zhang Z, Yu Z, He Q (2014) Cell-penetrating peptide based intelligent liposomal systems for enhanced drug delivery. Curr Pharm Biotechnol 15: 210–219.
22. Yu Z, Schmaltz RM, Bozeman TC, Paul R, Rishel MJ, et al. (2013) Selective tumor cell targeting by the disaccharide moiety of bleomycin. J Am Chem Soc 135: 2883–2886.
23. Cho K, Wang X, Nie S, Chen ZG, Shin DM (2008) Therapeutic nanoparticles for drug delivery in cancer. Clin Cancer Res 14: 1310–1316.
24. Ferrari M (2005) Cancer nanotechnology: opportunities and challenges. Nat Rev Cancer 5: 161–171.
25. Dobson PD, Kell DB (2008) Carrier-mediated cellular uptake of pharmaceutical drugs: an exception or the rule? Nat Rev Drug Discov 7: 205–210.
26. Hillaireau H, Couvreur P (2009) Nanocarriers' entry into the cell: relevance to drug delivery. Cell Mo Life Sci 66: 2873–2896.
27. Sahay G, Alakhova DY, Kabanov AV (2010) Endocytosis of nanomedicines. J Control Release 145: 182–195.
28. Torchilin VP (2005) Recent Advances with Liposomes as Pharmaceutical Carriers. Nat Rev Drug Discov 4: 145–160.
29. Liu Y, Ji M, Wong MK, Joo K-I, Wang P (2013) Enhanced therapeutic efficacy of iRGD-conjugated crosslinked multilayer liposomes for drug delivery. BioMed Research International 2013: 378380.
30. Joo K, Xiao L, Liu S, Liu Y, Lee C, et al. (2013) Crosslinked multilamellar liposomes for controlled delivery of anticancer drugs. Biomaterials 34: 3098–3109.
31. Liu Y, Fang J, Kim Y-J, Wong MK, Wang P (2014) Codelivery of doxorubicin and paclitaxel by cross-linked multilamellar liposome enables synergistic antitumor activity. Mol Pharmaceutics 11: 1651–1661.
32. Lee B, French K, Zhuang Y, Smith C (2003) Development of a syngeneic in vivo tumor model and its use in evaluating a novel P-glycoprotein modulator, PGP-4008. Oncol Res 14: 49–60.
33. Goutelle S, Maurin M, Rougier l, Barbaut X, Bourguignon L, et al. (2008) The Hill equation: a review of its capabilities in pharmacological modelling. Fundam Clin Pharmacol 22: 633–648.
34. Shen L, Peterson S, Sedaghat AR, McMahon MA, Callender M, et al. (2008) Dose-response curve slope sets class-specific limits on inhibitory potential of anti-HIV drugs. Nat Med 14: 762–766.
35. Robey RW, To KK, Polgar O, Dohse M, Fetsch P, et al. (2009) ABCG2: a perspective. Adv Drug Deliv Rev 61: 3–13.
36. Rahman AM, Yusuf SW, Ewer MS (2007) Anthracycline-induced cardiotoxicity and the cardiac-sparing effect of liposomal formulation. Int J Nanomedicine 2: 567–583.
37. Bird B, Swain S (2008) Cardiac toxicity in breast cancer survivors: review of potential cardiac problems. Clin Cancer Res 14: 14–24.

16

Metformin Protects Cardiomyocyte from Doxorubicin Induced Cytotoxicity through an AMP-Activated Protein Kinase Dependent Signaling Pathway: An *In Vitro* Study

Laura C. Kobashigawa, Yan Chun Xu, James F. Padbury, Yi-Tang Tseng*, Naohiro Yano*

Department of Pediatrics, Women & Infants Hospital, The Warren Alpert Medical School of Brown University, Providence, Rhode Island, United States of America

Abstract

Doxorubicin (Dox) is one of the most widely used antitumor drugs, but its cumulative cardiotoxicity have been major concerns in cancer therapeutic practice for decades. Recent studies established that metformin (Met), an oral anti-diabetic drug, provides protective effects in Dox-induced cardiotoxicity. Met has been shown to increase fatty acid oxidation, an effect mediated by AMP activated protein kinase (AMPK). Here we delineate the intracellular signaling factors involved in Met mediated protection against Dox-induced cardiotoxicity in the H9c2 cardiomyoblast cell line. Treatment with low dose Met (0.1 mM) increased cell viabilities and Ki-67 expressions while decreasing LDH leakages, ROS generations and $[Ca^{2+}]_i$. The protective effect was reversed by a co-treatment with compound-C, an AMPK specific inhibitor, or by an over expression of a dominant-negative AMPKα cDNA. Inhibition of PKA with H89 or a suppression of Src kinase by a small hairpin siRNA also abrogated the protective effect of the low dose Met. Whereas, with a higher dose of Met (1.0 mM), the protective effects were abolished regardless of the enhanced AMPK, PKA/CREB1 and Src kinase activity. In high dose Met treated cells, expression of platelet-derived growth factor receptor (PDGFR) was significantly suppressed. Furthermore, the protective effect of low dose Met was totally reversed by co-treatment with AG1296, a PDGFR specific antagonist. These data provide *in vitro* evidence supporting a signaling cascade by which low dose Met exerts protective effects against Dox via sequential involvement of AMPK, PKA/CREB1, Src and PDGFR. Whereas high dose Met reverses the effect by suppressing PDGFR expression.

Editor: Miguel López, University of Santiago de Compostela School of Medicine - CIMUS, Spain

Funding: This work was supported by the National Center for Research Resources (SP20RR018728-10) and the National Institute of General Medical Science (8 P20 GM103537-10) from the National Institute of Health (to Y-TT and JFP). The funders had no role in study design, data collection and analysis, decision to publish, or preparation of the manuscript.

Competing Interests: The authors have declared that no competing interests exist.

* Email: ytseng@wihri.org (YT); nyano@wihri.org (NY)

Introduction

Doxorubicin (Dox), an anthracycline antibiotic, has been established as an agent against a wide range of cancers [1]. However, the severe cardiotoxicity of Dox is a major factor limiting its use in the treatment of many malignancies [2].

Intensive investigations of Dox-induced cardiotoxicity have been carried out. The different lines of evidence have provided putative mechanisms, but the precise mechanism underlying Dox-induced cardiotoxicity is not fully elucidated. Most studies favor the hypothesis that free radical-induced oxidative stress plays a pivotal role. This is supported by the chemical structure of Dox and its tendency to generate reactive oxygen species (ROS) during drug metabolism [3–5]. Recent findings indicate that endothelial nitric oxide synthase (eNOS) reductase domain converts Dox to an unstable semiquinone intermediate that favors ROS generation [5]. Although gaining less attention than ROS has received, a number of studies suggested that Dox-mediated alteration of Ca^{2+} homeostasis is another possible mechanism of cardiotoxicity. Recent studies have demonstrated that Dox-mediated ROS generation induces increase of intracellular Ca^{2+} ($[Ca^{2+}]_i$), which plays a critical role in damage of cardiomyocytes [6].

Metformin (Met) is an oral biguanide anti-hyperglycemic drug that is widely used for the management of type 2 diabetes mellitus. The therapeutic effects of Met have been attributed to a combination of improved peripheral uptake and utilization of glucose, decreased hepatic glucose output, decreased rate of intestinal absorption of carbohydrate, and enhanced insulin sensitivity [7,8]. Beyond its glucose lowering effects, Met has been shown to exhibit antioxidant properties in various tissues and acts to decrease lipid peroxidation, an effect that is independent of its effect on insulin sensitivity [9. 10]. Further, Met has been demonstrated to exert cardioprotective effects that could be due to its direct beneficial effects on cellular and mitochondrial function and therefore be independent of its insulin-sensitizing effect [11].

Through its activation of 5′-adenosine monophosphate-activated protein kinase (AMPK), Met reduces the generation of ROS in cultured endothelial cells [12] and in animal models of heart failure [13,14] and protects cardiomyocytes from oxidative stress induced by H_2O_2 or TNFα [14,15]. However, the specific mechanism by which Met activates AMPK and the corresponding antioxidant effect has not been established. These antioxidant effects suggest that Met could offer a protection against the cardiotoxicity of Dox, although no data are available to support additional benefits of Met in patients being treated with the anthracycline.

The present study was undertaken to delineate signaling pathways by which Met treatment evokes protective effects against the Dox induced cardiotoxicity. For this purpose, we studied Dox-induced *in vitro* toxicity in a fetal rat cardiomyoblast cell line, H9c2, human fetal cardiomyocyte cell line, RL-14 and rat neonatal primary cardiomyocyte. The results of this study provide evidence that the cardioprotective effects of Met are mediated by activation of the AMPK, PKA Src and platelet-derived growth factor receptor (PDGFR). Furthermore, the protective effects are suppressed with high dose Met (1 mM) treatment secondary to reduced cellular PDGF-receptor (PDGFR) expression.

Materials and Methods

Reagents and antibodies

Unless otherwise specified, all materials were reagent grade and obtained from Sigma-Aldrich (St. Louis, MO, USA). Anti-Ki67 antibody was obtained from BD Biosciences (San Jose, CA, USA). Alkaline phosphatase (ALP) conjugated horse anti-mouse IgG antibody was obtained from Vector Laboratory (Burlingame, CA, USA). Anti-phosphorylated/total AMPKα, anti-phosphorylated/total acetyl-CoA carboxylase (ACC) and anti-phosphorylated PDGF receptor β (PDGFRβ) antibodies were obtained from Cell Signaling Technology (Danvers, MA, USA). Anti-phosphorylated/total CREB1, c-Src and total PDGFR-β antibodies were obtained from Santa Cruz Biotechnology (Santa Cruz, CA, USA). Anti-phosphorylated tyrosine antibody was obtained from Millipore (Billerica, MA, USA).

Cell culture

H9c2 rat fetal cardiomyoblasts (ATCC CRL-1446), RL14 human fetal cardiomyocytes (ATCC PTA-1499) and rat neonatal primary cardiomyocytes (Lonza, Allendale, NJ, USA) were grown in DMEM (Invitrogen, Carlsbad, CA, USA) supplemented with 10% (vol/vol) fetal bovine serum in a humidified atmosphere containing 5% CO_2 at 37°C. Cells were grown to 70% confluence and quietened overnight in serum-free medium before experiments.

Cell viability assay

Cell viabilities were estimated using CellTiter-Blue Cell Viability Assay (Promega, Fitchburg, WI, USA). Briefly, viable cells retain the ability to reduce resazurin into resorufin, which is highly fluorescent. Nonviable cells rapidly lose metabolic capacity, do not reduce the indicator dye, and thus do not generate a fluorescent signal. Buffered solution containing highly purified resazurin was added to cells growing on 96-well microplates. The spectral properties of the buffer changed upon reduction of resazurin to resorufin. Fluorescence which was emitted from resorufin was measured with maximum excitation and emission spectra of 560 nm and 590 nm, respectively.

Lactate dehydrogenase release

Lactate dehydrogenase (LDH) is a cellular enzyme released upon membrane damage and a recognized marker of cell damage or death [16]. LDH released into the incubation medium was estimated using an assay kit from Sigma-Aldrich. In brief, LDH reduces nicotinamide adenine dinucleotide, which is then converted a tetrazolium dye to a soluble, colored formazan derivative; this was measured using a micro plate reader (490 nm).

Reactive Oxygen Species Assay

Cellular ROS was measured using a detection assay kit (Abcam, Cambridge, MA, USA). In brief, 2′,7′-dichlorofluorescein diacetate (DCFDA), a fluorogenic dye that measures hydroxyl, peroxyl and other ROS activity within the cell, was added to the cells growing in the 96-well plates. After diffusion into the cells, DCFDA was deacetylated by cellular esterases to a non-fluorescent compound, which was later oxidized by ROS into 2′,7′-dichlorofluorescin (DCF), a highly fluorescent compound. Fluorescence from the DCF was detected by fluorescence micro plate reader with maximum excitation and emission spectra of 495 nm and 529 nm, respectively.

Determination of $[Ca^{2+}]_i$

Levels of $[Ca^{2+}]_i$ were measured using fluo-4 (Molecular Probe, Eugene, OR, USA), a fluorescent Ca^{2+}-indicator dye. Briefly, after removing the growth medium from the cells growing in 96-well microplates, 100 μL of dye loading solution (1× fluo-4 dye with 2.5 mM of probenecid) was added to each well. After incubation for one hour at 37°C, fluorescence from the fluo-4 was detected with a fluorescence micro plate reader with maximum excitation and emission spectra of 494 nm and 516 nm, respectively.

Immunohistochemistry

H9c2 cells were seeded on poly-L-lysine coated chamber slides. The cells were fixed with 2% formaldehyde and permeabilized by 0.2% TritonX-100, and incubated with a mouse monoclonal anti-Ki67 antibody overnight at 4°C in a humidified chamber. The cells were then incubated with an ALP conjugated anti-mouse IgG (H+L) secondary antibody for 30 min at room temperature. Bound antibody was detected using the ALP substrate kit (Vector Laboratories) and lightly counterstained with veronal acetate buffered 1% methyl green solution, pH 4.0. Permount (Fisher Scientific, Ottawa, Ontario, Canada) was used as the mounting media and sections were cover slipped. The immunohistochemical studies were repeated four times on samples prepared from independent cultures. The labeling index or the proportion of Ki67 positive cells was calculated according to the following formula: 100× (the number of Ki67-positive nuclei/total number of nuclei). Each image was analyzed four times to obtain an average labeling index.

AMPK activity assay

Cellular AMPK activities were measured using an AMPK kinase assay kit (Cyclex, Ina, Nagano, Japan). Briefly, cell lysate samples were added to plates coated with a substrate-peptide corresponding to surrounding mouse IRS-1 serine 789 (S789), which contains serine residues that can be phosphorylated by AMPK. After washing, anti-phosphorylated mouse IRS-1 S789 monoclonal antibody was added, then the colorimetric reaction was developed by peroxidase conjugated anti-mouse IgG and tetramethylbenzidine substrate (TMB). The absorbance was measured at 450 nm using a micro plate reader.

Western blotting

Protein levels of the cell lysates for Western blotting (50 μg/lane) were measured as described [17]. GelCode Blue (Thermo Scientific, Waltham, MA, USA) stain of the post transfer gel was used as the loading control for total and phosphorylated PDGFR-β blotting. The results were visualized with Super Signal West Pico chemiluminescent substrate (Thermo Scientific) and analyzed with the UN-SCAN-IT gel software for Windows (Silk Scientific Inc., Orem, UT, USA).

PKA activity assay

Cellular PKA activity was measured using a PKA kinase activity kit (Enzo Life Sciences, Farmingdale, NY, USA). Briefly, cell lysates to be assayed were added to PKA substrate coated micro plate wells, followed by the addition of ATP to initiate the phosphorylation reaction. After terminating the kinase reaction, a phosphorylated substrate specific antibody was added to the wells. The phosphor-specific antibody was subsequently bound by peroxidase conjugated secondary antibody. The assay was developed with TMB. The absorbance was measured at 450 nm using a micro plate reader.

Src activity assay

Protein lysates (1 mg) from H9c2 cells were immunoprecipitated with anti-cSrc antibody. Kinase activity was determined by measuring phosphorylation of a specific Src substrate (KVEKI-GEGTYGVVYK) using a Src assay kit (Millipore). Briefly, the cSrc immunoprecipitated beads were incubated with a [γ-^{32}P]ATP-ATP-Mg^{2+} mix at 30°C for 10 min. A sample without the substrate peptide was included as a background control. Reactions were terminated by adding 40% trichloroacetic acid. After centrifugation the supernatants that include phosphorylated substrate were transferred onto Whatman P81 ion-exchange cellulose chromatography paper circles (GE Healthcare, Little Chalfont, UK). The paper circles were washed five times in 0.75% phosphoric acid and once in acetone, and then counted in a liquid scintillation counter.

PI3K assay

PI3K activity was determined with *in vitro* immunoprecipitation lipid kinase assay. Briefly, cell lysates (0.5 mg) were immunoprecipitated with anti-phosphorylated tyrosine antibody-coated protein G-sepharose (GE Healthcare), and the beads were resuspend in assay buffer containing 300 µM adenosine to inhibit phosphoinositide 4-kinase (PI4K) activity [18]. L-α-phosphoinositide (Avanti Polar Lipid, Alabaster, AL, USA) was used as the lipid substrate (2 µg/reaction). After incubation, the final extracted reaction mixtures were spotted on to silica gel coated TLC plates (GE Healthcare), and were run in TLC buffer (65% n-propanol and 0.54 M acetic acid). The results were analyzed by phosphor-imaging. Densitometric analysis was performed by using the UN-SCAN-IT gel software.

Stable transfection

Constructs of wild type (WT), dominant-negative (DN) and constitutively active (CA) AMPKα1 in pcDNA3.1 expression vector were generously provided by Prof. David Carling (MRC Clinical Sciences Centre, Imperial College, London, UK). A construct of constitutive active Src (Y529F) in pUSEamp- was purchased from Millipore.

Short hairpin RNA (shRNA) against cSrc was constructed as follows. Two complementary short hairpin siRNA (shRNA) template oligonucleotides, containing 21-nucleotide target sequences of the rat cSrc tyrosine kinase (5′-AAG TAC AAC TTC CAT GGC ACT-3′, GenBank, AC122515.5), were annealed and ligated into the pScilencer 5.1-H1 Retro vector (Invitrogen, Carlsbad, CA, USA).

Stable transfections of these vectors were performed using Lipofectamine 2000 (Invitrogen), according to the manufacturer's instructions. Individual single cells were isolated and selected with G418 (AMPKα1s and active Src transfected cells, 500 µg/ml) or puromycin (shRNA transfected cells, 5 µg/ml). Phenotypes of the transfected cells were evaluated by AMPK and Src activities (Fig. S1, S2).

Statistical analysis

Statistics of the densitometric analysis were generated from four independent experiments. Statistical evaluations of the other assays (cell viability, LDH leakage, ROS generation, $[Ca^{2+}]_i$, AMPK activity, PKA activity, and Src activity) were performed from four independent experiments which tested at least 10 samples each time.

Statistical significance of the difference among groups was analyzed by the paired Student's t test or parametric ANOVA and Ryan's multiple comparison test using Microsoft Exel (Microsoft, Redmond, WA, USA) and ANOVA4 on the Web (http://www.hju.ac.jp/~kiriki/anova4/). All data were represented as the mean ± SD of at least four different experiments. A probability of $p<0.05$ was considered to represent a significant difference.

Results

Effects of Met on Dox-induced cardiomyocyte toxicity

H9c2 cells were seeded in 96-well microplates (3×10^3 cells/well) and quietened overnight in serum-free medium. In order to minimize the influence of serum on the metabolism of cells while keeping the cells in proliferative status, medium supplemented with reduced (1%, v/v) FBS was used in the experiment [19]. A concentration of Dox (10 nM) was determined to induce up to 40% of growth suppression after 72–96 hours (Fig.S3). The Met concentrations (0.1 and 1.0 mM) used in the experiments were adopted from published *in vitro* studies [20,21]. Cells were cultured in the reduced serum medium under various combinations of Dox and Met concentrations for up to 72 hours. After treatment with 10 nM of Dox for 72 hours, the cell viability was suppressed to 43.0±5.0% of the vehicle control level. Co-incubation with 0.1 mM of Met reduced the suppression level to 31.1±6.2%. Co-incubation with higher concentration (1.0 mM) of Met, however, did not affect the effect of Dox on cell viability (46.0±3.7% of the control level; Fig. 1A). Dox induced a significant increase in LDH leakage to culture supernatants, another index of cellular damage, after 24 hours of incubation (373.1±115.3% of the control level; Fig. 1B). The increase in LDH leakage was lessened by co-incubation of lower dose of Met (213.6±44.9%) but not by the higher dose of Met (347.8±104.6%). Furthermore, Dox induced a significant reduction of Ki-67 positive cells, (28.6±5.7% vs 5.1±1.4%, CTR vs Dox). The decrease in Ki-67 staining, again, was lessened by co-incubation of lower dose of Met (14.1±1.1%) but not by the higher dose of Met (5.8±2.8%; Fig. 1C). Since Dox-induced cardiotoxicity may be related to cellular ROS generation [3–5] or $[Ca^{2+}]_i$ [6], measurement of these factors could be informative to elucidate the mechanisms of how Met mediates protective effects against Dox-induced cardiotoxicity. Dox treatment significantly increased cellular ROS generation (770.5±154.4% of the control level after 6 hour incubation) and $[Ca^{2+}]_i$ (437.1±59.9% of the control level after 90 minute incubation). As expected, co-incubation of 0.1 mM of Met partially attenuated the Dox-induced effects (ROS, 295.4±35.6%, $[Ca^{2+}]_i$, 225.3±31.5%). Unexpectedly, co-incubation with 1.0 mM Met attenuated the effects as well (ROS, 279.8±31.7%, $[Ca^{2+}]_i$, 198.8±17.1%; Fig. 1D, E). Incubation with Met alone (0.1–1 mM) had no effects on H9c2 cell viability, LDH leakage, ROS generation and $[Ca^{2+}]_i$ (Fig.S4A-D).

In order to confirm the effects of Met on other cardiomyocytes in altered stages of differentiation, cell viability, LDH leakage,

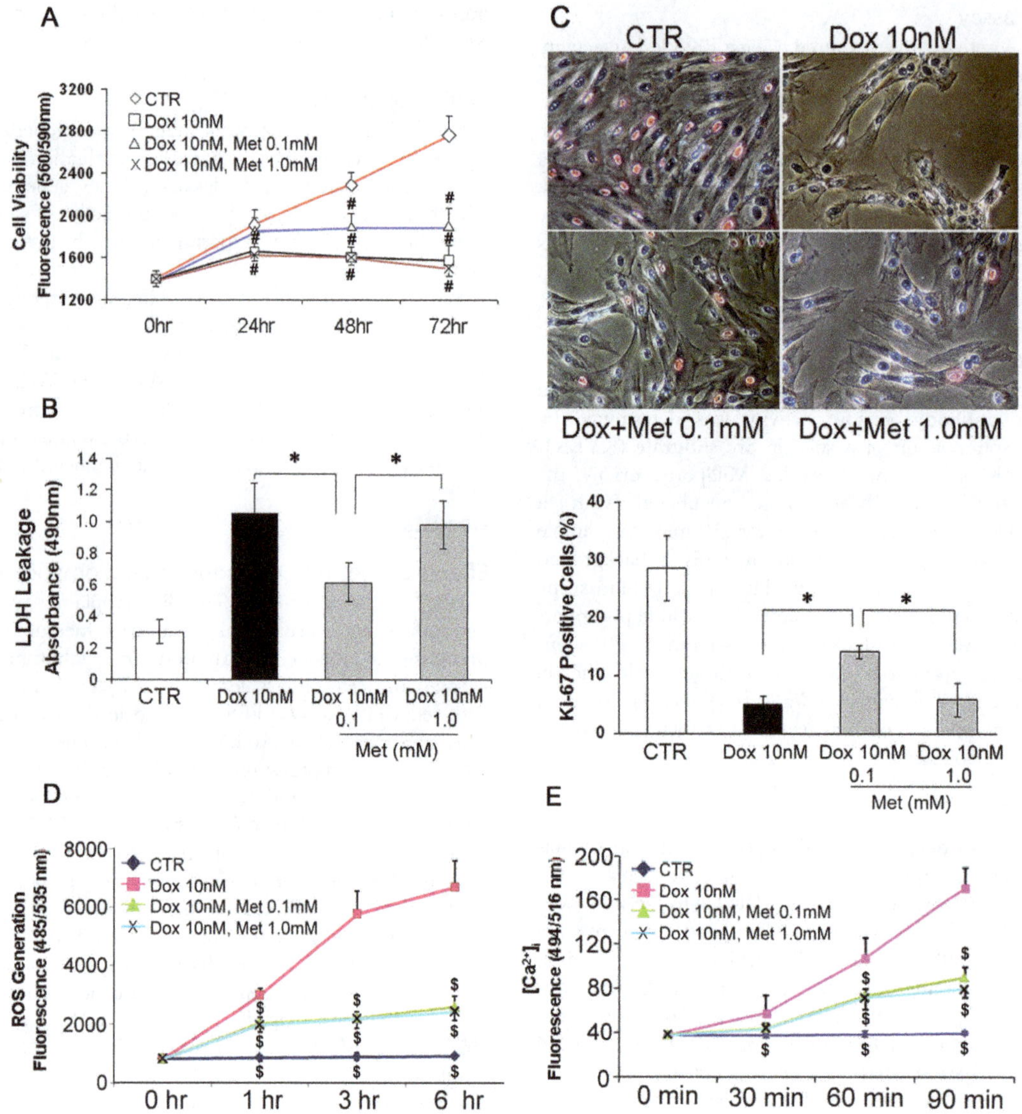

Figure 1. Low dose Met attenuates Dox induced cytotoxicity in H9c2 rat cardiomyoblasts. (A) H9c2 rat immortalized cardiomyoblasts were cultured with reduced FBS (1%) for up to 72 hours in 96-well culture plates under indicated conditions. Viability levels were estimated as described in Materials and Methods. (B) LDH leakages in H9c2 cells after Dox/Met treatment. Cells were treated with indicated conditions for 24 hours in serum free medium. LDH levels in culture supernatants were evaluated using LDH assay kit. (C) H9c2 cells were cultured on poly-L-lysine coated chamber slides for 24 hours under the conditions as indicated in reduced FBS medium. The slides were immunostained with anti-Ki-67 antibody (BD Biosciences) and ALP conjugated secondary antibody (Vector Laboratory). The numbers of Ki-67-positive vessels were counted in six randomized fields of the chambers. The total number of cells from each group was counted and normalized to each chamber. (D) H9c2 cells were cultured with conditions and for hours as indicated in serum free medium. Cellular ROS generations were measured using a detection assay kit. (E) H9c2 cells were cultured with serum free medium under the indicated conditions. Intra-cellular calcium levels ($[Ca^{2+}]_i$) were measured using fluo-4 (Molecular Probe), a fluorescent Ca^{2+}-indicator dye. Values represent mean ± S.D. (n = 4) from quadruplicate samples for each treatment at varying treatment conditions. * $p<0.05$; $^{\#}$ $p<0.05$ vs CTR; $^{\$}$ $p<0.05$ vs Dox 10 nM alone.

ROS generation and $[Ca^{2+}]_i$ were evaluated using RL14 human fatal cardiomyocytes and rat neonatal primary cardiomyocytes. As shown in Figure 2A-D, Met showed similar effects with these cells.

Effects of AMPK activity on protection against Dox-induced cardiomyocyte toxicity

Recent advances in the understanding of Met action have centered on the discovery that Met leads to increased phosphorylation and activation of AMPKα [22,23]. Therefore, the relationship between the protection against Dox-induced cardiomyocyte toxicity and AMPK activity were examined in this study.

Co-incubation of Met (0.1 and 1.0 mM) with 10 nM Dox significantly enhanced cellular AMPK activity in H9c2 cells after 72 hour incubation (0.1 mM Met; 584.0±88.3%, 1.0 mM Met; 1009.3±127.2% of the control level), while incubation with Dox alone showed no effect (91.2±1.6%; Fig.3A). AMPK phosphorylates and inhibits acetyl-CoA carboxylase (ACC), the key enzyme that controls generation of malonyl-CoA from acetyl-CoA. As malonyl-CoA decreases fatty acid oxidation through inhibition of carnitine palmitoyl transferase-1 (CPT-1), phosphorylation of ACC relieves the inhibition of CPT-1, favoring fatty acid oxidation. In the current study, Met increased AMPK (0.1 mM;

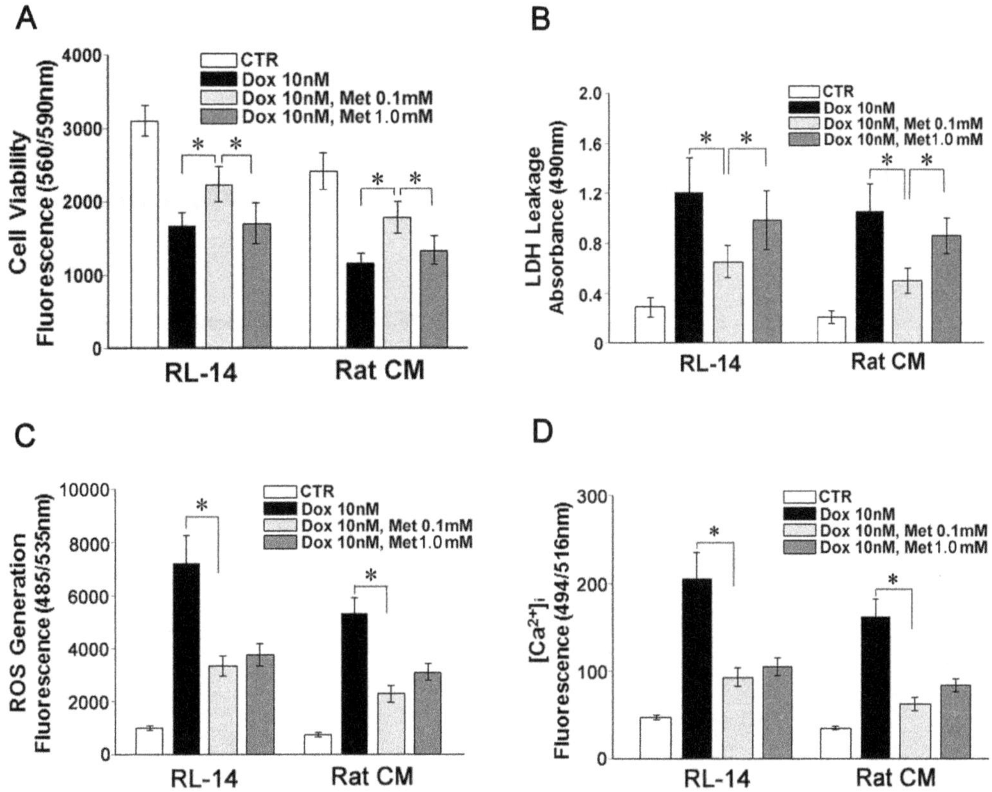

Figure 2. Effects of Met on Dox induced cytotoxicity in RL-14 human cardiomyocytes and rat primary cardiomyocytes. RL-14 human immortalized fetal cardiomyocytes and rat neonatal primary cardiomyocytes (Rat CM) were cultured with same conditions as we did for H9c2 cells, and (A) cell viabilities, (B) LDH leakages, (C) ROS generations and (D) $[Ca2+]_i$ were evaluated at 72 hour, 24 hour, 6 hour and 90 minute, respectively. Values represent mean ± S.D. (n = 4) from quadruplicate samples for each treatment at varying treatment conditions. * $p<0.05$.

1053.4±134.6%, 1.0 mM; 1224.3±299.2% of the control level) and ACC (0.1 mM; 4019.5±830.7%, 1.0 mM; 3501.5±1238.9% of the control level) phosphorylation in H9c2 cells after 72 hours of incubation (Fig. 3B). In order to verify the effects of AMPK activity on the Met induced effects, cells were co-incubated with of compound-C, an AMPK inhibitor. A concentration of the compound-C (10 μM) was determined that did not affect the cell viability while higher concentrations (20 μM, 40 μM) significantly reduce cell viability at 72-hour (Fig. S5). As shown in Fig. 3C, co-incubation of compound-C completely reversed the effects of Met in attenuating Dox-induced reduction in cell viability (compound C-; 68.4±6.9%, compound C+; 51.9±5.6% of the control level). Furthermore, H9c2 cells were stably transfected with plasmids with wild type (WT), dominant-negative (DN) or constitutively active (CA) AMPKα1 cDNAs (Fig. S1). In DN-AMPKα cells the protective effect of 0.1 mM Met was completely abrogated (Fig. 3D). These findings suggested that the 0.1 mM Met-mediated protective effects were dependent on the AMPK activity. Some clones of the CA-AMPKα1 transfected H9c2 cells showed extremely high AMPK activities which were comparable to those of cells treated with 1.0 mM of Met (Fig. S1). Interestingly, the CA-AMPKα1 transfected cells which obtained extremely high AMPK activities did not show protective effects against Dox-induced toxicity (Fig. 3D, Fig. S6). These results suggest that Met protected cardiomyocytes through moderately enhanced AMPK activities and the protective effect was reversed if the AMPK activity exceeded a certain threshold.

Effects of PKA activity on protection against Dox-induced cardiomyocyte toxicity

In previous studies, we described PKA as a crucial factor in cell survival of isoproterenol stimulated H9c2 cells [24,25]. To determine the involvement of PKA in the Met mediated protective effects, PKA activities were measured by *in vitro* kinase assay. In the cells co-incubated with Met, PKA activities were significantly elevated (Met 0.1 mM; 187.6±37.6%, Met 1.0 mM; 211.6±81.5% of the control level; Fig. 4A). Dox treatment alone had no effect on either PKA activity (108.2%±23.9% of the control level) or phosphorylation of CREB-1 (102.5±26.3% of the control level), a downstream transcription factor of the cAMP/PKA signaling pathway. Met also significantly increased CREB-1 phosphorylation (Met 0.1 mM; 1209.1±294.0%, Met 1.0 mM; 1298.1±439.3% of the control level; Fig. 4B). Inhibition of PKA activity with H89 (10 μM) abolished the protective effect of 0.1 mM Met (Met 0.1 mM, H89-; 64.5±8.4%, H89+; 36.5±4.0% cell viability of the control level; Fig. 4C). Forskolin (1 μM), an activator of adenylyl cyclase, attenuated Dox-induced toxicity on the cardiomyocyte (forskolin-; 39.6±6.9%, forskolin+; 57.5±8.5% cell viability of the control level), but did not enhance the effect of 0.1 mM Met on cell viability (forskolin-; 64.5±8.4, forskolin+; 61.7±9.0 cell viability of the control level; Fig.4D). Furthermore, the Met induced PKA activities were reversed by co-incubation with compound-C (compound C-; 187.6±37.6%, compound C+; 112.7±19.1% of the control level; Fig. 4E). These data suggested that the protective effect of Met was mediated by

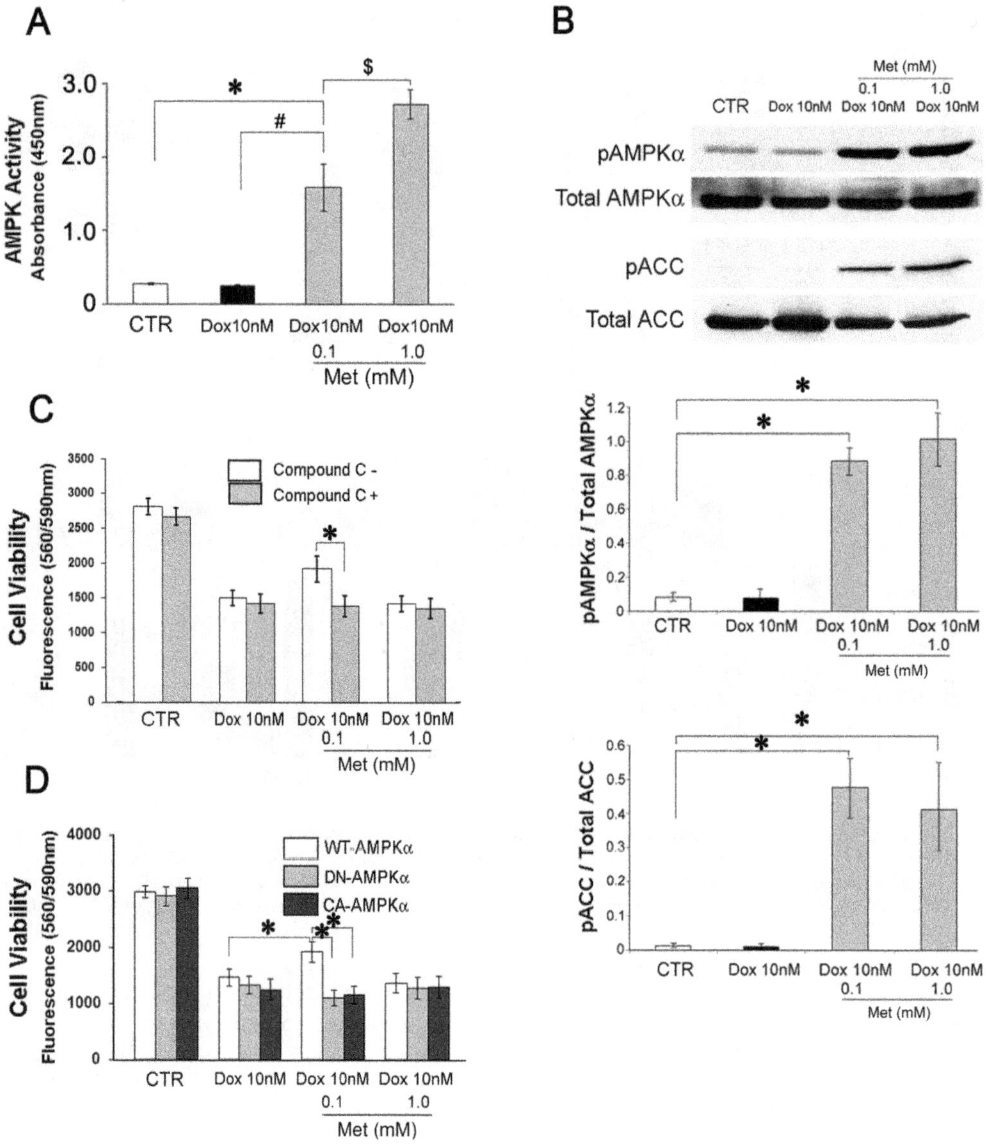

Figure 3. Protective effect of Met against Dox induced cytotoxicity depends on AMPK activity. (A) H9c2 cardiomyoblasts were cultured with reduced FBS (1%) for 72 hours, and then cell lysates were isolated with RIPA buffer supplemented with appropriate phosphatase inhibitors. AMP-activated protein kinase activities in the cell lysates were measured using an AMPK Kinase Assay Kit (Cyclex). (B) H9c2 cell lysates from 72 hour-culture were subject to western blotting using antibodies against phosphorylated or total AMPKα and acetyl-CoA carboxylase (ACC). The histograms show the densitometric scanning results. (C) H9c2 cells were cultured for 72 hours with reduced FBS (1%) in 96-well culture plates under indicated conditions with or without compound-C (10 μM). Cell viabilities were evaluated as described in Materials and Methods. (D) H9c2 cells stably over expressed wild type (WT), dominant negative (DN) or constitutively active (CA) AMPKα cDNA were cultured for 72 hours with reduced FBS (1%) under the indicated conditions. The cell viabilities were evaluated as described. Values represent mean ± S.D. from at least ten (A, C, D) or quadruplicate (B) samples for each treatment at varying treatment conditions. * $p<0.05$ vs CTR; # $p<0.05$ Dox 10 nM vs Dox 10 nM + Met 0.1 mM; $ $p<0.05$ Met 0.1 mM vs Met 1.0 mM (A), * $p<0.05$ (B, C, D).

the PKA activation, and the PKA activation was dependent on the AMPK activity.

Met-mediated protective effect is dependent on Src family tyrosine kinase

We have shown that the Src-family tyrosine kinase is involved in βAR-mediated anti-apoptosis in H9c2 cells [25]. In the present study, to explore the role of Src in Met-mediated cell protection, a series of experiments were initiated. First, cells were cultured with vehicle, Dox alone, or Dox in combination with Met for 72 hours, and then the cellular Src activity was measured. As shown in Fig. 5A, Met induced Src activation both in 0.1 and 1.0 mM of concentrations (189.9±51.9% and 203.3±42.0% of the control level, respectively).

Second, cSrc was knocked down by shRNA transfection. We have reported effective knockdown of Src at the RNA and protein levels in H9c2 cardiomyocyte with this approach [24,25]. In this study, H9c2 cells were stably transfected with a scrambled oligo control vector (pSilencer) or shSrc. Knock down of Src effectively obliterated the protective effect of 0.1 mM Met on the Dox-induced toxicity (pSilencer; 69.0±6.0%, shSrc; 35.7±6.0% cell viability of the control level; Fig. 5B).

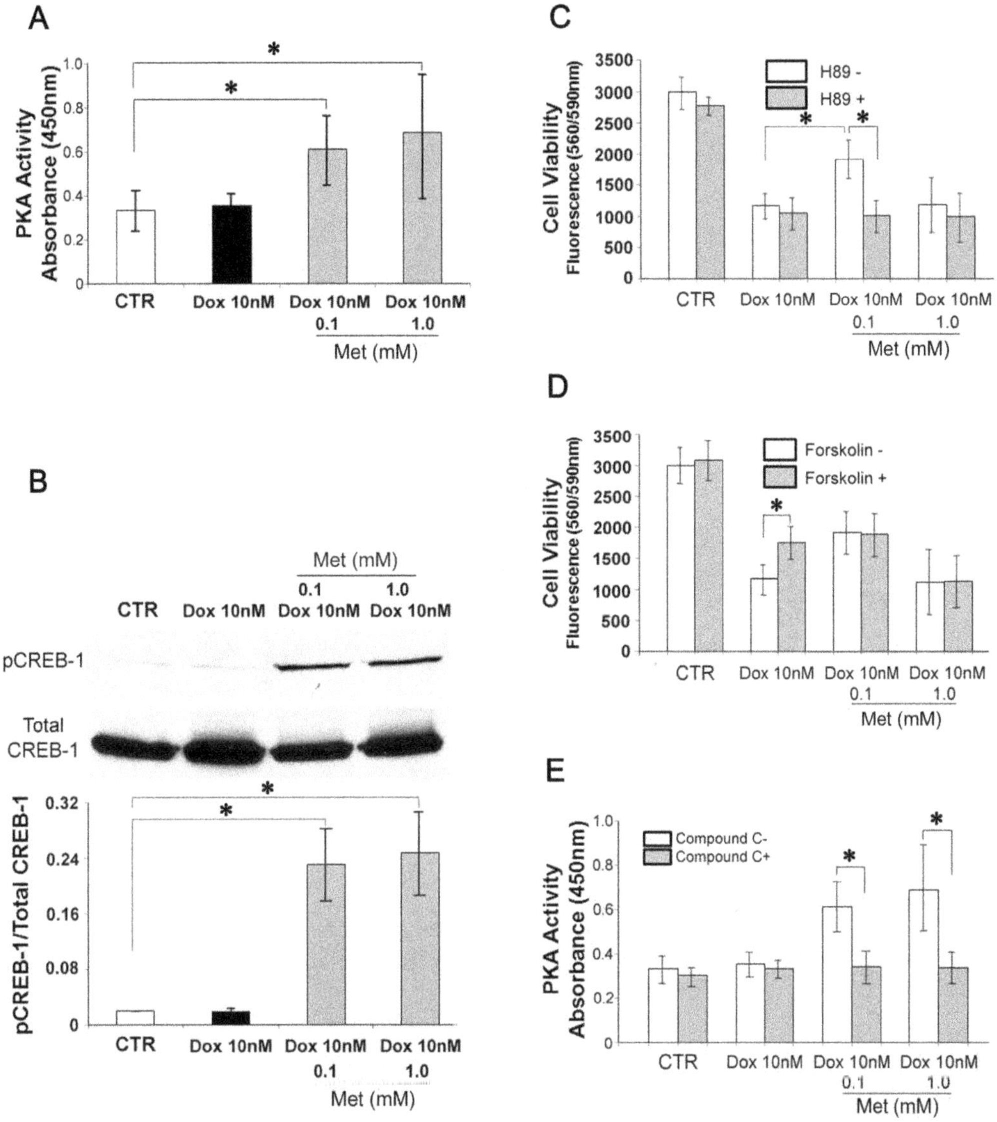

Figure 4. Protective effect of Met against Dox induced cytotoxicity is mediated by cAMP-PKA-CREB1 signaling pathway. (A) H9c2 cardiomyoblasts were cultured with reduced FBS (1%) for 72 hours, with indicated conditions and then cell lysates were isolated with RIPA buffer supplemented with appropriate phosphatase inhibitors. Protein kinase-A (PKA) activities in the cell lysates were measured as described in Materials and Methods. (B) H9c2 cell lysates from the 72 hour-culture were subject to Western blotting using antibodies against phosphorylated or total cAMP response element-binding protein-1 (CREB-1). The histograms show the densitometric scanning results. (C) H9c2 cells were cultured for 72 hours with reduced FBS (1%) under indicated conditions with or without H-89 (10 μM). The cell viabilities were evaluated as described. (D) H9c2 cells were cultured for 72 hours with reduced FBS (1%) for hours under indicated conditions with or without forskolin (1 μM). The cell viabilities were evaluated as described. (E) H9c2 cells were cultured for 72 hours with reduced FBS (1%), under indicated conditions with or without compound-C (10 μM) and then the cell lysates were evaluated for PKA activities. Values represent mean ± S.D. (n = 4) from quadruplicate samples for each treatment at varying treatment conditions. *, Statistically significant ($p<0.05$).

Third, constitutively active Src cDNA (Y529F) or a control vector (pUSEamp-) was stably transfected into H9c2 cells. Overexpression of the constitutively active Src significantly reduced Dox-induced cytotoxicity (pUSEamp-; 38.9±8.3%, active Src; 58.5±11.9% cell viability of the control level; Fig. 5C). The protective effect of 0.1 mM Met, however, was not further increased by overexpression of the constitutively active Src (pUSEamp-; 69.1±9.0%, active Src; 63.7±18.1% cell viability of the control level). Moreover, inhibition of PKA activity with H89 in these Src overexpressing cells did not abrogate the protective effect of 0.1 mM Met (active Src; 63.7±18.1%, active Src +H89; 72.6±10.1% cell viability of the control level; Fig.5D), which was observed in non-transfected H9c2 cells (Fig. 5C), suggesting PKA acts upstream of Src in this signaling pathway. These observations suggest that Src is a critical factor in the Met-induced anti-cytotoxic effect by functioning downstream of AMPK/PKA signaling pathway.

Expression of PDGFR is down regulated by co-incubation with 1.0 mM Met

We have shown that PDGFR plays a pivotal role in survival of H9c2 cells [24,25]. In order to explore the roles of PDGFR signaling in Met-induced survival in Dox-treated H9c2 cells,

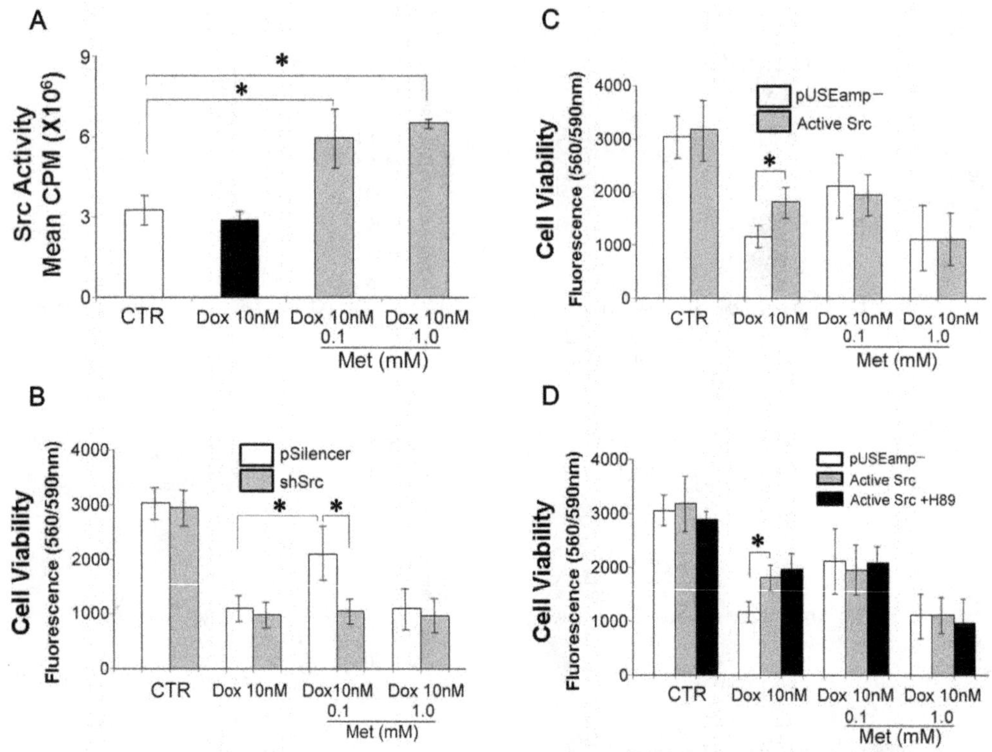

Figure 5. Protective effect of Met against Dox induced cytotoxicity is mediated by PKA dependent Src activation. (A) H9c2 cardiomyoblasts were cultured with reduced FBS (1%) for 72 hours, with indicated conditions. Src kinase activity was determined as described in Materials and Methods. The histograms show the average Src activity in CPM. (B) H9c2 cells stably transfected with short hairpin RNAi against cSrc (shSrc) or scrambled oligo encoded control plasmid (pSilencer) were cultured for 72 hours with reduced FBS (1%) the indicated conditions. The cell viabilities were evaluated as described. (C) H9c2 cells stably transfected with a constitutively active Src or a control empty vector (pUSEamp-) were cultured for 72 hours with reduced FBS (1%) under the indicated conditions. The cell viabilities were evaluated as described. (D) H9c2 cells stably transfected with an active Src or a control plasmid (pUSEamp-) were cultured for 72 hours under the indicated conditions with or without H89 (10 μM). Values represent mean ± S.D. (n = 4) from quadruplicate samples for each treatment at varying treatment conditions. *, Statistically significant ($p<0.05$).

experiments were performed as follows. Cellular expression and phosphorylation levels of PDGFR were evaluated by western blotting. As shown in Fig. 6A, the phosphorylation levels of PDGFRβ was increased in 0.1 mM Met treated rat neonatal primary cardiomyocytes and H9c2 cells. In contrast, the expression levels of the receptor were significantly suppressed in 1.0 mM Met treated cells. The PDGFR expression was also downregulated in the CA-AMPK transfected H9c2 cells which showed extremely high AMPK activity (Fig. S7). With the hypothesis that an AMPK/PKA/Src/PDGF sequence was a critical pathway for the Met induced cardiomyocyte protection and to verify the functional insufficiency of PDGFR response against PKA stimulation in 1.0 mM Met treated cells. We performed an experiment using activities of phosphoinositide 3-kinase (PI3K), a downstream molecule of PDGFR signaling, as an index for PDGFR sensitivities against forskolin. In 0.1 mM Met treated cells, forskolin stimulation induced a significant increase in PI3K activity while 1.0 mM Met treated cells showed no effect (Fig. 6B). Furthermore, co-incubation with AG1296, a PDGFR specific antagonist, abrogated 0.1 mM Met induced protective effect against Dox-mediated cytotoxicity in H9c2 cardiomyocytes (Fig. 6C). These findings suggested that PDGFR signaling is a crucial factor in Met-induced protective effect against Dox-mediated cytotoxicity of H9c2 cells. The reversal of the effect with the higher concentration (10 mM) of Met is a result of the down regulation and the functional loss of PDGFR.

Discussion

In this study, we demonstrated that metformin (Met), an anti-diabetic agent, has a clearly protective effect against doxorubicin-induced toxicity on cardiomyocytes through activation of AMPK. Whether Met, as a consequence of its modulated metabolism, influences cardiomyocyte survival remains unknown. We have previously reported a pro-survival/proliferation pathway in cardiomyocyte [24,25] and renal mesangial cells [26,27] involving G-protein coupled receptor (GPCR)-PKA-Src-receptor tyrosine kinase. The present study provides evidences that AMPK and PKA are activated sequentially following Met treatment. However, the mechanisms of AMPK dependent PKA activation are not fully clarified. A signaling interaction between AMPK and PKA was described in a hypothalamic cell line [28] and AMPK mediated CREB, a downstream transcription factor of a cAMP/PKA signaling pathway, activations were reported in hepatocyte [29] and neuronal cells [30]. Met/AMPK-induced transactivations of several GPCRs were also described in a pancreatic β-cell line [31]. All of the findings in the previous publications suggest high probability for the existence of AMPK/PKA/CREB or AMPK/GPCR/PKA/CREB signaling cascades in some cells.

Src has been identified as a key effector of PKA signaling [32,33]. In this study, we showed a pivotal role of the Src kinase as we have previously reported [24–26]. We have demonstrated that GPCR/PKA/Src to receptor tyrosine kinase (RTK) link is a

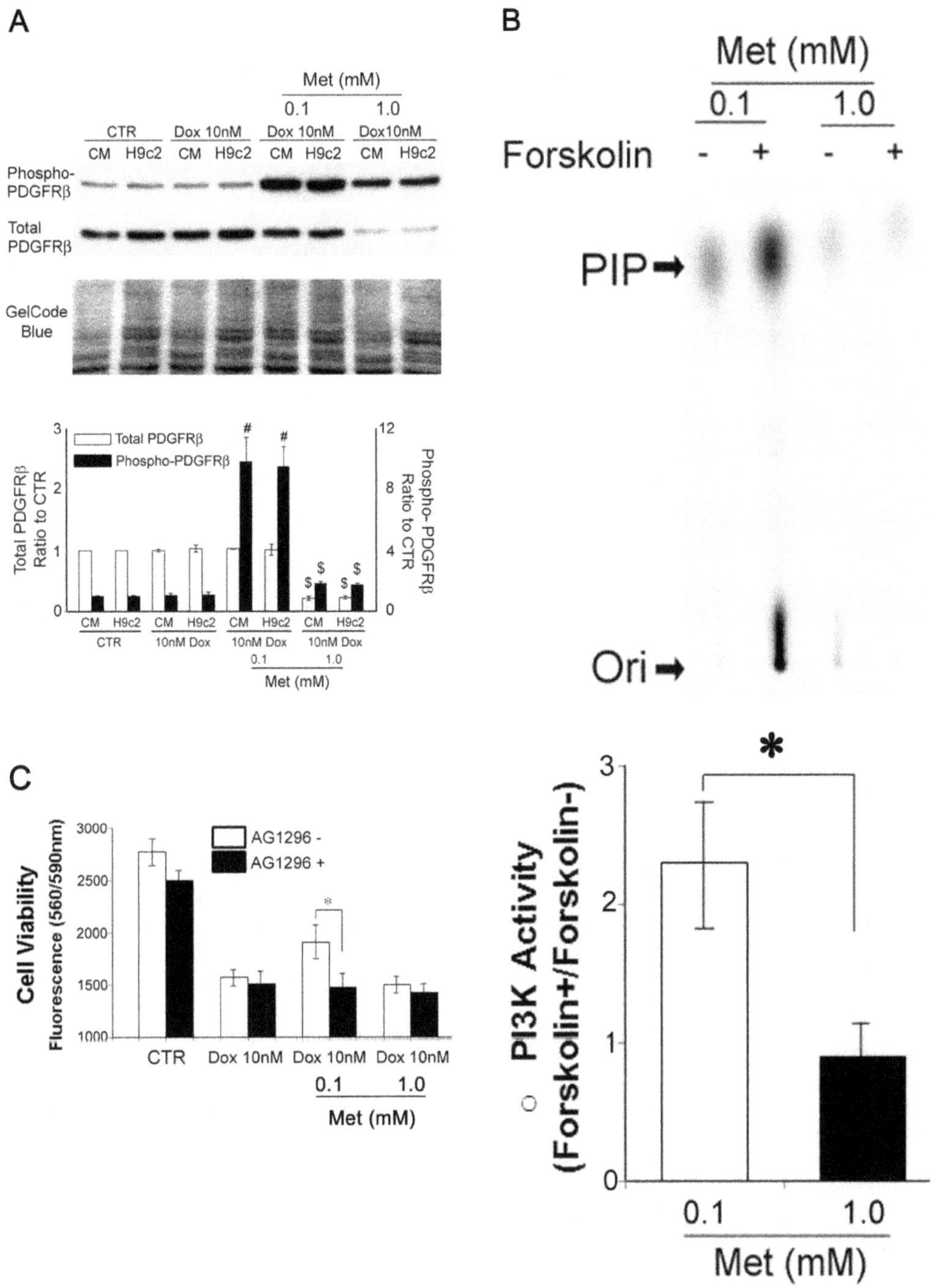

Figure 6. High dose Met abrogates the protective effects against Dox by suppressing the PDGFR expression. (A) Rat neonatal primary cardiomyocytes (CM) and H9c2 cardiomyoblasts were cultured with reduced FBS (1%) for 72 hours, with the indicated conditions. Cell lysates from the culture were subject to Western blotting using antibodies against phosphorylated or total platelet-derived growth factor receptor β-subunit (PDGFRβ). An image of the gel stained with GelCode Blue dye (Thermo) after transfer was shown as a loading monitor. The histograms show the densitometric scanning results. (B) Quiescent H9c2 cells were incubated with 0.1 or 1.0 mM metformin (Met) for 5 minutes with or without forskolin (1 μM). After the treatment, PI3K activities were determined as described in Materials and Methods. The histograms show the densitmetric scanning results. PIP, phosphoinositide 3-phosphate. Ori, origin of migration in thin-layer chromatography. (C) H9c2 cells were cultured for 72 hours with reduced FBS (1%), under the indicated conditions with or without AG1296 (10 μM). The cell viabilities were evaluated as described. * $p<0.05$, # $p<0.05$ vs CTR, $ $p<0.05$ vs Dox 10 nM + Met 0.1 mM. Values represent mean ± S.D. (n = 4) from quadruplicate samples for each treatment at varying treatment conditions.

notable pro-survival signaling pathway in cardiomyocytes and renal mesangial cells. In the present study, we provide convincing evidence that AMPK activation is critical in Met-mediated resistance against the Dox-induced cytotoxicity and that this protective effect was accomplished via sequential activation of PKA/Src/PDGFR.

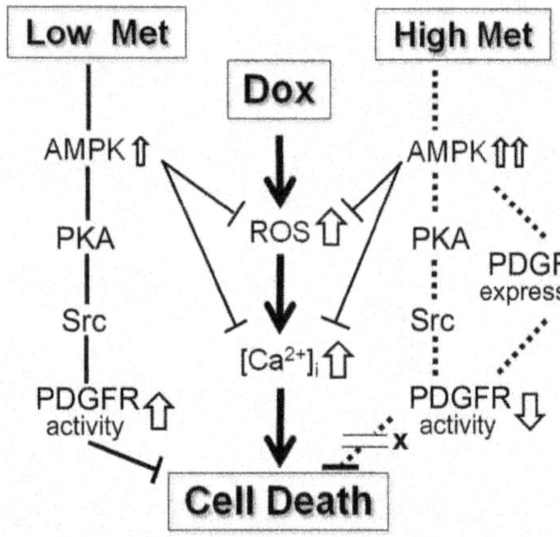

Figure 7. A hypothetical pathway for Met-mediated protection against Dox-induced toxicity in cardiomyocytes. Low dose (0.1 mM) Met induces moderate AMPK activation which is followed by sequential activations of PKA, Src and PDGFR and results in protection of the cells from Dox toxicity. High dose (1.0 mM) Met also leads to the sequential activations of AMPK, PKA and Src. With both dosages of the Met treatment, Dox induced ROS generations and $[Ca^{2+}]_i$ levels are suppressed. However, the excessive activities of AMPK with the high dose Met causes a suppression of PDGFR expression in cardiomyocytes and the protective effect of low dose Met is abrogated.

A very novel and interesting finding in this study is the dual effects of Met on cardiomyocyte survival. We showed that, at lower concentrations (0.1 mM), Met protected cardiomyocytes from the Dox-induced toxicity, whereas a higher concentration (1.0 mM) of Met failed to do so despite the fact that higher concentration of Met induced increases in many parameters we measured including AMPK. PKA, CREB1 and Src with even more potent manners than those with a lower concentration of Met. Moreover and most notably, a higher concentration of Met showed similar effects on ROS generations and $[Ca^{2+}]_i$ in Dox intoxicated cardiomyocytes. Our data suggested that the biphasic effect was caused by dose dependent alteration in PDGFR expression. Excessive AMPK activity in 1.0 mM Met treated cells may induce the suppression of the PDGFR expression. And the attenuated PDGFR signaling may be a factor to wipe out the Met induced effects of decreased ROS generation and $[Ca^{2+}]_i$ against Dox treatment. In the meanwhile, the elevated PDGFR activity in cells treated with the lower concentration of Met may overcome the Dox induced cardiotoxicity to maintain cell viabilities. However, this hypothesis is still premature because of lack of the bibliographical evidences to support it. Further investigations should be addressed to provide a logical explanation for these unexpected findings.

PDGF was originally identified in serum and platelets as a strong mitogen for fibroblasts, smooth muscle cells, and glial cells [34]. PDGF signaling plays important roles in the pathogenesis of several proliferative and degenerative diseases such as tumorigenesis, arteriosclerosis, and fibrosis [35]. In the present study, we demonstrated that the higher dose of Met resulted in a significant reduction of the levels of PDGFR. In contrast, lower dose of Met did not reduce the levels of PDGFR but enhanced the cellular activity of the receptor tyrosine kinase. More important, the protective effect of lower dose of Met is abrogated by PDGFR antagonist; clearly PDGFR signaling is important for the dual effect of Met-mediated protection against Dox toxicity.

In the last few years, several studies concerning about the protective effects of Met against the Dox toxicity has been published elsewhere [36–38]. Interestingly, in these papers, they demonstrated that even a dose of 4 mM of Met were able to protect cardiomyocytes in culture from the cytotoxic effect of doxorubicin. The cause of the discrepancy between our and their findings is not elucidated at present. Supposedly, differences in the lineage of the cells used (H9c2 vs HL-1) and dosage of Dox applied (10 nM vs 5 μM) may deduce to the inconsistency. Elucidating details in this discrepant action of Met on cardiomyocyte will benefit further understanding a mechanism of the protective effect of Met against cardiotoxicity of Dox.

The major proteolytic pathway involving the ubiquitin-proteasome system (UPS) is dependent on ATP [39]. Activation of AMPK results in the stimulation of a variety of cellular processes involved in the production of ATP, e. g., glucose uptake [40], protein synthesis [41] and UPS-mediated protein degradation [42]. In the present study, AMPK activity in 1.0 mM Met treated cells was significantly higher than those in 0.1 mM Met treated cells (Fig. 3A). Furthermore, constitutively active AMPKα cDNA transfected cells, which had even higher AMPK activities than those of 1.0 mM Met treated cells, showed suppressed PDGFR expression (Fig. S1, S6). Considering these findings, AMPK activities beyond a certain threshold may promote PDGFR degradation in H9c2 cardiomyocytes. Elucidating further details in this effect on PDGFR expression should be addressed in the future.

We have investigated the roles of AMPK and PKA as crucial factors in Met induced resistance against Dox toxicity on H9c2 cardiomyocytes. We demonstrated that PDGFR transactivation is involved in this pathway. We further established that Src played a pivotal role in the signaling pathway by functioning between PKA and PDGFR. We also described cellular PDGFR expression levels as regulatory factor for the protective effect of Met on cardiomyocytes. Based on these findings, despite the fact that bibliographic references to support this hypothesis are limited at present, we propose a hypothetical pathway for the Met-mediated protective effect against the Dox-induced toxicity on cardiomyocyte (Fig. 7). Although there are other components needed to be identified in this signaling pathway, our findings nonetheless provide important information for the protective effects of Met which has attracted attention recently. Elucidating further details in this signaling pathway should lead to better understanding over the conventional chemotherapy for malignant neoplasms.

Supporting Information

Figure S1 AMPK activities in empty vector (pcDNA3), wild type (WT), dominant negative (DN) or constitutively active (CA)-AMPKα transfected H9c2 cardiomyoblasts were as described in Materials and Methods. Three clones from each transfection were tested. Values represent mean ± S.D. (n = 4) from quadruplicate samples for each treatment. *, Significantly different from control (pcDNA3) ($p<0.05$).

Figure S2 Src activities in H9c2 cells stably transfected with empty control vector, shRNA against cSrc (sh-cSrc) or constitutively active Src cDNA H9c2 cardiomyocytes were evaluated as describes in Materials and Methods. Values represent mean ± S.D. (n = 4) from quadruplicate samples for each treatment. *, Significantly different from control (pSilencer for sh-cSrc and pUSEamp- for active Src) ($p<0.05$).

Figure S3 H9c2 cells were cultured for up to 96 hours with reduced FBS (1 with or without the indicated

concentrations of Dox. Cell viabilities were evaluated as described. Values represent mean (n = 4) from quadruplicate samples for each treatment.

Figure S4 H9c2 cells were cultured for indicated durations with reduced FBS (1%) with or without the indicated concentrations of Met. Cell viabilities (A), LDA leakages (B), ROS generations (C) and $[Ca^{2+}]_i$ (D) were evaluated as described. Values represent mean (n = 4) from quadruplicate samples for each treatment.

Figure S5 H9c2 cells were cultured for up to 72 hours with reduced FBS (1%) with or without the indicated concentrations of compound-C. Cell viabilities were evaluated as described. Values represent mean ± S.D. (n = 4) from quadruplicate samples for each treatment. *, Significantly different from control (CTR) ($p<0.05$).

Figure S6 H9c2 cells which were stably transfected with the indicated plasmids were cultured for 72 hours with reduced FBS (1%) with 10 nM Dox and 0.1 mM of Met. Cell viabilities and AMPK activities were evaluated as described.

Figure S7 Cell lysates from quiescent AMPKα plasmids transfected H9c2 cells were subject to Western blotting using antibodies against platelet-derived growth factor receptor β-subunit (PDGFRβ). An image of the gel stained after transfer was shown as a loading monitor. The histogram shows the densitometric scanning results. *, Significantly different from control (pcDNA3) ($p<0.05$).

Author Contributions

Conceived and designed the experiments: NY. Performed the experiments: NY LCK. Analyzed the data: NY LCK. Contributed reagents/materials/analysis tools: NY LCK. Wrote the paper: NY LCK. Review, and/or revision of the manuscript: LCK YCX YT JFP NY.

References

1. Wang JJ, Cortes E, Sinks LF, Holland JF (1971) Therapeutic effect and toxicity of adriamycin in patients with neoplastic disease. Cancer 28: 837–843.
2. Gottlieb JA, Gutterman JU, McCredie KB, Rodriguez V, Frei E III (1973) Chemotherapy of malignant lymphoma with adriamycin. Cancer Res 33: 3024–3028.
3. Iarussi D, Indolfi P, Casale F, Coppolino P, Tedesco MA, et al. (2001) Recent advances in the prevention of anthracycline cardiotoxicity in childhood. Curr Med Chem 8: 1649–1660.
4. Wallace KB (2003) Doxorubicin-induced cardiac mitochondrionopathy. Pharmacol Toxicol 93: 105–115.
5. Neilan TG, Blake SL, Ichinose F, Raher MJ, Buys ES, et al. (2007) Disruption of nitric oxide synthase 3 protects against the cardiac injury, dysfunction, and mortality induced by doxorubicin. Circulation 116: 506–514.
6. Kalivendi SV, Kotamraju S, Zhao H, Joseph J, Kalyanaraman B (2001) Doxorubicin-induced apoptosis is associated with increased transcription of endothelial nitric-oxide synthase. Effect of antiapoptotic antioxidants and calcium. J Biol Chem 276: 47266–47276.
7. Klip A, Leiter LA (1990) Cellular mechanism of action of metformin. Diabetes Care 13: 696–704.
8. Cusi K, Consoli A, DeFronzo RA (1996) Metabolic effects of metformin on glucose and lactate metabolism in noninsulin-dependent diabetes mellitus. J Clin Endocrinol Metab 81: 4059–4067.
9. Faure P, Rossini E, Wiernsperger N, Richard MJ, Favier A, et al. (1999) An insulin sensitizer improves the free radical defense system potential and insulin sensitivity in high fructose-fed rats. Diabetes 48: 353–357.
10. Kanigur-Sultuybek G, Guven M, Onaran I, Tezcan V, Cenani A, et al. (1995) The effect of metformin on insulin receptors and lipid peroxidation in alloxan and streptozotocin induced diabetes. J Basic Clin Physiol Pharmacol 6: 271–280.
11. Bhamra GS, Hausenloy DJ, Davidson SM, Carr RD, Paiva M, et al. (2008) Metformin protects the ischemic heart by the Akt-mediated inhibition of mitochondrial permeability transition pore opening. Basic Res Cardiol 103: 274–284.
12. Mahrouf M, Ouslimani N, Peynet J, Djelidi R, Couturier M, et al. (2006) Metformin reduces angiotensin-mediated intracellular production of reactive oxygen species in endothelial cells through the inhibition of protein kinase C. Biochem Pharmacol 72: 176–183.
13. Gundewar S, Calvert JW, Jha S, Toedt-Pingel I, Ji SY, et al. (2009) Activation of AMP-activated protein kinase by metformin improves left ventricular function and survival in heart failure. Circ Res 104: 403–411.
14. Sasaki H, Asanuma H, Fujita M, Takahama H, Wakeno M, et al. (2009) Metformin prevents progression of heart failure in dogs: role of AMP-activated protein kinase. Circulation 119: 2568–2577.
15. Kewalramani G, Puthanveetil P, Wang F, Kim MS, Deppe S, et al. (2009) AMP-activated protein kinase confers protection against TNF-α-induced cardiac cell death. Cardiovasc Res 84: 42–53.
16. Das A, Xi L, Kukreja RC (2005) Phosphodiesterase-5 inhibitor sildenafil preconditions adult cardiac myocytes against necrosis and apoptosis. Essential role of nitric oxide signaling. J Biol Chem 280: 12944–12955.
17. Tseng YT, Yano N, Rojan A, Stabila JP, McGonnigal BG, et al. (2005) Ontogeny of phosphoinositide 3-kinase signaling in developing heart: effect of acute β-adrenergic stimulation. Am J Physiol Heart Circ Physiol 289:H1834–H1842
18. Wong K, Cantley LC (1994) Cloning and characterization of a human phosphatidylinositol 4-kinase. J Biol Chem 269: 28878–28884.
19. Kalka D, Hoyer S (1998) Long-term cultivation of a neuroblastoma cell line in medium with reduced serum content as a model system for neuronal aging? Arch Gerontol Geriatr 27: 251–268.
20. An D, Kewalramani G, Chan JK, Qi D, Ghosh S, et al. (2006) Metformin influences cardiomyocyte cell death by pathways that are dependent and independent of caspase-3. Diabetologia 49: 2174–2184.
21. Yang J, Holman GD (2006) Long-term metformin treatment stimulates cardiomyocyte glucose transport through an AMP-activated protein kinase-dependent reduction in GLUT4 endocytosis. Endocrinology 147: 2728–2736.
22. Zhou G, Myers R, Li Y, Chen Y, Shen X, et al. (2001) Role of AMP-activated protein kinase in mechanism of metformin action. J Clin Invest 108: 1167–1174.
23. Fryer LG, Parbu-Patel A, Carling D (2002) The Anti-diabetic drugs rosiglitazone and metformin stimulate AMP-activated protein kinase through distinct signaling pathways. J Biol Chem 277: 25226–25232.
24. Yano N, Ianus V, Zhao TC, Tseng A, Padbury JF, et al. (2007) A novel signaling pathway for β-adrenergic receptor-mediated activation of phosphoinositide 3-kinase in H9c2 cardiomyocytes. Am J Physiol Heart Circ Physiol 293:H385–H393.
25. Yano N, Suzuki D, Endoh M, Tseng A, Stabila JP, et al. (2008) β-adrenergic receptor mediated protection against doxorubicin-induced apoptosis in cardiomyocytes: the impact of high ambient glucose. Endocrinology 149: 6449–6461.
26. Yano N, Suzuki D, Endoh M, Zhao TC, Padbury JF, et al. (2007) A novel phosphoinositide 3-kinase-dependent pathway for angiotensin II/AT-1 receptor-mediated induction of collagen synthesis in MES 13 mesangial cells. J Biol Chem 282: 18819–18830.
27. Yano N, Suzuki D, Endoh M, Cao TN, Dahdah JR, et al. (2009) High ambient glucose induces angiotensin-independent AT-1 receptor activation, leading to increases in proliferation and extracellular matrix accumulation in MES-13 mesangial cells. Biochem J 423: 129–143.
28. Damm E, Buech TR, Gudermann T, Breit A (2012) Melanocortin-induced PKA activation inhibits AMPK activity via ERK-1/2 and LKB-1 in hypothalamic GT1-7 cells. Mol Endocrinol 26: 643–654.
29. Yuan HD, Piao GC (2011) An active part of Artemisia sacrorum Ledeb. suppresses gluconeogenesis through AMPK mediated GSK3β and CREB phosphorylation in human HepG2 cells. Biosci Biotechnol Biochem 75: 1079–1084.
30. Choi IY, Ju C, Anthony Jalin AM, Lee d I, Prather PL, et al. (2013) Activation of cannabinoid CB2 receptor-mediated AMPK/CREB pathway reduces cerebral ischemic injury. Am J Pathol 182: 928–939.
31. Pan QR, Li WH, Wang H, Sun Q, Xiao XH, et al. (2009) Glucose, metformin, and AICAR regulate the expression of G protein-coupled receptor members in INS-1 β cell. Horm Metab Res 41: 799–804.
32. Ma YC, Huang J, Ali S, Lowry W, Huang XY (2000) Src tyrosine kinase is a novel direct effector of G proteins. Cell 102: 635–646.
33. Baker MA, Hetherington L, Aitken RJ (2006) Identification of SRC as a key PKA-stimulated tyrosine kinase involved in the capacitation-associated hyperactivation of murine spermatozoa. J Cell Sci 119: 3182–3192.
34. Heldin CH, Westermark B (1999) Mechanism of action and in vivo role of platelet-derived growth factor. Physiol Rev 79: 1283–1316.
35. Betsholtz C, Karlsson L, Lindahl P (2001) Developmental roles of platelet-derived growth factors. Bioessays 23: 494–507.
36. Asensio-López MC, Lax A, Pascual-Figal DA, Valdés M, Sánchez-Más J (2011) Metformin protects against doxorubicin-induced cardiotoxicity: involvement of the adiponectin cardiac system. Free Radic Biol Med 51: 1861–1871.

37. Asensio-López MC, Sánchez-Más J, Pascual-Figal DA, Abenza S, Pérez-Martínez, et al. (2013) Involvement of ferritin heavy chain in the preventive effect of metformin against doxorubicin-induced cardiotoxicity. Free Radic Biol Med 57: 188–200.
38. Asensio-López MC, Sánchez-Más J, Pascual-Figal DA, de Torre C, Valdes M, et al. (2014) Ferritin heavy chain as main mediator of preventive effect of metformin against mitochondrial damage induced by doxorubicin in cardiomyocytes. Free Radic Biol Med 67: 19–29.
39. Glickman MH, Ciechanover A (2002) The ubiquitin-proteasome proteolytic pathway: destruction for the sake of construction. Physiol Rev 82: 373–428.
40. Park H, Kaushik VK, Constant S, Prentki M, Przybytkowski E, et al. (2002) Coordinate regulation of malonyl-CoA decarboxylase, sn-glycerol-3-phosphate acyltransferase, and acetyl-CoA carboxylase by AMP-activated protein kinase in rat tissues in response to exercise. J Biol Chem 277: 32571–32577.
41. Bolster DR, Crozier SJ, Kimball SR, Jefferson LS (2002) AMP-activated protein kinase suppresses protein synthesis in rat skeletal muscle through down-regulated mammalian target of rapamycin (mTOR) signaling. J Biol Chem 277: 23977–23980.
42. Nakashima K, Yakabe Y (2007) AMPK activation stimulates myofibrillar protein degradation and expression of atrophy-related ubiquitin ligases by increasing FOXO transcription factors in C2C12 myotubes. Biosci Biotechnol Biochem 71: 1650–1656.

The Reversal Effects of 3-Bromopyruvate on Multidrug Resistance *In Vitro* and *In Vivo* Derived from Human Breast MCF-7/ADR Cells

Long Wu[1], **Jun Xu[1]**, **Weiqi Yuan[1]**, **Baojian Wu[2]**, **Hao Wang[3]**, **Guangquan Liu[1]**, **Xiaoxiong Wang[1]**, **Jun Du[3]***, **Shaohui Cai[1]***

1 Department of Clinical Pharmacology, College of Pharmacy, Jinan University, Guangzhou 510632, P. R. China, **2** Division of Pharmaceutics, College of Pharmacy, Jinan University, Guangzhou 510632, P. R. China, **3** School of Pharmaceutical Sciences, Sun Yat-sen University, Guang Zhou 510275, P. R. China

Abstract

Purpose: P-glycoprotein mediated efflux is one of the main mechanisms for multidrug resistance in cancers, and 3-Bromopyruvate acts as a promising multidrug resistance reversal compound in our study. To test the ability of 3-Bromopyruvate to overcome P-glycoprotein-mediated multidrug resistance and to explore its mechanisms of multidrug resistance reversal in MCF-7/ADR cells, we evaluate the *in vitro* and *in vivo* modulatory activity of this compound.

Methods: The *in vitro* and *in vivo* activity was determined using the MTT assay and human breast cancer xenograft models. The gene and protein expression of P-glycoprotein were determined using real-time polymerase chain reaction and the Western blotting technique, respectively. ABCB-1 bioactivity was tested by fluorescence microscopy, multi-mode microplate reader, and flow cytometry. The intracellular levels of ATP, HK-II, and ATPase activity were based on an assay kit according to the manufacturer's instructions.

Results: 3-Bromopyruvate treatment led to marked decreases in the IC_{50} values of selected chemotherapeutic drugs [e.g., doxorubicin (283 folds), paclitaxel (85 folds), daunorubicin (201 folds), and epirubicin (171 folds)] in MCF-7/ADR cells. 3-Bromopyruvate was found also to potentiate significantly the antitumor activity of epirubicin against MCF-7/ADR xenografts. The intracellular level of ATP decreased 44%, 46% in the presence of 12.5.25 μM 3-Bromopyruvate, whereas the accumulation of rhodamine 123 and epirubicin (two typical P-glycoprotein substrates) in cells was significantly increased. Furthermore, we found that the mRNA and the total protein level of P-glycoprotein were slightly altered by 3-Bromopyruvate. Moreover, the ATPase activity was significantly inhibited when 3-Bromopyruvate was applied.

Conclusion: We demonstrated that 3-Bromopyruvate can reverse P-glycoprotein-mediated efflux in MCF-7/ADR cells. Multidrug resistance reversal by 3-Bromopyruvate occurred through at least three approaches, namely, a decrease in the intracellular level of ATP and HK-II bioactivity, the inhibition of ATPase activity, and the slight decrease in P-glycoprotein expression in MCF-7/ADR cells.

Editor: Aamir Ahmad, Wayne State University School of Medicine, United States of America

Funding: This work was funded by the National Natural Science Foundation of China (No. 30973565, No. 81273538 and No. 81202461) and the Fundamental Research Funds for the Central Universities (No. 21612115) as well as China Postdoctoral Science Foundation (No. 2013M531906). The funders had no role in study design, data collection and analysis, decision to publish, or preparation of the manuscript.

Competing Interests: The authors have declared that no competing interests exist.

* Email: dujun2345@yahoo.cn (JD); csh5689@sina.com (SHC)

These authors contributed equally to this work.

Introduction

Breast cancer is one of the most critical threats to women, and its incidence is increasing year by year [1]. Chemotherapy and endocrine therapy are still predominantly used for the treatment of breast cancer. While advancements in breast cancer treatment and prevention have emerged over the last decade, multidrug resistance (MDR) has been a main cause of breast cancer chemotherapy failure [2]. The mechanisms underlying MDR are rather complex, and among them, transporter-mediated efflux is a major one that has received enormous attention [3,4]. The efflux transporters, including P-glycoprotein (ABCB-1/P-gp)[5], multidrug resistance proteins (MRPs) [6], and breast cancer resistance protein (BCRP) [7] are over-expressed in many cancer cells, limiting the entry of the drug into the inside of cells and conferring the resistance of cells to the drugs [4]. P-gp belongs to the ABC transporter family (ABC) with seventeen trans-membrane helices and two ATP-binding domains [2]. The physiological expression of P-gp protein has been found in liver, intestine, and

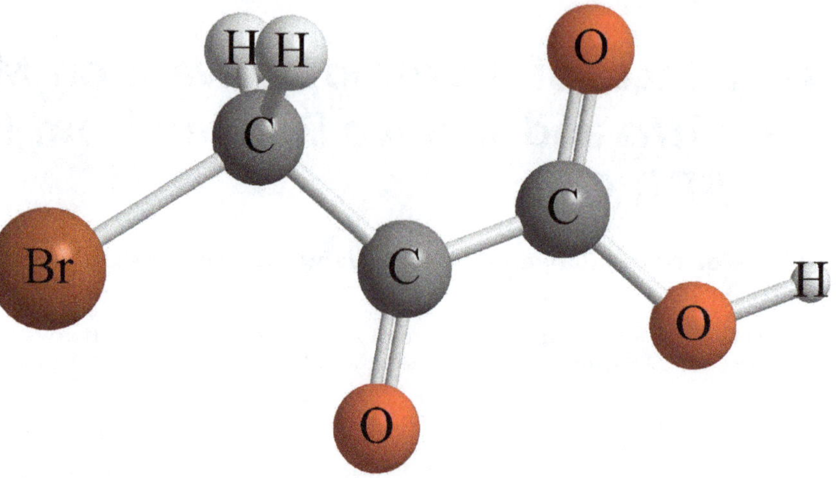

Figure 1. Chemical structure of 3-BrPA.

blood-brain barrier. Many anticancer drugs (e.g., doxorubicin, paclitaxel, daunorubicin, and epirubicin) are substrates of P-gp [8]. However, it is still difficult to predict P-gp activity toward a new compound, although many structure-activity relationships have been established.

3-Bromopyruvate (3-BrPA; Fig. 1) is a hexokinase II (HK-II) inhibitor, showing potent inhibitory activity in the glycolysis process [9]. 3-BrPA demonstrates anticancer activity in a panel of cancer cell lines and animal tumor models [10]. Most of the known targets are thus involved in energy metabolism, and the anticancer effect of 3-BrPA is accordingly proposed to be due to the high dependence of tumor cells on glycolysis [26]. It is also reasonable to deduce that 3-BrPA can efficiently reverse the MDR of ABCB-1/P-gp overexpressing tumor cells, which with a high demand for ATP produced by glycolysis. Therefore, the objective of the present study is to characterize the biochemical changes caused by 3-BrPA using MCF-7/ADR cells in an attempt to elucidate the mechanisms underlying MDR reversal. The biochemical characterization was centered on the P-gp function and the ATP level. Our study should be beneficial to the ultimate elucidation of the mechanisms of MDR reversal by 3-BrPA.

Materials and Methods

Chemicals and reagents

3-BrPA, verapamil (VRP), paclitaxel, MTT and rhodamine 123(Rh123) were purchased from Sigma-Aldrich (Deisenhofen, Germany). Doxorubicin (Dox) and epirubicin (EPI) were purchased from Zhejiang HISUN Pharmaceuticals Co (Zhejiang, China). Daunorubicin was supplied by National Institute for the Food and Drug Control (Beijing, China). Mouse anti-ABCB-1/P-gp was obtained from Santa Cruz (CA, USA). Other antibodies were purchased from Cell Signaling Technology (Beverly, MA, USA). Alexa Fluor 488 goat anti-mouse IgG (H+L) was purchased from Life Technologies (Gaithersburg, MD, USA).

Cell culture and cell viability

The breast cancer cell line MCF-7 and its drug-resistant variant MCF-7/ADR were kindly provided by Cancer institute & Hospital. Chinese Academy of Medical Sciences (Beijing, China).

These cell lines were maintained in RPMI1640 medium (Sigma, U.S.A.) supplemented with 10% fetal bovine serum (HyClone, U.S.A.), 100 units/mL penicillin G (Sigma, U.S.A.) and 100 μg/mL streptomycin (Sigma, U.S.A.). Cells were incubated in a humidified atmosphere with 5% CO_2 at 37°C [12].

Cell viability was determined using the MTT assay. Cells were seeded in 96-well plates for 24h for cell attachment and were then incubated for 48 h with various concentrations (0.005–50 μM) of doxorubicin, paclitaxel, daunorubicin, and epirubicin in the presence or absence of 3-BrPA or VRP. MTT was then added into each well, and the cells were incubated for 4h [13]. Finally, the plates were centrifuged (1,000 rpm, 5 min) and the supernatant removed. The cell pellets were dissolved in 150 μL DMSO. The colored formazan products were quantified photometrically at 490 nm in a multi-mode microplate reader (Bio-Rad Laboratories, U.S.A.), and IC_{50} was then calculated using Graphpad Prism 5.0 [14].

Animals and xenograft model

Female Balb/c nude, 4–6 weeks, 18–22 g weight were housed in a specific pathogen-free room using the MCF-7 and MCF-7/ADR xenografts. All experiment animals were purchased from the Guangdong Medical Laboratory Animal Center.

In our study, the models of xenografts of MCF-7 and MCF-7/ADR were established as follows: the breast cancer cell line MCF-7 and its drug-resistant variant MCF-7/ADR cells were collected and resuspended in PBS with an equal volume of Matrigel (BD,USA) and then were inoculated into the mice for chemotherapeutic studies. Mice received a subcutaneous (s.c.) injection of the cells under the armpit (10^7 cells in 200μL). After s.c. implantation of the cells, the mice were randomized into four groups after the tumors reached approximately 100 mm^3 in size, and then they received various regimens: control (normal saline, q2d×11, iv); 3-BrPA (q2d×11, iv, 5 mg/kg); EPI (q2d×11, iv, 0.5 mg/kg); 3-BrPA (q2d×11, iv, 5 mg/kg) and EPI (q2d×11, iv, 0.5 mg/kg) (3-BrPA and EPI were dissolved in normal saline and given 1 h before EPI was injected). The animals' weight was measured every 2 days. We monitored tumor growth starting on the first day of treatment and measured the volume of the xenograft every 2 days. The tumor volume (V) was calculated using the formula $V = \pi a*b^2/6$, where a and b are the longest and shortest diameters, respectively. Experiments were approved by the Laboratory Animal Ethics Committee Jinan University, China (Permit Number: 20131225001).

Table 1. Primers used for real-time PCR.

Gene	Forward primer 5′-3′	Reverse primer 5′-3′
ABCA-1	CAATCTCACCACTTCGGTCTCCA	CTCTTCTCATCACTTTCCTCGCC
ABCB-1[29]	TGGTGTTTGGAGAAATGACAGATAT	ACCAATTCCACTGTAATAATAGGCA
ABCC-1	AAATAGAGACTGAGAGTGAGCAACC	CATGAGAGGGAAAGAAAAGAGG
ABCC-2	CCTATGTCCCACAGCAGTCCT	ATTTATACCCTTCTCTCCAATCTCA
ABCC-3	CTGTTTTCTTTGTCACCCCCTTG	CAGAAGATAATGAGGACCCCCG
ABCG-1	AAGGGGGTCGCTCCATCATTT	GGTTGTGGTAGGTTGGGCAGTT
ABCG-2	AAAGGAACCCAAGGAGATAGGAG	GCAGGAGAAAGAATGAGAGAGGAAA
β-actin [30]	GTTGCGTTACACCCTTTCTTGAC	CTCGGCCACATTGTGAACTTTG

Drug accumulation and efflux assay

For visualization of the effects of 3-BrPA on the intracellular retention of Rh123, 5×10^5 cells were seeded on 6-well plate slides on the day prior to the assay and treatment with 3-BrPA (12.5, 25 μM) or 10 μM VRP for 4 h at 37°C. Then cells were incubated with either 5 μM Rh123 alone or a 5 μM Rh123 complex with 3-BrPA or VRP in fresh RPMI1640 medium for 1 h in darkness at 37°C. After the cells were washed for three times with cold PBS, images were acquired by fluorescence microscopy (Olympus, Japan) 488 nm excitation and 535 nm emission [15] wavelength [16].

To make a further quantitative analysis of Rh123 retention, 1×10^4 cells/well were seeded in 96-well black plates, cultured overnight, and treated with 3-BrPA (12.5, 25 μM) or 10 μM VRP for 4 h at 37°C. Cells were then incubated with either 5 μM Rh123 alone or in the presence of 3-BrPA or VRP in fresh RPMI1640 medium for 1 h at 37°C. After washing cells for three times with cold PBS, the fluorescent intensity was detected by multi-mode microplate reader at 488 nm excitation and 535 nm emission wavelengths.

Simultaneously, Rh123 efflux was also quantified in this study, 1×10^4 cells/well were seeded in 96-well black plates and cultured overnight. Cells were treated with 3-BrPA (12.5, 25 μM) or 10 μM VRP for 4 h at 37°C. Then 5 μM Rh123 or 5 μM Rh123 with 3-BrPA as well as VRP was cultured in fresh RPMI1640 medium for 1 h at 37°C. After the removal of Rh123, an exclusion step was performed in the presence or absence of 3-BrPA or VRP, and then the cells were washed three times with cold PBS at the desired time (0, 30, 60, 90, or 120 min) and measured spectrofluorometrically

Table 2. Effect of 3-BrPA on reversing ABCB-1/P-gp mediated drug resistance in MCF-7 and MCF-7/ADR.

Drug	Combined medication		IC_{50}± SD[a] (μM) (fold-reversal)[b]	
			MCF-7	MCF-7/ADR
doxorubicin	3-BrPA (μM)	0	0.41±0.021(1.00)	9.35±0.039(1.00)
		12.5	0.62±0.004(0.66)	0.46±0.032(20.33)**
		25	0.40±0.054(1.02)	0.03±0.001(283.33)**,#
	VRP (μM)	10	0.38±0.017(1.08)	0.45±0.040(20.92)**
Paclitaxel	3-BrPA (μM)	0	0.05±0.001(1.00)	4.08±0.032(1.00)
		12.5	0.047±0.007(1.06)	0.477±0.095(8.55)**
		25	0.046±0.005(1.09)	0.048±0.007(85)**,#
	VRP (μM)	10	0.045±0.001(1.01)	0.463±0.015(8.81)**
daunorubicin	3-BrPA (μM)	0	0.078±0.003(1.00)	22.47±0.033(1.00)
		12.5	0.077±0.003(1.01)	0.112±0.003(200.6)**
		25	0.078±0.008(1.00)	0.105±0.004(214)**
	VRP (μM)	10	0.079±0.009(0.99)	0.112±0.001(200.6)**
epirubicin	3-BrPA (μM)	0	0.153±0.008(1.00)	18.49±0.097(1.00)
		12.5	0.245±0.071(0.62)	0.122±0.042(151.6)**
		25	0.213±0.036(0.72)	0.108±0.003(171.2)**
	VRP (μM)	10	0.105±0.018(1.46)	0.196±0.001(96.4)**

Cell survival was determined by MTT assay as described in Materials and Methods.
[a]Data in the table are shown as the means ± SD (n = 6) of at least three independent experiments.
[b]RR value indicating the fold reversal of MDR.
**$P<0.01$,*$P<0.05$ for the IC_{50} versus that absence of 3-BrPA.
#$P<0.05$ for the IC_{50} versus that VRP.

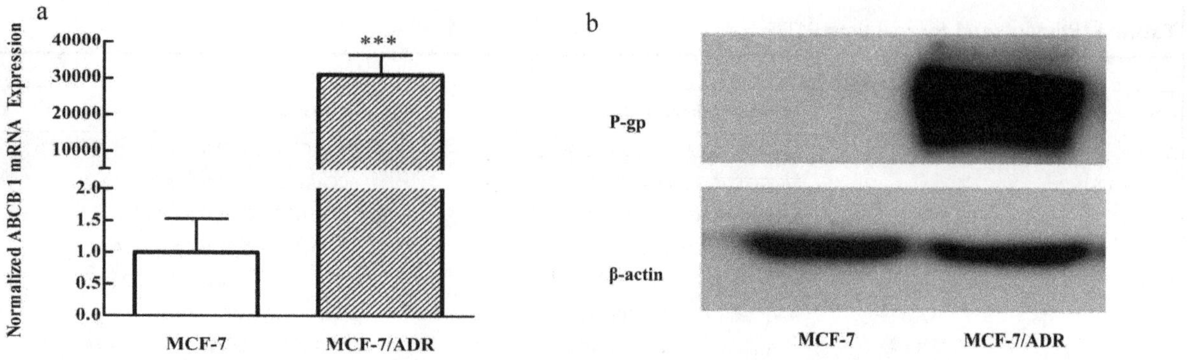

Figure 2. P-gp overexpression in MCF-7/ADR cell lines. a: ABCB-1 expression level in MCF-7 vs. MCF-7/ADR cells by real-time PCR b: P-gp expression level in MCF-7 vs. MCF-7/ADR cells by Western blotting ***$P<0.001$ versus the parental cells.

at 488 nm excitation and 535 nm emission wavelength using a multi-mode microplate reader [17].

The intracellular amount of EPI was quantitatively determined by flow cytometry (Beckman Coulter, U.S.A.). One milliliter of cell suspension (1×10^6 cells/mL) was treated with various concentrations of 3-BrPA (12.5, 25 μM) or 10 μM verapamil for 4 h at 37°C and then incubated with 10 μM EPI for an additional 1 h in darkness at 37°C, respectively. After that, cells were collected by

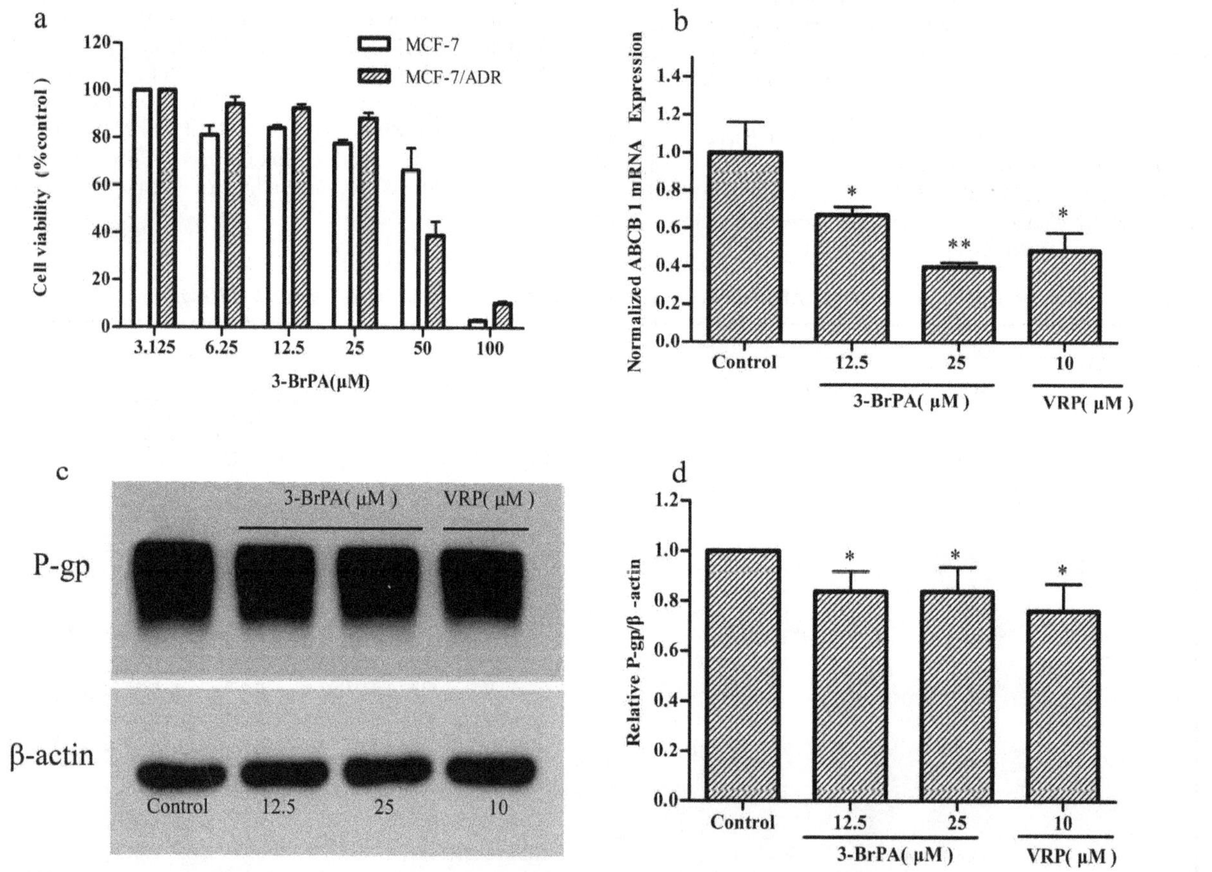

Figure 3. The cytotoxicity of 3-BrPA, effect of 3-BrPA on the mRNA and protein expression levels of ABCB-1/P-gp. These cell lines were exposed to the indicated concentration of 3-BrPA for 48 h, and cell viability was determined by MTT assay. Each points represents the mean ± SD (n = 6). Each experiment was performed three times. a: The cytotoxicity of 3-BrPA in MCF-7, MCF-7/ADR,After treated with desired concentrations of 3-BrPA for 48 h b: The mRNA level of P-gp in MCF-7/ADR cells treated with or without 3-BrPA was determined by real –time PCR, β-actin served as internal controls for real-time PCR respectively. c, d: The protein expression level of P-gp in MCF-7/ADR cells treated with or without 3-BrPA was determined by Western blotting analysis, β-actin served as internal controls Western blotting, respectively. *$P<0.05$ compared with the control, **$P<0.01$compared with the control.

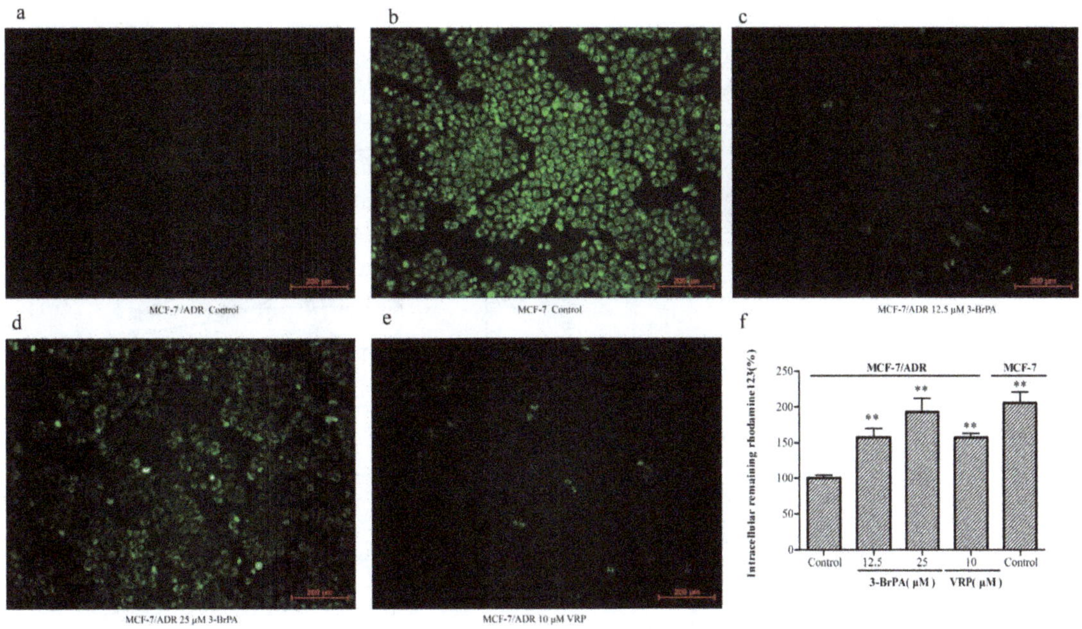

Figure 4. 3-BrPA and VRP increase the accumulation of Rh123 in MCF-7/ADR cells. Cells were treated with 12.5, 25 μM 3-BrPA and 10 μμ VRP for 4 h at 37°C. Then Rh123 (5 μM) was added and incubated in the dark at 37°C for an additional 1 h. After washing cells three times with cold PBS, images were acquired by a fluorescence microscopy at 488 nm extraction and 535 nm emission wavelength for Rh123. The fluorescence intensity was quantitatively detected by multi-mode microplate reader. a-e: 3-BrPA and VRP increase the accumulation of Rh123 in MCF-7/ADR by fluorescence microscopy f: 3-BrPA and VRP increase the accumulation of Rh123 in MCF-7/ADR by multi-mode microplate reader $^{**}P<0.05$ compared with the control.

centrifugation at 1,000 rpm and washed for three times with cold PBS. Finally, the cells were re-suspended in PBS buffer and analyzed by flow cytometry (Beckman Coulter, U.S.A.) equipped at an excitation wavelength of 488 nm and an emission wavelength 590 nm, respectively [18].

Intracellular ATP measurement

Intracellular ATP levels were measured using a firefly luciferase based ATP Assay Kit (Beyotime, China) according to the manufacturer's instructions. In brief, 5×10^4 cells/well were seeded in 12-well plates for 24 h to allow for cell attachment and were then incubated with or without 3-BrPA (12.5, 25 μM) in RPMI1640 medium for 48 h at 37°C. After every well plate, 100 μL of each supernatant was mixed with 100 μL ATP detection working dilution. Luminance (RLU) was measured by multi-mode microplate reader. The protein of each treatment group was determined by the BCA Protein Assay Kit (Beyotime, China). The total ATP levels were expressed as n mol/mg protein [19].

Hexokinase-II bioactivity

The activity of Hexokinase-II (HK-II) was examined by HK Assay Kit (Nanjinjiancheng, China). In brief, cells were seeded in plates cultured overnight to allow for cell attachment and were then incubated with or without 3-BrPA (12.5, 25 μM) in RPMI1640 medium for 48 h at 37°C. After that, the activities of HK-II bioactivity were detected by ultraviolet spectrophotometry (Thermo, USA) [20].

Real-time PCR detection of mRNA

The expression of a cancer resistance protein gene was analyzed at the mRNA and the protein level in this study. The mRNA expression was determined by real-time PCR. Total RNA was isolated from cells and tumor tissues using the Trizol reagent (Takara, Japan) according to the manufacturer's instructions [21]. Complementary DNA (cDNA) corresponding to 0.8 μg of total RNA was used per reaction (20 μL) in a real-time quantitative PCR reaction performed on a Roche Light Cycler (Mannheim, Germany) and using Power SYBER Green Master Mix (Takara, Japan). The primers as shown in Table 1.

Western blotting

Protein lysates collected from cells and tumor tissues were resolved by SDS-PAGE and transferred onto PVDF membranes (0.22 μm). The membranes were incubated with the desired primary antibody for P-gp (1:1,000) and β-actin (1:1,000) overnight at 4°C, followed by incubation with the appropriate secondary antibody for 2 h at room temperature. The detection of β-actin was used as a loading control [22].

ATPase activity

The ATPase activity was determined by P-gp-Glo Assay Systems with P-glycoprotein (Promega, U.S.A.). Sodium vanadate (Na_3VO_4) was used as a P-gp ATPase inhibitor. The activity of P-gp ATPase was measured in the presence of 3-BrPA, in accordance with the instructions. The sample luminescence reflects the ATP level, which is negatively correlated with the activity of P-gp ATPase and recorded using the multi-mode microplate readers [17]. The activity detected in cells treated with the test compound is expressed as the percentage of basal activity. By comparing the basal activity to the activity after exposure to test compounds, the compounds can be ranked as stimulating, inhibiting, or having no effect on basal P-gp ATPase activity.

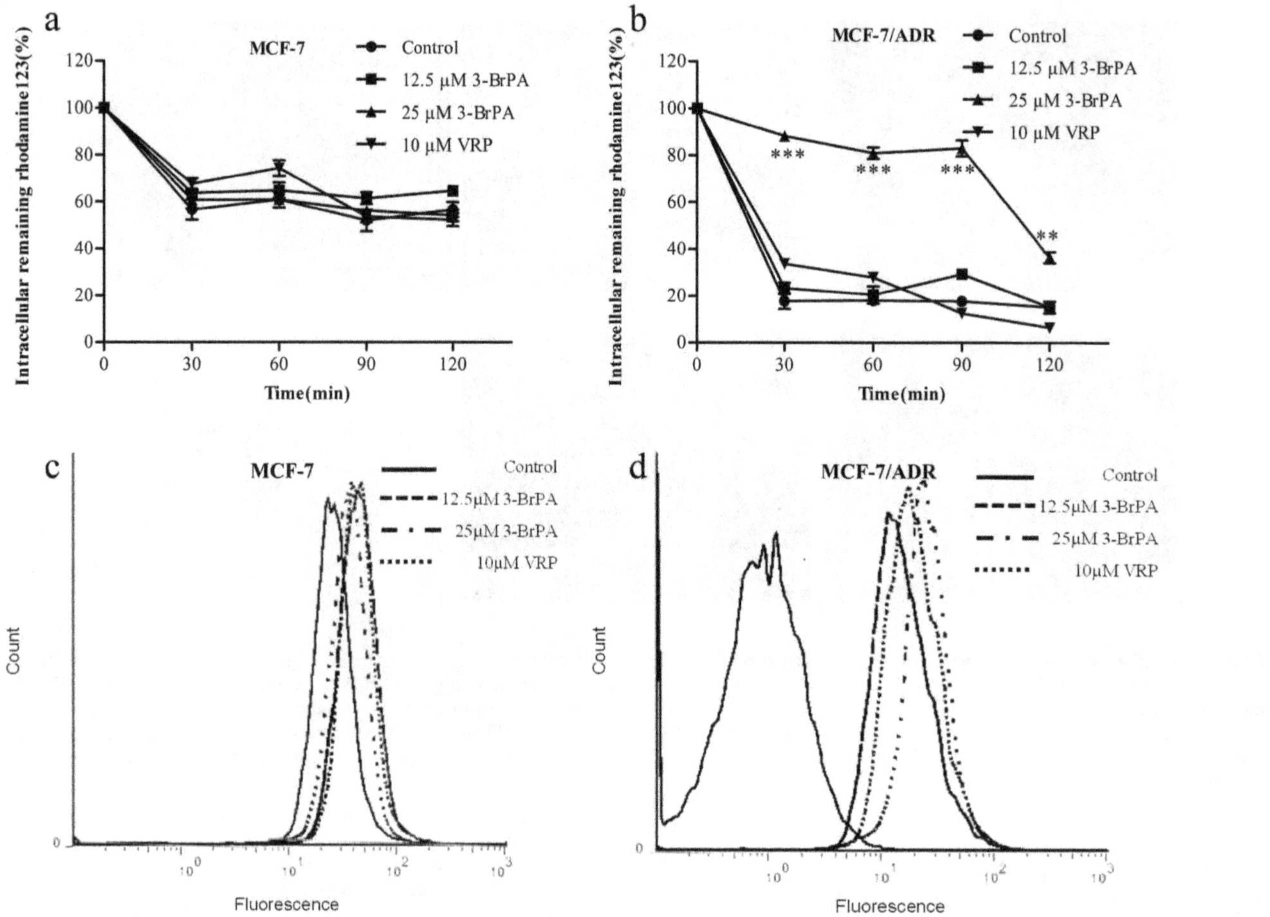

Figure 5. Inhibition of Rh123 efflux from MCF-7/ADR cells by 3-BrPA and VRP. 3-BrPA and VRP increase the accumulation of EPI in cells. a,b: After incubation 1 h in the presence of Rh123 (5 μM) and 3-BrPA (12.5, 25 μM) and VRP (10 μM),the cells were washed and incubated in fresh medium for indicated times. Each point represents the mean ± SD (n = 6). Each experiment was performed three times. c,d: These cells were incubated with 3-BrPA (12.5, 25 μM) at 37°C for 4 h, then 10 μM EPI was added for another 1 h incubation. Intracellular fluorescence was analyzed by flow cytometry. Control cells that were not exposed to any 3-BrPA, and VRP (10 μM) were used as positive control. The change of intracellular fluorescence in MCF-7 and MCF-7/ADR ***$P<0.01$ compared with the control.

Data analysis

Each experiment was conducted at least three times, and the data are expressed as mean ± SD. A significant difference was determined using one-way ANOVA analysis. A value of $P<0.05$, $P<0.01$, or $P<0.001$ was considered statistically significant.

The multidrug resistance ratio (MR) was defined to evaluate the extent of cell resistance to the anti-cancer drugs:

$$MR = \frac{IC_{50,(\text{the P-gp overexpressing cell lines})}}{IC_{50,(\text{the corresponding parental lines})}}.$$

The reversal ratio (RR) was defined to evaluate the ability of a reversing agent to reverse the multidrug resistance:

$$RR = \frac{IC_{50,(\text{the P-gp overexpressing cell lines})}}{IC_{50,(\text{the presence of reverser the P-gp overexpressing cell lines})}}.$$

Results

MDR characterization in MCF-7/ADR cells

We determined the IC_{50} values of several anti-cancer drugs in both MCF-7/ADR cells and their parental cells (Table 2). The multidrug resistance ratios (MRs) were 23, 82, 288, and 121 for doxorubicin, paclitaxel, daunorubicin, and epirubicin, respectively. The results indicated that MCF-7/ADR was a suitable cell line for the evaluation of the MDR reversal capability of 3-BrPA.

ABCB-1/P-gp overexpression in MCF-7/ADR cells

The mRNA level of ABCB-1 in MCF-7/ADR cells was significantly higher (about 30,000 times) than that in MCF-7 (Fig. 2a). In addition, the P-gp protein was overexpressed in the multidrug resistance cell line, whereas it was hardly found in the parental cells (Fig. 2b).

MDR reversal by 3-BrPA in MCF-7/ADR cells

The cytotoxicity of 3-BrPA was evaluated using MTT assay. 3-BrPA showed significant cytotoxicity when the dose was 50 μM or higher (Fig. 3a). Therefore, two dosing levels (12.5 μM and 25 μM) that did not show obvious cytotoxicity were chosen to

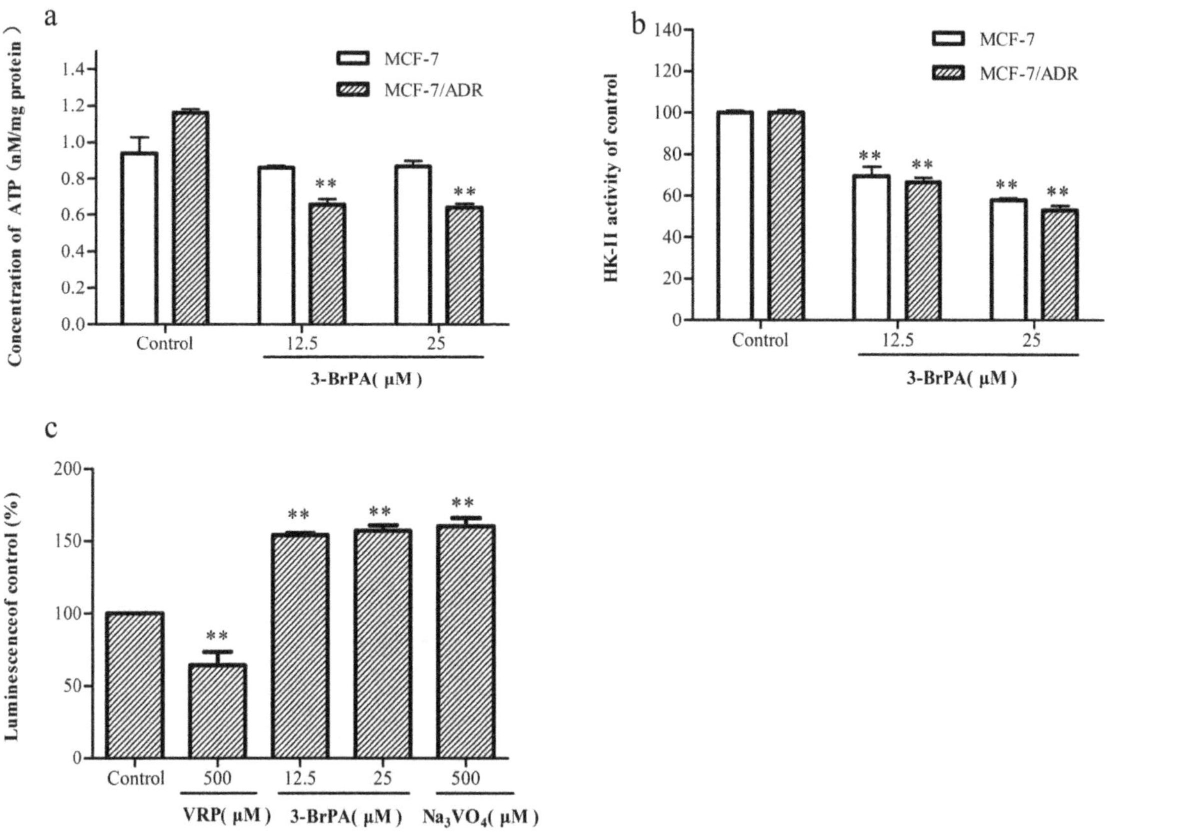

Figure 6. Reduction in ATP production and inhibition of HK-II and ABCB-1 ATPase activity of cells by 3-BrPA. After the treatment with 3-BrPA (12.5, 25 μM), the ATP levels and HK-II activity were determined by ATP Assay Kit and HK Assay Kit respectively. Each point represents the mean ± SD (n = 6). The ATPase activity of ABCB-1 was determined in recombinant human ABCB-1 membranes treated with 3-BrPA compared with Na_3VO_4. Each point represents the mean ± SD (n = 6) for at least three replicates. a: The effect of 3-BrPA on ATP level in MCF-7 and MCF-7/ADR b: The effect of 3-BrPA on HK-II activity in MCF-7 and MCF-7/ADR c: The effect of 3-BrPA on ABCB-1 ATPase activity in MCF-7 and MCF-7/ADR $^{**}P<0.01$ compared with the control.

assess their MDR reversal ability. 3-BrPA significantly decreased the IC_{50} values of doxorubicin, paclitaxel, daunorubicin, and epirubicin in MCF-7/ADR cells, whereas it did not alter the IC_{50} values in MCF-7 cells (Table 2). The reversal ratios (RRs) were 20–283, 9–85, 201–214 and 152–171 for doxorubicin, paclitaxel, daunorubicin, and epirubicin, respectively. The results indicated that 3-BrPA significantly reversed the resistance of the cells to the typical chemotherapeutics that are P-gp substrates [23].

The changes of ABCB-1/P-gp expression caused by 3-BrPA *in vitro*

The use of 3-BrPA led to slight decreases (of 0.3–0.6 times) in the mRNA level of ABCB-1 in MCF-7/ADR cells (Fig. 3b). Meanwhile, the expression of P-gp protein was also slightly reduced by 0.17 and 0.2 in the presence of 3-BrPA (12.5, 25 μM) (Fig. 3c and 3d).

3-BrPA enhancement of the uptake of Rh123 and EPI in MCF-7/ADR cells

The accumulation of Rh123 was greatly enhanced by 3-BrPA in the resistant cells, evidenced by the increased fluorescent intensity in the presence of the compound (Fig. 4a). The extent of enhancement was 1.8 times, as revealed by the quantitative analysis (Fig. 4b). To be specific, the percentage of remaining intracellular Rh123 at 30, 60, 90, and 120 min in MCF-7/ADR is 88%, 83%, 81%, and 37% of control, respectively, after incubation with 25 μM 3-BrPA (Fig. 5b). These results suggested that 3-BrPA can modify the transport property of Rh123, which may result from the inhibition of ABCB-1/P-gp functioning.

The EPI uptake in MCF-7/ADR cells was measured using flow cytometric analysis [24]. The results showed that the location of the fluorescence peak gradually shifted to the right (about 90%) in the presence of 3-BrPA in relation to its absence (Fig. 5c). However, the changes in EPI uptake were negligible in MCF-7.

3-BrPA decreased the intracellular level of ATP and inhibited the HK-II bioactivity in MCF-7/ADR cells

The ATP levels, which were only 0.13 and 0.14 n mol/mg protein in the parental cells, were significantly decreased inside of the resistant cells by 0.51 and 0.52 n mol/mg protein by 3-BrPA (Fig. 6a). Furthermore, 3-BrPA (12.5–25 μM) inhibited almost half of the HK-II activity in both resistant and parental cells (Fig. 6b).

The biological actions of 3-BrPA appear to be rather complex [25,26]. The important intracellular proteins that interacted with 3-BrPA included HK-II [27], GAPDH, and mitochondrial succinate dehydrogenase. The decrease in the ATP level was most likely resulted from HK-II inhibition associated with the reduced ATP production from glycolysis [28]. This is supported by

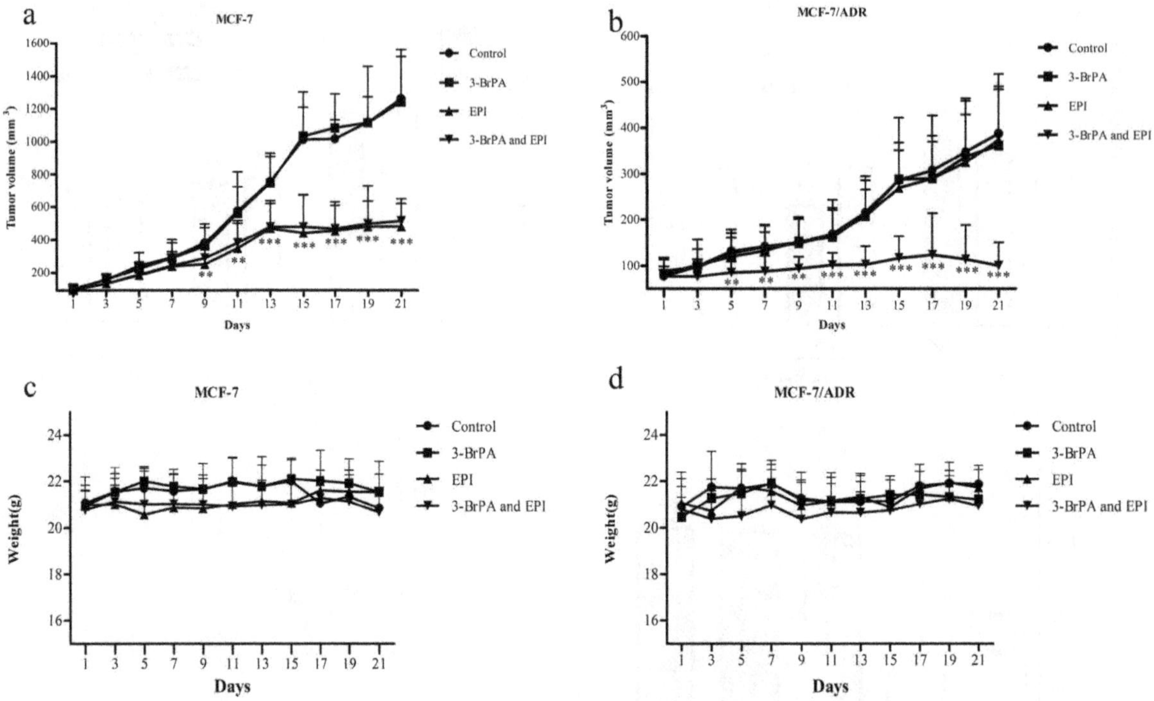

Figure 7. The MDR reversal effect of 3-BrPA on MCF/ADR xenograft model. The treatments were as follows: control (normal saline, q2d×11, iv); 3-BrPA (q2d×11, iv, 5 mg/kg); EPI (q2d×11, iv, 0.5 mg/kg); 3-BrPA (q2d×11, iv, 5 mg/kg) and EPI (q2d×11, iv, 0.5 mg/kg), 3-BrPA and EPI were dissolved in normal saline, and was given 1 h before EPI was injected, mean of tumor volume for each group (n = 6) after implantation. Each point on line graph represents the mean of tumor volume (mm^3) at a particular day after implantation, and each bar represents SD. Potentiation of antitumor effects of EPI by 3-BrPA in ABCB-1/P-gp overexpressing MCF-7/ADR xenograft model is shown. a: Changes in the mean of tumor volume over the time course of the experiment in MCF-7 xenograft model. b: Changes in tumor volume over the time course of the experiment in ABCB-1/P-gp overexpressing MCF-7/ADR xenograft model are shown. c: Changes in the mean of body weight over the time course of the experiment in MCF-7 xenograft model are shown. d: Changes in the mean of body weight over the time course of the experiment in ABCB-1/P-gp overexpressing MCF-7/ADR xenograft model are shown. ***$P<0.001$ versus the control group; **$P<0.01$ versus the control group.

the fact that the HK-II activity was inhibited by 3-BrPA in the resistant cells (Fig. 6b).

3-BrPA showed inhibitory effects on ATPase activity

The inhibitory effects of 3-BrPA on ATPase activity was assessed using the ATPase Assay Kit. 3-BrPA showed strong inhibition on ATPase activity, and the inhibitory potency of 3-BrPA (12.5 and 25 μM) was comparable to that of sodium vanadate (Fig. 6c).

Reversal of MDR by 3-BrPA in MCF-7/ADR xenografts

The MCF-7/ADR cells were exposed to 25 μM 3-BrPA, achieving the maximum potentiation of EPI cytotoxicity (171-fold, Table 2). 3-BrPA was also found to potentiate significantly the antitumor activity of EPI against MCF-7/ADR xenografts *in vivo* (Fig. 7).

No significant difference was observed in tumor size between experimental animals treated with saline and EPI in MCF-7/ADR. However, the mean tumor size in the EPI group was significantly smaller than that of the saline groups in MCF-7 (Fig. 7a and 7b). The results indicated that it is a suitable *in vivo* model for evaluation of the MDR reversal capability of 3-BrPA.

Treatment of 3-BrPA tumor-bearing nude mice with EPI (0.5 mg/kg, i.v.) or 3-BrPA (5 mg/kg, i.v.) alone had little or no effect on the growth rate of the tumors (Fig. 7b and Fig. 8). However, 3-BrPA plus EPI reduced the growth rate of the tumors significantly (Fig. 7b and Fig. 8). Remarkably, the regimen of the combination of EPI and 3-BrPA did not cause any deaths in the experimental process. There was no substantial or reproducible increase in body weight loss in animals treated with EPI plus 3-BrPA compared with the drug-alone groups (Fig. 7c and 7d). This suggests that this regimen did not result in increased toxic side effects. Therefore, the toxicity of co-administration of EPI and 3-BrPA was tolerable.

Down-regulation of ABCB-1/P-gp expression caused by 3-BrPA *in vivo*

To investigate the significance of ABCB-1/P-gp down-regulation *in vivo*, we assessed ABCB-1/P-gp expression in tumor tissues. Real-time PCR and Western blotting results demonstrated that treatment with 3-BrPA resulted in 30% ABCB-1 mRNA and 40% P-gp protein reduction of normal saline in MCF-7/ADR xenografts, respectively (Fig. 9a and 9b). Interestingly, the increased ABCB-1 mRNA and P-gp protein levels in the EPI group's tumor tissue were confirmed by real-time PCR and Western blotting. However, the ABCB-1/P-gp expression of the 3-BrPA plus EPI group was significantly smaller than that of the EPI group in MCF-7/ADR tumor tissue. These data indicate that 3-BrPA inhibits the expression of ABCB-1/P-gp *in vivo*.

Discussion

A broad range of MDR reversal modulators that interact with ABC transporters have been reported in preclinical or clinical trials since the advent of the first-generation MDR reversal agents (e.g., VRP and cyclosporine A). However, there are two major

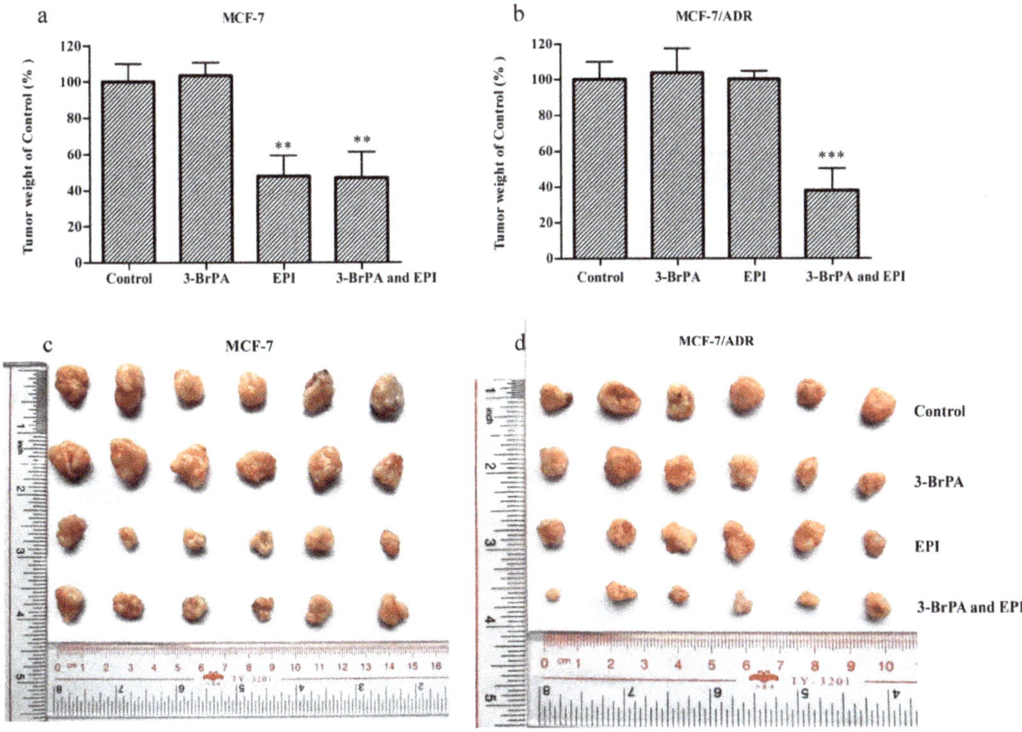

Figure 8. The changes of tumor weight by 3-BrPA on MCF/ADR xenograft model. a: The bar graph represents the mean of tumor weights (mice, n = 6) of the excised MCF-7 tumor from different mice. b: The bar graph represents the mean of tumor weights (mice, n = 6) of the excised ABCB-1/P-gp overexpressing MCF-7/ADR tumor from different groups. c:A representative picture of the excised MCF-7 tumor sizes from different groups is shown on the 21th day after implantation. d: A representative picture of the excised ABCB-1/P-gp overexpressing MCF-7/ADR tumor sizes from different groups is shown on the 21th day after implantation. Each group represents the mean of determinations, and the bar represents SD. ***$P<0.001$ versus the control group; **$P<0.01$ versus the control group.

defects as that enhancing the toxicity of the cytotoxic drugs and relative non-specificity with weak effect. All of these obstacles clearly indicate that the development of potential MDR reversal modulators with low toxicity is an important approach to the research on modulators. Recently, Ayako Nakano found that glycolysis inhibition restores the susceptibility of ABC transporter-expressing cells to chemotherapeutic agents [11]. 3-BrPA is a potent inhibitor of HK-II and effectively inhibits glycolysis. Most of the known targets are thus involved in energy metabolism, and the anti-cancer effect of 3-BrPA is accordingly proposed to be due to the high dependence of tumor cells on glycolysis [26]. It is also reasonable to deduce that 3-BrPA can efficiently reverse the MDR of ABCB-1/P-gp overexpressing tumor cells, which with a high demand for ATP produced by glycolysis.

The present *in vitro* and *in vivo* studies demonstrated that 3-BrPA is a more potent modulator of P-gp mediated MDR than the first-generation positive modulator VRP. The *in vitro* and *in vivo* potency were evaluated by several assays using a drug-resistant variant MCF-7/ADR with a high level of ABCB-1/P-gp special expression (*Fig. S1*), which was confirmed by real-time PCR in our studies. MTT assay was used to assess quantitatively the effect of 3-BrPA by calculating the IC_{50} and the reversal ratios (RRs) after the post addition of cytotoxic drugs. To preclude the intrinsic cytotoxicity of 3-BrPA, a non-cytotoxic concentration of 3-BrPA was selected to be used in our studies, and the results showed that 3-BrPA was very potent in reversing the resistance of MCF-7/ADR cell lines. The same assay was also used for MCF-7 to determine whether 3-BrPA could function with the cytotoxic drugs to reverse MDR or not. As the results showed, 3-BrPA did not influence the IC_{50} of the wild-type MCF-7 cells, confirming the combined sensitizing effect of 3-BrPA. Based on the above results, further experiments were conducted *in vivo*. The ability of 3-BrPA to reverse P-gp-mediated MDR *in vivo* was evaluated using MCF-7 and MCF-7/ADR xenograft models in combination with cytotoxic drug EPI to investigate the effect of 3-BrPA *in vivo*. As the data showed, EPI alone significantly reduced the growth rate of the parental sensitive MCF-7 cell line xenograft and that the co-administration of 3-BrPA did not enhance the activity of EPI. In contrast, EPI used alone had no effect on the growth rate of the MCF-7/ADR resistant cell line tumors, while the co-administration of 3-BrPA restored the antitumor activity of cytotoxic agent. 3-BrPA showed great promise in reversing cancer cell resistance to chemotherapeutics in the present data.

Given the results shown above, we investigated whether 3-BrPA could inhibit the efflux of ABCB-1 to enhance the cytotoxicity of the agents by increasing the intracellular drug concentration as following two parts. We first observed the accumulation Rh123 a substrate of ABCB-1 by spectrofluorometrically, multi-mode microplate reader, and flow cytometry, suggesting that the intracellular accumulation of Rh123 and EPI was enhanced under the presence of 3-BrPA. However, we also found that the degree of the fluorescence decay of Rh123 in the presence of 3-BrPA was significantly slower than in the control group, which showed that the effect of 3-BrPA on enhancing the accumulation of Rh123 in resistant cells was closely related to its power in inhibiting the efflux of Rh123. As much evidence has shown, the resistant cell lines frequently ABCB-1/P-gp overexpress cells,

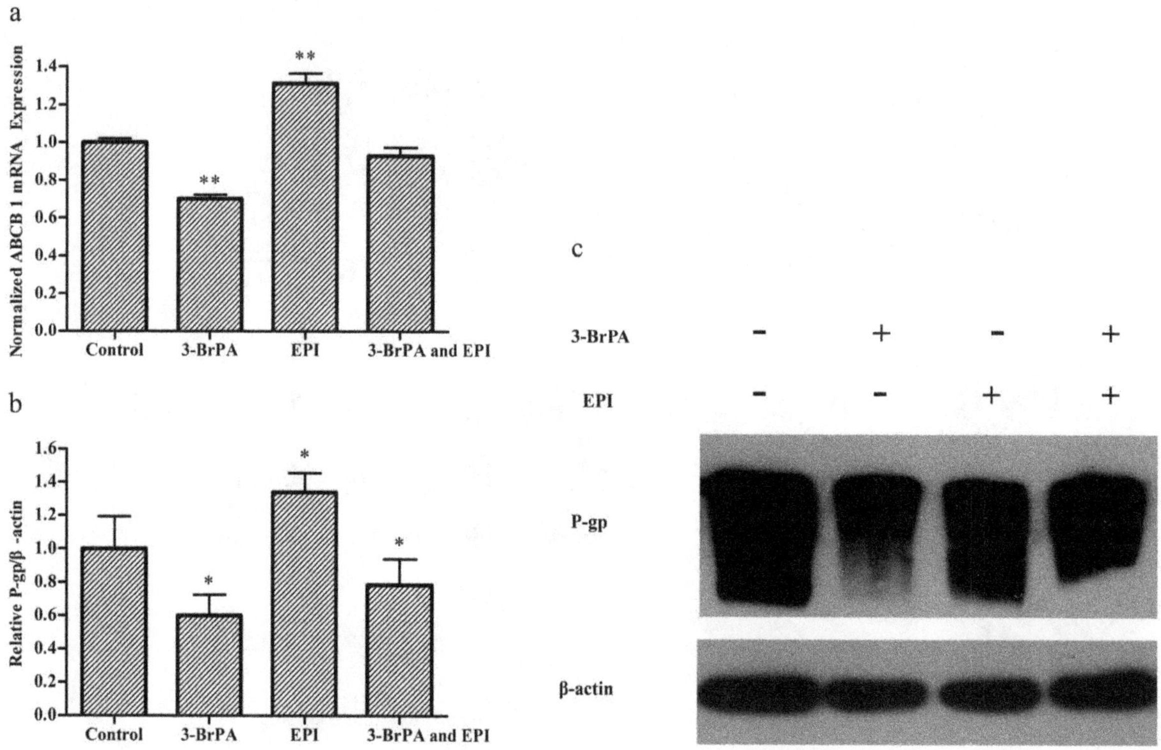

Figure 9. ABCB-1/P-gp expression changes caused by 3-BrPA *in vivo*. a: The mRNA level of ABCB-1 in MCF-7/ADR tumor tissue treated with different groups was determined by real-time PCR, β-actin served as internal controls for real-time PCR respectively. b, c: The protein expression level of P-gp in MCF-7/ADR tumor tissue treated with different groups was determined by Western blotting analysis, β-actin served as internal controls Western blotting, respectively. **P*<0.05 compared with the control, ***P*<0.01 compared with the control.

showing a positive correlation with the degree of resistance of the cells.

Many compounds show the power to reverse resistance in tumor cells by down the expression of ABCB-1/P-gp. In our previous studies, the real-time PCR and Western blotting results showed that ABCB-1/P-gp did drop slightly at the mRNA and protein levels in MCF-7/ADR cells and tumor tissue. More interestingly, this is the first time we have found that 3-BrPA could influence the distribution of P-gp (*Fig. S2*). We speculate that 3-BrPA ubiquitin ligases affect protein turnover. What is worth more attention is that 3-BrPA could reverse the resistance of tumor cells by depleting ATP and inhibiting the activity of HK-II at the same time.

One of the major reason to inhibit the activity of ABCB-1/P-gp activity is to deplete ATP. Thus, we investigated the effect of 3-BrPA on the function of ABCB-1/P-gp. ABCB-1 is a transporter protein with two trans-membrane domains (TMD) and two nucleotide binding domains (NBD). A substrate can get into the substrate-binding region favorably when it enters the cell through the phospholipid bilayer, which will stimulate the release of ATP. ATP hydrolysis plays an important role in this process, so ATPase plays a key role in influencing the ABCB-1 function on transporting drugs. The data from our studies indicated that 3-BrPA had a direct inhibitory effect on ATPase activity, which also illustrated that 3-BrPA could influence ABCB-1 function by inhibiting the ATPase.

3-BrPA was shown to be a great modulator of P-gp-mediated MDR *in vitro* and *in vivo* with glorious potential. *In vivo*, 3-BrPA appeared to be well tolerated, whether used alone or in combination with cytotoxic agents, as indicated by the minimal change in body weight and the zero mortality rates. Meanwhile, the HE assay also showed that there was no apparent tissue necrosis in all major organs (*data not shown*). However, in our research on 3-BrPA, we also found that the most prominent feature of 3-BrPA was the low stability. Therefore, further research will be conducted on 3-BrPA to reform its structure, trying to obtain a stable, targeted MDR reversal agent with low-toxicity. To the best of our knowledge, the great reversal activity of 3-BrPA may remind us not only that the macromolecule compounds have great reversal activity but also that a small molecule is likely to be achieved easily with high efficiency and sometimes low toxicity. Finally, it is expected that all the workon 3-BrPA will provide useful clues for further research on MDR reversal agents. Elucidation of the MDR reversal mechanism is of interest to pharmacologists, as the information would provide guidance on whether it is possible to develop 3-BrPA as an adjuvant MDR-reversing agent in chemotherapy.

Supporting Information

Figure S1 ABC family genes expression *in vitro* and *in vivo*. a: The mRNA level of ABCA-1,ABCB-1, ABCC-1, ABCC-2, ABCC-3,ABCG-1,ABCG-2 in MCF-7 and MCF-7/ADR cells. b: The mRNA level of ABCA-1,ABCB-1, ABCC-1, ABCC-2, ABCC-3,ABCG-1,ABCG-2 in MCF-7 and MCF-7/ADR tumor tissues.

Figure S2 3-BrPA could influence the distribution of P-gp.

Author Contributions

Conceived and designed the experiments: LW JX JD SHC. Performed the experiments: LW JX WQY GQL HW XXW. Analyzed the data: LW JX. Contributed reagents/materials/analysis tools: BJW JD SHC. Contributed to the writing of the manuscript: LW JX BJW.

References

1. Fernandes AF, Cruz A, Moreira C, Santos MC, Silva T (2014) Social Support Provided to Women Undergoing Breast Cancer Treatment: A Study Review. Advances in Breast Cancer Research 3: 47–53.
2. Aller SG, Yu J, Ward A, Weng Y, Chittaboina S, et al. (2009) Structure of P-glycoprotein reveals a molecular basis for poly-specific drug binding. Science 323: 1718–1722.
3. Zahreddine H, Borden KL (2013) Mechanisms and insights into drug resistance in cancer. Frontiers in pharmacology 4: 1–8.
4. Ling V (1997) Multidrug resistance: molecular mechanisms and clinical relevance. Cancer Chemoth Pharm 40: S3-S8.
5. Ni L-N, Li J-Y, Miao K-R, Qiao C, Zhang S-J, et al. (2011) Multidrug resistance gene (MDR1) polymorphisms correlate with imatinib response in chronic myeloid leukemia. Med Oncol 28: 265–269.
6. Choudhuri S, Klaassen CD (2006) Structure, function, expression, genomic organization, and single nucleotide polymorphisms of human ABCB1 (MDR1), ABCC (MRP), and ABCG2 (BCRP) efflux transporters. Int J Toxicol 25: 231–259.
7. Natarajan K, Xie Y, Baer MR, Ross DD (2012) Role of breast cancer resistance protein (BCRP/ABCG2) in cancer drug resistance. Biochem Pharmacol 83: 1084–1103.
8. Thomas H, Coley HM (2003) Overcoming multidrug resistance in cancer: an update on the clinical strategy of inhibiting p-glycoprotein. Cancer control 10: 159–159.
9. Chen Z, Zhang H, Lu W, Huang P (2009) Role of mitochondria-associated hexokinase II in cancer cell death induced by 3-bromopyruvate. Biochimica et Biophysica Acta (BBA)-Bioenergetics 1787: 553–560.
10. Ko YH, Smith BL, Wang Y, Pomper MG, Rini DA, et al. (2004) Advanced cancers: eradication in all cases using 3-bromopyruvate therapy to deplete ATP. Biochem Biophys Res Commun 324: 269–275.
11. Nakano A, Tsuji D, Miki H, Cui Q, El Sayed SM, et al. (2011) Glycolysis inhibition inactivates ABC transporters to restore drug sensitivity in malignant cells. PloS one 6: e27222.
12. Jiang G-M, He Y-W, Fang R, Zhang G, Zeng J, et al. (2010) Sodium butyrate down-regulation of indoleamine 2, 3-dioxygenase at the transcriptional and post-transcriptional levels. Int J Biochem Cell B 42: 1840–1846.
13. Zhang J, Guo H, Zhang H, Wang H, Qian G, et al. (2011) Putative tumor suppressor miR-145 inhibits colon cancer cell growth by targeting oncogene friend leukemia virus integration 1 gene. Cancer 117: 86–95.
14. Marks DC, Belov L, Davey MW, Davey RA, Kidman AD (1992) The MTT cell viability assay for cytotoxicity testing in multidrug-resistant human leukemic cells. Leukemia Res 16: 1165–1173.
15. Trivedi ER, Blumenfeld CM, Wielgos T, Pokropinski S, Dande P, et al. (2012) Multi-gram synthesis of a porphyrazine platform for cellular translocation, conjugation to Doxorubicin and cellular uptake. Tetrahedron Lett: 5475–5478.
16. Skowronek P, Haferkamp O, Rödel G (1992) A fluorescence-microscopic and flow-cytometric study of HeLa cells with an experimentally induced respiratory deficiency. Biochem Biophys Res Commun 187: 991–998.
17. Touil Y, Zuliani T, Wolowczuk I, Kuranda K, Prochazkova J, et al. (2013) The PI3K/AKT Signaling Pathway Controls the Quiescence of the Low-Rhodamine123-Retention Cell Compartment Enriched for Melanoma Stem Cell Activity. Stem Cells: 641–651.
18. Zhang D-M, Shu C, Chen J-J, Sodani K, Wang J, et al. (2012) BBA, a derivative of 23-hydroxybetulinic acid, potently reverses ABCB1-mediated drug resistance in vitro and in vivo. Molecular pharmaceutics 9: 3147–3159.
19. Chen K, Zhang Q, Wang J, Liu F, Mi M, et al. (2009) Taurine protects transformed rat retinal ganglion cells from hypoxia-induced apoptosis by preventing mitochondrial dysfunction. Brain Res 1279: 131–138.
20. Allam AB, Brown MB, Reyes L (2012) Disruption of the S41 Peptidase Gene in Mycoplasma mycoides capri Impacts Proteome Profile, H2O2 Production, and Sensitivity to Heat Shock. PloS one 7: e51345.
21. Hayashida S, Arimoto A, Kuramoto Y, Kozako T, Honda S-i, et al. (2010) Fasting promotes the expression of SIRT1, an NAD+-dependent protein deacetylase, via activation of PPARα in mice. Mol Cell Biochem 339: 285–292.
22. Fang R, Zhang G, Guo Q, Ning F, Wang H, et al. (2013) Nodal promotes aggressive phenotype via Snail-mediated epithelial–mesenchymal transition in murine melanoma. Cancer Lett 333: 66–75.
23. Chen JJ, Sun YL, Tiwari AK, Xiao ZJ, Sodani K, et al. (2012) PDE5 inhibitors, sildenafil and vardenafil, reverse multidrug resistance by inhibiting the efflux function of multidrug resistance protein 7 (ATP-binding Cassette C10) transporter. Cancer science 103: 1531–1537.
24. Luk CK, Tannock IF (1989) Flow cytometric analysis of doxorubicin accumulation in cells from human and rodent cell lines. J Natl Cancer I 81: 55–59.
25. Shoshan MC (2012) 3-bromopyruvate: Targets and outcomes. J Bioenerg Biomembr 44: 7–15.
26. Pedersen PL (2012) 3-bromopyruvate (3BP) a fast acting, promising, powerful, specific, and effective "small molecule" anti-cancer agent taken from labside to bedside: introduction to a special issue. J Bioenerg Biomembr 44: 1–6.
27. Mathupala SP, Ko YH, Pedersen PL. Hexokinase-2 bound to mitochondria: cancer's stygian link to the "Warburg Effect" and a pivotal target for effective therapy; 2009. Elsevier. pp. 5475–5478.
28. Bayley J-P, Devilee P (2012) The Warburg effect in 2012. Current opinion in oncology 24: 62–67.
29. Albermann N, Schmitz-Winnenthal FH, Z'graggen K, Volk C, Hoffmann MM, et al. (2005) Expression of the drug transporters MDR1/ABCB1, MRP1/ABCC1, MRP2/ABCC2, BCRP/ABCG2, and PXR in peripheral blood mononuclear cells and their relationship with the expression in intestine and liver. Biochem Pharmacol 70: 949–958.
30. Glare E, Divjak M, Bailey M, Walters E (2002) β-Actin and GAPDH housekeeping gene expression in asthmatic airways is variable and not suitable for normalising mRNA levels. Thorax 57: 765–770.

MHC-I Molecules Selectively Inhibit Cell-Mediated Cytotoxicity Triggered by ITAM-Coupled Activating Receptors and 2B4

Rubén Corral-San Miguel, Trinidad Hernández-Caselles, Antonio José Ruiz Alcaraz, María Martínez-Esparza, Pilar García-Peñarrubia*

Department of Biochemistry and Molecular Biology B and Immunology, School of Medicine, University of Murcia, Campus of International Excellence "Campus Mare Nostrum" and IMIB (Instituto Murciano de Investigaciones Biosanitarias)-Arrixaca, Murcia, Spain

Abstract

NK cell effector functions are controlled by a combination of inhibitory receptors, which modulate NK cell activation initiated by stimulatory receptors. Most of the canonical NK cell inhibitory receptors recognize allelic forms of classical and non-classical MHC class I molecules. Furthermore, high expression of MHC-I molecules on effector immune cells is also associated with reverse signaling, giving rise to several immune-regulatory functions. Consequently, the inhibitory function of MHC class I expressed on a human NKL cell line and activated primary NK and T cells on different activating receptors are analyzed in this paper. Our results reveal that MHC-I molecules display specific patterns of "selective" inhibition over cytotoxicity and cytokine production induced by ITAM-dependent receptors and 2B4, but not on NKG2D. This contrasts with the best known "canonical" inhibitory receptors, which constitutively inhibit both functions, regardless of the activating receptor involved. Our results support the existence of a new fine-tuner inhibitory function for MHC-I molecules expressed on cytotoxic effector cells that could be involved in establishing self-tolerance in mature activated NK cells, and could also be important in tumor and infected cell recognition.

Editor: Jacques Zimmer, Centre de Recherche Public de la Santé (CRP-Santé), Luxembourg

Funding: This work was supported by the Fundación Séneca (CARM) project number 03112/PI/05 to PGP (http://fseneca.es/). The funders had no role in study design, data collection and analysis, decision to publish, or preparation of the manuscript.

Competing Interests: The authors have declared that no competing interests exist.

* Email: pigarcia@um.es

Introduction

The mechanisms that control the activity of NK and other cytotoxic effector cells are determined by a fine balance between signals triggered by activating and inhibitory receptors, which ultimately determine the activation of the effector cell [1–2]. Regarding cytotoxicity, several NK cell-activating receptors may directly recognize ligands expressed on the surface of infected or stressed tumor target cells [1–2]. In addition to cytolytic activity, NK cells produce immunoregulatory cytokines such as IFN-γ, TGF-β, IL-1, IL-10, GM-CSF and chemokines when triggered by activating receptors [1–2]. The role of inhibitory receptors in this human NK cell immunoregulatory function has not been totally established. Inhibitory receptors antagonize NK cell responses through the recruitment of the protein tyrosine phosphatases, SHP-1 and SHP-2, to their ITIM (Immunoreceptor Tyrosine-based Inhibitory Motif) sequences [1–2]. Despite the complexity of the target recognition process, NK cells maintain self-tolerance, a function that is also achieved by a combination of inhibitory receptors that modulate the NK cell activation process initiated by activating receptors [3–4]. The best studied human (canonical) NK cell inhibitory receptors, Killer Ig-like receptors, (KIRs), Leukocyte Ig-like receptors (LILRs) and lectins-like receptors such as CD94/NKG2A, mediate self-tolerance through chronic cognate interaction with their ligands, mainly MHC (Major Histocompatibility Complex) class I molecules expressed on target cells. Thus, loss of MHC-I expression by virus-infected or tumor cells leads to NK cell activation as proposed by the "missing-self hypothesis" [1–3]. Additionally, it seems that the MHC-I environment redesigns NK cell receptor expression and reactivity [4]. Hence, mouse NK cells that express inhibitory receptors specific for self-MHC are more responsive than their non-expressing counterparts [5]. On the other hand, MHC-I-deficient mice display reduced responsiveness despite having self-tolerant NK cells [6].

Beside their classical function concerning antigen presentation and self-tolerance, MHC class I molecules can also mediate reverse signaling after aggregation, and display non-classical functions [7–9]. In this respect, previous studies from our laboratory have shown that crosslinking MHC-I on the membrane of human cytolytic effector cells induces intracellular tyrosine phosphorylation and inhibits the cytotoxicity directed against tumor cells [10–12]. Furthermore, constitutively expressed MHC class I molecules on macrophages protect mice from sepsis by attenuating TLR-triggered inflammatory responses [13]. These findings demonstrate that MHC class I molecules can act not only as ligands, but also as signaling receptors able to mediate reverse signaling through direct aggregation or association with other receptors.

This work further explores the role of MHC-I molecules expressed on human activated NK and T cells triggered by different activating receptors. The results show that MHC class I proteins exert an inhibitory function on both NK cell-mediated cytotoxicity and IFN-γ production, depending on the particular killer activating receptor triggered in the activated effector cells. Therefore, besides the well known role of MHC-I molecules expressed on target cells, NK cell upregulation of MHC class I could constitute a novel mechanism of immune-regulation, tolerance and evasion of tumor or infected cells.

Materials and Methods

Antibodies

The anti-HLA class I mAb used were: W6/32 (IgG2a, obtained from ATCC), BB7.7 (IgG2b, which recognizes a combinatorial determinant of HLA-A, B and C and β_2- microglobulin; obtained from ATCC), KD1 (IgG2a, anti-CD16), HP-3B1 (IgG2a, anti-CD94), Z199 (IgG2b, anti-heterodimer CD94/NKG2A) and HP-F1 (IgG1, anti-ILT2) were kindly provided by Dr. A. Moretta (Milan, Italy) and Dr. M. López-Botet (Barcelona, Spain). All of them were supernatants from hybridoma cultures. 3D12 (IgG1, anti-HLA-E obtained from eBioScience, San Diego, CA). Anti-NKG2D (clone 1D11, IgG1) was from eBioscience, anti-NKp46 (IgG2b) was from RD Systems and anti-2B4 (C1.7, IgG1) was from Immunotech. Isotype control Abs were from Sigma-Aldrich. HLA-G membrane expression was assessed with an MEM-G9 mAb specific for HLA-G H chain associated with β_2-microglobulin, and MEM-G1 mAb, specific for the HLA-G free H chain molecule were from Exbio (Praha, CZ). The conjugated mAb FITC-anti-CD3, FITC-anti-CD25, PE-anti-CD56 and PE- and Cy5-anti-CD16 were from Becton Dickinson.

Effector and target cells

The human NK cell line NKL (kindly provided by Dr Michael J. Robertson, Indiana University (Bloomington, IN)) [14] was cultured at a growth rate ranging from plateau to exponential phase (approx. from 0.05×10^6 cells/ml to 0.6×10^6 cells/ml) for up to 24–48 h, using complete tissue culture medium (RPMI 1640, 10% heat-inactivated FBS and antibiotics; Gibco) supplemented with 100 U/ml rIL-2 (Proleukin; Chiron). Additionally, to increase NKL killer activity, cells were grown in the presence of 1000 U/ml rIL-2 for 24–48 h.

Polyclonal primary NK cells were obtained from the blood of healthy volunteers. Protocols were approved by the Ethics Committee of the University of Murcia and complied with the Helsinki Declaration and the Good Clinical Practice guidelines. Volunteers always gave written informed consent. Peripheral blood lymphocytes (PBL) were stimulated with irradiated allogeneic cells as previously described [15], in the presence of IL-15 (25 ng/ml) (R&D systems). After stimulation, activated cells were maintained in IL-2-supplemented (100 U/ml) TCM until cellular quiescence (low expression of CD25). NK cells were then purified by negative selection using anti-CD3 (OKT3) and goat anti-mouse-coated magnetic beads (Dynabeads, Invitrogen). The resulting populations were shown to be >95% $CD3^-CD16^+CD56^+$ by flow cytometry.

Target cells used were mouse mastocytoma FcR^+ P815 (ATCC) grown in TCM.

Immunofluorescence analysis

Phenotypic analysis of cells was carried out by direct or indirect immunofluorescence staining, depending on whether or not the primary mAb was fluorochrome-conjugated or unconjugated, respectively, on a FACScan cytometer (Becton-Dickinson) as previously described [10]. Cytofluorometer data were analysed using the CellQuest program (Becton-Dickinson). A minimum of 4000 events per sample was analyzed.

Cytotoxicity assays

The cytotoxic activity of human NK cells was tested in 4 h ^{51}Cr release assays [10]. Target cells were labeled with $Na^{51}{}_2CrO_4$ (100 μCi^-[3.7 MBq]/10^6 cells; PerkinElmer) for 1.5 hour at 37°C. Target cells were washed and seeded on U-bottom 96-well plates at 5000 cells per well. Effector cells were then added in 100 µL medium at different E/T (Effector/Target) ratios.

The redirected lysis assays were performed using ^{51}Cr-labeled P815 target cells pre-incubated with optimized concentrations of the following mAb against activating and/or inhibitory receptors or control Ig: anti-CD16 (culture supernatant), anti-NKp46 (0.34 µg/ml), NKG2D (0.34 µg/ml), 2B4 (0.17 µg/ml), anti-MHC-I (culture supernatant), anti-ILT2, anti-NKG2A or anti-CD94 (culture supernatants) and isotype control Ig (1.25 µg/ml). Effector cells were added at different E/T ratios and incubated for 4 h at 37°C. Then, supernatants were collected to determine ^{51}Cr release, and the percentage of lysis was calculated as follows:

$$\%\,\text{lysis} = \left(cpm_{exp.} - cpm_{spont.}\right)100/\left(cpm_{max.} - cpm_{spont.}\right)$$

The cpm_{spont} was <15% of cpm_{max} in all experiments.

Cytokine production assays

For cytokine production studies, NKL (25000 cells/well, grown in 100 U/ml rIL-2) or purified polyclonal NK cells (50000 cells/well) were co-cultured with P815 cells at a 1:1 E/T ratio in the presence of the same combination of mAb, using twice the Ab concentration used for the cytotoxicity assay. After 22–24 h incubation, cell free supernatants were collected and tested for IFN-γ concentration by ELISA (eBioscience).

Calculating the percentages of inhibition of cytotoxicity and cytokine production

The results, reported as the percentage of inhibition, were calculated as follows:

$$\%\,\text{inhibition of cytotoxic function} = \left(\%\,lysis_{(Activ.+\,isotype\ control)} - \%\,lysis_{(Activ.+\,Inhib.)}\right)100\,/\left(\%\,lysis_{(Activ.+isotype\ control)} - \%\,lysis_{(isotype\ control)}\right)$$

$$\%\,\text{inhibition of IFN-}\gamma\text{ secretion} = \left([\text{IFN-}\gamma]_{(Activ.+isotype\ control)} - [\text{IFN-}\gamma]_{(Activ.+Inhib.)}\right)100\,/\left([\text{IFN-}\gamma]_{(Activ.+isotype\ control)} - [\text{IFN-}\gamma]_{(isotype\ control)}\right)$$

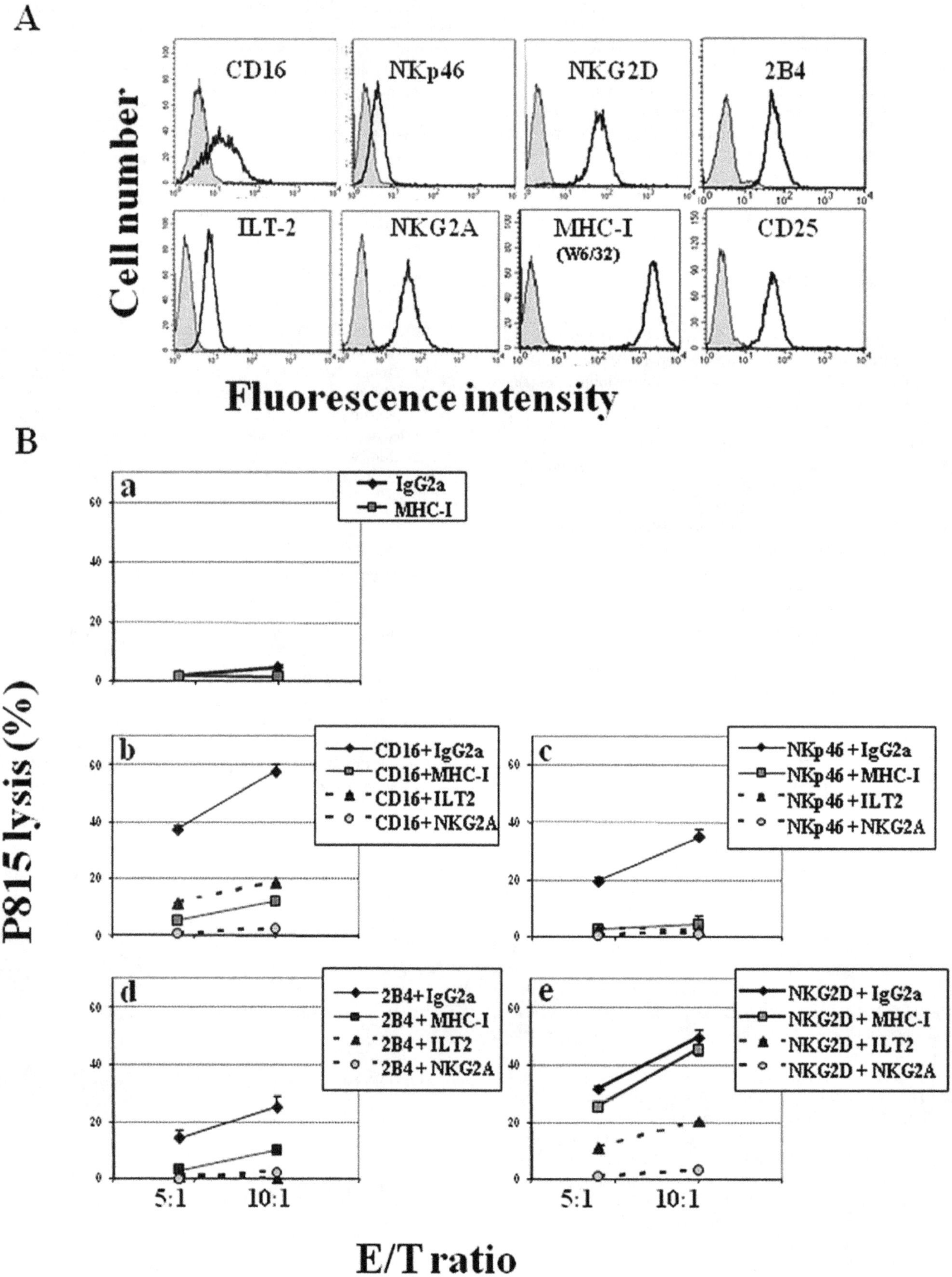
A
Cell number
CD16
NKp46
NKG2D
2B4
ILT-2
NKG2A
MHC-I
(W6/32)
CD25
Fluorescence intensity
B
P815 lysis (%)
a
IgG2a
MHC-I
b
CD16+IgG2a
CD16+MHC-I
CD16+ILT2
CD16+NKG2A
c
NKp46+IgG2a
NKp46+MHC-I
NKp46+ILT2
NKp46+NKG2A
d
2B4+IgG2a
2B4+MHC-I
2B4+ILT2
2B4+NKG2A
e
NKG2D+IgG2a
NKG2D+MHC-I
NKG2D+ILT2
NKG2D+NKG2A
5:1
10:1
E/T ratio

Figure 1. MHC-I engagement selectively inhibits cytotoxicity on NKL cells. (**A**) Exponentially growing NKL cells (see *Material and Methods* section) were phenotyped by flow cytometry. Filled histograms represent isotype control and open histograms represent surface receptor stained cells. (**B**) NKL cells were co-cultured with ^{51}Cr-P815 cells in the presence of mAb: IgG2a isotype control or anti-MHC-I (**a**), against KAR (CD16 (**b**), NKp46 (**c**), 2B4 (**d**), and NKG2D (**e**)), plus control IgG2a or anti-MHC-I, anti-ILT2 or anti-NKG2A inhibitory receptors. The figure depicts one representative assay out of three performed with similar results.

Statistical analysis

Data are reported as mean ±SD. Statistical differences were analyzed using the Mann-Whitney U test, and p values lower than 0.05 were considered to indicate statistical significance. Calculations were performed using the SPSS 21.0 software (Chicago, IL, USA).

Results

The co-ligation of MHC-I expressed on NKL cells with different activating receptors selectively inhibits their cytolytic activity

We have previously shown that MHC-I can transduce inhibitory signals upon engagement with putative ligands expressed on the surface of K562 target cells [10,12]. Here, we study the inhibitory effect of NK cell-expressed MHC-I molecules on the cytolytic activity triggered by different Killer Activating Receptors (KARs). To accomplish this, we use the redirected cytotoxicity assay against the FcR$^+$ P815 murine cell line. To validate this assay, we first determined the basal level of P815 target cells killing by NKL (3.6±2.7% lysis at 20:1 E/T ratio). The low level observed indicated that any interaction of NKL cell-activating receptors with putative murine ligand(s) was not significant in this experimental setting. Next, taking advantage of the fact that two different receptors may be co-ligated on the membrane of effector cells, NKL cells were triggered with optimal concentrations of mAb against CD16, NKp46 (CD335), NKG2D (CD314) or 2B4 (CD244) KARs, together with one of the following: isotype control Ab, anti-MHC-I (W6/32) or mAb specific for the canonical inhibitory receptors ILT2 or CD94/NKG2A (as positive controls of inhibition). Constitutive NKL cell expression of these cell markers is shown in **Figure 1A**. As negative control we previously determined that co-ligation of CD16, NKG2D and NKp46 with other NKL cell membrane receptors, such as CD2, CD58, CD54, CD50, CD29, CD44 and CD25, had no significant effect in this assay compared with mAb W6/32 (Figure S1 in File S1). **Figure 1B (panel a)** shows that anti-MHC-I, or its isotype-matched mAb alone, did not affect NKL-mediated P815 killing. However, anti-MHC-I mAb W6/32 was able to strongly reduce the killing of P815 triggered by anti-CD16 (91.3±8.3% inhibition, **Fig. 1B, panel b**), anti-NKp46 (90.8±5.3% inhibition, **Fig. 1B, panel c**), at 5:1 and 10:1 E/T ratio, or anti-2B4 mAb (70.3±18.0% inhibition **Fig. 1B, panel d**) at 5:1 and 10:1 E/T ratio. In contrast, the same concentration of anti-MHC-I mAb could not significantly reduce the killing triggered by NKG2D (**Fig. 1B, panel e**), which produced only 12.6±15.9% inhibition, when the E/T ratio was 5:1 and 10:1. As expected, anti-ILT2 or anti-CD94/NKG2A mAb completely neutralized the lysis of P815 induced by every single activating mAb used (**Fig. 1B, panels b–e**). Altogether, these results confirm that MHC-I molecules play an inhibitory role in the membrane of NKL cells.

To discard the possibility of an artefactual inhibition due to competition between activating and inhibitory mAb for P815 FcR, the percentages of NKL/P815 conjugation under the experimental conditions described above were determined. The results shown in Figure S2 in File S1 supported that the selective inhibition exerted by MHC-I molecules over CD16-, NKG2D- and NKp46-mediated NKL cytotoxicity in the reverse assays is not caused by a FcR competition phenomenon.

Co-engagement of MHC-I with different activating receptors selectively inhibits the cytolytic activity of activated primary human NK and T cells

Whether or not the inhibitory capacity of MHC class I molecules expressed on NKL cells is a general mechanism of inhibition in activated human NK cells was further studied. For this, polyclonal populations of activated NK cells from PBMC obtained from six healthy donors were expanded by co-culture with allogeneic cells in the presence of IL-15. Under these experimental conditions we were able to obtain a population of activated NK cells (from 40 to 85% of CD3$^-$CD16^{++}CD56$^+$ cells among different donors) which were sub-cultured in IL-2 supplemented culture medium until quiescence (very low expression of CD25 antigen after 3–4 weeks of sub-cultures). NK cells were further enriched by negative selection, and then tested for the surface expression of every receptor included in the current study by flow cytometry analysis. **Figure 2A** shows the results obtained from a representative donor out of six performed with similar results. Most of these cells expressed CD16, CD56, CD94, NKG2D and 2B4 antigen (**Fig. 2A**) although, as has been described in freshly isolated PBLs [16], the expression of NKG2D varied among donors, with mean percentages of 67.2±23.5% from the six individuals tested. The percentages of NKp46$^+$ cells also varied among individuals and were lower (34.2±24.5%) than those reported for resting human NK cells [17]. The percentages of ILT2$^+$ cells were very low (6.7±5.7%), while NKG2A$^+$ cells reached 48.1±11.9% in these NK cells (**Fig. 2A**). Furthermore, we found that these quiescent NK cells were mainly CD16^{bright}CD56^{dim} and CD16^{bright}CD56$^-$ (**Fig. 2A**). Therefore, they could be phenotypically similar to the described CD56^{dim} subset of resting NK cells, which displays high natural cytotoxic ability after activation [18].

The results obtained in cytotoxicity assays were consistent with those obtained for NKL cells. Thus, MHC-I engagement could inhibit the cytotoxicity triggered by CD16 depending on the concentration of CD16 mAb assayed (**Fig. 2B panel b-c and 2C**). In agreement with results obtained with NKL, MHC-I could only slightly counteract (13.2±6.9% inhibition at E/T ratio of 5:1) the effect of NKG2D-activating receptor (**Fig. 2B panel d and 2C**), whereas NKG2A effectively inhibited the specific P815 killing mediated by this activating receptor (66.3±24%). Furthermore, P815 lysis induced by NKp46 was highly decreased by co-ligation with MHC-I (69.9±16.2%), (**Fig. 2B panel e, and 2C**). Finally, 2B4 triggered cytotoxic activity was almost completely neutralized by NKG2A (88.9±8.9%), and anti-MHC-I was also able to notably decrease the killing effect (76.7±10.3%), (**Fig. 2B panel f and 2C**). These results demonstrate and confirm that, contrarily to classic MHC-I recognizing inhibitory receptors, the inhibition of cytotoxicity after the engagement of MHC-I molecules on activated human NK cells is a selective phenomenon that depends on the specific activating receptor triggered.

To further study the inhibitory ability of MHC-I molecules on the activity triggered by ITAM-bearing activating receptors, we

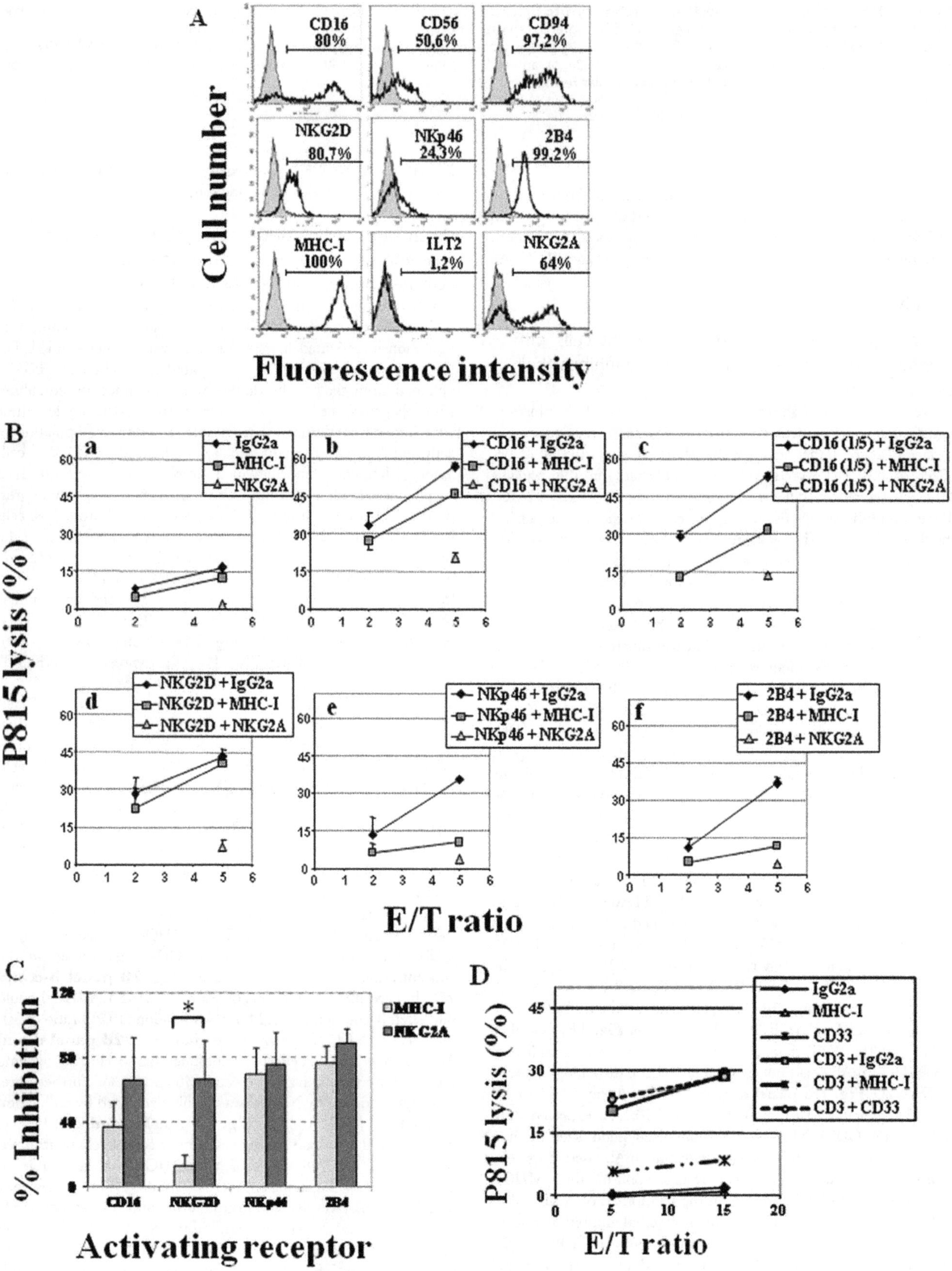
A
CD16
80%
CD56
50,6%
CD94
97,2%
NKG2D
80,7%
NKp46
24,3%
2B4
99,2%
MHC-I
100%
ILT2
1,2%
NKG2A
64%
Cell number
Fluorescence intensity
B
a
IgG2a
MHC-I
NKG2A
b
CD16 + IgG2a
CD16 + MHC-I
CD16 + NKG2A
c
CD16 (1/5) + IgG2a
CD16 (1/5) + MHC-I
CD16 (1/5) + NKG2A
d
NKG2D + IgG2a
NKG2D + MHC-I
NKG2D + NKG2A
e
NKp46 + IgG2a
NKp46 + MHC-I
NKp46 + NKG2A
f
2B4 + IgG2a
2B4 + MHC-I
2B4 + NKG2A
P815 lysis (%)
E/T ratio
C
*
MHC-I
NKG2A
% Inhibition
CD16
NKG2D
NKp46
2B4
Activating receptor
D
IgG2a
MHC-I
CD33
CD3 + IgG2a
CD3 + MHC-I
CD3 + CD33
P815 lysis (%)
E/T ratio

Figure 2. MHC-I engagement selectively inhibits cytotoxicity on activated human primary NK cells triggered by CD16, NKp46 or 2B4 but not by NKG2D activating receptors. (**A**) Phenotype of activated but quiescent polyclonal NK cells. Filled histograms represent isotype control and open histograms represent surface receptor stained cells. Numbers are percentages of positive cells in each panel. Data show one representative donor out of six tested in this study. (**B**) Purified quiescent NK cells were co-cultured with ^{51}Cr-P815 cells at 2:1 and 5:1 E/T ratios in the presence of mAb IgG2a isotype control, anti-MHC-I or anti-NKG2A (**a**), or against KAR (CD16 undiluted (**b**), CD16 diluted 1/5 (**c**), NKG2D (**d**), NKp46 (**e**) and 2B4 (**f**)), plus control Ig, anti-MHC-I or anti-NKG2A mAb. One representative donor (n = 6) is shown. (**C**) Inhibition percentages (mean ±SD) for each inhibitory receptor in all performed assays. Statistically significant difference comparing MHC-I *versus* NKG2A inhibitory effect is presented, *p = 0.034. (D) **MHC-I engagement selectively inhibits cytotoxicity on activated human T cells triggered by anti-CD3 activating receptor.** Purified activated T cells were co-cultured with P815 cells at 5:1 and 15:1 E/T ratios in the presence of mAb against CD3 plus control IgG2a, CD33 (WM53) or MHC-I (W6/32) mAb. One representative donor (n = 5) is shown.

studied P815 redirected lysis by activated T cells from five donors, after co-ligation of MHC-I with CD3/TcR molecules (**Fig 2D**). Ab isotype and anti-CD33 mAb were used as negative control of inhibition since we found that mAb anti-CD33 is able to inhibit the cytotoxicity triggered by DAP10-coupled NKG2D, but not by receptors transducing through ITAM-bearing adaptors (manuscript submitted). As shown in primary NK cells, MHC-I engagement strongly reduced the CD3 triggered cytotoxicity (76.52±11.86 at E/T ratio of 5:1) compared with the anti-CD33 mAb (WM53) (15.37±14.07) and the isotype control (0.28±0.46) at the same ratio. These results indicated that MHC-I molecules play an inhibitory role on ITAM-dependent cytotoxic activating signaling pathways.

Co-engagement of MHC-I by others anti-MHC-I mAb with different NK activating receptors selectively inhibits cytolytic activity of NKL cells

Next we determined whether different MHC-I, classical and non-classical, molecules were expressed on NKL cells, and whether they exerted an inhibitory function in NK cell-mediated cytotoxicity. For this purpose, besides W6/32 (which recognizes the α3 domain of MHC-I) we used mAb BB7.7 (which recognizes a combinatorial determinant of the HLA-A, B and C and β2-microglobulin), the anti-HLA-E 3D12 mAb and anti-HLA-G mAb. Flow cytometry analyses revealed that the NKL cells were BB7.7^{+}, HLA-E^{+} and HLA-G^{-} (**Figure 3A**). Redirected lysis experiments (**Figure 3B**) revealed that the mAb BB7.7 behaved similarly to W6/32, since both inhibited the cytotoxic activity mediated by CD16 and NKp46, although the inhibitory activity of BB7.7 on signals initiated by NKp46 was even stronger than that of W6/32 mAb. Consistent with the above results, none of them acted as inhibitor on cytotoxicity triggered by NKG2D. These results also suggest that the inhibitory function of MHC-I molecules involves the presence of β2-microglobulin and excludes the involvement of the HLA-E non-classical MHC-I protein.

Inhibition of IFN-γ secretion by NK cells after co-ligation of MHC-I with different NK activating receptors

NK cells regulate cell–mediated immune responses by secreting a wide array of cytokines [1–2,18]. Consequently, we next evaluated the secretion of IFN-γ by NKL cells co-cultured with P815 after co-ligation of either MHC-I or CD94/NKG2A with the activating receptors used above. First, it was checked that NKL cells did not produce IFN-γ when cultured alone or mixed with equal amounts of P815 cells (data not shown). **Figure 4A** displays the results obtained from one representative experiment out of four performed with similar results and **Figure 4B** shows the mean ±SD of percentages from four experiments. As expected, IFN-γ production was almost undetectable when cells were triggered by anti-CD94 mAb, unlike when IgG2a isotype control was used alone (**Fig. 4A**). In agreement with reported data [19] IFN-γ secretion was weakly induced by anti-NKG2D mAb in NKL cells, but it was secreted when cells were stimulated through CD16-, NKp46- or 2B4-activating receptors (**Fig. 4A**). Anti-CD94 mAb drastically inhibited the IFN-γ secretion induced by every activating receptor studied (from 94.0±11.1% to 98.7±1.6% of inhibition (**Fig. 4A and B**)). Regarding MHC-I molecules, W6/32 mAb was also able to partially inhibit the secretion of the IFN-γ induced by anti-CD16, anti-NKp46 or anti-2B4 mAb (75.1±12.5% to 80.1±19.0%), and occasionally induced a slight increase in IFN-γ production triggered by anti-NKG2D mAb (**Fig 4A-B**). In line with the results obtained with anti-CD94 mAb, anti-ILT2 mAb almost completely inhibited the IFN-γ production induced by all activating receptors studied on the NKL cell line (data not shown).

Next, we evaluated the ability of MHC-I to inhibit the secretion of IFN-γ in purified polyclonal activated NK cells. **Figure 4C** shows that anti-CD16 mAb was the best inducer of IFN-γ secretion as previously described for resting human NK cells [20]. The results indicated that, in this experimental setting, anti-MHC-I mAb almost completely inhibited the secretion of IFN-γ induced by every single activating receptor studied. In turn, anti-CD94/NKG2A mAb only partially inhibited the secretion of IFN-γ induced by the same activating receptors (**Figure 4C and D**). This diminished inhibition could be explained by the partial expression of NKG2A on these activated NK cell populations (**Figure 2A**).

Taken together, our results showed that, a) MHC-I molecules are selective inhibitors of both cytotoxicity and IFN-γ secretory function of NK cells, whereas b) canonical inhibitory receptors, such as CD94/NKG2A and ILT2, are able to prevent the secretion of this cytokine induced by most human activating receptors.

Discussion

The present results further reinforce and extend experimental evidence from our laboratory concerning the inhibitory function triggered by MHC-I molecules expressed on NKL, human primary NK cells and a CD8^{+}αβ T cell clone, K14B06 [10–12]. Herein we demonstrate that, similarly to the best known human inhibitory receptors, ILT2 and CD94/NKG2A, the inhibitory activity of MHC-I is strongly exerted on activating receptors, CD16 and NKp46, which transduce intracellular signals by association with ITAM-bearing adaptor molecules (which depend on Syk and ZAP-70). MHC-I engagement also inhibited, although more weakly, the activating signals triggered by the SAP-associated 2B4 activating receptor. Notably and unlike canonical inhibitory receptors, MHC-I has no inhibitory effect on the activating signals triggered by NKG2D (a DAP10-coupled specific activating receptor recruiting PI3K). In contrast to canonical inhibitory receptors, the MHC-I cytoplasmic tail is short and lacks consensus inhibitory signaling motifs. Nevertheless, it has been

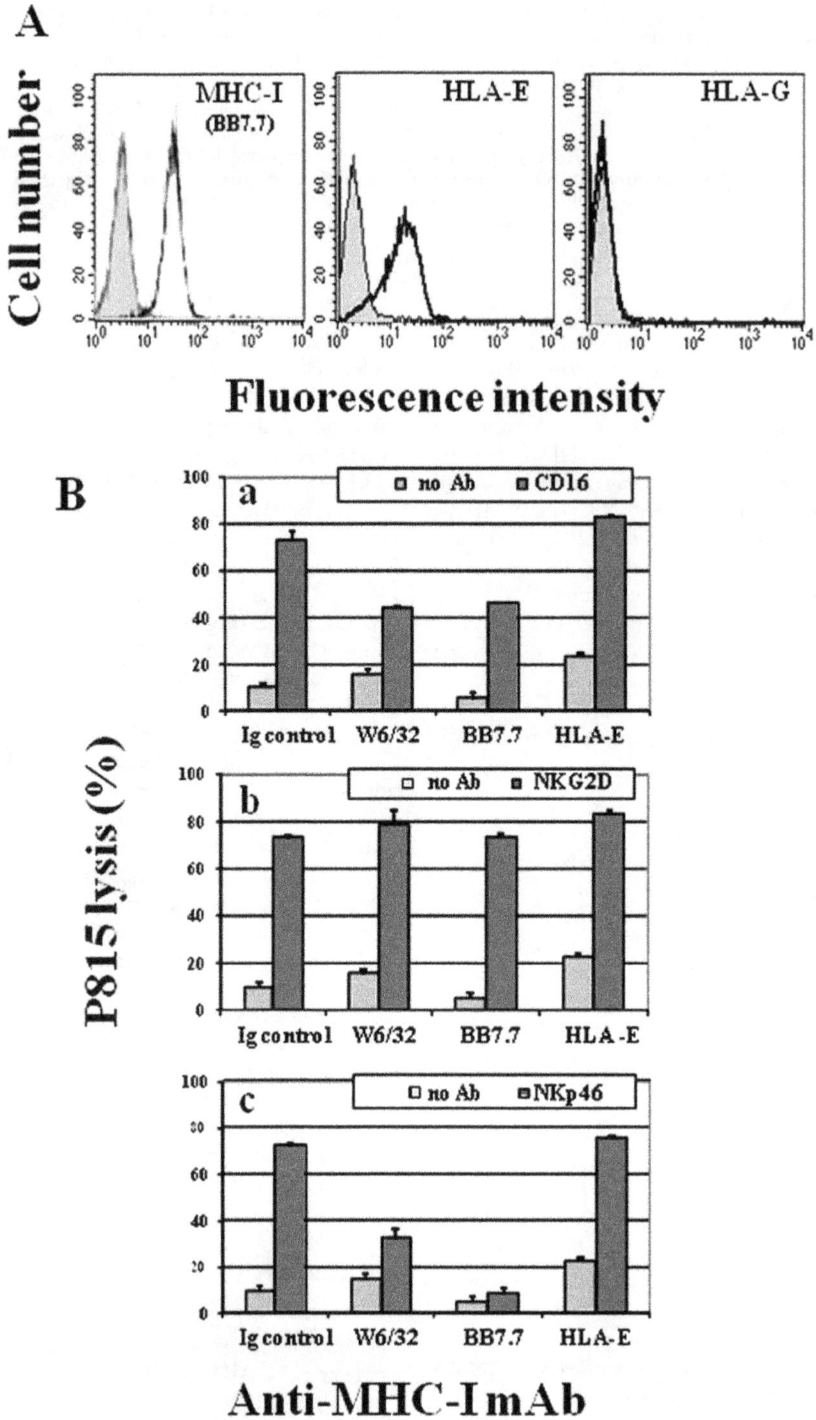

Figure 3. Classical MHC-I molecules are involved in selective killing inhibition of NKL cells triggered by CD16 and NKp46 activating receptors. (**A**) Classical and non-classical MHC-I expression on NKL cells. Filled histograms represent isotype control and open histograms represent surface receptor stained cells. (**B**) Exponentially growing NKL cells were co-cultured with ^{51}Cr-P815 cells at 5:1 E/T ratio in the presence of mAb against KAR (CD16 (**a**), NKG2D (**b**) or NKp46 (**c**)), plus control Ig, or different anti-MHC-I mAb (W6/32, BB7.7 or HLA-E clone 3D12). One representative experiment (n = 3) is shown.

largely suggested that the aggregation of MHC-I proteins is able to induce positive and negative intracellular signals in T, B and NK cells [7–12,21–28]. In our previous work, we detected that MHC-I crosslinking with anti-mouse IgG F(ab')$_2$ on NKL cells induced tyrosine phosphorylation [10]. Moreover, the constitutive location of MHC-I proteins within lipid rafts on NKL cells [10,29], as well as the MHC-I-specific inhibition of CD94-induced MTOC reorientation towards the P815:K14B06 contact area [11–12], strongly suggested that the inhibition of non-restricted cytotoxicity by aggregation of MHC class I molecules is mediated by

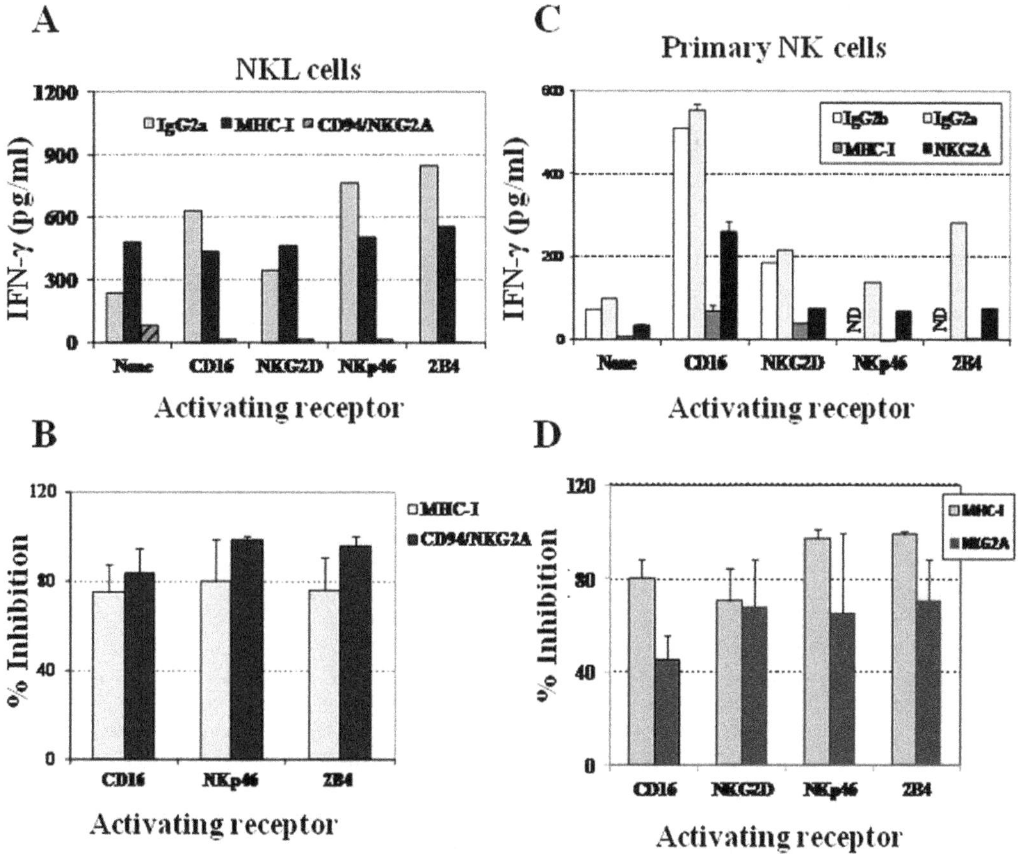

Figure 4. Inhibition of IFN-γ secretion by MHC-I in NKL and human activated NK cells. Exponentially growing NKL cells (**A and B**) were co-cultured with P815 cells at 1:1 E/T ratio as described in *Materials and Methods.* (**A**) IFN-γ secretion is efficiently inhibited by anti-CD94 mAb in all cases. Anti-MHC-I mAb partially inhibits the secretion of IFN-γ induced by CD16, NKp46 and 2B4. Figure shows (**A**) one representative assay and (**B**) percentage of inhibition (mean ±SD) from the four experiments performed. (**C and D**) IFN-γ secretion by purified quiescent human activated primary NK cells is inhibited by anti-MHC-I mAb. Panel **C** shows one representative assay out of five (three different donors), and **D** the percentages of inhibition (mean ±SD) of anti-MHC-I and anti-NKG2A mAb. ND: not determined.

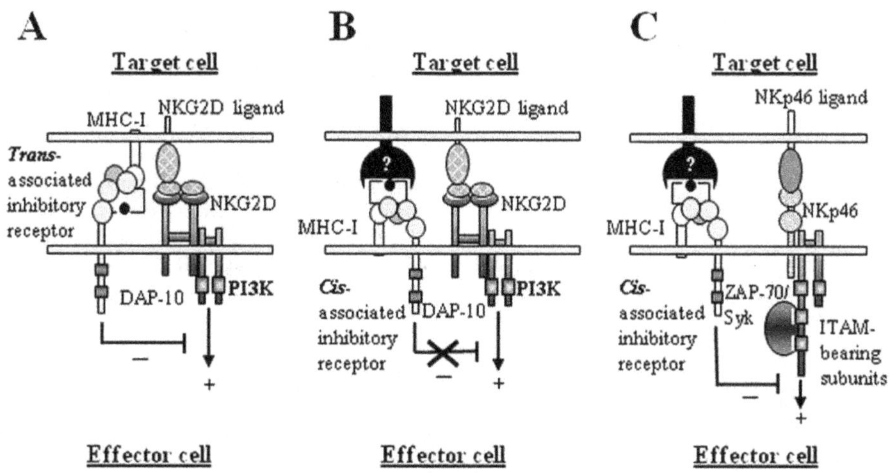

Figure 5. Model for MHC-I selective inhibition. (**A**) *Trans*-associated inhibitory receptors to MHC-I molecules are always inhibitory for effector cells. (**B**) and (**C**) *Cis*-associated inhibitory receptor/MHC-I selectively inhibits activating receptor signaling. It is proposed that LIRL receptors which bind to α3-β2m domains, and KIR or CD94-NKG2 receptors which bind to α1–α2 domains on MHC-I molecules [31] could participate in these interactions (shown as unknown receptors).

intracellular inhibitory signals triggered by MHC-I. Consistent with these findings, it has recently been described that the constitutive expression of MHC class I molecules on murine macrophages inhibits the TLR4-triggered inflammatory response by association with the src kinase ftp and SHP-2 [13]. It has been reported that the cytoplasmic domain of MHC class I molecules is not needed for T cell signaling through these receptors, while the transmembrane region is indispensable for this effect [30]. Thus, it seems most likely that the MHC-I inhibitory function exerted upon ITAM-mediated NK cell cytotoxicity and IFN-γ secretion is mediated by either a lateral or *cis* association with some of the long list of cell surface molecules reported to physically associate with MHC-I proteins [31–32]. To date, it is unclear whether any type of MHC class I molecule is able to transduce inhibitory signals, or whether this property is limited to certain classical, non-classical, or even to their MHC-I open conformers bearing the monomorphic determinant recognized by anti-MHC-I mAb W6/32. MHC-I open conformers are unfolded molecules highly expressed on activated effector cells, where they form clusters through lateral or *cis* interaction with β2m-associated forms of MHC-I, as well as with non-classical HLA-F molecules, a feature that is likely to increase the avidity of any receptor recognition [33–35]. Moreover, open conformers are tyrosine phosphorylated probably mediated by Lck, since this src kinase is associated with HC-10 immunocomplexes [36]. Because KIR3DL2 and KIR2DS4 physically and functionally interact *in trans* with HLA-F and MHC-I open conformers [35], it is possible that these interactions also take place in *cis*, regulating KIR availability and activity. At this moment, we cannot totally exclude the involvement of open conformers in the inhibitory effect described here since we have not been able to obtain the specific mAbs. Nevertheless, our previous data from primary unstimulated human NK cells (in which the expression of open conformers is probably low) [10], together with the results obtained here with mAb that recognize β2m and those for the anti-HLAB27 mAb inhibition of CD94-redirected lysis of P815 by a $CD8^{+}\alpha\beta$ T cell clone [11–12] point to the involvement of classical trimeric human MHC-I molecules. Regarding *cis* interactions between MHC-I and inhibitory receptors, it has been reported from a murine model, that MHC-I molecules are recognized by Ly49 inhibitory receptors in *cis* and *trans* [32]. Furthermore, approximately 75% of the Ly49A receptors are masked by *cis* interaction with endogenous $H\text{-}2D^{d}$ ligands [37] and, interestingly, the licensing of NK cells requires both *cis* and *trans* recognition of MHC class I molecules [38]. Although it is unclear whether this is a general feature in human NK cells, recent evidence has shown the *cis* association of LIR1/ILT2 with the MHC-I molecules that modulates the accessibility to antibodies and binding to the human CMV MHC-I homolog UL18 [39].

Our results suggest that a putative MHC-I/inhibitory receptor association in *cis* could dually regulate the activity of both inhibitory and activating receptors, in agreement with Held and Mariuzza [31]. Thus, constitutive MHC I/Inhibitory receptor *cis* interactions could weaken inhibitory signals by reducing the ability of KIRs, LILRs and/or CD94/NKG2A to detect self ligands on target cells, as previously shown in murine NK cells [32], while selectively up-regulating their inhibitory capacity, as shown in **Figure 5C**. Our model proposes that inhibitory receptor-MHC-I interaction *in trans* would always be inhibitory for NK cells (**Fig. 5A**), whereas the same interaction *in cis* might be inhibitory, depending on the activating pathway triggered (**Fig. 5B *vs* 5C**). The experimental approach used here could mimic a synaptic trimolecular complex that would be integrated by an effector MHC-I molecule associated *in cis* to a hypothetical LIRL or KIR receptor through the α3-β2m domains, and a KIR or CD94-NKG2 receptor (shown as unknown receptors) bound to the α1-α2 domains of the MHC-I molecule (reviewed in ref. [31]), as shown in **Fig. 5B and 5C**.

Related to these findings, we have recently identified that CD33 (either in *cis* or *trans*) acts as a unique fine-tune inhibitory receptor with the capacity to efficiently antagonize the cytotoxic response mediated by NKG2D (a DAP10-coupled specific activating receptor recruiting PI3K), or the SAP-associated 2B4 activating receptor, but not by CD16 or NKp46 receptors coupled to ITAM bearing subunits (depending on Syk and ZAP-70) (manuscript submitted). In addition, CD33 does not inhibit the IFN-γ production of NKL cells. Here, we show that, unlike but complementary to CD33, MHC-I inhibits both cytotoxicity and IFN-γ secretion on NK cells triggered by CD16, NKp46, and 2B4, but not by NKG2D. Consequently, we propose that CD33 and MHC-I belong to a new group of selective inhibitory receptors (**Figure 5B *vs* 5C**), distinct from the best known canonical inhibitory receptors such as ILT2 or CD94/NKG2A, which efficiently regulate both the cytotoxicity and cytokine production triggered by all activating receptors, independently of the specific intermediates recruited.

Previously, we suggested that ILT2 (LILRB1, CD85j) and ILT4 (LILRB2, CD85d) proteins could be the principal MHC-I ligands candidates on APC to confer a suppressive effect on activated NK cells after ligation [10,12]. It is possible that the resistance of mature DC to NK lysis could be related not only to the described up-regulation of MHC class I expression on their surface [40], but also to a hypothetically increased expression of LILRs.

In conclusion, this work describes for the first time a group of Killer cell selective inhibitory receptors in NK and activated T cells, which may be strongly involved in the regulation of immune responses against cancer and infected cells, in protecting self-cells and, probably, in avoiding autoimmunity. The selective nature of the inhibitory effect described provides new tools for dissecting the molecular mechanisms involved in cytotoxic cell inhibition. Further work is necessary to understand the integration of these multiple signals, the results of which will certainly improve our knowledge and ability to manipulate NK cell signaling pathways.

Supporting Information

File S1 Supporting figures. Figure S1, Crosslinking the NKL cell surface receptors CD58, CD54 (ICAM-1), CD50 (ICAM-3), CD29, CD44, CD2 and CD25 with the killer activating receptors, CD16, NKG2D and NKp46 did not significantly decrease the NKL cell-mediated cytotoxicity against P815 cells. Figure S2, MHC-I engagement augments NKL/P815 cell conjugation. Exponentially growing Ca-AM-stained (calcein acetoxymethylester) NKL cells were co-cultured with HE-stained (hydroethidine) P815 cells plus mAb against Killer Activating Receptors or Inhibitory receptors at 1:2 E/T ratio.

Acknowledgments

The authors thank Dr. M. J. Robertson for the NKL cell line and Drs. A. Moretta and M. López-Botet for the gifts of antibodies.

Author Contributions

Conceived and designed the experiments: PGP THC. Performed the experiments: RCSM THC AJRA MME. Analyzed the data: RCSM THC AJRA PGP. Contributed to the writing of the manuscript: PGP THC.

References

1. Long EO, Kim HS, Liu D, Peterson ME, Rajagopalan S (2013) Controlling natural killer cell responses: integration of signals for activation and inhibition. Annu Rev Immunol 31: 227–58.
2. Lanier LL (2008) Up to the tightrope: natural killer cell activation and inhibition. Nat Immunol 9 (5): 495–502.
3. Yokoyama WM, Kim S (2006) How do Natural Killer cells find self to achieve tolerance? Immunity 24: 249–257.
4. Höglund P, Brodin P (2010) Current perspectives of natural killer cell education by MHC class I molecules. Nat Rev Immunol 10 (10): 724–34.
5. Fernandez NC, Treiner E, Vance RE, Jamieson AM, Lemieux S, et al. (2005) Subset of natural killer cells achieves self-tolerance without expressing inhibitory receptors specific for self-MHC molecules. Blood 105: 4416–4423.
6. Liao N, Bix M, Zijlstra M, Jaenisch R, Raulet D (1991) MHC class I deficiency: susceptibility to natural killer (NK) cells and impaired NK activity. Science 253: 199–202.
7. Tscherning T, Claesson MH (1994) Signal transduction via MHC class-I molecules in T cells. Scand J Immunol 39: 117–121.
8. Skov S (1998) Intracellular signal transduction mediated by ligation of MHC class I molecules. Tissue Antigens 51: 215–223.
9. Pedersen AE, Skov S, Bregenholt S, Ruhwald M, Claesson MH (1999) Signal transduction by the major histocompatibility complex class I molecule. APMIS 107: 887–895.
10. Rubio G, Férez X, Sánchez-Campillo M, Gálvez J, Martí S, et al. (2004) Cross-linking of MHC class I molecules on human NK cells inhibits NK cell function, segregates MHC I from the NK cell synapse, and induces intracellular phosphotyrosines. J Leukoc Biol 76: 116–124.
11. Caparros E, de Heredia AB, Carpio E, Sancho D, Aguado E, et al. (2004) Aggregation of MHC class I molecules on a CD8+ alphabeta T cell clone specifically inhibits non-antigen-specific lysis of target cells. Eur J Immunol 34: 47–55.
12. Aparicio Alonso P, Rubio Pedraza G, Caparrós Cayuela E, Férez X, Beltrán de Heredia A, et al. (2004) Inhibition of non MHC-restricted cytotoxicity of human NK cells and a CD8+αβ T cell clone by MHC class I cross-linking. Inmunología 23 (3): 284–292.
13. Xu S, Liu X, Bao Y, Zhu X, Han C, et al. (2012) Constitutive MHC class I molecules negatively regulate TLR-triggered inflammatory responses via the Fps-SHP-2 pathway. Nat Immunol 13: 551–60.
14. Robertson MJ, Cochran KJ, Cameron C, Le JM, Tantravahi R, et al. (1996) Characterization of a cell line, NKL, derived from an aggressive human natural killer cell leukemia. Exp Hematol 24: 406–415.
15. Hernández-Caselles T, Martínez-Esparza M, Pérez-Oliva AB, Quintanilla-Cecconi AM, García-Alonso A, et al. (2006) A study of CD33 (SIGLEC-3) antigen expression and function on activated human T and NK cells: two isoforms of CD33 are generated by alternative splicing. J Leukoc Biol 79: 46–58.
16. Bauer S, Groh V, Wu J, Steinle A, Phillips JH, et al. (1999) Activation of NK cells and T cells by NKG2D, a receptor for stress-inducible MICA. Science 285: 727–729.
17. Sivori S, Vitale M, Morelli L, Sanseverino L, Augugliaro R, et al. (1997) p46, a novel natural killer cell-specific surface molecule that mediates cell activation. J Exp Med 186 (7): 1129–1136.
18. Cooper MA, Fehniger TA, Caligiuri MA (2001) The biology of human natural killer-cell subsets. Trends Immunol 22(11): 633–640.
19. André P, Castriconi R, Espéli M, Anfossi N, Juarez T, et al. (2004) Comparative analysis of human NK cell activation induced by NKG2D and natural cytotoxicity receptors. Eur J Immunol 34: 961–971.
20. Bryceson YT, March ME, Ljunggren HG, Long EO (2006) Synergy among receptors on resting NK cells for the activation of natural cytotoxicity and cytokine secretion. Blood 107: 159–166.
21. Dasgupta JD, Granja CB, Yunis EJ, Relias V (1993) MHC class I antigens regulate CD3-induced tyrosine phosphorylation of proteins in T cells. Int Immunol 6: 481–489.
22. Skov S, Bregenholt S, Claesson MH (1997) MHC class I ligation of human T cells activates the ZAP70 and $p56^{lck}$ tyrosine kinases, leads to an alternative phenotype of the TcR/CD3ζchain, and induces apoptosis. J Immunol 158: 3189–3196.
23. Gilliland LK, Norris NA, Grosmaire LS, Ferrone S, Gladstone P, et al. (1989) Signal transduction in lymphocyte activation through crosslinking of HLA class I molecules. Human Immunol 25: 269–289.
24. Gepper TD, Wacholtz MC, Patel SS, Lightfoot E, Lipsky PE (1989) Activation of human T cells clones and Jurkat cells by cross-linking class I MHC molecules. J Immunol 142: 3763–3772.
25. Woodle ES, Smith DM, Bluestone JA, Kirkman WM III, Green DR, et al. (1997) Anti-Human Class I MHC antibodies induce apoptosis by a pathway that is distinct from the Fas antigen-mediated pathway. J Immunol 158: 2156–2164.
26. Smith DM, Bluestone JA, Jeyarajah DR, Newberger MH, Engelhard VH, et al. (1994) Inhibition of T cell activation by a monoclonal antibody reactive against the α3 domain of human MHC class I molecules. J Immunol 153: 1054–1067.
27. Taylor DS, Nowell PC, Kornbluth J (1987) Anti-HLA class I antibodies inhibit the T cell-independent proliferation of human B lymphocytes. J Immunol 139: 1792–1796.
28. Petersson MGE, Gronberg A, Kiessling R, Ferm MT (1995) Engagement of MHC I proteins on natural killer cells inhibits their killing capacity. Scand J Immunol 42: 34–38.
29. García-Peñarrubia P, Férez X, Gálvez J (2005) Quantitative analysis of the factors that affect the determination of colocalization coefficients in dual-color confocal images. IEEE T Image Processing 14(8): 1151–1158.
30. Gur H, el-Zaatari F, Geppert TD, Wacholtz MC, Taurog JD, et al. (1990) Analysis of T cell signaling by class I MHC molecules: the cytoplasmic domain is not required for signal transduction. J Exp Med 172: 1267–1270.
31. Held W, Mariuzza RA (2008) Cis interactions of immunoreceptors with MHC and non-MHC ligands. Nat Rev Immunol 8: 269–279.
32. Doucey MA, Scarpellino L, Zimmer J, Guillaume P, Luescher IF, et al. (2004) Cis-association of Ly49A with MHC class I restricts natural killer cell inhibition. Nat Immunol 5: 328–336.
33. Raine T, Allen R (2005) MHC-I recognition by receptors on myelomonocytic cells: new tricks for old dogs? BioEssays 27: 542–550.
34. Arosa FA, Santos SG, Powis SJ (2007) Open conformers: the hidden face of MHC-I molecules. Trends Immunol 28(3): 115–23.
35. Goodridge JP, Burian A, Lee N, Geraghty DE (2010) HLA-F Complex without Peptide Binds to MHC Class I Protein in the Open Conformer Form. J Immunol 184: 6199–6208.
36. Santos SG, Powis SJ, Arosa FA (2004) Misfolding of Major Histocompatibility Complex Class I Molecules in Activated T Cells Allows cis-Interactions with Receptors and Signaling Molecules and Is Associated with Tyrosine Phosphorylation. J Biol Chem 279: (51) 53062–53070.
37. Andersson KE, Williams GS, Davis DM, Höglund P (2007) Quantifying the reduction in accessibility of the inhibitory NK cell receptor Ly49A caused by binding MHC class I proteins in cis. Eur J Immunol 37: 516–527
38. Bessoles S, Angelov GS, Back J, Leclercq G, Vivier E, et al. (2013) Education of Murine NK Cells Requires Both cis and trans Recognition of MHC Class I Molecules. J Immunol 191(10): 5044–5051.
39. Li NL, Fu L, Uchtenhagen H, Achour A, Burshtyn DN (2013) Cis association of leukocyte Ig-like receptor 1 with MHC class I modulates accessibility to antibodies and HCMV UL18. Eur J Immunol 43: 1042–1052.
40. Ferlazzo G, Tsang ML, Moretta L, Melioli G, Steinman RM, et al. (2002) Human Dendritic Cells Activate Resting Natural Killer (NK) Cells and Are Recognized via the NKp30 Receptor by Activated NK Cells. J Exp Med 195: 343–351.

Cytotoxicity of Polyaniline Nanomaterial on Rat Celiac Macrophages *In Vitro*

Yu-Sang Li[9], Bei-Fan Chen[9], Xiao-Jun Li, Wei Kevin Zhang, He-Bin Tang*

Department of Pharmacology, College of Pharmacy, South-Central University for Nationalities, Wuhan, PR China

Abstract

Polyaniline nanomaterial (nPANI) is getting popular in many industrial fields due to its conductivity and stability. The fate and effect of nPANI in the environment is of paramount importance towards its technological applications. In this work, the cytotoxicity of nPANI, which was prepared by rapid surface polymerization, was studied on rat celiac macrophages. Cell viability of macrophages treated with various concentrations of nPANI and different periods ranging from 24 to 72 hours was tested by a MTT assay. Damages of nPANI to structures of macrophages were evaluated according to the exposure level of cellular reactive oxygen species (ROS) and change of mitochondrial membrane potential (MMP). We observed no significant effects of nPANI on the survival, ROS level and MMP loss of macrophages at concentrations up to 1 µg/ml. However, higher dose of nPANI (10 µg/ml or above) induced cell death, changes of ROS level and MMP. In addition, an increase in the expression level of caspase-3 protein and its activated form was detected in a Western blot assay under the high dose exposure of nPANI. All together, our experimental results suggest that the hazardous potential of nPANI on macrophages is time- and dose-dependent and high dose of nPANI can induce cell apoptosis through caspase-3 mediated pathway.

Editor: Myon-Hee Lee, East Carolina University, United States of America

Funding: This study was supported by the National Natural Science Foundation of China (81373842, 81101538), and Natural Science Foundation of China Hubei (2013CFB451). The funders had no role in study design, data collection and analysis, decision to publish, or preparation of the manuscript.

Competing Interests: The authors have declared that no competing interests exist.

* Email: hbtang2006@mail.scuec.edu.cn

[9] These authors contributed equally to this work.

Introduction

Nano-conductive-polymer materials develop rapidly in recent years. They have been widely applied in chemical, electronic, aerospace and medical field thanks to the combined excellent characteristics of both nanomaterial and conductive polymer. Along with the increasing production and use of nanomaterials, there has been a growing concern about the hazardous of inevitable unintended human exposure [1–3]. These nanometer-sized materials can access, mostly through the lungs, gastrointestinal tract, skin, injection and implantation, into human body posing significantly serious health threats [4–6].

As one of the most famous conductive polymer, nano-structured PANI (nPANI) was rapidly developed in industries and clinical fields with a lot of advantages, including availability of its raw materials, easy preparation, maneuverability of particle size and morphology, good electrical conductivity, environmental stability, biocompatibility and the reversible doping-dedoping process [7–10]. Recently, limited researches [11–14] had been carried out on the biocompatibility and cytotoxicity of PANI and its composites, but there was no definite answer whether the use of nPANI is safe or not. Therefore, the uncertainty of its toxicity is still a big problem for wide range of bioapplications [15].

Macrophages are important cells of the immune system that are responsive to cell debris and pathogens. Its applicability in immuno-toxicology has been established for cytotoxicity of exogenous chemicals [16]. In the present study, nPANI was prepared in the form of nano fibers by the rapid surface polymerization process [17–19]. Its cytotoxicity and toxic mechanism on rat celiac macrophages were examined by cell death, cellular reactive oxygen species (ROS) level, loss of mitochondrial membrane potential (MMP) and apoptosis-associated caspase activation.

Materials and Methods

Preparation of nPANI

Typically, nPANI was prepared with a surface polymerization method, by using ammonium persulfate (APS; Sinopharm, China) as the oxidant and hydrochloric acid as the doping agent. The procedures were described in details in our previous report [20]. After polymerization, the prepared neutral nPANI solution was then further dialyzed by saline to remove hypertoxic oligomer. The well cleaned nPANI was stocked in the form of neutral aqueous suspension (15 mg/ml) prior to use.

Characterization of nPANI

The morphology of nPANI was observed with a scanning electron microscope (SEM, Hitachi S-4800, Japan). The UV-Vis absorption spectra of nPANI suspensions were measured on a

Varian Cary 50 UV-Vis spectrophotometer (Varian Cary 50, Agilent). The Fourier infrared spectra of nPANI were recorded on a Bruker VERTEX 70 infrared spectrometer in a transmission mode.

Animal care

The care and use of animals for this study were performed according to the Guide for Animal Experimentation, South-Central University for Nationalities and the Committee of Research Facilities for Laboratory Animal Sciences, South-Central University for Nationalities, China. The protocols were approved by the Committee on the Ethics of Animal Experiments of the South-Central University for Nationalities, China (Permit Number: 2011-SCUEC-AEC-002). All efforts were made to minimize suffering.

Cell culture

The isolated primary macrophages from adult Wistar rat abdominal cavity (6–9 weeks of age) were maintained in Dulbecco's-modified eagle's medium (DMEM, Gibco, USA) containing 10% (v/v) fetal bovine serum (Gibco, USA), 1% penicillin-streptomycin solution, and suspended to a density of 6.0×10^5 cells/ml. Cells were seeded in a 96-well plates with 200 μl per well. Eight wells were supplied for each exposing nPANI concentration, three of them were used as background correction, and the rest were experimental group. Cells were allowed to attach for 12 hours onto the 96-well plate under 5% CO_2 at 37°C. Then, they were exposed with regular growth medium containing nPANI at different concentrations ranging from 0.1 to 100 μg/ml or pure water as a negative control unless otherwise instructed.

Cell morphology and viability assays

Cell viability was measured by a MTT assay. After being exposed to different concentrations of nPANI for 24 to 72 hours, cells were imaged by an inverted phase contrast microscope (Nikon Eclipse Ti-S, Japan). Then cells were rinsed with PBS and recovered by incubating with fresh culture medium without serum for an hour. After that, 5 mg/ml MTT (3-(4,5-dimethylthiazol-2-yl)-2,5-diphenyltetrazolium bromide, Sigma, USA) was added directly to the medium. After adding MTT, all samples were incubated for 4 hours at 37°C. Medium was then removed from cells, and DMSO was added to the wells to dissolve the formazan crystals. The absorbance was measured at 490 nm after oscillation of 15 minutes. All of the experiments were performed in triplicates. The results were expressed as percentages of the control (without nPANI).

Reactive oxygen species (ROS) assay

The generation of superoxide radical and hydrogen peroxide were detected by 2,7-dichlorodihydrofluorescein diacetate (DCF-DA) staining. For ROS assay, 6.0×10^5 cells per well were cultured in 35 mm dishes, and incubated with nPANI at different concentrations for 6 hours. Then ROS detection kit (Beyotime, China) was used for the assay. ROSup (50 μg/ml) was used as the positive control. Fluorescent intensity was detected by Enzyme-labeled meter (TECAN infinite M200, Switzerland) at an excitation wavelength of 488 nm and an emission wavelength of 525 nm.

Mitochondrial membrane potential assay

JC-1 fluorescent probe was used to determine the mitochondrial membrane potential change. Cells in this assay were cultured as the former. Cells treated with carbonyl cyanide 3-chlorophenylhydrazone (CCCP; 0.01 mM) were considered as the positive control. All the processes were conducted following the test kit (Beyotime, China). Fluorescent intensity of JC-1 monomer was detected by Enzyme-labeled meter (TECAN infinite M200, Switzerland) at an excitation wavelength of 490 nm and an emission wavelength of 530 nm, while that of JC-1 polymer was detected at an excitation wavelength of 525 nm and an emission wavelength of 590 nm. In this study, the ratio of JC-1 monomers and polymers was used as a representation of MMP (mitochondrial membrane potential).

Western blot assay

After incubating with control, 10 and 100 μg/ml nPANI for 24 hours, cells were lysed with protein lysis buffer (Beyotime, China). The concentration of total protein was detected by Lowry method. Equal amounts of protein were fractionated by 10% SDS gels and transferred to polyvinylidene difluoride membranes (Millipore Corporation, USA). After blocked with 5% nonfat dry milk, the membranes were incubated with an anti-caspase3 antibody (1:1000 dilution, Boster, China) or anti-actin antibody (1:1000 dilution, Boster, China) at 4°C overnight. After removing primary antibodies, the membranes were washed 3 times for 5 minutes by TBST (Tris-Buffered Saline, 0.1% Tween-20) solution and followed by exposure of secondary antibodies (1:5000 dilution, goat anti-rabbit or goat anti-mouse, Boster, China) for 2 hours at 4°C. Finally, after wash, bands on the membranes were visualized by developer and fixing solution [21]. The protein bands were quantified using the ImageJ software (NIH).

Statistical analysis

One-way analysis of variance (ANOVA) was used as the statistical test. Results shown in the figures are expressed as means ± standard error of mean (SEM). A value of $P<0.05$ was considered statistically significant.

Results

Characterization of nPANI

The nPANI was prepared by oxidative polymerization of aniline, resulting in the production of a mixture containing polymer, aniline oligomer, diphenylamine and benzidine. The polymerization was initiated by adding APS into aniline solution. Once started, the solution turned from initial colorless to weak green, and finally to dark blue. After the polymerization, the nPANI product was cleaned by dialysis, and the suspension was neutralized with diluted ammonia water, resulted in a pure neutral water solution.

Scanning electron microscopy revealed the morphology of polymerized nPANI, as shown in Fig. 1A. Polymers presented a typical nanofiber structure, being in consistent with the previous report [20]. Fig. 1B showed the UV-vis absorption spectra of nPANI aqueous solutions at different pHs. At acidic pH, nPANI is in its acid doped state. The absorptions of acid doped PANI at pH 2 were located at 350 and 750 nm, which are attributed to π-π^* and π-polaron transitions, respectively. This suggested that the nPANI material at pH 2 had a higher level of proton doping [22]. When the suspension was adjusted to neutral or alkaline, the aforementioned bands were blue shifted to 330 and 580 nm at pH 7, and 330 and 550 nm at pH 12, respectively, representing the dedoping of nPANI. The state of nPANI changed from emeraldine salt to emeraldine base during such a dedoping process, which is consistent with the observation for conventional PANI reported by Wan and Yang [23].

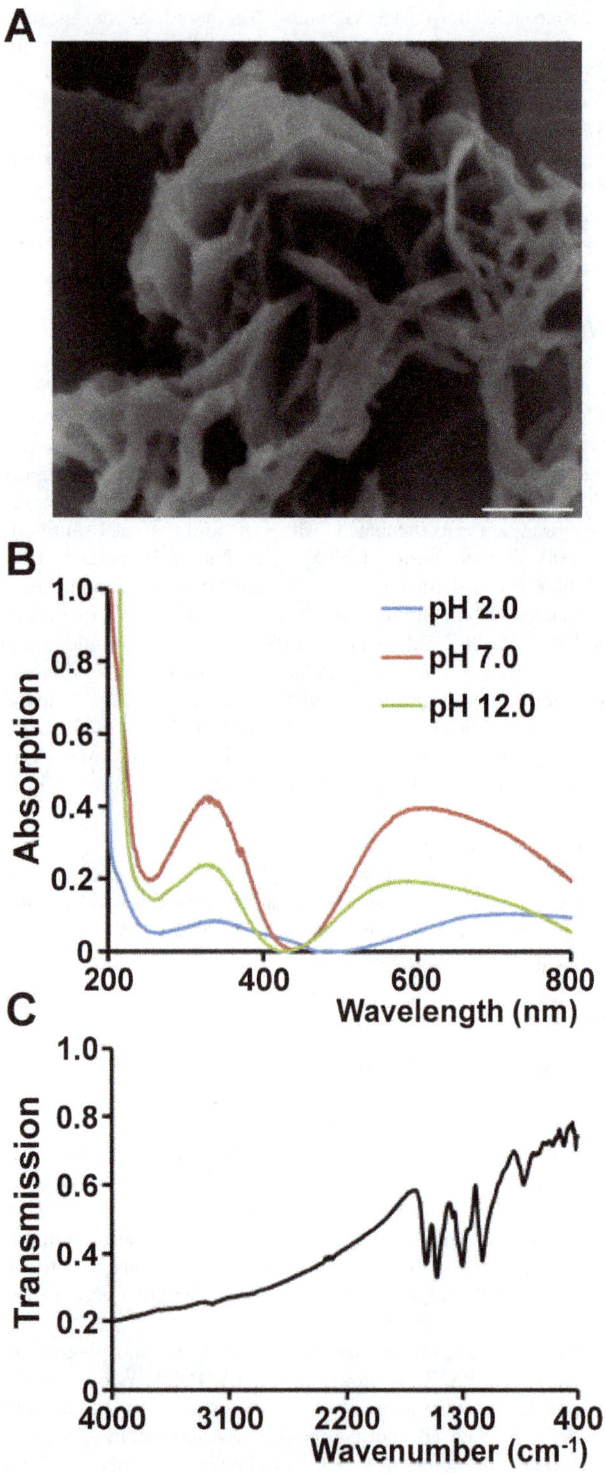

Figure 1. Characterization of nPANI. (A) The scanning electron microscope image of nPANI. Scale bar is 500 nm. (B) UV-vis absorption spectra of nPANI aqueous solutions at pH 2.0, pH 7.0, and pH 12.0. Ultra DI-water was used as a background solution. (C) FTIR spectrum of nPANI. KBr was used as a background.

Fig. 1C showed the FTIR spectrum of nPANI, where the characteristic bands of PANI were observed [24,25]. For example, the C=C stretching vibration of quinoid, C=C stretching vibration of benzene rings, C-N stretching of secondary aromatic ring, and out-of-plane bending vibrations of C-H occurred at 1580, 1498, 1303 and 828 cm^{-1}, respectively.

Cell damage and proliferation

To investigate the cytotoxicity of nPANI, rat celiac macrophages were selected. Cell death, loss of mitochondrial membrane potential (MMP), cellular reactive oxygen species (ROS) level and apoptosis-associated caspase activation were quantified in the present study.

As we know, morphological features played a leading role in the description of cell death. In Fig. 2A, the control macrophages adherent to the culture dish firmly with clear and smooth contour. The density and morphological features of cells exposed in 0.1 and 1 μg/ml nPANI for 24 hours showed no significant difference from the control group. However, in groups treated with 10 and 100 μg/ml nPANI, the density of cells was less and the cells were more transparent with vaguer rims compared with the control group. Moreover, vacuoles of different sizes could be visualized in these cells, and we also noticed tiny blue particles in the vacuoles.

Next, we quantified the cytotoxicity of nPANI on the macrophages, using concentrations of 0.1–100 μg/ml and treatment time of 24–72 hours. As shown in Fig. 2B, the cytotoxicity of nPANI on macrophages was dose- and time-dependent. When the concentration of nPANI was less than 1 μg/ml, cell viability remained to be 100% ($P>0.05$) in 72 hours. However, when the concentration went beyond 10 μg/ml, cell apoptosis existed in 24 hours after the incubation of nPANI ($P<0.05$, $P<0.001$, respectively). With the exposure time extended, more cells were dying in these two groups. In one word, the cytotoxicity of nPANI is dose- and time-dependent.

ROS generation

Environmental stress, such as UV exposure or heat, can increase ROS levels dramatically due to significant damage to cell structures. Therefore, to characterize the cytotoxicity of nPANI, ROS production of cells was also monitored. In Fig. 2C, hardly any change of ROS production was detected in low concentration (less than 1 μg/ml) treated group, while in the ROSup (positive control) treated group a huge increase was seen ($p<0.001$). Consistent with the cell viability assay, nPANI with concentration more than 10 μg/ml could promote intracellular active oxygen level and hence induce oxidative stress reaction and cell death.

Mitochondrial depolarization

Mitochondrial depolarization impairs the efficacy of the electron transport chain leading to massive ROS production. In order to further characterize the cytotoxicity of nPANI, we measured mitochondrial membrane potential (MMP) of cells. As shown in Fig. 2D, After 6-hour incubation, the ratio of JC-1 monomers to polymers in macrophages exposed in 0.1 and 1 μg/ml nPANI was not significant compare with the control group, suggesting that low concentration of nPANI could not alter MMP level of macrophages. However, 10 and 100 μg/ml nPANI could significantly change the mitochondrial membrane potential of macrophages.

Increased caspase-3 expression

Since high dose nPANI could induce cell apoptosis, we examined the expression and activation of caspase-3, an apoptosis related protein, under such condition. In Fig. 3, high dose nPANI (10, 100 μg/ml) induced more expression of caspase-3 protein in macrophages 24 hours. In addition, activated caspase-3 could be

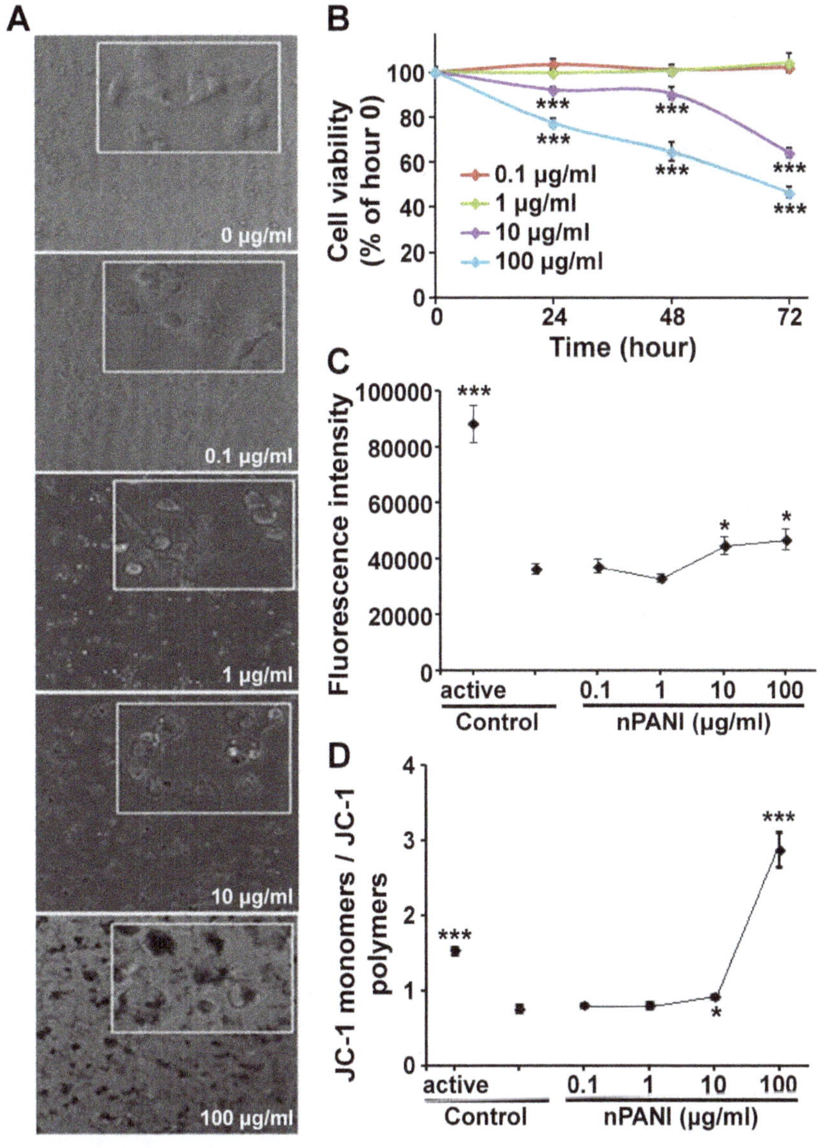

Figure 2. Cytotoxicity of nPANI. (A) Morphology of macrophages under phase-contrast microscope (20× objective, inset: 40×) treated with nPANI at different concentrations. (B) Cell viability of macrophages treated with nPANI at different concentrations for different time periods. (C) ROS production by macrophages after being incubated with nPANI at different concentrations for 6 hours. (D) Effect of 6 hours incubation of nPANI on the mitochondrial membrane potential of macrophages. All data were expressed by mean ± S.E.M. of six measurements and each experiment was performed in triplicate. * and *** denote $p<0.05$ and 0.001 versus the corresponding control.

observed, suggesting that caspase-3 was activated to different degrees in both treated groups. Therefore we speculated that caspase-3 might play a regulatory role in nPANI induced apoptosis of macrophages.

Discussion

In the present study, we have explored the toxicity of nPANI at different concentrations (0.1~100 μg/ml) on macrophages. The results showed that when concentration of nPANI was higher than 10 μg/ml, macrophage's survival was significantly threatened, and the harm was dose- and time-dependent. In general, expose of low concentration of nPANI did not show serious toxicity on macrophage in our research, which is consistent with the results of Yslas et al [13]. However, the upper limit of safety threshold of nPANI towards macrophages (less than 10 μg/ml) is lower than that towards lung fibroblast cells (25 μg/ml) [14], suggesting a necessity of studying cytotoxicity of nPANI towards different cell types.

It has been demonstrated that biological effects (such as eukaryotic cell toxicity, anti bacteria effect, and light toxicity of Lolium perenne) of nanomaterials (all kinds of nanometer metal oxide and carbon nanomaterials) are mediated by ROS [26]. Since nanomaterials are usually conductors or semi-conductors, their electric charge would interfere with electronic transduction of cells and thus increase the intracellular level of ROS and affect the permeability of cell membrane. As a result, these nanomaterials would enter cells, accumulate to form a vicious spiral, and destroy cell's osmotic balance [11]. Finally, the normal function of cells is absolutely restricted, resulting in cell lysis or apoptosis. As shown in Fig. 2C, we have shown that oxidative stress responses in

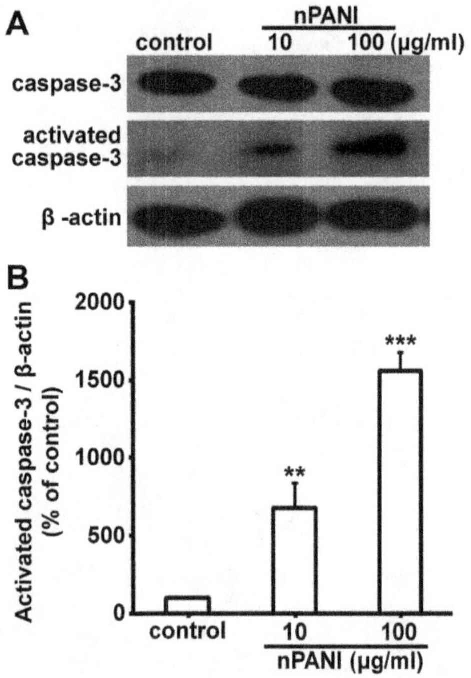

Figure 3. The effects of nPANI on the expressions of caspase-3 and activated caspase-3 expressions in macrophages. (A) Representative Western blots of the caspase-3 and β-actin expressions. (B) The relative levels were analyzed by determining the ratio of the activated caspase-3/β-actin. The values are the means ±S.E.M. of three replicates. ** and *** denote $p<0.01$ and 0.001 versus the control, respectively.

macrophages were elevated when the nPANI concentration go beyond 10 μg/ml.

In order to maintain a certain level of membrane potential, the permeability of mitochondrial membrane to outer electrolyte and foreign material is usually limited. From the early observations, we could clearly see that the macrophages swallow extracellular polyaniline nanoparticles. Microscopic examination also showed that when the nPANI concentration was more than 10 μg/ml, granular nPANI was visible in cells. This led to a speculation that nPANI could contact mitochondria directly after entering into cytoplasm and made the mitochondrial membrane porous, resulting in an increased permeability and unbalanced electrolytes inside the mitochondria. Therefore, the mitochondrial membrane potential would be lost and hence destroy the normal mitochondrial function, and cut off the respiratory chain. As a result, there would be peroxide accumulation in mitochondria and cytosol and cause oxidative stress reaction [27,28]. In addition, too-low mitochondrial membrane potential would bring about DNA fragmentation, eventually leading to cell death [29]. In accordance with this notion, the mitochondrial membrane potential showed decrease when the concentration of nPANI exceeded 10 μg/ml.

Caspase-3 is an important member of the caspase family. It is expressed widely in different tissue and cell types, and plays a crucial role in the final steps of cell apoptosis [30]. Here we have shown that the expression of active form of Caspase-3 was increased under the treatment of 10 and 100 μg/ml nPANI in a dose-dependent manner, further confirming the involvement of cell apoptosis process in nPANI induced cytotoxicity.

Conclusion

In this report, we have prepared nanometer-sized organic polyaniline, and this nPANI appeared to cause cytotoxicity on rat celiac macrophages in a time- and dose-dependent manner. We also demonstrated that the cytotoxicity of nPANI was triggered by generation of oxidative stress and change of intracellular mitochondrial membrane potential. In addition, we have shown that the pro-apoptotic protein caspase-3 took part in the nPANI-induced cell apoptosis. All together, we conclude that the safety upper limit for nPANI is less than 10 μg/ml.

Author Contributions

Conceived and designed the experiments: YSL HBT. Performed the experiments: BFC YSL HBT. Analyzed the data: XJL WKZ YSL HBT. Contributed to the writing of the manuscript: YSL HBT.

References

1. Service RF (2004) Nanotoxicology. Nanotechnology grows up. Science 304: 1732–1734.
2. Nel A, Xia T, Madler L, Li N (2006) Toxic potential of materials at the nanolevel. Science 311: 622–627.
3. Fischer HC, Chan WC (2007) Nanotoxicity: the growing need for in vivo study. Curr Opin Biotechnol 18: 565–571.
4. Pang C, Selck H, Misra SK, Berhanu D, Dybowska A, et al. (2012) Effects of sediment-associated copper to the deposit-feeding snail, Potamopyrgus antipodarum: a comparison of Cu added in aqueous form or as nano- and micro-CuO particles. Aquat Toxicol 106–107: 114–122.
5. Patil G, Khan MI, Patel DK, Sultana S, Prasad R, et al. (2012) Evaluation of cytotoxic, oxidative stress, proinflammatory and genotoxic responses of micro- and nano-particles of dolomite on human lung epithelial cells A(549). Environ Toxicol Pharmacol 34: 436–445.
6. Radad K, Al-Shraim M, Moldzio R, Rausch WD (2012) Recent advances in benefits and hazards of engineered nanoparticles. Environ Toxicol Pharmacol 34: 661–672.
7. Kawasumi M (2004) The discovery of polymer-clay hybrids. Journal of Polymer Science Part A: Polymer Chemistry 42: 819–824.
8. Kim HS, Hobbs HL, Wang L, Rutten MJ, Wamser CC (2009) Biocompatible composites of polyaniline nanofibers and collagen. Synthetic Metals 159: 1313–1318.
9. Kurian M, Dasgupta A, Galvin ME, Ziegler CR, Beyer FL (2006) A Novel Route to Inducing Disorder in Model Polymer-Layered Silicate Nanocomposites. Macromolecules 39: 1864–1871.
10. Yang C, Du J, Peng Q, Qiao R, Chen W, et al. (2009) Polyaniline/Fe3O4 nanoparticle composite: synthesis and reaction mechanism. J Phys Chem B 113: 5052–5058.
11. Humpolicek P, Kasparkova V, Saha P, Stejskal J (2012) Biocompatibility of polyaniline. Synthetic Metals 162: 722–727.
12. Khan JA, Qasim M, Singh BR, Khan W, Das D, et al. (2014) Polyaniline/CoFe2O4 nanocomposite inhibits the growth of Candida albicans 077 by ROS production. Comptes Rendus Chimie 17: 91–102.
13. Yslas EI, Ibarra LE, Peralta DO, Barbero CA, Rivarola VA, et al. (2012) Polyaniline nanofibers: acute toxicity and teratogenic effect on Rhinella arenarum embryos. Chemosphere 87: 1374–1380.
14. Oh WK, Kim S, Kwon O, Jang J (2011) Shape-dependent cytotoxicity of polyaniline nanomaterials in human fibroblast cells. J Nanosci Nanotechnol 11: 4254–4260.
15. Villalba P, Ram MK, Gomez H, Bhethanabotla V, Helms MN, et al. (2012) Cellular and in vitro toxicity of nanodiamond-polyaniline composites in mammalian and bacterial cell. Materials Science and Engineering: C 32: 594–598.
16. Ross M, Matthews A, Mangum L (2014) Chemical Atherogenesis: Role of Endogenous and Exogenous Poisons in Disease Development. Toxics 2: 17–34.
17. Ayad M, El-Hefnawy G, Zaghlol S (2013) Facile synthesis of polyaniline nanoparticles; its adsorption behavior. Chemical Engineering Journal 217: 460–465.
18. Huang YF, Lin CW (2012) Facile synthesis and morphology control of graphene oxide/polyaniline nanocomposites via in-situ polymerization process. Polymer 53: 2574–2582.
19. Li Y, Gong J, He G, Deng Y (2011) Synthesis of polyaniline nanotubes using Mn2O3 nanofibers as oxidant and their ammonia sensing properties. Synthetic Metals 161: 56–61.

20. Li J, Tang H, Zhang A, Shen X, Zhu L (2007) A New Strategy for the Synthesis of Polyaniline Nanostructures: From Nanofibers to Nanowires. Macromolecular Rapid Communications 28: 740–745.
21. Lewis CW, Taylor RG, Kubara PM, Marshall K, Meijer L, et al. (2013) A western blot assay to measure cyclin dependent kinase activity in cells or in vitro without the use of radioisotopes. FEBS Lett 587: 3089–3095.
22. Singh K, Ohlan A, Pham VH, Balasubramaniyan R, Varshney S, et al. (2013) Nanostructured graphene/Fe(3)O(4) incorporated polyaniline as a high performance shield against electromagnetic pollution. Nanoscale 5: 2411–2420.
23. Wan M, Yang J (1995) Mechanism of proton doping in polyaniline. Journal of Applied Polymer Science 55: 399–405.
24. Chiang JC, MacDiarmid AG (1986) 'Polyaniline': Protonic acid doping of the emeraldine form to the metallic regime. Synthetic Metals 13: 193–205.
25. Macdiarmid AG, Chiang JC, Richter AF, Epstein AJ (1987) Polyaniline: a new concept in conducting polymers. Synthetic Metals 18: 285–290.
26. Artetxe U, García-Plazaola JI, Hernández A, Becerril JM (2002) Low light grown duckweed plants are more protected against the toxicity induced by Zn and Cd. Plant Physiology and Biochemistry 40: 859–863.
27. Jones CF, Grainger DW (2009) In vitro assessments of nanomaterial toxicity. Adv Drug Deliv Rev 61: 438–456.
28. Kroll A, Dierker C, Rommel C, Hahn D, Wohlleben W, et al. (2011) Cytotoxicity screening of 23 engineered nanomaterials using a test matrix of ten cell lines and three different assays. Part Fibre Toxicol 8: 9.
29. Chiu WH, Luo SJ, Chen CL, Cheng JH, Hsieh CY, et al. (2012) Vinca alkaloids cause aberrant ROS-mediated JNK activation, Mcl-1 downregulation, DNA damage, mitochondrial dysfunction, and apoptosis in lung adenocarcinoma cells. Biochem Pharmacol 83: 1159–1171.
30. Alnemri ES, Livingston DJ, Nicholson DW, Salvesen G, Thornberry NA, et al. (1996) Human ICE/CED-3 protease nomenclature. Cell 87: 171.

Permissions

All chapters in this book were first published in PLOS ONE, by The Public Library of Science; hereby published with permission under the Creative Commons Attribution License or equivalent. Every chapter published in this book has been scrutinized by our experts. Their significance has been extensively debated. The topics covered herein carry significant findings which will fuel the growth of the discipline. They may even be implemented as practical applications or may be referred to as a beginning point for another development.

The contributors of this book come from diverse backgrounds, making this book a truly international effort. This book will bring forth new frontiers with its revolutionizing research information and detailed analysis of the nascent developments around the world.

We would like to thank all the contributing authors for lending their expertise to make the book truly unique. They have played a crucial role in the development of this book. Without their invaluable contributions this book wouldn't have been possible. They have made vital efforts to compile up to date information on the varied aspects of this subject to make this book a valuable addition to the collection of many professionals and students.

This book was conceptualized with the vision of imparting up-to-date information and advanced data in this field. To ensure the same, a matchless editorial board was set up. Every individual on the board went through rigorous rounds of assessment to prove their worth. After which they invested a large part of their time researching and compiling the most relevant data for our readers.

The editorial board has been involved in producing this book since its inception. They have spent rigorous hours researching and exploring the diverse topics which have resulted in the successful publishing of this book. They have passed on their knowledge of decades through this book. To expedite this challenging task, the publisher supported the team at every step. A small team of assistant editors was also appointed to further simplify the editing procedure and attain best results for the readers.

Apart from the editorial board, the designing team has also invested a significant amount of their time in understanding the subject and creating the most relevant covers. They scrutinized every image to scout for the most suitable representation of the subject and create an appropriate cover for the book.

The publishing team has been an ardent support to the editorial, designing and production team. Their endless efforts to recruit the best for this project, has resulted in the accomplishment of this book. They are a veteran in the field of academics and their pool of knowledge is as vast as their experience in printing. Their expertise and guidance has proved useful at every step. Their uncompromising quality standards have made this book an exceptional effort. Their encouragement from time to time has been an inspiration for everyone.

The publisher and the editorial board hope that this book will prove to be a valuable piece of knowledge for researchers, students, practitioners and scholars across the globe.

List of Contributors

EK Radhakrishnan and Eppurathu Vasudevan Soniya
Division of Plant Molecular Biology, Rajiv Gandhi Centre for Biotechnology, Thiruvananthapuram, Kerala, India

Smitha V. Bava, Sai Shyam Narayanan, Lekshmi R. Nath, Ruby John Anto and Arun Kumar T. Thulasidasan
Division of Cancer Research, Rajiv Gandhi Centre for Biotechnology, Thiruvananthapuram, Kerala, India

Ziqing Wang, Yi Luo, Qiujia Shao, Ballington L. Kinlock, James E. K. Hildreth and Bindong Liu
Center for AIDS Health Disparities Research, School of Medicine, Meharry Medical College, Nashville, Tennessee, United States of America

Hua Xie
Department of Oral Biology and Research, School of Dentistry, Meharry Medical College, Nashville, Tennessee, United States of America

Chenliang Wang
Center for AIDS Health Disparities Research, School of Medicine, Meharry Medical College, Nashville, Tennessee, United States of America
Institute of Gastroenterology and Institute of Human Virology, Sun Yat-sen University, Guangzhou, Guangdong, Peoples of Republic of China

Xiangru Wen
Jiangsu Key Laboratory of Brain Disease Bioinformation, Xuzhou Medical College, Xuzhou, Jiangsu Province, China
School of Basic Education Sciences, Xuzhou Medical College, Xuzhou, Jiangsu Province, China

Yuanjian Song
Jiangsu Key Laboratory of Brain Disease Bioinformation, Xuzhou Medical College, Xuzhou, Jiangsu Province, China
Research Center for Neurobiology and Department of Neurobiology, Xuzhou Medical College, Xuzhou, Jiangsu Province, China

Kai Wang, Yifang Zhang and Tingting Sun
College of Animal Science and Technology, Yunnan Agricultural University, Yunnan, Kunming Province, China

Ziming Zhao
School of Pharmacy, Xuzhou Medical College, Xuzhou, Jiangsu Province, China

Fang Zhang, Jian Wu, Yanyan Fu, Yang Du and Hongzhi Liu
Research Center for Neurobiology and Department of Neurobiology, Xuzhou Medical College, Xuzhou, Jiangsu Province, China

Lei Zhang, Ying Sun and YongHai Liu
Department of Neurology, Affiliated Hospital of Xuzhou Medical College, Xuzhou, Jiangsu Province, China

Kai Ma
School of Basic Education Sciences, Xuzhou Medical College, Xuzhou, Jiangsu Province, China
Department of Medical Information, Xuzhou Medical College, Xuzhou, Jiangsu Province, China

Kemal Alpay, Kaappo Aittokallio and Sakari Hietanen
Department of Obstetrics and Gynecology and Joint Clinical Biochemistry Laboratory of Turku University Hospital, Medicity Research Laboratory, University of Turku, Turku, Finland

Mehdi Farshchian, Elina Siljamäki and Veli-Matti Kähäri
Department of Dermatology and MediCity Research Laboratory, University of Turku and Turku University Hospital, Turku, Finland

Johanna Tuomela
Department of Cell Biology and Anatomy, University of Turku, Turku, Finland

Jouko Sandholm
Cell Imaging Core, Turku Centre for Biotechnology, University of Turku and Åbo Akademi University, Turku, Finland

Marko Kallio
VTT Health, VTT Technical Research Centre of Finland, Turku, Finland

Radka Křikavová, Jan Hošek, Ján Vančo, Jakub Hutyra and Zdeněk Trávníček
Regional Centre of Advanced Technologies and Materials & Department of Inorganic Chemistry, Faculty of Science, Palacky´ University, Olomouc, Czech Republic

Zdeněk Dvořák
Regional Centre of Advanced Technologies and Materials & Department of Cell Biology and Genetics, Faculty of Science, Palacky´ University, Olomouc, Czech Republic

Bo-hyun Choi, In-geun Ryoo, Han Chang Kang and Mi-Kyoung Kwak
College of pharmacy, The Catholic University of Korea, Bucheon, Gyeonggi-do, Republic of Korea

Flávia C. Costa, Halyna Fedosyuk, Renee Y. Neades, Allen M. Chazelle, Lesya Zelenchuk, Andrea H. Fonteles and Parmita Dalal
Department of Biochemistry and Molecular Biology, University of Kansas Medical Center, Kansas City, Kansas, United States of America

Kenneth R. Peterson
Department of Biochemistry and Molecular Biology, University of Kansas Medical Center, Kansas City, Kansas, United States of America
Department of Anatomy and Cell Biology, University of Kansas Medical Center, Kansas City, Kansas, United States of America

Anuradha Roy and Rathnam Chaguturu
High Throughput Screening Laboratory, University of Kansas, Lawrence, Kansas, United States of America

Biaoru Li
Department of Pediatrics, Georgia Regents University, Augusta, Georgia, United States of America

Betty S. Pace
Department of Pediatrics, Georgia Regents University, Augusta, Georgia, United States of America
Department of Molecular and Cell Biology, Georgia Regents University, Augusta, Georgia, United States of America

Yi Cao, Martin Roursgaard, Pernille Høgh Danielsen, Peter Møller and Steffen Loft
Section of Environmental Health, Department of Public Health, University of Copenhagen, Copenhagen, Denmark

Nikolai Siebert, Diana Seidel, Christin Eger, Madlen Jüttner and Holger N. Lode
Department of Pediatric Oncology and Hematology, University Medicine Greifswald, Greifswald, Germany

Debanjana Chakraborty, Arindam Maity and Nirup Bikash Mondal
Department of Chemistry, Indian Institute of Chemical Biology, Council of Scientific and Industrial Research, Jadavpur, Kolkata, West Bengal, India

Tarun Jha
Department of Pharmaceutical Technology, Division of Medicinal and Pharmaceutical Chemistry, Jadavpur University, Kolkata, West Bengal, India

Fawzi Ebrahim, Jayanth Suryanarayanan Shankaranarayanan, Jagat R. Kanwar,
Sneha Gurudevan and Rupinder K. Kanwar
Nanomedicine-Laboratory of Immunology and Molecular Biomedical Research, School of Medicine, Faculty of Health, Deakin University, Geelong, Victoria, Australia

Uma Maheswari Krishnan
Centre for Nanotechnology & Advanced Biomaterials (CeNTAB), School of Chemical & Biotechnology, SASTRA University, Thanjavur, India

Hye Jin Jung, Pyo June Pak, Sung Hyo Park, Jae Eun Ju and Namhyun Chung
Department of Biosystems and Biotechnology, College of Life Sciences and Biotechnology, Korea University, Seoul, Korea

Joong-Su Kim
Bioindustry Process Center, Jeonbuk Branch Institute, Korea Research Institute of Bioscience and Biotechnology, Jeoneup, Korea

Hoi-Seon Lee
College of Agriculture and Life Science, Chonbuk National University, Jeonju, Korea

Tao Zhou, Lili Ye and Yu Bai
School of life Sciences, Anhui University, Hefei, China

Bryan Cox
Department of Chemistry, Emory University, Atlanta, Georgia, United States of America

Aiming Sun, Dennis Liotta and James P. Snyder
Department of Chemistry, Emory University, Atlanta, Georgia, United States of America
Emory Institute for Drug Development (EIDD), Emory University, Atlanta, Georgia, United States of America

Haian Fu
Department of Pharmacology and Emory Chemical Biology Discovery Center, Emory University, Atlanta, Georgia, United States of America

Bei Huang, Dahai Liu and Yong Li
School of life Sciences, Anhui University, Hefei, China
Center for Stem Cell and Translational Medicine, Anhui University, Hefei, China

Tsunehito Higashi, Yosuke Mai, Takahiro Horinouchi, Koji Terada, Akimasa Hoshi,
Prabha Nepal, Takuya Harada, Mika Horiguchi, Chizuru Hatate and Soichi Miwa
Department of Cellular Pharmacology, Graduate School of Medicine, Hokkaido University, Sapporo, Hokkaido, Japan

Yoichi Noya and Yuji Kuge
Central Institute of Isotope Science, HokkaidoUniversity, Sapporo, Hokkaido, Japan

Yarong Liu, Jinxu Fang and Kye-Il Joo
Mork Family Department of Chemical Engineering and Materials Science, University of Southern California, Los Angeles, California, United States of America

Michael K. Wong
Division of Medical Oncology, Norris Comprehensive Cancer Center, Keck School of Medicine, University of Southern California, Los Angeles, California, United States of America

Pin Wang
Mork Family Department of Chemical Engineering and Materials Science, University of Southern California, Los Angeles, California, United States of America
Department of Biomedical Engineering, University of Southern California, Los Angeles, California, United States of America
Department of Pharmacology and Pharmaceutical Sciences, University of Southern California, Los Angeles, California, United States of America

Laura C. Kobashigawa, Yan Chun Xu, James F. Padbury, Yi-Tang Tseng and Naohiro Yano
Department of Pediatrics, Women & Infants Hospital, The Warren Alpert Medical School of Brown University, Providence, Rhode Island, United States of America

Long Wu, Jun Xu, Weiqi Yuan, Guangquan Liu, Xiaoxiong Wang and Shaohui Cai
Department of Clinical Pharmacology, College of Pharmacy, Jinan University, Guangzhou 510632, P. R. China

Baojian Wu
Division of Pharmaceutics, College of Pharmacy, Jinan University, Guangzhou 510632, P. R. China

Hao Wang and Jun Du
School of Pharmaceutical Sciences, Sun Yat-sen University, Guang Zhou 510275, P. R. China

Rubén Corral-San Miguel, Trinidad Hernández-Caselles, Antonio José Ruiz Alcaraz,
María Martínez-Esparza and Pilar García-Peñarrubia
Department of Biochemistry and Molecular Biology B and Immunology, School of Medicine, University of Murcia, Campus of International Excellence "Campus Mare Nostrum" and IMIB (Instituto Murciano de Investigaciones Biosanitarias)-Arrixaca, Murcia, Spain

Yu-Sang Li, Bei-Fan Chen, Xiao-Jun Li, Wei Kevin Zhang and He-Bin Tang
Department of Pharmacology, College of Pharmacy, South-Central University for Nationalities, Wuhan, PR China

Index

www.ingramcontent.com/pod-product-compliance
Lightning Source LLC
Chambersburg PA
CBHW061251190326
41458CB00011B/3642
* 9 7 8 1 6 3 2 4 1 4 4 7 2 *